Nursing Theories and Nursing Practice

Marilyn E. Parker

Professor
College of Nursing
Florida Atlantic University
Boca Raton, Florida

F. A. DAVIS COMPANY • Philadelphia

F. A. Davis Company
1915 Arch Street
Philadelphia, PA 19103

Printed in the United States of America

Last digit indicates print number: 10 9 8 7 6 5 4 3 2 1

Acquisitions Editor: Joanne P. DaCunha, RN, MSN
Cover Designer: Louis J. Forgione

As new scientific information becomes available through basic and clinical research, recommended treatments and drug therapies undergo changes. The authors and publisher have done everything possible to make this book accurate, up to date, and in accord with accepted standards at the time of publication. The authors, editors, and publisher are not responsible for errors or omissions or for consequences from application of the book, and make no warranty, expressed or implied, in regard to the contents of the book. Any practice described in this book should be applied by the reader in accordance with professional standards of care used in regard to the unique circumstances that may apply in each situation. The reader is advised always to check product information (package inserts) for changes and new information regarding dose and contraindications before administering any drug. Caution is especially urged when using new or infrequently ordered drugs.

Library of Congress Cataloging-in-Publication Data

Nursing theories and nursing practice / [edited by] Marilyn E. Parker.
    p. ; cm.
    Includes bibliographical references and index.
    ISBN 0-8036-0604-4
      1. Nursing—Philosophy. 2. Nursing. I. Parker, Marilyn E.
     [DNLM: 1. Nursing Theory—Biography. 2. Nurses—Biography. WY 86 N9737 2000]
    RT84.5 .N8793 2000
    610.73'01—dc21

                              00-030335

This book is dedicated to my mother,
Lucile Marie Parker

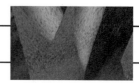

This book offers the perspective that nursing theory is essentially connected with nursing practice, research, education, and development. Nursing theories, regardless of complexity or abstraction, reflect nursing and are used by nurses to frame their thinking, action, and being in the world. As guides for nursing endeavors, nursing theories are practical in nature and facilitate communication with those being nursed as well as with colleagues, students, and persons practicing in related health and illness services. At the same time, all aspects of nursing are essential for developing and evolving nursing theory. It is hoped that these pages make clear the interrelations of nursing theory and various nursing endeavors, and that the discipline and practice of nursing will thus be advanced.

This very special book is intended to honor the work of nursing theorists and nurses who use these theories in their day-to-day nursing care, by reflecting and presenting the unique contributions of eminent nursing thinkers and doers of our lifetimes. Our foremost nursing theorists have written for this book, or their work has been described by nurses who have thorough knowledge of the work of the theorist and deep respect for the theorist as person, nurse, and scholar. Indeed, to the extent possible, contributing authors have been selected by theorists to write about their theoretical work. The pattern for each chapter was developed by each author or team of authors according to their individual thinking and writing styles, as well as the scientific perspectives of the chapter. This freedom of format has helped to encourage the latest and best thinking of contributing authors; several authors have shared the insight that in preparing a chapter for this book, their work has become more full and complete.

This book is intended to assist nursing students in undergraduate and graduate nursing programs to explore and appreciate nursing theories and their use in nursing practice. In addition and in response to calls from practicing nurses, this book is intended for use by those who desire to enrich their practice by the study of nursing theories and related illustrations of nursing practice and scholarship. The first section of the book provides an overview of nursing theory and a focus for thinking about evaluating and choosing nursing theory for use in nursing practice. An

outline at the beginning of each chapter provides a map for the chapter. Selected points are highlighted in each chapter and space for notes is provided. The book concludes with an appendix of nursing theory resources. An instructor's manual has been prepared for this book; it reflects the experiences of many who have both met the challenges and have had such a good time teaching and learning nursing theory in undergraduate and graduate nursing programs.

The design of this book highlights work of nurses who were thinking and writing about nursing up to fifty years ago or more. Building, then, as now, on the writing of Florence Nightingale, these nurse scholars have provided essential influences for the evolution of nursing theory. These influences can be seen in the theory presentations in the section of the book that includes the nursing theories that are most in use today. The last section of this book features two theorists who initially developed nursing theories at the middle range. These scholars describe processes and perspectives on theory development, giving us views of the future of nursing theory as we move into the twenty-first century. Each chapter of the book includes both descriptions of a particular theory and the use of the theory in nursing practice, research, education, administration, or governance.

For the latest and best thinking of some of nursing's finest scholars, all nurses who read and use this book will be grateful. For the continuing commitment of these scholars to our discipline and practice of nursing, we are all thankful. Continuing to learn and share what you love keeps the work and the love alive, nurtures the commitment, and offers both fun and frustration along the way. This has been illustrated in the enthusiasm for this book shared by many nursing theorists and contributing authors who have worked to create this book and by those who have added their efforts to make it live. For me, it has been a joy to renew friendships with colleagues who have joined me in preparing this book, and to find new friends and colleagues as contributing authors.

Nursing Theories and Nursing Practice has roots in a series of nursing theory conferences held in South Florida beginning in 1989 and ending when efforts to cope with the aftermath of Hurricane Andrew interrupted the energy and resources needed for planning and offering the 5th South Florida Nursing Theory Conference. Many of the theorists in this book addressed audiences of mostly practicing nurses at these conferences. Two books stimulated by those conferences and published by the National League for Nursing are *Nursing Theories in Practice* (1990) and *Patterns of Nursing Theories in Practice* (1993). It is the intention of the contributing authors of the current edition of *Nursing Theories and Nursing Practice* to contribute some earnings from this book to future conferences about nursing theory and nursing practice.

Even deeper roots of this book are found early in my nursing career, when I seriously considered leaving nursing for the study of pharmacy, because, in my fatigue and frustration mixed with youthful hope and desire for more education, I could not answer the question "What is nursing?" and could not distinguish the work of nursing from other tasks I did everyday. Why should I continue this work? Why should I seek degrees in a field that I could not define? After reflecting on these questions and using them to examine my nursing, I could find no one who would consider the questions with me. I remember being asked "Why would you ask that question? You're a nurse; you must surely know what nursing is." Such responses, along with a drive for serious consideration of my questions, led me to the library. I clearly remember reading several descriptions of nursing that, I thought, could have just as well have been about social work or physical therapy. I then found nursing defined and explained in a book about education of practical nurses written by Dorothea Orem. During the weeks that followed, as I did my work of nursing in the hospital, I explored Orem's ideas about why people need nursing, nursing's purposes, and what nurses do. I found a fit of her ideas, as I understood them, with my practice, and learned that I could go even further to explain and design nursing according to these ways of thinking about nursing. I discovered that nursing shared some knowledge and practices with other services, such as pharmacy and medicine, and I began to distinguish nursing from these related fields of practice. I decided to stay in nursing and made plans to study and work with Dorothea Orem. In addition to learning about nursing theory and its meaning in all we do, I learned from Dorothea that nursing is a unique discipline of knowledge and professional practice. In many ways, my earliest questions about nursing have guided my subsequent study and work. Most of what I have done in nursing has been a continuation of my initial experience of the interrelations of all aspects of nursing scholarship, including the scholarship

that is nursing practice. Over the years, I have been privileged to work with many nursing scholars, some of whom are featured in this book. My love for nursing and my respect for our discipline and practice have deepened, and knowing now that these values are so often shared is a singular joy.

Many faculty colleagues and students continue to help me study nursing and have contributed to this book in ways I would never have adequate words to acknowledge. I have been fortunate to hold faculty appointments in universities where nursing theory has been honored and am especially fortunate today to be in a College of Nursing where both faculty and students ground our teaching, scholarship, and practice in nursing theory. I am grateful to my knowledgeable colleagues who reviewed and offered helpful suggestions for chapters of this book, and to those who contributed as chapter authors. It is also our good fortune that many nursing theorists and other nursing scholars live in or willingly visit our lovely state of Florida.

During the last year of our work on this book, nursing lost three of the theorists acclaimed in this book as essential influences on the evolution of nursing theory. Ernestine Wiedenbach died in the spring of 1998. As this book was being prepared for production, word came of the death of Dorothy Johnson. Hildegard Peplau died in March of 1999. Typical of their commitments to nursing, both Dorothy Johnson and Hildegard Peplau had told me of their interests in this project, had advised me on the authors they would like to have prepare the chapters on their contributions, and had asked to be given updates on our progress.

Perhaps we should expect that a work of love and commitment, such as this book, and the contributors who have devoted so much to it, would be affected by major life events taking place during its development. In addition to the recent loss of three of our nursing theorists and mentors, several of us have experienced more personal life transitions and major losses during preparation of this work. Illnesses and deaths of spouses and parents have touched us in profound ways. There can be no doubt that our experiences of transition are reflected within the pages of this book. I am grateful for the tender sharing and deep understanding of author colleagues in so many lovely and loving ways. I have written the dedication of this book for my mother and hope this extends to other loved ones we may choose to remember in this way.

This book began during a visit with Joanne DaCunha, an expert nurse and editor for F. A. Davis Company, who has seen it to publication with what I believe is her love of nursing. I am grateful for her wisdom, kindness, and understanding of nursing. Peg Waltner's respect for the purposes of this book and for the special contributions of the authors has been matched only by her fine attention to detail. Without the reliable and expert assistance of Marguerite Purnell, this manuscript might still be on my dining room table. I thank my husband, Terry Worden, for his abiding love and for always being willing to help, and my niece, Cherie Parker, who, as a nursing graduate student, represents many nurses who inspire the work of this book.

Marilyn E. Parker
West Palm Beach, Florida

Nursing Theorists

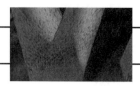

Anne Boykin
Dean and Professor
College of Nursing
Florida Atlantic University
Boca Raton, Florida

Lydia Hall†

Virginia Henderson†

Dorothy Johnson*†

Imogene King
Professor Emeritus
College of Nursing
University of South Florida
Tampa, Florida

Madeleine Leininger
Professor Emeritus
College of Nursing
Wayne State University
Detroit, Michigan

Myra Levine†

Betty Neuman
Beverly, Ohio

Margaret Newman*
St. Paul, Minnesota

Florence Nightingale†

Dorothea E. Orem
Orem & Shields, Inc.
Savannah, Georgia

Ida Jean Orlando (Pelletier)*
Belmont, Massachusetts

Josephine Paterson*

Rosemarie Rizzo Parse
Founder and Editor, *Nursing Science Quarterly*
Professor and Niehoff Chair
Loyola University
Chicago, Illinois

Hildegard Peplau†

Marilyn Anne Ray
Professor
College of Nursing
Florida Atlantic University
Boca Raton, Florida

Martha Rogers†

Sister Callista Roy
Professor of Nursing
Boston College
Boston, Massachusetts

Savina Schoenhofer
Professor of Nursing
Alcorn State University
Natchez, Mississippi

Kristen Swanson
Associate Professor
School of Nursing
University of Washington
Seattle, Washington

Jean Watson
Distinguished Professor
Founder, Center for Human Caring
School of Nursing
University of Colorado Health Science Center
Denver, Colorado

Ernestine Wiedenbach†

Loretta Zderad*

†Deceased
*Retired

Contributing Authors

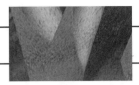

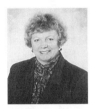

Patricia D. Aylward, MSN
Sante Fe Community College
Gainesville, Florida

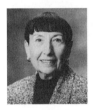

Sandra Schmidt Bunkers, Ph.D.
Chair of Nursing and Kohlmeyer
Distinguished Teaching Professor
Augustana College
Sioux Falls, South Dakota

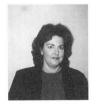

Nettie Birnbach, Ed.D., FAAN
Professor Emeritus
College of Nursing
State University of New York at
    Brooklyn
Brooklyn, New York

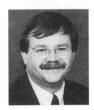

Howard Butcher, Ph.D.
Assistant Professor
College of Nursing
University of Iowa
Iowa City, Iowa

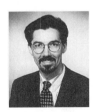

William K. Cody, Ph.D.
Associate Professor and Chair
School of Nursing
University of North Carolina
    at Charlotte
Charlotte, North Carolina

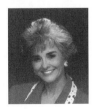

Marcia Dombro, Ed.D.
Chairperson, Continuing
Professional/Community
    Education Alliance
Miami-Dade Community College
Miami, Florida

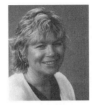

Lynne Dunphy, Ph.D.
Associate Professor
College of Nursing
Florida Atlantic University
Boca Raton, Florida

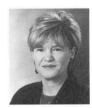

Maureen Frey, Ph.D.
Nurse Researcher
Children's Hospital of Michigan
Detroit, Michigan

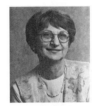

Theresa Gesse, Ph.D.
Associate Professor
Founder and Director, Nurse
Midwifery Program
School of Nursing
University of Miami
Miami, Florida

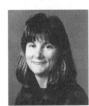

Shirley Countryman Gordon, Ph.D.
Assistant Professor
College of Nursing
Florida Atlantic University
Boca Raton, Florida

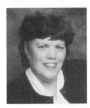

Bonnie Holoday, DNS, FAAN
Dean, Graduate School and
    Associate Vice Provost for
    Research
Professor of Nursing
Clemson University
Clemson, South Carolina

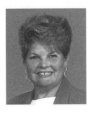

Marjorie Isenberg, DNS, FAAN
Professor
College of Nursing
Wayne State University
Detroit, Michigan

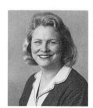

Renee Jester, MSN
Advanced Practice Nurse
Jensen Beach, Florida

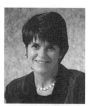

Gail J. Mitchell, Ph.D.
Chief Nursing Officer
Sunnybrook Health Science Centre
Toronto, Ontario, Canada

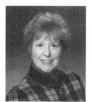

Mary Killeen, Ph.D.
Associate Professor
Department of Nursing
University of Michigan-Flint
Flint, Michigan

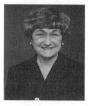

Ruth M. Neil, Ph.D.
Assistant Professor
School of Nursing
University of Colorado Health
   Science Center
Denver, Colorado

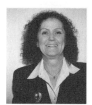

Susan Kleiman, MS
Clinical Specialist
Centerport, New York

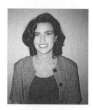

Cherie M. Parker, MS
Advanced Practice Nurse
West Palm Beach, Florida

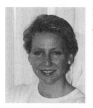

Danielle Linden, MSN
Advanced Practice Nurse
Deerfield Beach, Florida

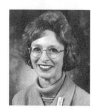

Ann R. Peden, DSN
Associate Professor
College of Nursing
University of Kentucky
Lexington, Kentucky

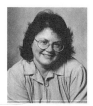

Violet Malinski, Ph.D.
Associate Professor
Hunter-Bellevue School of Nursing
City University of New York
New York, New York

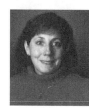

**Margaret Dexheimer Pharris,
   Ph.D.**
Faculty, Adolescent Teaching
   Project
Assistant Director Sexual Assault
   Resource Service
School of Nursing
University of Minnesota
Minneapolis, Minnesota

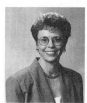

Marilyn R. McFarland, Ph.D.
Adjunct Faculty
College of Nursing and Allied
   Health
Saginaw Valley State University
University Center, Michigan

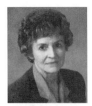
Marguerite J. Purnell, MSN
Doctoral Student
University of Miami
Miami, Florida

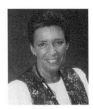
Theris A. Touhy, ND
Assistant Professor
College of Nursing
Florida Atlantic University
Boca Raton, Florida

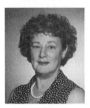
Maude Rittman, Ph.D.
Associate Chief of Nursing Service
    for Research
Gainesville Veteran's Administration
Medical Center
Gainesville, Florida

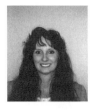
Marian C. Turkel, Ph.D.
Assistant Professor
College of Nursing
Florida Atlantic University
Boca Raton, Florida

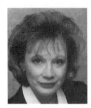
Karen Schaeffer, DNSc
Nursing Education/Research
Bethlehem, Pennsylvania

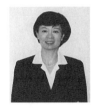
Lyn Zhan, Ph.D.
Assistant Professor
College of Nursing
University of Massachusetts,
    Boston
Boston, Massachusetts

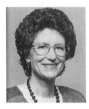
Christina Leibold Sieloff, Ph.D.
Assistant Professor
School of Nursing
Oakland University
Rochester, Michigan

Consultants

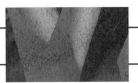

Nancy Nightengale Gillispie, RN, Ph.D.
Chairperson and Associate Professor
Saint Francis College
Fort Wayne, Indiana

Marilyn Loen, Ph.D., RN
Metropolitan State University
St. Paul, Minnesota

Mary Taylor Martof, RN, Ed.D.
Associate Professor
Louisiana State University Medical Center School
    of Nursing
New Orleans, Louisiana

Erin E. Mullins-Rivera, Ph.D., RN
Assistant Professor
Saint Francis College
Fort Wayne, Indiana

Anne T. Pithian, MSN, RN
Assistant Professor
St. Luke's College of Nursing
Sioux City, Iowa

Patsy Ruchala RN, Ph.D.
St. Louis University
School of Nursing
St. Louis, Missouri

Overview of Contents

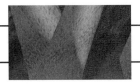

SECTION I
Perspectives on Nursing Theory
An introduction to nursing theory includes: definitions of nursing theory, nursing theory and nursing knowledge, types of nursing theory, and nursing's need for theory. Choosing, analyzing, and evaluating nursing theory focuses on questions from practicing nurses about studying and using nursing theory, a guide for choosing a theory to study, and several frameworks for theory analysis and evaluation. A guide for the study of nursing theory for use in nursing practice is presented, along with questions for selecting theory for use in nursing administration.

SECTION II
Evolution of Nursing Theory: Essential Influences
This section opens with a chapter on Florence Nightingale and a description of her profound influence on the discipline and practice of nursing. Subsequent chapters present major nursing theories that have both reflected and influenced nursing practice, education, research, and ongoing theory development in nursing during the last half of the twentieth century.

SECTION III
Nursing Theory in Nursing Practice, Education, Research, Administration, and Governance
The major nursing theories in use at the end of the twentieth century are presented in this section. Most chapters about particular nursing theories are written by the theorists themselves. Some chapters are written by nurses with advanced knowledge about particular nursing theories; these authors have been acknowledged by specific theorists as experts in presenting their work. Each chapter also includes a section illustrating the use of the theory in nursing practice, research, education, administration, or governance.

SECTION IV
Nursing Theory: Illustrating Processes of Development
Two nursing theorists' unique processes of developing nursing theory are presented in this section. Each theorist has written about research and development of middle-range theory as well as about further exploration of theory in the contexts of programs of research and theory development. The political and economic dimensions of one of the theories in contemporary nursing practice is illustrated.

APPENDIX
Evaluating Nursing Theory Resources

SUBJECT INDEX

Contents

Section I

Perspectives on Nursing Theory

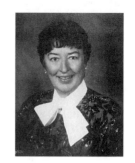

Chapter *1*

Introduction to Nursing Theory

❖ Definitions of Nursing Theory

❖ Nursing Theory in the Context of Nursing Knowledge

❖ Types of Nursing Theory

❖ Nursing's Need for Nursing Theory

❖ Nursing Theory and the Future

❖ Summary

❖ References

Marilyn E. Parker

Florence Nightingale taught us that nursing theories describe and explain what is and what is not nursing (Nightingale, 1859/1992). Today knowledge development in nursing is taking place on several fronts, with a variety of scholarly approaches contributing to advances in the discipline. Nursing practice increasingly takes place in interdisciplinary community settings, and the form of nursing in acute care settings is rapidly changing. Various paradigms and value systems that express perspectives held by several groups within the discipline ground the knowledge and practice of nursing. Because the language of nursing is continually being formed and distinguished, it often seems confusing, as does any language that is new to the ears and eyes. Nurses who have active commitments to the work of the discipline, whether in nursing practice, research, education, or administration, are essential for the continuing development of nursing theory. This chapter offers an approach to understanding nursing theory within three contexts: nursing knowledge, nursing as a discipline, and nursing as a professional practice. The chapter closes with an invitation to share with contributing authors of this book their visions of nursing theory in the future.

DEFINITIONS OF NURSING THEORY

A *theory,* as a general term, is a notion or an idea that explains experience, interprets observation, describes relationships, and projects outcomes. Theories are mental patterns or constructs created to help understand and find meaning from our experience, organize and articulate our knowing, and ask questions leading to new insights. As such, theories are not discovered in nature but are human inventions. They are descriptions of our reflections, of what we observe, or of what we project and infer. For these reasons, theory and related terms have been defined and described in a number of ways according to individual experience and what is useful at the time. Theories, as reflections of understanding, guide our actions, help us set forth desired outcomes, and give evidence of what has been achieved. A theory, by traditional definition, is an organized, coherent set of concepts and their relationships to each other that offers descriptions, explanations, and predictions about phenomena.

Early writers about nursing theory brought definitions of theory from other disciplines to direct future work within nursing. A theory is a "conceptual sys-

> **Theories are not discovered in nature but are human inventions.**

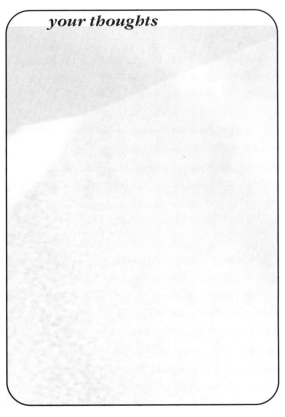

your thoughts

tem or framework invented for some purpose" (Dickoff & James, 1968, p. 198). Ellis (1968, p. 117) defined theory as "a coherent set of hypothetical, conceptual, and pragmatic principles forming a general frame of reference for a field of inquiry." McKay (1969, p. 394) asserted that theories are the capstone of scientific work, and that the term refers to "logically interconnected sets of confirmed hypotheses. Barnum (1998, p. 1) later offers a more open definition of theory as a "construct that accounts for or organizes some phenomenon," and states simply that a nursing theory describes or explains nursing.

Definitions of theory emphasize various aspects of theory and demonstrate that even the conceptions of nursing theory are various and changing. Definitions of theory developed in recent years are more open and less structured than definitions created before the last decade. Not every nursing theory will fit every definition of what is a nursing theory. For purposes of nursing practice, a definition of nursing theory that has a focus on the meaning or possible impact of the theory on practice is desirable. The following definitions of theory are consistent with general ideas of theory in nursing as well as in other disciplines. They are inclusive enough to be used for purposes of nursing practice, education, and administration, as well as nursing research, but can also provide a focus on one main nursing endeavor.

> Theory is a set of concepts, definitions, and propositions that projects a systematic view of phenomena by designating specific interrelationships among concepts for purposes of describing, explaining, predicting, and/or controlling phenomena. (Chinn & Jacobs, 1987, p. 70)

> Theory is a creative and rigorous structuring of ideas that projects a tentative purposeful and systematic view of phenomena. (Chinn & Kramer, 1995, p. 71)

> Nursing theory is a conceptualization of some aspect of reality (invented or discovered) that pertains to nursing. The conceptualization is articulated for the purpose of describing, explaining, predicting or prescribing nursing care. (Meleis, 1997, p. 12)

> Nursing theory is an inductively and/or deductively derived collage of coherent, creative, and focused nursing phenomena that frame, give meaning to, and help explain specific and selective aspects of nursing research and practice. (Silva, 1997, p. 55)

NURSING THEORY IN THE CONTEXT OF NURSING KNOWLEDGE

The notion of paradigm can be useful as a basis for understanding nursing knowledge. *Paradigm* is a global, general framework made up of assumptions about aspects of the discipline held by members to be essential in development of the discipline. The concept of paradigm comes from the work of Kuhn (1970, 1977), who used the term to describe models that guide scientific activity and knowledge development in disciplines. Kuhn set forth the view that science does not evolve as a smooth, regular, continuing path of knowledge development over time, but that there are periodic times of revolution when traditional thought is challenged by new ideas, and "paradigm shifts" occur. In addition, Kuhn's work has meaning for nursing and other practice disciplines because of his recognition that science is the work of a community of scholars in the context of society. Because paradigms are broad, shared perspectives held by members of the discipline, they are often called "worldviews." Paradigms and worldviews of nursing are subtle and powerful, permeating all aspects of the discipline and practice of nursing.

Kuhn's (1970, 1977) description of scientific development is particularly relevant to nursing today as new perspectives are being articulated, some traditional views are being strengthened, and some views are taking their places as part of our history. As we continue to move away from the historical conception of nursing as a part of medical science, developments in the nursing discipline are directed by several new worldviews. Among these are fresh and innovative perspectives on person, nursing, and knowledge development. Changes in the nursing paradigm are being brought about by nursing scholars addressing disciplinary concerns based on values and beliefs about nursing as a human science, caring in nursing, and holistic nursing.

The literature offers additional ways to describe and understand nursing theory. Fawcett (1993) asserts that nursing theory is one component of a hierarchical structure of nursing knowledge development that includes metaparadigm, philosophy, conceptual models, nursing theory, and empirical indicators. These conceptual levels of knowledge development in nursing are interdependent; each level of development is influenced by work at other levels. Walker and Avant (1995) describe the importance of relating theories that have been developed at these various levels of abstraction.

Theoretical work in nursing must be dynamic; that is, it must be continually in process and useful for the purposes and work of the discipline. It must be open to adapt and extend in order both to guide nursing endeavors and to reflect development within nursing. Although there is diversity of opinion among nurses about terms used to describe theoretical development, the following discussion of types of theoretical development in nursing is offered as a context for further understanding nursing theory.

Metaparadigm for Nursing

The metaparadigm for nursing is a framework for the discipline that sets forth the phenomena of interest and the propositions, principles, and methods of the discipline. The metaparadigm is very general and is intended to reflect agreement among members of the discipline about the field of nursing. This is the most abstract level of nursing knowledge and closely mirrors beliefs held about nursing. The metapara-

> As we continue to move away from the historical conception of nursing as part of medical science, developments in the nursing discipline are directed by several new worldviews.

digm offers a context for developing conceptual models and theories. Dialogue on the metaparadigm of nursing today is dynamic because of the range of considerations about what comprises the essence and form of nursing.

All nurses have some awareness of nursing's metaparadigm by virtue of being nurses. However, because the term may not be familiar, it offers no direct guidance for research and practice (Walker & Avant, 1995; Kim, 1997). Historically, the metaparadigm of nursing described concepts of person, environment, health, and nursing. Modifications and alternative concepts for this framework are being explored throughout the discipline (Fawcett, 1993). An example of alternative concepts is the work of Kim (1987, 1997), which sets forth four domains focusing on client, client-nurse encounters, practice, and environment. In recent years, increasing attention has been directed to the nature of nursing's relationship with the environment (Schuster & Brown, 1994; Kleffel, 1996). Newman, Sime, and Corcoran-Perry (1991, p. 3) propose that a single focus statement, "nursing is the study of caring in the human health experience," guide the overall direction of the discipline. Reed (1995) challenges nurses to continue the dialogue about perspectives on knowledge development in the discipline.

Nursing Philosophy

Developments in the metaparadigm of nursing are accompanied by changes in statements of values and beliefs written as nursing philosophies. A philosophy comprises statements of enduring values and beliefs held by members of the discipline. These statements address the major concepts of the discipline, setting forth beliefs about what nursing is, how to think about and do nursing, the relationships of nursing, and the environment of nursing. Philosophical statements are practical guides for examining issues and clarifying priorities of the discipline. Nurses use philosophical statements to examine fit among personal, professional, organizational, and societal beliefs and values.

Conceptual Models of Nursing

Conceptual models are sets of general concepts and propositions that provide perspectives on the major concepts of the metaparadigm, such as person, health and well-being, and the environment. Conceptual models also reflect sets of values and beliefs, as in philosophical statements as well as preferences for practice and research approaches. Fawcett (1993, 1999) points out that direction for research must be described as part of the conceptual model in order to guide development and testing of nursing theories. Conceptual models are less abstract than the metaparadigm and more abstract than theories, offering guidance to nursing endeavors but no distinct direction. Conceptual models may also be called "conceptual frameworks" or "systems."

Nursing Theories

In general, nursing theory describes and explains the phenomena of interest to nursing in a systematic way in order to provide understanding for use in nursing practice and research. Theories are less abstract than conceptual models or systems, although they vary in scope and levels of abstraction. Grand theories of nursing are those general constructions about the nature and goals of nursing. Middle-range nursing theories point to practice and are useful in a defined set of nursing situations. Theories developed at the mid-

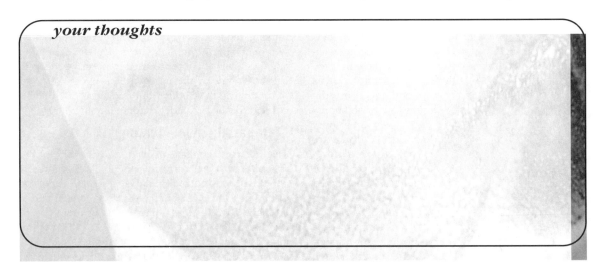

your thoughts

dle range include specific concepts and are less abstract than grand theories. At the next level, nursing
practice theories address issues and questions in a
particular practice setting in which nursing provides
care for a specific population. In addition to considering the scope and levels of abstraction of nursing
theories, they are also sometimes described by the
content or focus of the theory, such as health promotion, and caring and holistic nursing theories.

TYPES OF NURSING THEORY

Nursing theories have been organized into categories and types. George (1995) sets forth categories
of theories according to the orientation of the theorist: nursing problems, interactions, general systems,
and energy fields. Another view is that nursing theory forms a continuum of grand theories at one end
and theories focused on practice at the other (Chinn
& Kramer, 1995; Walker & Avant, 1995; Fitzpatrick,
1997). Meleis (1997) describes types of nursing theory based on their levels of abstraction and goal orientation. Barnum (1998) divides theories into those
that *describe* and those that *explain* nursing phenomena. Types of nursing theories generally include
grand theory, middle-range theory, and practice theory. These will be described below.

Grand Nursing Theory

Grand theories have the broadest scope and present
general concepts and propositions. Theories at this
level may both reflect and provide insights useful for
practice but are not designed for empirical testing.
This limits the use of grand theories for directing, explaining, and predicting nursing in particular situations. Theories at this level are intended to be perti-
nent to all instances of nursing.

Development of grand theories resulted from the
deliberate effort of committed scholars who have engaged in thoughtful reflection on nursing practice
and knowledge and the many contexts of nursing
over time. Nursing theorists who have worked at this
level have had insights guided by nursing and related
metaparadigms and sometimes have experienced
leaps of knowing grounded in these insights. Although there is debate about which nursing theories
are grand in scope, the following are usually considered to be at this level: Leininger's Theory of Culture
Care Diversity and Universality, Newman's Theory of
Health as Expanding Consciousness, Rogers' Science
of Unitary Human Beings, Orem's Self-Care Deficit
Nursing Theory, and Parse's Theory of Human Becoming. These theories are presented in the third
section of this book.

Middle-range Nursing Theory

Middle-range theory was proposed by Robert Merton (1968) in the field of sociology to provide theories that are both broad enough to be useful in complex situations and appropriate for empirical testing.
Nursing scholars proposed using this level of theory
because of the difficulty in testing grand theory (Jacox, 1974). Middle-range theories are more narrow
in scope than grand theories and offer an effective
bridge between grand theories and nursing practice.
They present concepts and propositions at a lower
level of abstraction and hold great promise for increasing theory-based research and nursing practice
strategies.

The literature presents a growing number of reports of nurses' experiences of developing and using
middle-range theory. The nursing practice issues to
which these nurses are responding are complex and
represent a wide range of practice arenas (Chinn,
1994). The methods used for developing middle-
range theories are many and represent some of the
most exciting work being published in nursing today.
Many of these new theories are built on content of
related disciplines and brought into nursing practice
and research (Lenz, Suppe, Gift, Pugh, & Milligan,
1995; Polk, 1997; Eakes, Burke, & Hainsworth, 1998).
The literature also offers middle-range nursing theories that are directly related to grand theories of nursing (Olson & Hanchett, 1997; Ducharme, Ricard, Duquette, Levesque, & Lachance, 1998). Reports of
nursing theory developed at this level include implications for instrument development, theory testing
through research, and nursing practice strategies. Illustrations of the process and product of nursing theory developed at the middle range are presented in
Section IV of this book.

Nursing Practice Theory

Nursing practice theory has the most limited scope
and level of abstraction and is developed for use
within a specific range of nursing situations. Theories developed at this level have a more direct impact
on nursing practice than do theories that are more
abstract. Nursing practice theories provide frameworks for nursing interventions, and predict outcomes and the impact of nursing practice. At the
same time, nursing questions, actions, and procedures may be described or developed as nursing
practice theories. Ideally, nursing practice theories
are interrelated with concepts from middle-range
theories, or may be deduced from theories at the
middle range. Practice theories should also reflect
concepts and propositions of more abstract levels of

nursing theory. Theory developed at this level is also termed prescriptive theory (Dickoff, James, & Wiedenbach, 1968; Crowley, 1968), situation-specific theory (Meleis, 1997), and micro theory (Chinn & Kramer, 1995).

The day-to-day experience of nurses is a major source of nursing practice theory. The depth and complexity of nursing practice may be fully appreciated as nursing phenomena and relations among aspects of particular nursing situations are described and explained. Benner (1984) demonstrated that dialogue with expert nurses in practice is fruitful for discovery and development of practice theory. Research findings on various nursing problems offer data to develop nursing practice theories as nursing engages in research-based development of theory and practice. Nursing practice theory has been articulated using multiple ways of knowing through reflective practice (Johns & Freshwater, 1998). The process includes quiet reflection on practice, remembering and noting features of nursing situations, attending to one's own feelings, reevaluating the experience, and integrating new knowing with other experience (Gray & Forsstrom, 1991).

NURSING'S NEED FOR NURSING THEORY

Nursing theories address the phenomena of interest to nursing, including the focus of nursing; the person, group, or population nursed; the nurse; the relationship of nurse and nursed; and the hoped-for goal or purposes of nursing.

> The day-to-day experience of nurses is a major source of nursing practice theory.

Based on strongly held values and beliefs about nursing, and within contexts of various worldviews, theories are patterns that guide the thinking about, being, and doing of nursing. They provide structure for developing, evaluating, and using nursing scholarship and for extending and refining nursing knowledge through research. Nursing theories either implicitly or explicitly direct all avenues of nursing, including nursing education and administration. Nursing theories provide concepts and designs that define the place of nursing in health and illness care. Through theories, nurses are offered perspectives for relating with professionals from other disciplines who join with nurses to provide human services. Nursing has great expectations of its theories. Theories must, at the same time, provide structure and substance to ground the practice and scholarship of nursing and also be flexible and dynamic to keep pace with the growth and changes in the discipline and practice of nursing.

> Theories are patterns that guide the thinking about, being, and doing of nursing.

Nursing Is a Discipline

Nursing has taken its place as a discipline of knowledge that includes networks of facts, concepts, and approaches to inquiry. The discipline of nursing is also a community of scholars, including nurses in all venues where nursing occurs, which shares commitment to values, concepts, and processes to guide the thought and work of the discipline. Consistent with thinking of nursing scholars about the discipline of nursing (Donaldson & Crowley, 1978; Meleis, 1997) is the classic work of King and Brownell (1976). These authors have set forth attributes of all disciplines. These have particular relevance for nursing and illustrate the need for nursing theory. The attributes of King and Brownell are used as a framework to address the need of the discipline for nursing theory. Each of the attributes is described below from the perspective of the discipline of nursing.

> The discipline of nursing is a community of scholars, including nurses in all venues where nursing occurs.

Expression of Human Imagination

Nursing theory requires curiosity and wonder, as well as critical thinking on the part of the theorists and students of theory. Nursing theory is dependent on the imagination and questioning of nurses in practice and on their creativity to bring ideas of nursing theory into practice. In order to remain dynamic and useful, our discipline requires openness to new ideas and innovative approaches that grow out of members' reflections and insights. There must be support for creative exploration and expression in new theoretical ways.

Domain

A discipline of knowledge and professional practice must be clearly defined by statements of the *domain*—the theoretical and practical boundaries of that discipline and practice. The domain of nursing includes the phenomena of interest, problems to be addressed, main content and methods used, and roles required of members of the discipline (Kim,

1997; Meleis, 1997). The processes and practices claimed by members of the discipline community grow out of these domain statements. Nursing theories containing descriptions of nursing's domain may incorporate a statement of focus of the discipline. The focus may be set in statements about human, social, and ecological concerns addressed by nursing. The focus of the discipline of nursing is a clear statement of social mandate and service used to direct the study and practice of nursing (Newman, Sime, & Corcoran-Perry, 1991).

Nightingale (1859/1992) may have led the call for domain and focus by distinguishing nursing from medicine and other services. Later, Donaldson and Crowley (1978) stated that a discipline has a special way of viewing phenomena and a distinct perspective that defines the work of the discipline. The call for clarity of focus continues in the current environment of nursing practice (Parse, 1997). Nursing theories set forth focus statements or definitions of the discipline and practice of nursing and direct thought and action to fulfill the unique purposes of nursing. This enhances autonomy, and accountability and responsibility are defined and supported. The domain of nursing is also called the "metaparadigm of nursing," as described in the previous section of this chapter.

Syntactical and Conceptual Structures

These structures essential to the discipline are inherent in each of the nursing theories. The conceptual structure delineates the proper concerns of nursing, guides what is to be studied, and clarifies accepted ways of knowing and using content of the discipline. This structure is grounded in the metaparadigm and philosophies of nursing. The conceptual structure relates concepts within nursing theories, and it is from this structure that we learn what is and is not nursing. The syntactical structures help nurses and other professionals understand the talents, skills, and abilities that must be developed within the community. This structure directs descriptions of data needed from research as well as evidence required to demonstrate the impact of nursing practice.

In addition, these structures guide nursing's use of knowledge, research, and practice approaches developed by related disciplines. It is only by being thoroughly grounded in the concepts, substance, and modes of inquiry of the discipline that the boundaries of the discipline, however tentative, can be understood and possibilities for creativity across interdisciplinary borders can be created and explored.

Specialized Language and Symbols

As nursing theory has evolved, so has the need for concepts, language, and forms of data that reflect new ways of thinking and knowing in nursing. The complex concepts used in nursing scholarship and practice require language that can be used and understood. The language of nursing theory facilitates communication among members of the discipline. Expert knowledge of the discipline is often required for full understanding of the meaning of special terms. At the same time, it is often realized that nursing chooses to use commonly understood language in order to communicate more fully with those served.

Heritage of Literature and Networks of Communication

This attribute calls attention to the array of books, periodicals, artifacts, and aesthetic expressions, as well as audio, visual, and electronic media that have

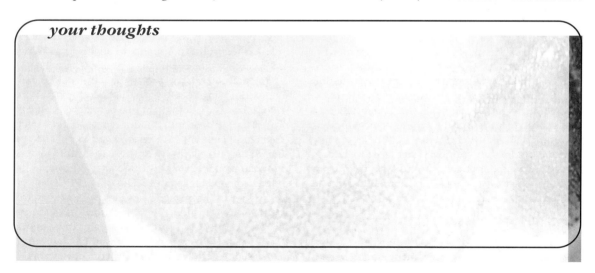

your thoughts

developed over centuries to communicate the nature and development of nursing. Conferences and other forums on every aspect of nursing and for nurses of all interests occur frequently throughout the world. Nursing organizations and societies also provide critical communication links. Nursing theories form the bases for many of the major contributions to the literature, conferences, societies, and other communication networks of the discipline of nursing.

Tradition

The tradition and history of the discipline of nursing is evident in study of nursing theories that have been developed over time. There is recognition that theories most useful today often have threads of connection with theoretical developments of past years. For example, many theorists have acknowledged the influence of Florence Nightingale and have acclaimed her leadership in influencing nursing theories of today. In addition, nursing has a rich heritage of practice. Nursing's practical experience and knowledge have been shared, transformed into content of the discipline, and are evident in the work of many nursing theorists (Gray & Pratt, 1991).

Values and Beliefs

Nursing has distinctive views of persons and strong commitments to compassionate and knowledgeable care of persons through nursing. Nurses often express their love and passion for nursing. Nurses in small groups and in larger nursing organizations express values, hopes, and dreams for the future of their discipline and offer recognition of and appreciation for achievements in the field. The statements of values and beliefs are expressed in the philosophies of nursing that are essential underpinnings of theoretical developments in the discipline.

Systems of Education

Nursing holds the stature and place of a discipline of knowledge and professional practice within institutions of higher education because of the grounding of articulated nursing theories that have set forth the unique contribution of nursing to human affairs. A distinguishing mark of any discipline is the education of future and current members of the community. Nursing theories, by setting directions for the substance and methods of inquiry for the discipline, provide the basis for nursing education and often the framework to organize nursing curricula.

Nursing Is a Professional Practice

Closely aligned with attributes of nursing as a discipline described above is consideration of nursing as a professional practice. Professional practice includes clinical scholarship and processes of nursing persons, groups, and populations who need the special human service that is nursing. The major reason for structuring and advancing nursing knowledge is for the sake of nursing practice. The primary purpose of nursing theories is to further the development and understanding of nursing practice. Theory-based research is needed in

> The major reason for structuring and advancing nursing knowledge is for the sake of nursing practice.

order to explain and predict nursing outcomes essential to the delivery of nursing care that is both humane and cost-effective (Gioiella, 1996). Because nursing theory exists to improve practice, the test of nursing theory is a test of its usefulness in professional practice (Fitzpatrick, 1997). The work of nursing theory is moving from academia into the realm of nursing practice. Chapters in the remaining sections of this book highlight use of nursing theories in nursing practice.

Nursing practice is both the source of and goal for nursing theory. From the viewpoint of practice, Gray and Forsstrom (1991) suggest that through use of theory, nurses find different ways of looking at and assessing phenomena, have rationale for their practice and criteria for evaluating outcomes. Recent studies reported in the literature affirm the importance of use of nursing theory to guide practice (Baker, 1997; Olson & Hanchett, 1997; Barrett, 1998; O'Neill & Kenny, 1998; Whitener, Cox, & Maglich, 1998). Further, these studies illustrate that nursing theory can stimulate creative thinking, facilitate communication, and clarify purposes and relationships of practice. The practicing nurse has an ethical responsibility to use the theoretical knowledge base of the discipline, just as it is the nurse scholars' ethical responsibility to develop the knowledge base specific to nursing practice (Cody, 1997).

Integral to both the professional practice of nursing and nursing theory is the use of empirical indicators. These are developed to meet demands of clinical decision making in the context of rapidly changing needs for nursing and the knowledge required for nursing practice. These indicators include procedures, tools, and instruments to determine the impact of nursing practice and are essential to research and management of outcomes of practice (Jennings & Staggers, 1998). Resulting data form the basis for improving quality of nursing care and influencing health-care policy. Empirical indicators, grounded carefully in nursing concepts, provide clear demonstration of the utility of nursing theory in practice, research, administration, and other nursing endeavors (Hart & Foster, 1998; Allison & McLaughlin-Renpenning, 1999). Fawcett (1993) has placed empirical indicators in the hierarchy of nursing knowledge and relates them to nursing theory when they are an outgrowth of particular aspects of nursing theories.

Meeting the challenges of systems of care delivery and interdisciplinary work demands practice from a theoretical perspective. Nursing's disciplinary focus is essential within an interdisciplinary environment (Allison & McLaughlin-Renpenning, 1999). Nursing actions reflect nursing concepts and thought. Careful, reflective, and critical thinking is the hallmark of expert nursing and nursing theories should undergird these processes. Appreciation and use of nursing theory offer opportunity for successful collaboration with related disciplines and practices, and provide definition for nursing's overall contribution to health care. Nurses must know what they are doing, why they are doing what they are doing, what may be the range of outcomes of nursing, and indicators for measuring nursing's impact. These nursing theoretical frameworks serve in powerful ways as guides for articulating, reporting, and recording nursing thought and action.

One of the assertions referred to most often in the nursing theory literature is that theory is given birth in nursing practice and, following examination and refinement through research, must be returned to practice (Dickoff, James, & Wiedenbach, 1968). Within nursing as a practice discipline, nursing theory is stimulated by questions and curiosities arising from nursing practice. Development of nursing knowledge is a result of theory-based nursing inquiry. The circle continues as data, conclusions, and recommendations of nursing research are evaluated and developed for use in practice. Nursing theory must be seen as practical and useful to practice and the insights of practice must in turn continue to enrich nursing theory.

NURSING THEORY AND THE FUTURE

Nursing theory in the future will be more fully integrated with all domains of the discipline and practice of nursing. New, more open and inclusive ways to theorize about nursing will be developed. These new ways will acknowledge the history and traditions of nursing but will move nursing forward into new realms of thinking and being. Gray and Pratt (1991,

p. 454) project that nursing scholars will continue to develop theories at all levels of abstraction, and that theories will be increasingly interdependent with other disciplines such as politics, economics, and aesthetics. These authors expect a continuing emphasis on unifying theory and practice that will contribute to validation of the discipline of nursing. Reed (1995) notes the "ground shifting" with reforming of philosophies of nursing science and calls for a more open philosophy, grounded in nursing's values, which connects science, philosophy, and practice. Theorists will work in groups to develop knowledge in an area of concern to nursing, and these phenomena of interest, rather than the name of the author, will define the theory (Meleis, 1992).

> It is important to question to what extent theories developed and used in one major culture are appropriate for use in other cultures.

Nursing's philosophies and theories must increasingly reflect nursing's values for understanding, respect, and commitment to health beliefs and practices of cultures throughout the world. It is important to question to what extent theories developed and used in one major culture are appropriate for use in other cultures. To what extent must nursing theory be relevant in multicultural contexts? Despite efforts of many international scholarly societies, how relevant are our nursing theories for the global community? Can nursing theories inform us how to stand with and learn from peoples of the world? Can we learn from nursing theory how to come to know those we nurse, how to be with, to truly listen and hear? Can these questions be recognized as appropriate for scholarly work and practice for graduate students in nursing? Will these issues offer direction for studies of doctoral students? If so, nursing theory will offer new ways to inform nurses for humane leadership in national and global health policy.

Perspectives of various time worlds in relation to present nursing concerns were described by Schoenhofer (1994). Faye G. Abdellah, one of nursing's finest international leaders, offers the advice that we must maintain focusing on those we nurse (McAuliffe, 1998). Abdellah notes that nurses in other countries have often developed their systems of education, practice, and research based on learning from our mistakes. She further proposes an international electronic "think tank" for nurses around the globe to dialogue about nursing (McAuliffe, 1998). Such opportunities could lead nurses to truly listen, learn, and adapt theoretical perspectives to accommodate cultural variations. We must somehow come to appreciate the essence and beauty of nursing, just as Nightingale knew it to be. Perhaps it will be realized that the essence of nursing is universal, and only the ways of expressing nursing vary.

Many of the chapters of this book contain insights and projections about nursing theory in the coming century. It is somewhat frightening to write about nursing theory in the twenty-first century and it takes courage and perhaps more than a bit of humor to do so. All of us have ways to look back to the year 1900; even if we were not present or cannot remember the context of our lives then, we have heard and read about those times. All can realize the vast changes that have taken place during the twentieth century. Nurses and nursing have participated in these changes. Nursing theorists and scholars who are contributing authors for this book have not only reflected and projected about the future, they have also been willing to share with us their thoughts on the future of nursing theory as we enter the new millennium.

Summary

One challenge of nursing theory is the perspective that theory is always in the process of developing and that, at the same time, it is useful for the purposes and work of the discipline. This may be seen as ambiguous or as full of possibilities. Continuing students of the discipline are required to study and know the basis for their contributions to nursing and to those we serve, while at the same time be open to new ways of thinking, knowing, and being in nursing. Exploring structures of nursing knowledge and understanding the nature of nursing as a discipline of knowledge and professional practice provides a frame of reference to clarify nursing theory. The wise study and use of nursing theory can be a helpful companion in the new millennium.

References

Allison, S. E., & McLaughlin-Renpenning, K. E. (1999). *Nursing administration in the 21st century: A self-care theory approach.* Thousand Oaks, CA: Sage Publications.

Baker, C. (1997). Cultural relativism and cultural diversity: Implications for nursing practice. *Advances in Nursing Science, 20*(1), 3–11.

Barnum, B. S. (1998). *Nursing theory: Analysis, application, evaluation* (5th ed.). Philadelphia: Lippincott.

Barrett, E. A. (1998). A Rogerian practice methodology for health patterning. *Nursing Science Quarterly, 11*(4), 136–138.

Benner, P. (1984). *From novice to expert: Excellence and power in clinical nursing practice.* New York: Addison-Wesley.

Chinn, P. (1994). *Developing substance: Mid-range theory in nursing.* Gaithersburg, MD: Aspen Publications.

Chinn, P., & Jacobs, M. (1987). *Theory and nursing: A systematic approach.* St. Louis: C. V. Mosby.

Chinn, P., & Kramer, M. (1995). *Theory and nursing: A systematic approach* (4th ed.). St. Louis: Mosby-Year Book.

Cody, W. K. (1997). Of tombstones, milestones, and gemstones: A retrospective and prospective on nursing theory. *Nursing Science Quarterly, 10*(1), 3–5.

Crowley, D. (1968). Perspectives of pure science. *Nursing Research, 17*(6), 497–501.

Dickoff, J., & James, P. (1968). A theory of theories: A position paper. *Nursing Research, 17*(3), 197–203.

Dickoff, J., James, P., & Wiedenbach, E. (1968). Theory in a practice discipline. *Nursing Research, 17*(5), 415–435.

Donaldson, S. K., & Crowley, D. M. (1978). The discipline of nursing. *Nursing Outlook, 26*(2), 113–120.

Ducharme, F., Ricard, N., Duquette, A., Levesque, L., & Lachance, L. (1998). Empirical testing of a longitudinal model derived from the Roy Adaptation Model. *Nursing Science Quarterly, 11*(4), 149–159.

Eakes, G., Burke, M., & Hainsworth, M. (1998). Middle-range theory of chronic sorrow. *Image: Journal of Nursing Scholarship, 30*(2), 179–184.

Ellis, R. (1968). Characteristics of significant theories. *Nursing Research, 17*(3), 217–222.

Fawcett, J. (1993). *Analysis and evaluation of nursing theory.* Philadelphia: F. A. Davis Company.

Fawcett, J. (1999). *The relationship of theory and research* (2nd ed.). Philadelphia: F. A. Davis Company.

Fitzpatrick, J. (1997). Nursing theory and metatheory. In King, I., & Fawcett, J. (Eds.), *The language of nursing theory and metatheory.* Indianapolis, IN: Center Nursing Press.

George, J. (1995). *Nursing theories: The base for professional nursing practice.* Norwalk, CT: Appleton & Lange.

Gioiella, E. C. (1996). The importance of theory-guided research and practice in the changing health care scene. *Nursing Science Quarterly, 9*(2), 47.

Gray, J., & Forsstrom, S. (1991). Generating theory for practice: The reflective technique. In Gray, J., & Pratt, R. (Eds.). (1991). *Towards a discipline of nursing.* Melbourne: Churchill Livingstone.

Gray, J., & Pratt, R. (Eds.) (1991). *Towards a discipline of nursing.* Melbourne: Churchill Livingstone.

Hart, M., & Foster, S. (1998). Self-care agency in two groups of pregnant women. *Nursing Science Quarterly, 11*(4), 167–171.

Jacox, A. (1974). Theory construction in nursing: An overview. *Nursing Research, 23*(1), 4–13.

Jennings, B. M., & Staggers, N. (1998). The language of outcomes. *Advances in Nursing Science, 20*(4), 72–80.

Johns, C., & Freshwater, D. (1998). *Transforming nursing through reflective practice.* London: Oxford Science Ltd.

Kim, H. (1987). Structuring the nursing knowledge system: A typology of four domains. *Scholarly Inquiry for Nursing Practice: An International Journal, 1*(1), 99–110.

Kim, H. (1997). Terminology in structuring and developing nursing knowledge. In King, I. & Fawcett, J. (Eds.), *The language of nursing theory and metatheory.* Indianapolis, IN: Center Nursing Press.

King, A. R., & Brownell, J. A. (1976). *The curriculum and the disciplines of knowledge.* Huntington, NY: Robert E. Krieger Pub. Co.

Kleffel, D. (1996). Environmental paradigms: Moving toward an ecocentric perspective. *Advances in Nursing Science, 18*(4), 1–10.

Kuhn, T. (1970). *The structure of scientific revolutions* (2nd ed.). Chicago: University of Chicago Press.

Kuhn, T. (1977). *The essential tension: Selected studies in scientific tradition and change.* Chicago: University of Chicago Press.

Lenz, E., Suppe, F., Gift, A., Pugh, L., & Milligan, R. (1995). Collaborative development of middle-range theories: Toward a theory of unpleasant symptoms. *Advances in Nursing Science, 17*(3), 1–13.

McAuliffe, M. (1998). Interview with Faye G. Abdellah on nursing research and health policy. *Image: Journal of Nursing Scholarship, 30*(3), 215–219.

McKay, R. (1969). Theories, models and systems for nursing. *Nursing Research, 18*(5), 393–399.

Meleis, A. (1992). Directions for nursing theory development in the 21st century. *Nursing Science Quarterly, 5,* 112–117.

Meleis, A. (1997). *Theoretical nursing: Development and progress.* Philadelphia: Lippincott.

Merton, R. (1968). *Social theory and social structure.* New York: The Free Press.

Newman, M., Sime, A., & Corcoran-Perry, S. (1991). The focus of the discipline of nursing. *Advances in Nursing Science, 14*(1), 1–6.

Nightingale, F. (1859/1992). *Notes on nursing: What it is and what it is not.* Philadelphia: Lippincott.

Olson, J., & Hanchett, E. (1997). Nurse-expressed empathy, patient outcomes, and development of a middle-range theory. *Image: Journal of Nursing Scholarship, 29*(1), 71–76.

O'Neill, D. P., & Kenny, E. K. (1998). Spirituality and chronic illness. *Image: Journal of Nursing Scholarship, 30*(3), 275–280.

Parse, R. (1997). Nursing and medicine: Two different disciplines. *Nursing Science Quarterly, 6*(3), 109.

Polk, L. (1997). Toward a middle-range theory of resilience. *Advances in Nursing Science, 19*(3), 1–13.

Reed, P. (1995). A treatise on nursing knowledge development for the 21st century: Beyond postmodernism. *Advances in Nursing Science, 17*(3), 70–84.

Schoenhofer, S. (1994). Transforming visions for nursing in the timeworld of *Einstein's Dreams. Advances in Nursing Science, 16*(4), 1–8.

Schuster, E., & Brown, C. (1994). *Exploring our environmental connections.* New York: National League for Nursing.

Silva, M. (1997). Philosophy, theory, and research in nursing: A linguistic journey to nursing practice. In King, I., & Fawcett, J. (Eds.), *The language of nursing theory and metatheory.* Indianapolis, IN: Center Nursing Press.

Walker, L., & Avant, K. (1995). *Strategies for theory construction in nursing.* Norwalk, CT: Appleton-Century-Crofts.

Whitener, L. M., Cox, K. R., & Maglich, S. A. (1998). Use of theory to guide nurses in the design of health messages for children. *Advances in Nursing Science, 20*(3), 21–35.

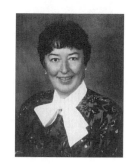

Chapter 2

Studying Nursing Theory: Choosing, Analyzing, Evaluating

❖ Reasons for Studying Nursing Theory

❖ Questions from Practicing Nurses about Using Nursing Theory

❖ Choosing a Nursing Theory to Study

❖ An Exercise for the Study of Nursing Theory

❖ Analysis and Evaluation of Nursing Theory

❖ Summary

❖ References

Marilyn E. Parker

The primary purpose for nursing theory is to advance the discipline and professional practice of nursing. One of the most urgent issues facing the discipline of nursing is the need to bring together nursing theory and practice. Their continuing separation is artificial. Nursing can no longer afford to see these endeavors as disconnected and belonging to either scholars or practitioners. The examination and use of nursing theories are essential for closing the gap between nursing theory and nursing practice. Nurses in practice have a responsibility to study and value nursing theories, just as nursing theory scholars must understand and appreciate the day-to-day practice of nursing.

This issue is highlighted by considering a brief encounter during a question period at a conference. A nurse in practice, reflecting her experience, asked a nurse theorist: "What is the meaning of this theory to my practice? I'm in the real world! I want to connect—but how can connections be made between your ideas and my reality?" The nurse theorist responded by describing the essential values and assumptions of her theory. The nurse said: "Yes, I know what you are talking about. I just didn't know I knew it and I need help to use it in my practice" (Parker, 1993, p. 4). To remain current in the discipline, all nurses must be continuing students, must join in community to advance nursing knowledge and practice, and must accept their obligations to an ongoing investigation of nursing theories.

> One of the most urgent issues of the discipline is the need to bring together nursing theory and practice.

This chapter provides a focus on the study of nursing theories with the idea of review and selection of nursing theory for use in any nursing endeavor: practice, education, administration, research, and development. Methods of analysis and evaluation of nursing theory set forth in the literature will be presented. Although nursing theory is essential for all nursing, the main focus of theory analysis and evaluation in this chapter is the use of nursing theories in nursing practice. The chapter begins with responses to the questions: Why study nursing theory? What does the practicing nurse want from nursing theory?

REASONS FOR STUDYING NURSING THEORY

Nursing practice is essential for developing, testing, and refining nursing theory. The everyday practice of nursing enriches nursing theory. When nurses are thinking about nursing, their ideas are about the content and structure of the discipline of nursing. Even if nurses do not conceptualize them in this way, their ideas are about nursing theory. The development of many nursing theories has been enhanced by reflection and dialogue about actual nursing situations. We might consider that aspects of nursing theories are explored and refined in the day-to-day practice of nursing. Creative nursing practice is the direct result of ongoing theory-based thinking, decision making, and action of nurses. Nursing practice must continue to contribute to thinking and theorizing in nursing, just as nursing theory must be used to advance understanding and the impact of practice.

Nursing practice and nursing theory are guided by the same abiding values and beliefs. Nursing practice is guided by enduring values and beliefs as well as by knowledge held by individual nurses. These values, beliefs, and knowledges echo those held by other nurses in the discipline, including nurse scholars and those who study and write about nursing's metaparadigm, philosophies, and theories. In addition, nursing theorists and nurses in practice think about and work with the same phenomena, including the person nursed, the actions and relationships in the nursing situation, and the context of nursing.

Many nurses practice according to ideas and directions from other disciplines, such as medicine, psychology, and public health. This is not uncommon to nursing historically and is deeply ingrained in the medical system, as well as in many settings in which nurses practice today. The depth and scope of the practice of nurses who follow notions about nursing held by other disciplines are limited to practices understood and accepted by those disciplines. Nurses who learn to practice from nursing perspectives are awakened to the challenges and opportunities of practicing nursing more fully and with a greater sense of autonomy, respect, and satisfaction for themselves and those they nurse. These nurses learn to reframe their thinking about nursing knowledge and practice and are then able to bring knowledge from other disciplines into their practice—not to direct their practice, but in order to meet goals of nursing.

> Creative nursing practice can be the direct result of ongoing, theory-based thinking, decision making, and action of nurses.

Nurses who understand nursing's theoretical base are free to see beyond immediate facts and delivery systems, and are able to choose to bring the full range of health sciences and technologies into their practice. These nurses can envision and contribute to the many possibilities of the discipline. Nurses who study nursing theory realize that although no group actually owns ideas, disciplines do claim ideas for their use. In the same way, no group actually owns techniques, though disciplines do claim them for their practice. For example, before World War II, nurses rarely took blood pressure readings. This was not because they were unable, but because they did not claim the use of this technique to facilitate their nursing. Such realization can also lead to understanding that the things nurses do that are often called nursing are not nursing at all. The techniques used by nurses, such as taking blood pressure readings, are actually activities that give the nurse access to persons for nursing. Nursing theories inform the nurse about what nursing is and guide the use of other ideas and techniques for nursing purposes.

If nursing theory is to be useful, it must be brought into practice. Nurses can be guided by nursing theory in a full range of nursing situations. Nursing theory can change nursing practice. Nurses should no longer ignore the possibilities of theory-based practice, withholding this quality of nursing so that persons they nurse never experience theory-based nursing. Chapters of this book affirm the use of nursing theory in practice and the study and assessment of theory for ultimate use in practice.

QUESTIONS FROM PRACTICING NURSES ABOUT USING NURSING THEORY

Study of nursing theory may either precede or follow selection of a nursing theory for use in nursing practice. Analysis and evaluation of nursing theory are key ways to study theory. These activities are demanding and deserve the full commitment of nurses who undertake the work. Because it is understood that study of nursing theory is not a simple, short-term endeavor, nurses often question doing such work. The following questions about studying and using nursing theory have been collected from many conversations with nurses about nursing theory. These queries also identify specific issues that are important to nurses who consider study of nursing theory.

My Nursing Practice

- Does this theory reflect nursing practice as I know it? Can it be understood in relation to my nursing practice? Will it support what I believe to be excellent nursing practice?
- Is the theory specific to my area of nursing? Can the language of the theory help me explain, plan, and evaluate my nursing? Will I be able to use the terms to communicate with others?
- Can this theory be considered in relation to a wide range of nursing situations? How does it relate to more general views of nursing people in other settings?
- Will my study and use of this theory support nursing in my interdisciplinary setting?
- Will those from other disciplines be able to understand, facilitating cooperation?
- Will my work meet the expectations of patients and others? Will other nurses find my work helpful and challenging?

My Personal Interests, Abilities, and Experiences

- Is the study of nursing theories in keeping with my talents, interests, and goals? Is this something I want to do?
- Will I be stimulated by thinking about and trying to use this theory? Will my study of nursing be enhanced by use of this theory?
- What will it be like to think about nursing theory in nursing practice?
- Will my work with nursing theory be worth the effort?
- What must I do? Am I able?

Resources and Support

- Will this be useful to me outside the classroom?
- What resources will I need to understand more fully the terms of the theory?
- Will I be able to find the support I need to study and use the theory in my practice?

The Theorist, Evidence, and Opinion

- Who is the author of this theory? What is the background of nursing education and experience brought to this work by the theorist? Is the author an authoritative nursing scholar?
- What are the opinions of knowledgeable nurses about the work of the theorist?
- What is the evidence that use of the theory may lead to improved nursing care? Has the theory been useful to guide nursing organizations and administrations? What about influencing nursing and health-care policy?

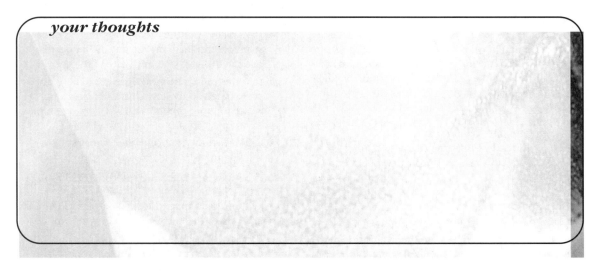

your thoughts

- What is the evidence that this nursing theory has led to nursing research, including questions and methods of inquiry? Did the theory grow out of nursing research reports? Out of nursing practice issues and problems?
- Does the theory reflect the latest thinking in nursing? Has the theory kept pace with the times in nursing? Is this the nursing theory for the future?

CHOOSING A NURSING THEORY TO STUDY

It is important to give adequate attention to selection of theories for study. Results of this work may have lasting influences on one's nursing practice. For all the reasons already offered in this book, aspects of one's personal and professional life may encounter challenges and growth. It is not unusual for nurses who begin to work with nursing theory to realize their practice is changing and that their future efforts in the discipline and practice of nursing are markedly altered.

There is always some measure of hope mixed with anxiety as nurses seriously explore nursing theory for the first time. Individual nurses who practice with a group of colleagues often wonder how to select and study nursing theories. Nurses and nursing students in courses considering nursing theory have similar questions. Nurses in new practice settings designed and developed by nurses have the same concerns about getting started as do nurses in hospital organizations who want more from their nursing.

The following exercise is grounded in the belief that the study and use of nursing theory in nursing

practice must have roots in the practice of the nurses involved. Moreover, the nursing theory used by particular nurses must reflect elements of practice that are essential to those nurses while at the same time bringing focus and freshness to that practice. This exercise calls on the nurse to think about the major components of nursing, and calls forth the values and beliefs nurses hold most dear. In these ways, the exercise begins to parallel knowledge development reflected in the nursing metaparadigm and nursing philosophies as described in Chapter 1. From this point on, the nurse is guided to connect nursing theory and nursing practice in the context of nursing situations. It is from these experiences that decisions about nursing theory and practice are derived.

AN EXERCISE FOR THE STUDY OF NURSING THEORY

Select a comfortable, private, and quiet place to reflect and write. Begin to be quiet and relaxed by taking some deep, slow breaths. Think about the reasons you went into nursing in the first place. Bring your nursing practice into focus. Consider your practice today. Continue to reflect and, without being distracted, make notes, so you won't forget your thoughts and feelings. If you are doing this exercise with a group of colleagues, make an effort to wait until later to share your reflections, and only then as you wish to do so. When you have been still for a time and have taken the opportunity to reflect on your practice, you may proceed with the following questions. Continue to reflect and to make notes as you consider each question about your beliefs and values.

Enduring Values

- What are the enduring values and beliefs that brought me to nursing?
- What beliefs and values keep me in nursing today?
- What are those values I hold most dear?
- What are the ties of these values with my personal values?
- How do my personal and nursing values connect with what is important to society?

Nursing Situations

Reflect on a nursing situation, that is, an instance of nursing in which you interacted with a person for nursing purposes. This can be a situation from your current practice or may come to your memory from your nursing in years past. Consider the purpose or hoped for outcome of the nursing.

- Who was my patient as a person?
- What were the needs for nursing the person?
- Who was I as a person in the nursing situation?
- Who was I as a nurse in the situation?
- What was the interaction like between the patient and myself?
- What nursing responses did I offer to the needs of the patient?
- What other nursing responses might have been possible?
- What was the environment of the nursing situation?
- What about the environment was important to the needs for nursing and to my nursing responses?

Connecting Values and the Nursing Situation

Nursing can change when we bring to awareness the connections of values and beliefs and nursing situations. Consider that values and beliefs are the basis for our nursing. Briefly describe the connections of your values and beliefs with your chosen nursing situation.

- How are my values and beliefs reflected in the nursing situation?
- Are my values and beliefs in conflict in the situation?
- Do my values come to life in the nursing situation?
- Are my values frustrated?

Verifying Awareness and Appreciation

In reflecting and writing about values and situations of nursing that are important to us, we often come to a fuller awareness and appreciation of nursing. Make notes about your insights. You might consider these initial notes the beginning of a journal in which you record your study of nursing theories and their use in nursing practice. This is a great way to follow your progress and is a source of nursing questions for future study. You may want to share this process and experience with your colleagues. These are ways to clarify and verify views about nursing and to seek and offer support for nursing values and situations that are critical to our practice. If you are doing this exercise in a group, this is the time to share your essential values and beliefs with your colleagues.

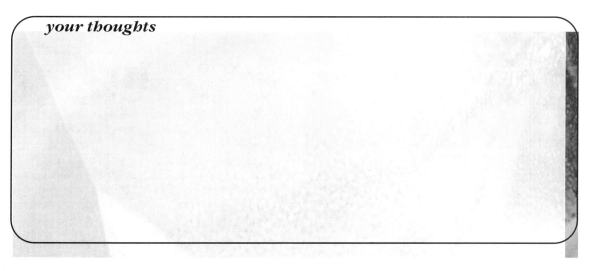

your thoughts

Using Insights to Choose Theory

The notes describing your experience will help in selecting a nursing theory to study and consider for guiding practice. You will want to answer these questions:

- What nursing theory seems consistent with the values and beliefs that guide my practice?
- What theories do I believe are consistent with my personal values and society's beliefs?
- What do I want from the use of nursing theory?
- Given my reflection on a nursing situation, do I want theory to support this description of my practice?
- Do I hope to use nursing theory to improve my experience of practice for myself and for my patients?

Using Authoritative Sources

Use your questions and new insights to begin a literature search. Gather and use library resources, such as CINAHL. Search the Internet and use on-line resources for information on nursing theories and their use in practice, research, education, and administration. Join an on-line group dialogue about a particular nursing theory. You and your colleagues may seek consultation for assistance with analysis and evaluation of specific nursing theories.

Using a Guide to Select a Nursing Theory

This is the time to explore using the following guides for analysis and evaluation of nursing theory. Done individually or as a group, this is an additional opportunity to learn and to share. This is demanding work, but along with the challenge, this can also be fun, gratifying, and a good way to strengthen bonds with colleagues.

> The whole theory must be studied. Parts of the theory without the whole will not be fully meaningful and could lead to misunderstanding.

ANALYSIS AND EVALUATION OF NURSING THEORY

It is important to understand definitions of nursing theory, as described in Chapter 1, before moving to theory analysis and evaluation. These definitions direct examination of structure, content, and purposes of theories. Although each of these definitions is adequate for study of any nursing theory, the definition that seems to best fit with the particular purpose for study of theory should be chosen. For example, one of the definitions by Chinn and Jacobs (1987) and Chin and Kramer (1995) may be chosen for using theory in research. The definition by Silva (1997) may be more appropriate for study of nursing theory for use in practice. Another way to think about this is to consider whether the definition of nursing theory in use fits the theory being analyzed and evaluated. Look carefully at the theory, read the theory as presented by the theorist, and read what others have written about the theory. The whole theory must be studied. Parts of the theory without the whole will not be fully meaningful and may lead to misunderstanding.

Before selecting a guide for analysis and evaluation, consider the level and scope of the theory, as discussed in the previous chapter. Is the theory a grand nursing theory? A philosophy? A middle-range nursing theory? A practice theory? Not all aspects of theory described in an evaluation guide will be evident in all levels of theory. For example, questions about the metaparadigm are probably not appropriate to use in analyzing middle-range theories. Whall (1996) recognizes this in offering particular guides for analysis and evaluation that vary according to three types of nursing theory: models, middle-range theories, and practice theories.

Theory analysis and evaluation may be thought of as one process or as a two-step sequence. It may be helpful to think of analysis of theory as necessary for adequate study of a nursing theory and evaluation of theory as the assessment of the utility of a theory for particular purposes. Guides for theory evaluation are intended as tools to inform us about theories, and to encourage further development, refinement, and use of theory. There are no guides for theory analysis and evaluation that are adequate and appropriate for every nursing theory.

Johnson (1974) wrote about three basic criteria to guide evaluation of nursing theory. These have continued in use over time and offer direction for guides in use today. These criteria are that the theory should

- define the congruence of nursing practice with societal expectations of nursing decisions and actions;
- clarify the social significance of nursing, or the impact of nursing on persons receiving nursing; and
- describe social utility, or usefulness of the theory in practice, research, and education.

Following are outlines of the most frequently used guides for analysis and evaluation. These guides are components of the entire work about nursing theory of the individual nursing scholar and offer various interesting approaches to the study of nursing theory. Each guide should be studied in more detail than is offered in this introduction and should be examined in context of the whole work of the individual nurse scholar.

The approach to theory analysis set forth by Chinn and Kramer (1995) is to use guidelines for describing nursing theory that are based on their definition of theory that is presented in Chapter 1. The guidelines set forth questions that clarify the facts about aspects of theory: purpose, concepts, definitions, relationships, structure, assumptions, and scope. These authors suggest that the next step in the process of evaluation is critical reflection about whether and how the nursing theory works. Questions are posed to guide this reflection:

- Is the theory clearly stated?
- Is it stated simply?
- Can the theory be generalized?
- Is the theory accessible?
- How important is the theory?

Fawcett (1993) developed a framework of questions that separates the activities of analysis and evaluation. Questions for analysis in this framework flow from the structural hierarchy of nursing knowledge proposed by Fawcett and defined in Chapter 1. The questions for evaluation guide examination of theory content and use for practical purposes. Following is a summary of the Fawcett (1993) framework.

For Theory Analysis, Consideration Is Given To:

- scope of the theory
- metaparadigm concepts and propositions included in the theory
- values and beliefs reflected in the theory
- relation of the theory to a conceptual model and to related disciplines
- concepts and propositions of the theory

For Theory Evaluation, Consideration Is Given To:

- significance of the theory and relations with structure of knowledge
- consistency and clarity of concepts, expressed in congruent, concise language
- adequacy for use in research, education, and practice

- feasibility to apply the theory in practical contexts

Meleis (1997) states that the structural and functional components of a theory should be studied prior to evaluation. The structural components are assumptions, concepts, and propositions of the theory. Functional components include descriptions of the following: focus, client, nursing, health, nurse-client interactions, environment, and nursing problems and interventions. After studying these dimensions of the theory, critical examination of these elements may take place, as summarized below:

- Relations between structure and function of the theory, including clarity, consistency, and simplicity
- Diagram of theory to understand further the theory by creating a visual representation
- Contagiousness, or adoption of the theory by a wide variety of students, researchers, and practitioners, as reflected in the literature
- Usefulness in practice, education, research, and administration
- External components of personal, professional, and social values, and significance

Summary

Nursing theory, knowledge development through research, and nursing practice are closely linked and interrelated. In so many ways, the connections of nursing practice with nursing theory bring the practicing nurse to the challenge of studying nursing theory. Considering a commitment to study nursing theory raises many questions from nurses about to undertake this important work. Analysis and evaluation of nursing theory are the main ways of studying nursing theory.

References

Chinn, P., & Jacobs, M. (1987). *Theory and nursing: A systematic approach*. St. Louis: C. V. Mosby.

Chinn, P., & Kramer, M. (1995). *Theory and nursing: A systematic approach* (4th ed.). St. Louis: Mosby Year-Book.

Fawcett, J. (1993). *Analysis and evaluation of nursing theory*. Philadelphia: F. A. Davis.

Johnson, D. (1974). Development of theory: A requisite for nursing as a primary health profession. *Nursing Research, 23*(5), 372–377.

Meleis, A. (1997). *Theoretical nursing: Development and progress*. Philadelphia: Lippincott.

Parker, M. (1993). *Patterns of nursing theories in practice.* New York: National League for Nursing.

Silva, M. (1997). Philosophy, theory, and research in nursing: A linguistic journey to nursing practice. In King, I., & Fawcett, J. (Eds.), *The language of nursing theory and metatheory*. Indianapolis, IN: Center Nursing Press.

Whall, A. (1996). The structure of nursing knowledge: Analysis and evaluation of practice, middle-range, and grand theory. In Fitzpatrick, J., & Whall, A. (Eds.), *Conceptual models of nursing: Analysis and application* (3rd ed.). Stamford, CT: Appleton & Lange.

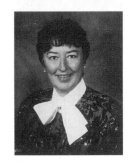

Chapter 3

Guides for Study of Theories for Practice and Administration

❖ Study of Theory for Nursing Practice

❖ A Guide for Study of Nursing Theory for Use in Practice

❖ Study of Theory for Nursing Administration

❖ Summary

❖ References

Marilyn E. Parker

Nurses, individually and in groups, are affected by rapid and dramatic change throughout health and medical systems. Nurses practice in increasingly diverse settings. Nurses often develop organized nursing practices through which accessible health care to communities can be provided. Community members may be active participants in selecting, designing, and evaluating the nursing they receive. Interdisciplinary practice is frequently the norm.

Theories and practices from related disciplines are brought to nursing to use for nursing purposes. The scope of nursing practice is continually being expanded to include additional knowledge and skills from related disciplines, such as medicine and psychology. Although the majority of nurses practice in hospitals, an increasing number of nurses practice elsewhere in the community, taking the venue of their practice closer to those served by nursing.

Groups of nurses working together as colleagues to provide nursing often realize that they share the same values and beliefs about nursing. The study of nursing theories can clarify the purposes of nursing and facilitate building a cohesive practice to meet these purposes. Regardless of the setting of nursing practice, nurses may choose to study nursing theories together in order to design and articulate theory-based practice. The exercise in Chapter 2 is offered to facilitate this work.

> The scope of nursing practice is continually being expanded to include knowledge and skills from related disciplines.

This chapter offers guides for continuing study of nursing theory for use in nursing practice. Because many nurses are creating new practice organizations and settings, a guide for study of nursing theory for use in nursing administration has been developed. The guides are intended for use in conjunction with the overall study of nursing theory, including the methods of analysis and evaluation outlined in Chapter 2. The first guide is a set of questions for consideration in study and selection of a nursing theory for use in practice. The second guide is an outline of factors to consider when studying nursing theory for use in nursing organization and administration.

Responses to questions offered and points summarized in the guides may be found in nursing literature as well as by use of audiovisual and electronic resources. Primary source material, including the writing of nurses who are recognized authorities in specific nursing theories and the use of nursing theory, should be used. Subsequent chapters of this book offer such sources. Users of this guide are invited to examine each question carefully and add questions from other theory analysis and evaluation guides to meet their particular purposes.

STUDY OF THEORY FOR NURSING PRACTICE

Four main questions have been developed and refined to facilitate study of nursing theories for use in nursing practice (Parker, 1993). These questions are intended to focus on concepts within the theories as well as points of interest and general information about each theory. This guide was developed for use by practicing nurses and students in undergraduate and graduate programs of nursing education. Many nurses and students have used these questions and have contributed to their continuing development. The guide may be used to study most of the nursing theories developed at all levels. It has been used to create surveys of nursing theories. An early motivation for developing this guide was the work by the Nursing Development Conference Group (1973).

A GUIDE FOR STUDY OF NURSING THEORY FOR USE IN PRACTICE

1. **How is nursing conceptualized in the theory?**

   Is the focus of nursing stated?
   - *What does the nurse attend to when practicing nursing?*
   - *What guides nursing observations, reflections, decisions, and actions?*
   - *What does the nurse think about when considering nursing?*
   - *What are illustrations of use of the theory to guide practice?*

   What is the purpose of nursing?
   - *What do nurses do when they are practicing nursing?*
   - *What are exemplars of nursing assessments, designs, plans, and evaluations?*
   - *What indicators give evidence of quality and quantity of nursing practice?*
   - *Is the richness and complexity of nursing practice evident?*

   What are the boundaries or limits for nursing?
   - *How is nursing distinguished from other health and medical services?*
   - *How is nursing related to other disciplines and services?*

- What is the place of nursing in interdisciplinary settings?
- What is the range of nursing situations in which the theory is useful?

How can nursing situations be described?
- What are attributes of the one nursed?
- What are characteristics of the nurse?
- How can interactions of the nurse and the one nursed be described?
- Are there environmental requirements for the practice of nursing?

2. **What is the context of development of the theory?**

Who is the nursing theorist as person and as nurse?
- Why did the theorist develop the theory?
- What is the background of the theorist as nursing scholar?
- What are central values and beliefs set forth by the theorist?

What are major theoretical influences on this theory?
- What nursing models and theories influenced this theory?
- What are relationships of this theory with other theories?
- What nursing-related theories and philosophies influenced this theory?

What were major external influences on development of the theory?
- What were the social, economic, and political influences?
- What images of nurses and nursing influenced the theory?
- What was the status of nursing as a discipline and profession?

3. **Who are authoritative sources for information about development, evaluation, and use of this theory?**

Who are nursing authorities who speak about, write about, and use the theory?
- What are the professional attributes of these persons?
- What are the attributes of authorities, and how does one become one?
- Which other nurses should be considered authorities?

What major resources are authoritative sources on the theory?

- Books? Articles? Audiovisual media? Electronic media?
- What nursing societies share and support work of the theory?
- What service and academic programs are authoritative sources?

4. **How can the overall significance of the theory to nursing be described?**

What is the importance of the theory of nursing over time?
- What are exemplars of the use to structure and guide individual practice?
- Is the theory used to guide programs of nursing education?
- Is the theory used to guide nursing administration and organizations?
- Does published nursing scholarship reflect significance of the theory?

What is the experience of nurses who report consistent use of the theory?
- What is the range of reports from practice?
- Has nursing research led to further theory formulations?
- Has the theory been used to develop new nursing practices?
- Has the theory influenced design of methods of nursing inquiry?
- What has been the influence of the theory on nursing and health policy?

What are projected influences of the theory on the future of nursing?
- How has nursing as a community of scholars been influenced?
- In what ways has nursing as a professional practice been strengthened?
- What future possibilities for nursing are open because of this theory?
- What will be the continuing social value of the theory?

STUDY OF THEORY FOR NURSING ADMINISTRATION

Literature on nursing delivery systems and administration have addressed the value of nursing theory for use in administration of nursing and health-care organizations (Huckaby, 1991; Walker, 1993; Young & Hayne, 1988). Nurses in group practice may seek to use a nursing theory that will not only guide their practice, but also provide visions for the organization and administration of their practice. A shared understanding of the focus of nursing can facilitate goal-setting and achievement as well as day-to-day communication among nurses in practice and administration. Allison and McLaughlin-Renpenning (1999) describe the need for a vision of nursing shared by all throughout health care and nursing organizations. These authors, using Orem's general Self-Care Deficit Nursing Theory (see Chapter 13), offer demonstration that a theory of nursing can guide practice as well as the organization and administration.

The above guide for the study of nursing theories for use in nursing practice can be extended to consider essential aspects of nursing in organizations. The following questions are derived from components of a model for nursing administration (Allison & McLaughlin-Renpenning, 1999). The questions are intended to guide descriptions of the nursing organization. Responses to these questions can be used to evaluate nursing theory for use in a nursing practice organization.

- What are purposes of the organization? Mission? Goals?
- What are the purposes of nursing? How do these purposes contribute to the purposes of the organization?
- How can the range of nursing situations be described? What is the population served?
- What nursing and related technologies are required for nursing?
- What are the projections for nursing situations and technological needs for the future?
- How is communication facilitated? In nursing? Among disciplines and services?

- How are services for those nursed coordinated?
- In what ways is nursing professional development achieved? Career advancement?
- How are research and development of nursing practice and theory advanced?

Summary

This chapter has presented a guide designed for use by nurses to study nursing theory for use in practice. The guide is intended to be used along with more general formats of analysis and evaluation of nursing theory. This guide provides additional evaluative components for use by nurses who are focusing on nursing practice. An additional set of questions is offered for nurses who are considering nursing organization and administration. These questions are intended to further guide the study of nursing theory for use in the organization and administration of nursing.

References

Allison, S. E., & McLaughlin-Renpenning, K. E. (1999). *Nursing administration in the 21st century: A self-care theory approach.* Thousand Oaks, CA: Sage Publications.

Huckaby, L. (1991). The role of conceptual frameworks in nursing practice, administration, education, and research. *Nursing Administration Quarterly, 15* (3), 17–28.

Nursing Development Conference Group. (1973). *Concept formalization in nursing: Process and product.* Boston: Little, Brown & Co.

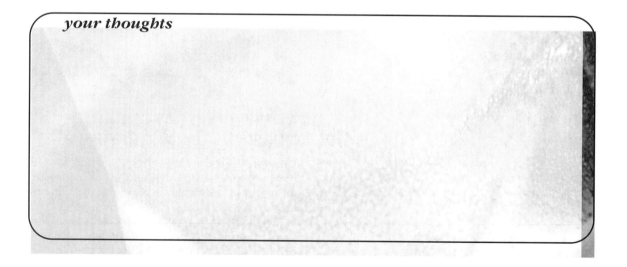

your thoughts

Orem, D. (1995). *Nursing: Concepts of practice* (5th ed.). St. Louis: Mosby-Year Book.

Parker, M. (1993). *Patterns of nursing theories in practice*. New York: National League for Nursing.

Walker, D. (1993). A nursing administration perspective on use of Orem's self-care nursing theory. In Parker, M., *Patterns of nursing theories in practice* (pp. 253–263). New York: National League for Nursing.

Young, L., & Hayne, A. (1988). *Nursing administration: From concepts to practice*. Philadelphia: W. B. Saunders.

Section II

Evolution of Nursing Theory:
Essential Influences

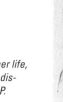

Florence Nightingale at Embley in 1857: pencil drawing of her by G. Scharf. This was one of the most active and fruitful periods of her life, but as happened so often, she reacted with symptoms of nervous distress. From Elspeth Huxley: Florence Nightingale *(1975), p. 139, G. P. Putnam's Sons, New York.*

Chapter 4

Florence Nightingale
Caring Actualized:
A Legacy for Nursing

Lynne Hektor Dunphy

But out of suffering may come the cure. Better have pain than paralysis! A hundred struggle and drown in the breakers. One discovers the new world. But rather, ten times rather, die in surf, heralding the way to the new world, than stand idly on the shore!

—Florence Nightingale, "Cassandra" (1852/1979)

INTRODUCING THE THEORIST

Florence Nightingale transformed a "calling from God" and an intense spirituality into a new social role for women: that of nurse. Her caring was a public one, expressed in and committed to people improving the quality of their lives. "Work your true work," she wrote, "and you will find God within you." A reflection on this statement is to be found in a well-known quote from *Notes on Nursing* (1859/1992), "Nature [i.e., the manifestation of God] alone cures . . . what nursing has to do . . . is put the patient in the best condition for nature to act upon him" (Macrae, 1995, p. 10). Although Nightingale never defined human care or caring in *Notes on Nursing,* there can be no doubt that her life in nursing exemplified and personified an ethos of caring. Jean Watson (1992, p. 83), in the 1992 commemorative edition of *Notes on Nursing,* observed, "Although Nightingale's feminine-based caring-healing model has transcended time and is prophetic for this century's health reform, the model is yet to truly come of age in nursing or the health care system."

This chapter reiterates Nightingale's life from the years 1820 to 1860, delineating the formative influences on her ideas about nursing. A biographical approach was used to examine her education, travel, and spiritual background, her Crimean experiences, the medical milieu, and her views on women, all providing historical context for her ideas about nursing as we recall them today. Part of what follows is a well-known tale, yet it remains a tale that is irresistible, casting an age-old spell on the reader, like the flickering shadow of Nightingale and her famous lamp in the dark and dreary halls of the Barrack Hospital, Scutari, on the outskirts of Constantinople, circa 1854–1856. And it is a tale that still carries much relevance for our nursing practice today.

EARLY LIFE AND EDUCATION: THE SEEDS OF CARING PLANTED

A profession, a trade, a necessary occupation, something to fill and employ all my faculties, I have always felt essential to me, I have always longed for, consciously or not. . . . The first thought I can remember, and the last, was nursing work. . . .

—Florence Nightingale, cited in Cook (1913, p. 106)

Nightingale, the second and youngest daughter born to Fanny Smith, age 32, and William Edward Nightingale, age 25, came into this world on May 12, 1820. She was born in Florence, Italy, the city she was named for, in Villa Colombia, and christened in its drawing room. The Nightingales were on an extended European tour, begun in 1818 shortly after their marriage. This was a common journey for those of their class and wealth. Their first daughter, Parthenope, had been born in the city of that name in the previous year.

W. E. N., as Nightingale's father was referred to affectionately, was by nature retiring and studious. He had fallen for his opposite in the vivacious Fanny Smith, who was ambitious and socially minded with great aspirations for both daughters. Fanny was from a distinguished, wealthy, liberal family, Unitarian in religious outlook. Fanny's father, William Smith, was a well-known politician of the age, who sat for 46 years as a member of Parliament, in the House of Commons. Sir Thomas Cook (1913), Nightingale's first and official biographer, describes William Smith as follows: "A stout defender of liberty of thought and conscience, a persistent opponent of religious tests and disabilities," and in religion, a Unitarian (Cook, Vol. I, 1913, p. 5). He is also described as "a leading Abolitionist; he championed the seated factory workers; he did battle for the rights of Dissenters and Jews" (Woodham-Smith, 1983, p. 2). These themes were to resonate throughout Nightingale's life. Smith's daughter, Fanny, however, was of a more outgoing nature. She chose to attend the Anglican Church, rather than the Unitarian, primarily for social reasons, and when recalling her upbringing as one of 10 siblings, she noted, "We Smiths never thought of anything all day but our own ease and pleasure."

Nightingale's father was also a professed Unitarian. Both parents were part of the class known as the "landed gentry," rich though not titled. Her family on both sides was enormously wealthy, educated, well traveled, and part of an elite inner circle of influential people of the day.

The Nightingales owned several homes—a country home called Lea Hurst in Derbyshire; a town house in London; and Embley Park, a large and lavish home located in Hampshire, outside of London. It was Fanny's opinion that Lea Hurst was too small. "Why, it only has 15 bedrooms!" she was heard to observe. W. E. N., an amateur architect, took an active hand in the design of his houses (Cook, 1913; Huxley, 1975).

A legacy of humanism, liberal thinking, and love of speculative thought was bequeathed to Nightingale by her father. His views on the education of women were far ahead of his time. W. E. N. undertook the education of both his daughters. Florence and her sister studied music; grammar; composition; modern languages; Ancient Greek and Latin; constitutional history; and Roman, Italian, German, and Turkish history; as well as mathematics (Barritt, 1973). Cook describes the following:

> Among Florence's papers were preserved many sheets in her father's handwriting, containing the heads of admirable outlines of the political history of England and some foreign states. Her own note-books show that in her teens she had mastered the elements of Greek and Latin. She analyzed the *Tusculan Disputations*. She translated portions of the *Phaedo*, the *Crito* and the *Apology*. She had studied Greek, Roman, and Turkish history. She had analyzed Dugald Stewart's *Philosophy of the Human Mind*. Her father was in the habit, too, of suggesting themes on which his daughters were to write compositions. It was the system of the College Essay. "Florence has now taken mathematics," wrote her sister in 1840, "and, like everything else she undertakes, she is deep in them and working very hard." (Cook, Vol. I, 1913, p. 13)

From an early age, Florence exhibited independence of thought and action. The sketch (Figure 4–1) of W. E. N. and his daughters was done by one of Fanny's sisters, a beloved aunt, Julia Smith. It is Parthenope, the older sister, who clutches her father's hand and Florence who, as described by her aunt, "independently stumps along by herself" (Woodham-Smith, 1983, p. 7).

Travel also played a part in Nightingale's education. Eighteen years after Florence's birth, the Nightingales and both daughters made an extended tour of the Continent, covering France, Italy, and Switzerland between the years of 1837 and 1838. In 1847, Nightingale went to Italy and France with close friends, the Bracebridges, where they were to witness the revolutions of 1848. In 1849, again with the Bracebridges, Nightingale traveled to Egypt and then on to Athens in 1850 (Sattin, 1987). From there, Nightingale visited Germany, making her first acquaintance with Kaiserswerth, a Protestant religious community that contained the Institution for the

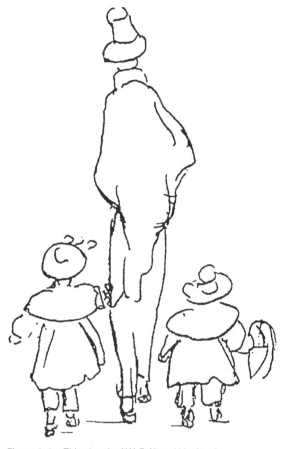

Figure 4–1 *This sketch of W. E. N. and his daughters was done by one of his wife Fanny's sisters, Julia Smith. From Woodham-Smith, p. 9, permission of Sir Harry Verney, Bart.*

Training of Deaconesses, with a hospital school, penitentiary, and orphanage. A Protestant pastor, Theodore Fleidner, and his young wife had established this community in 1836, in part to provide training for women deaconesses (Protestant "nuns") who wished to nurse. Nightingale was to return there in 1851 against much family opposition to stay from July through October, participating in a period of "nurses training" (Cook, Vol. I, 1913; Woodham-Smith, 1983).

Life at Kaiserswerth was spartan. The trainees were up at 5 A.M., ate bread and gruel, and then worked on the hospital wards until 12 noon. Then they had a 10-minute break for broth with vegetables. Three P.M. saw another 10-minute break for tea and bread. They worked until 7 P.M., had some broth, and then Bible lessons until bed. What the Kaiserswerth training lacked in expertise it made up in a spirit of reverence and dedication. Florence wrote,

"The world here fills my life with interest and strengthens me in body and mind" (Huxley, 1975).

In 1852, Nightingale visited Ireland, touring hospitals and keeping notes on various institutions along the way. Nightingale took two trips to Paris; in 1853, hospital training again was the goal, this time with the sisters of St. Vincent de Paul, an order of nursing sisters. In August 1853, she accepted her first "official" nursing post as superintendent of an "Establishment for Gentlewomen in Distressed Circumstances during Illness," located at 1 Harley Street, London. After 6 months at Harley Street, Nightingale wrote in a letter to her father: "I am in the hey-day of my power" (Nightingale, cited in Woodham-Smith, 1983, p. 77).

By October 1854, larger horizons beckoned.

> Her religious convictions made service to God, through service to humankind, a driving force in her life.

SPIRITUALITY: THE ROOTS OF NIGHTINGALE'S CARING

Today I am 30—the age Christ began his Mission. Now no more childish things, no more vain things, no more love, no more marriage. Now, Lord let me think only of Thy will, what Thou willest me to do. O, Lord, Thy will, Thy will. . . .

—**Florence Nightingale, private note, 1850, cited in Woodham-Smith (1983, p. 130)**

By all accounts, Nightingale was an intense and serious child, always concerned with the poor and the ill, mature far beyond her years. A few months before her 17th birthday, Nightingale recorded in a personal note dated February 7, 1837, that she had been called to God's service. What that service was to be was unknown at that point in time. This was to be the first of four such experiences that Nightingale documented.

The fundamental nature of her religious convictions made service to God, through service to humankind, a driving force in her life. She wrote: "The kingdom of Heaven is within; but we must make it without" (Nightingale, private note, cited in Woodham-Smith, 1983).

It would take 15 long and torturous years, from 1837 to 1853, for Nightingale to actualize her calling to the role of nurse. This was a revolutionary choice for a woman of her social standing and position, and her desire to nurse met with vigorous family opposition for many years. Along the way, she turned down several proposals of marriage, potentially, in her mother's view, "brilliant matches," such as that of Richard Monckton Milnes. However, her need to serve God and to demonstrate her caring through meaningful activity proved stronger. She did not think that she could be married and also do God's will.

This lengthy and protracted period, experienced by a number of great young individuals who go onto achieve a historic identity, was identified by Erik Erikson as a "moratorium." Erikson, noted most commonly in nursing for his developmental model of the "Eight Stages of Man" (Erikson, 1950), also postulated an extended identity crisis and resolution for certain individuals. These "great" young adults, unable to fit into existing societal roles, structures, and ideologies, resolve their own crisis of identity by evolving a new form of social organization, a new way of looking at the world, or a new ideology (Erikson, 1958, 1974). In the case of the historic individual, his or her developmental "task" of identity is usually a role that is new, a life's work that is original:

> Still others [young adults], although suffering and deviating dangerously through what appears to be a prolonged adolescence, eventually come to contribute an original bit to an emerging style of life: the very danger which they have sensed has forced them to mobilize capacities to see and say, to dream and plan, to design and construct, in new ways. (Erikson, 1958, pp. 14–15)

Nightingale indeed fit this model, with well-documented sufferings, confusion, and "searchings for truth" during the years between 1837 and 1853 (Hektor, 1984). This period ended for Nightingale when she assumed her first official post as "nurse administrator" in 1853, followed by her Crimean years, 1854 to 1856.

Joann G. Widerquist (1992, p. 49) identifies Nightingale's spirituality as a "belief in perfectionism" and perceives this as closely tied to underlying Unitarian ideas. Although they were not unified by doctrine or creed, the Unitarians, like the Quakers, were a small group that wielded influence beyond their numbers. Among other things, the Unitarians believed in salvation by character as well as the progress of humankind onward and upward forever. Their belief about salvation included both health and wholeness (Widerquist, 1992, p. 50). Strains of these ideas are also prevalent in Nightingale's writings about nursing.

Calabria and Macrae (1994) note that for Nightingale there was no conflict between science and spirituality; actually, in her view, science is necessary for the development of a mature concept of God. The development of science allows for the concept of one perfect God who regulates the universe through universal laws as opposed to random happenings. Nightingale referred to these laws, or the organizing principles of the universe as "Thoughts of God" (Macrae, 1995, p. 9). As part of God's plan of evolution, it was the responsibility of human beings to discover the laws inherent in the universe and apply them to achieve well-being. In *Notes on Nursing* (1860/1969, p. 25), she wrote:

> God lays down certain physical laws. Upon his carrying out such laws depends our responsibility (that much abused word). . . . Yet we seem to be continually expecting that He will work a miracle—i.e. break his own laws expressly to relieve us of responsibility.

Nightingale elaborated her thoughts on this matter in a letter to Benjamin Jowett, a religious advisor: "It is a religious act to clean out a gutter and to prevent cholera, and that it is not a religious act to pray (in the sense of asking)" (Quinn & Prest, 1981, p. 18).

Influenced by the Unitarian ideas of her father and her extended family, as well as by the more traditional Anglican church she attended, Nightingale remained for her entire life a searcher after religious truth, studying a variety of religions and reading widely. She was a devout believer in God. Nightingale wrote: "I believe that there is a Perfect Being, of whose thought the universe in eternity is the incarnation" (Calabria & Macrae, 1994, p. 20). Dossey (1998) recasts Nightingale in the mode of "religious mystic." However, to Nightingale, mystical union with God was not an end in itself, but the source of strength and guidance for doing one's work in life. For Nightingale, service to God was service to humanity (Calabria & Macrae, 1994, p. xviii).

During the 1850s Nightingale produced an 829-page work in three volumes, which she had privately printed in 1860. The first volume was entitled *Suggestions for Thought to the Searchers after Truth among the Artisans of England*; the second and third volumes were entitled simply *Suggestions for Thought to Searchers after Religious Truth*. In a letter to John Stuart Mill (September 5, 1860), framing her thoughts on this work, Nightingale wrote the following:

> Many years ago, I had a large and very curious acquaintance among the artisans of the North of England and London. I learned that they were without any religion whatever—though diligently seeking after one, principally in

Comte and his school. Any return to what is called Christianity appeared impossible. It is for them that this book is written. (Calabria & Macrae, 1994, p. ix)

A census completed in England in 1851 revealed that most of the poor and working class had no faith, and that religion was espoused primarily by the middle class (Widerquist, 1992, p. 52). Nightingale viewed the ideas presented in her religious treatise as an alternative to atheism. Nightingale was also an empiricist, but instead of abolishing God as did Comte, she sought to unify religion and science in a way that would bring order, meaning, and purpose to human life. She viewed spirituality as a science and wrote that our knowledge of God, as revealed in the laws of the universe, should be continually evolving (Macrae, 1995, p. 10). Given this unusual (for the time) evolutionary view, Nightingale, ever the freethinker, was decidedly against a single set of teachings as a final authority. In *Suggestions for Thought* (cited in Calabria & Macrae, 1994, p. 126) she wrote:

> [b]ut man's capabilities of observation, thought, and feeling exercised on the universe, past, present, and to come, are the sources of religious knowledge.

In Nightingale's view, nursing should be a search for the truth, it should be a discovery of God's laws of healing and their proper application. This is what she was referring to in *Notes on Nursing* when she wrote about the Laws of Health, as yet unidentified. It was the Crimean War that provided the stage for her to actualize these foundational beliefs, rooting forever in her mind certain "truths."

WAR: CARING ACTUALIZED

I stand at the altar of those murdered men and while I live I fight their cause
—**Nightingale, cited in Woodham-Smith (1983)**

Nightingale had powerful friends and had gained prominence through her study of hospitals and health matters during her travels. When Great Britain became involved in 1854 in the Crimean War, Nightingale was ensconced in her first official nursing post at 1 Harley Street. Britain had joined France and Turkey to ward off an aggressive Russian advance in the Crimea (Figure 4-2). The interests of all was the preservation of the balance of power. A successful advance of Russia through Turkey could threaten the peace and stability of the European continent.

The first actual battle of the war, the Battle of Alma, was fought in September 1854. It was written

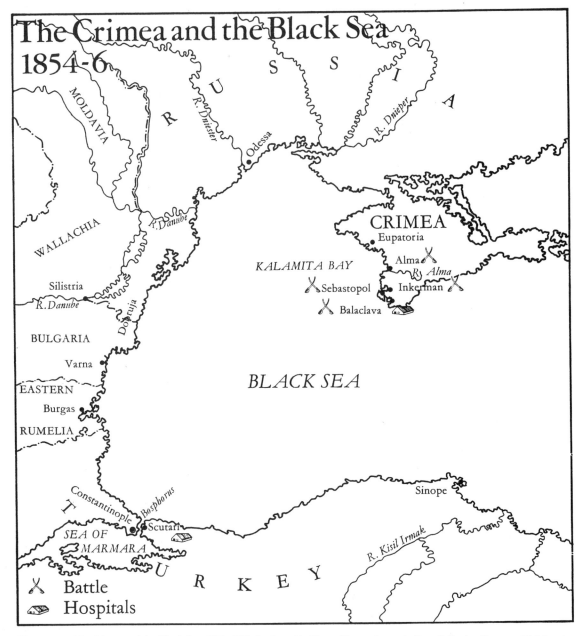

Figure 4–2 *The Crimea and the Black Sea, 1854–1856. Designed by Manuel Lopez Parras in Elspeth Huxley,* Florence Nightingale *(1975), p. 998, G. P. Putnam's Sons, New York.*

of that battle that it was a "glorious and bloody victory." The best technology of the times, the telegraph, was to have an effect on what was to follow. In prior wars, news from the battlefields trickled home slowly. However, the invention of the telegraph enabled war correspondents to telegraph reports home with rapid speed. The horror of the battlefields was relayed to a concerned citizenry. De-

scriptions of wounded men, disease, and illness abounded. Who was to care for these men? The French had the Sisters of Charity to care for their sick and wounded. What were the British to do? (Woodham-Smith, 1983; Goldie, 1987).

The minister of war was Sidney Herbert, Lord Herbert of Lea, who was the husband of Liz Herbert; both were close friends of Nightingale. He had an

innovative solution: appoint Miss Nightingale and charge her to head a contingent of nurses to the Crimea, to provide help and organization to the deteriorating battlefield situation. It was a brave move on the part of Sidney Herbert. Medicine and war were exclusively male domains. To send a woman into these hitherto uncharted waters was risky at best. But, as is well known, Nightingale was no ordinary woman, and she more than rose to the occasion. In a passionate letter to Nightingale, requesting her to accept this post, Sidney Herbert, minister of war, wrote:

> Your own personal qualities, your knowledge and your power of administration, and among greater things, your rank and position in society, give you advantages in such a work that no other person possesses. (Dolan, 1971, p. 2)

At the very same time, such that their letters actually crossed, Nightingale wrote to Sidney Herbert, offering her services.

The unique blend of Nightingale's background, family friends, and connections in high places, combined with her own interests and proclivities, provided the impetus for the famous mission to the Crimea, led by her. Accompanied by 38 hand-picked "nurses" who had no formal training, she arrived on November 4, 1854, to "take charge," and did not return to England until August 1856.

Biographer Woodham-Smith and Nightingale's own correspondence, as cited in a number of sources (Cook, 1913; Huxley, 1975; Goldie, 1987; Summers, 1988; Vicinus & Nergaard, 1990), paint the most vivid picture of the experiences that Nightingale sustained there, experiences that cemented her views on disease and contagion, as well as her commitment to an environmental approach to health and illness:

> The filth became indescribable. The men in the corridors lay on unwashed floors crawling with vermin. As the Rev. Sidney Osborne knelt to take down dying messages, his paper became thickly covered with lice. There were no pillows, no blankets; the men lay, with their heads on their boots, wrapped in the blanket or greatcoat stiff with blood and filth which had been their sole covering for more than a week . . . [S]he [Miss Nightingale] estimated . . . there were more than 1000 men suffering from acute diarrhea and only 20 chamber pots. . . . [T]here was liquid filth which floated over the floor an inch deep. Huge wooden tubs stood in the halls and corridors for the men to use. In this filth lay the men's food—Miss Nightingale saw the skinned carcass of a sheep lie in a ward all night . . . the stench from the hospital could be smelled *outside* the walls. (Woodham-Smith, 1983)

The immediate priority of Nightingale and her small band of nurses on her arrival in the Crimea was not in the sphere of medical or surgical nursing as currently known; rather, their order of business was *domestic management*. This is evidenced in the following exchange between Nightingale and one of her party as they approached Constantinople: "Oh, Miss Nightingale, when we land don't let there be any red-tape delays, let us get straight to nursing the poor fellows!" Nightingale's reply: "The strongest will be wanted at the wash tub" (Cook, 1913; Dolan, 1971).

Although the bulk of this work continued to be done by orderlies after Nightingale's arrival (with the laundry farmed out to the soldiers' wives), it was accomplished only with Nightingale's persistence: "She insisted on the huge wooden tubs in the wards being emptied, standing [obstinately] by the side of each one, sometimes for an hour at a time, never scolding, never raising her voice, until the orderlies gave way and the tub was emptied" (Cook, 1913; Summers, 1988; Woodham-Smith, 1983).

Nightingale set up her own extra "diet kitchen." Small portions, helpings of such things as arrowroot, port wine, lemonade, rice pudding, jelly, and beef tea, whose purpose was to tempt and revive the appetite, were able to be provided to the men. It was therefore a logical sequence from cooking to feeding, from administering food to administering medicines. Because no antidote to infection existed at this time, the provision, by Nightingale and her nurses, of cleanliness, order, encouragement to eat, feeding, clean bed linen, clean bodies, and clean wards, was essential to recovery (Summers, 1988). Following is such a description:

> Those who remember the cooking for the sick which prevailed at Scutari before, and that introduced after the kitchen department underwent the "female revolution," will be able to appreciate the difference which attention to this point must make on the results of treatment . . . it was in the management of those cases of such frequent occurrence in the East, where a lingering convalescence—most liable to relapse—has succeeded—that the extras from those special kitchens came to tell in the treatment. Nourishment, properly and judiciously administered, was the sole medication on which we could rely in such cases. It was often of itself sufficient to cure, and it was in attending to this that the female nurses saved so many lives. (Woodham-Smith, 1983)

Mortality rates at the Barrack Hospital in Scutari fell. Some attribute the decline to the onset of warmer weather in March 1855, thus ensuring freer ventilation. Before this, in February, at Nightingale's insistence, the prime minister had sent to the Crimea a sanitary commission to investigate the mortality rates. Beginning their work in March, they described the conditions at the Barrack Hospital as "murderous." Setting to work immediately, they opened the channel through which the water supplying the hospital flowed, where a dead horse was found. During the first two weeks of their work, the commission cleared "556 handcarts and large baskets full of rub-

bish . . . 24 dead animals and 2 dead horses buried." In addition, they flushed and cleansed sewers, limewashed walls, tore out shelves that harbored rats, and got rid of vermin. The Commission, Nightingale said, "saved the British Army." Miss Nightingale's anti-contagionism was sealed as the mortality rates began showing dramatic declines (Rosenberg, 1979).

Figure 4–3 illustrates Nightingale's own hand-drawn "coxcombs," as they were referred to, as Nightingale, being always aware of the necessity of documenting outcomes of care, kept copious records of all sorts (Cook, 1913; Rosenberg, 1979; Woodham-Smith, 1983).

It was these events that set the stage for the solidification of the "Nightingale legend" and that recurring icon, "The Lady with the Lamp." Lytton Strachey, noted biographer of the Victorian age, provides us with some of the most vivid descriptions of Miss Nightingale, capturing the complexity of the real woman:

> Certainly she was heroic. Yet her heroism was not that simple sort so dear to readers of novels and the compilers of hagiologies. . . . It was made of sterner stuff. To the wounded soldier on his couch of agony she might well appear in the guise of a gracious angel of mercy; but the military surgeons, and the orderlies, and her own nurses, and the "Purveyor," and Dr. Hall, and even Lord Stratford himself could tell a different story. It was not by gentle sweetness and womanly self-abnegation that she had brought order out of the chaos in the Scutari Hospital, that, from her own resources, she had clothed the British Army, that she had spread her dominion over the serried and re-

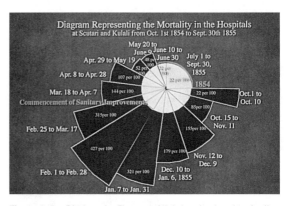

Figure 4–3 *Diagram by Florence Nightingale showing declining mortality rates. From Cohen, I. B. (1981).* Florence Nightingale: The passionate statistician. *Scientific American, 250(3): 128–137.*

luctant powers of the official world; it was by strict method, by stern discipline, by rigid attention to detail, by ceaseless labor, by the fixed determination of indomitable will. (Strachey, 1918, p. 156)

He goes on to describe her physical demeanor:

Beneath her cool and calm demeanor lurked fierce and passionate fires. As she passed through the wards in her plain dress, so quiet, so unassuming, she struck the casual observer simply as the pattern of the perfect lady; but the keener eye [saw] something more than that—the serenity of high deliberation in the scope of the capricious brow, the sign of power in the dominating curve of the thin nose, and the traces of a harsh and dangerous temper—something peevish, something mocking, and yet something precise—in the small and delicate mouth. (Strachey, 1918, p. 156)

Strachey extends his description to Miss Nightingale's voice:

As for her voice, it was true of it, even more than her countenance, that it "had that in it one must fain call master." Those clear tones were in no need of emphasis: "I never heard her raise her voice," said one of her companions. Only, when she had spoken, it seemed as if nothing could follow but obedience. Once, when she had given some direction, a doctor ventured to remark that the thing could not be done. "But it must be done," said Miss Nightingale. A chance bystander, who heard the words, never forgot through all his life the irresistible authority of them. And they were spoken quietly—very quietly indeed. (Strachey, 1918, pp. 156-157)

Florence Nightingale possessed *moral authority,* so firm because it was grounded in caring, and in a larger mission that came from her spirituality. For Miss Nightingale, spirituality was a much broader, more unitive concept than that of religion. Her spirituality involved the sense of a presence higher than human presence, the divine intelligence that creates, sustains, and organizes the universe, and an awareness of our inner connection to this higher reality. Through this inner connection flows creative endeavors and insight, a sense of purpose and direction. For Miss Nightingale, spirituality was intrinsic to human nature, and the deepest, most potent resource for healing. Nightingale was to write in *Suggestions for Thought* (cited in Calabria & Macrae, 1994, p. 58) that "human consciousness is tending to

become what God's consciousness is—to become One with the consciousness of God." This progression of consciousness to unity with the divine was an evolutionary view and not typical of either the Anglican or Unitarian views of the time (Rosenberg, 1979; Welch, 1986; Widerquist, 1992; Slater, 1994; Calabria & Macrae, 1994; Macrae, 1995).

There were 4 miles of beds in the Barrack Hospital at Scutari, a suburb of Constantinople. A letter to the London Times dated February 24, 1855, reported the following:

When all the medical officers have retired for the night and silence and darkness have settled upon those miles of prostrate sick, she may be observed, alone with a little lamp in her hand, making her solitary rounds. (Kalisch & Kalisch, 1987)

In April 1855, after having been in Scutari for 6 months, Florence wrote to her mother, "[A]m in sympathy with God, fulfilling the purpose I came into the world for" (Woodham-Smith, 1983). Henry Wadsworth Longfellow authored "Santa Filomena" to commemorate Miss Nightingale:

Lo! In that house of misery
A lady with a lamp I see
    Pass through the glimmering gloom
    And flit from room to room
And slow as if in a dream of bliss
The speechless sufferer turns to kiss
    Her shadow as it falls
    Upon the darkening walls
As if a door in heaven should be
Opened and then closed suddenly
    The vision came and went
    The light shone and was spent.
A lady with a lamp shall stand
In the great history of the land
    A noble type of good
    Heroic womanhood
        (Longfellow, cited in Dolan, 1971, p. 5)

Miss Nightingale slipped home quietly, arriving at Lea Hurst in Derbyshire on August 7, 1856, after 22 months in the Crimea, after sustained illness from which she was never to recover, after ceaseless work, and after witnessing suffering, death, and despair that would haunt her for the remainder of her life. Her hair was shorn; she was pale and drawn (Figure 4-4). She took her family by surprise. The next morning, a peal of the village church bells and a prayer of Thanksgiving were, her sister wrote, " 'all the innocent greeting' except for those provided by the spoils of war that had proceeded her—a one-

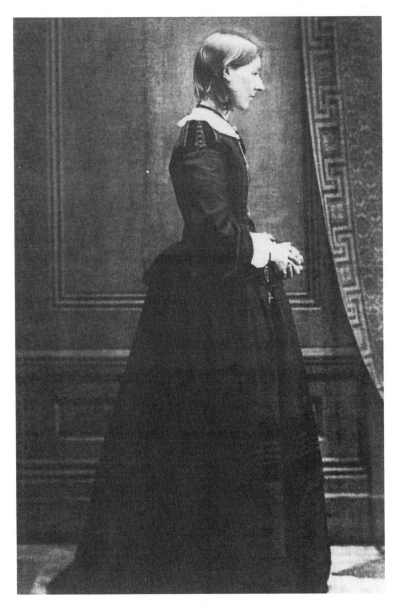

Figure 4–4 *A rare photograph of Florence taken on her return from the Crimea. Although greatly weakened by her illness, she refused to accept her friends' advice to rest, and pressed on relentlessly with her plans to reform the army medical services. From Elspeth Huxley,* Florence Nightingale *(1975), p. 139, G. P. Putnam's Sons, New York.*

legged sailor boy, a small Russian orphan, and a large puppy found in some rocks near Balaclava. All England was ringing with her name, but she had left her heart on the battlefields of the Crimea and in the graveyards of Scutari" (Huxley, 1975, p. 147).

THE MEDICAL MILIEU

In watching disease, both in private homes and public hospitals, the thing which strikes the experienced observer most forcefully is this, that the symptoms or the sufferings generally considered to be inevitable and incident to the disease are very often not symptoms of the disease at all, but of something quite different—of the want of fresh air, or light, or of warmth, or of quiet, or of cleanliness, or of punctuality and care in the administration of diet, of each or of all of these.

—**Florence Nightingale,** *Notes on Nursing*
(1860/1969, p. 8)

To gain a better understanding of Nightingale's ideas on nursing, one must enter the peculiar world of nineteenth-century medicine and its views on health and disease. Considerable new medical knowledge had been gained by 1800. Gross anatomy

Section II *Evolution of Nursing Theory: Essential Influences*

was well known; chemistry promised to throw light on various body processes. Vaccination against smallpox existed. There were some established drugs in the pharmacopoeia: cinchona bark, digitalis, and mercury. Certain major diseases, such as leprosy and the bubonic plague, had almost disappeared. The crude death rate in western Europe was falling, largely related to decreasing infant mortality as a result of improvement in hygiene and standard of living (Ackernecht, 1982; Shyrock, 1959).

Yet physicians at the turn of the century, in 1800, still had only the vaguest notion of diagnosis. Speculative philosophies continued to dominate medical thought, although inroads and assaults continued to be made that eventually gave way to a new outlook on the nature of disease: from belief in general states common to all illnesses to an understanding of disease-specificity resultant symptomatology. It was this shift in thought—a paradigm shift of the first order—that gave us the triumph of twentieth-century medicine, with all its attendant glories and concurrent sterility.

The eighteenth century was host to two major traditions or paradigms in the healing arts: one based on "empirics," or "experience," trial and error, with an emphasis on curative remedies; the other based on Hippocratic notions and learning. Evidence of both these trends persisted into the nineteenth century and can be found in Nightingale's philosophy.

Consistent with the speculative and philosophical nature of her superior education (Barritt, 1973), Nightingale, like many of the physicians of her time, continued to emphatically disavow the reality of specific states of disease. She insisted on a view of sickness as an "adjective," not a substantive noun. Sickness was not an "entity" somehow separable from the body. Consistent with her more holistic view, sickness was an aspect, or quality of the body as a whole. Some physicians, as she phrased it, taught that diseases were like cats and dogs, distinct species necessarily descended from other cats and dogs. She found such views misleading (Nightingale, 1860/1969).

At this point in time, in the mid-nineteenth century, there were two competing theories regarding the nature and origin of disease. One view was known as "contagionism," postulating that some diseases were communicable, spread via commerce and population migration. The strategic consequences of this explanatory model was *quarantine* and its attendant bureaucracy aimed at shutting down commerce and trade to keep disease away from noninfected areas. To the new and rapidly emerging merchant classes, quarantine represented government interference and control (Ackernecht, 1982; Arnstein, 1988).

The second school of thought on the nature and origin of disease, of which Nightingale was an ardent champion, was known as "anticontagionism." It postulated that disease resulted from local environmental sources and arose out of "miasmas"—clouds of rotting filth and matter, activated by a variety of things such as meteorologic conditions (note the similarity to elements of water, fire, air, and earth on humors); the filth must be eliminated from *local* areas to prevent the spread of disease. Commerce and "infected" individuals were left alone (Rosenberg, 1979).

William Farr, another Nightingale associate and avid anticontagionist, was Britain's statistical superintendent of the General Register Office. Farr categorized epidemic and infectious diseases as *zygomatic*, meaning pertaining to or caused by the process of fermentation. The debate as to whether fermentation was a chemical process or a "vitalistic" one had been raging for some time (Swazey & Reed, 1978). The familiarity of the process of fermentation helps to explain its appeal. Anyone who had seen bread rise could immediately grasp how a minute amount of some contaminating substance could in turn "pollute" the entire atmosphere, the very air that was breathed. What was at issue was the *specificity* of the contaminating substance. Nightingale, and the anticontagionists, endorsed the position that a "sufficiently intense level of atmospheric contamination could induce both endemic and epidemic ills in the crowded hospital wards [with particular configurations of environmental circumstances determining which]" (Rosenberg, 1979).

Anticontagionism reached its peak prior to the political revolutions of 1848; the resulting wave of conservatism and reaction brought contagionism back into dominance, where it remained until its reformulation into the germ theory in the 1870s. Leaders of the contagionists were primarily high-ranking military physicians, politically united. These divergent worldviews accounted in some part for Nightingale's clashes with the military physicians she encountered during the Crimean War.

Given the intellectual and social milieu in which Nightingale was raised and educated, her stance on contagionism seems preordained and logically consistent. Likewise, the eclectic religious philosophy she evolved contained attributes of the philosophy of Unitarianism with the fervor of Evangelicalism, all based on an organic view of humans as part of nature. The treatment of disease and dysfunction was inseparable from the nature of man as a whole, and likewise, the environment. And all were linked to God.

The emphasis on "atmosphere" (read "environment") in the Nightingale model is consistent with the views of the "anticontagionists" of her time. This worldview was reinforced by Nightingale's Crimean experiences, as well as her liberal and progressive political thought. Additionally, she viewed all ideas as being distilled through a distinctly *moral* lens (Rosenberg, 1979). As such, Nightingale was typical of a number of intellectuals of her generation. These thinkers struggled to come to grips with an increasingly complex and changing world order, and frequently combined a language of two disparate realms of authority: the moral realm and the emerging scientific paradigm that has assumed dominance in the twentieth century. Traditional religious and moral assumptions were garbed in a mantle of "scientific objectivity," often spurious at best, however more

in keeping with the increasingly rationalized and bureaucratic society accompanying the growth of science.

THE FEMINIST CONTEXT OF NIGHTINGALE'S CARING

I have an intellectual nature which requires satisfaction and that would find it in him. I have a passionate nature which requires satisfaction and that would find it in him. I have a moral, an active nature which requires satisfaction and that would not find it in his life.

—**Florence Nightingale, private note, 1849, cited in Woodham-Smith (1983, p. 51)**

Florence Nightingale wrote the following tortured note upon her final refusal of Richard Monckton Milnes's proposal of marriage: "I know I could not bear his life," she wrote, "that to be nailed to a continuation, an exaggeration of my present life without hope of another would be intolerable to me—that voluntarily to put it out of my power ever to be able to seize the chance of forming for myself a true and rich life would seem to be like suicide" (Nightingale, personal note cited in Woodham-Smith, 1983, p. 52). For Miss Nightingale there was no compromise. Marriage and pursuit of her "mission" were not compatible. She chose the mission, a clear repudiation of the mores of her time, which were rooted in the time-honored role of family and "female duty."

The census of 1851 revealed that there were 365,159 "excess women" in England, meaning women who were not married. These women were viewed as redundant, as described in an essay about the census entitled, "Why Are Women Redundant?" (Widerquist, 1992, p. 52). Many of these women had no acceptable means of support, and the development of a suitable occupation for women by Nightingale, that of nursing, was a significant historical development and a major contribution by Nightingale to the plight of women in the nineteenth century. However, in other ways, her views on women and the question of the rights of women were quite mixed.

The book *Notes on Nursing: What It Is and What It Is Not* (1859/1969) was written not as a manual to teach nurses to nurse, but rather to help all women to learn how to nurse. Nightingale believed all

> *Notes on Nursing* was written not to teach nurses to nurse, but to help all women learn how to nurse.

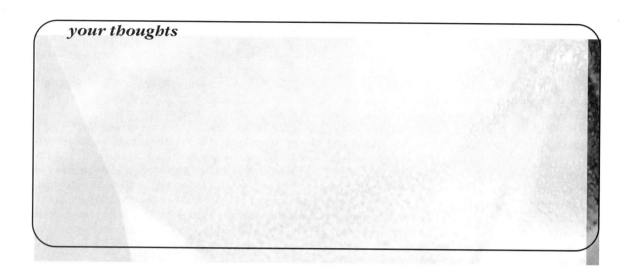

women required this knowledge in order to take proper care of their families during times of sickness and to promote health, specifically what Nightingale referred to as "the health of houses," that is, the "health" of the environment, which she espoused. Nursing, to her, was clearly situated within the context of female duty.

Susan Reverby, historian, in *Ordered to Care: The Dilemma of American Nursing* (1987, p. 43) traces contemporary conflicts within the profession of nursing back to Nightingale herself. She asserts that Nightingale's ideas about female duty and authority, along with her views on disease causality, brought about an independent field—that of nursing—that was separate, and in the view of Nightingale, equal if not superior, to that of medicine. But this field was dominated by a female hierarchy and insisted on both deference and loyalty to the authority of the physician. Reverby sums it up as follows: "Although Nightingale sought to free women from the bonds of familial demand, in her nursing model she rebound them in a new context."

Does the record support this evidence? Was Nightingale a champion for women's rights or a regressive force? As noted earlier, the answer is far from clear.

The economic policy of laissez-faire permeated the day. The theory held that ultimately it was the law of supply and demand that would promote competition, which in turn would produce the maximum number of goods and thus benefit society. In this dog-eat-dog world, what would hold society together? In another paradox of the age, the solution was a common set of moral standards, in the "unfettered energetic actions of persons together with the uniform subjugation of all to the national code of Duty" (Arnstein, 1988, p. 91).

The shelter for all moral and spiritual values, threatened by the crass commercialism that was flourishing in the land, as well as the spirit of critical inquiry that accompanied this age of expanding scientific progress, was agreed upon: the home. This was considered by all a "sacred place, a Temple" (Houghton, 1957, p. 343). And who was the head of this home? Woman. Although the Victorian family was patriarchal in nature in that women had virtually no economic and/or legal rights, they nonetheless yielded a major *moral* role (Houghton, 1957; Perkins, 1987; Arnstein, 1988).

There was hostility on the part of men as well as some women to women's emancipation. Many intelligent women—for example, Beatrice Webb, George Eliot, and, at times, Nightingale herself—viewed the emancipation of their sex with apprehension. In Nightingale's case, the best word might be "ambivalence." There was a fear of weakening women's moral influence, coarsening the feminine nature itself.

This stance is best equated with *cultural feminism,* defined as a belief in inherent gender differences. Women, in contrast to men, are viewed as morally superior, the holders of family values and continuity, refined, delicate, and in need of protection. This school of thought, important in the nineteenth century, used arguments for women's suffrage such as the following: "[W]omen must make themselves felt in the public sphere because their *moral* perspective would improve corrupt masculine politics." In the case of Nightingale, these cultural feminist attitudes "made her impatient with the idea of women seeking rights and activities just

Chapter 4 *Florence Nightingale   Caring Actualized: A Legacy for Nursing*

because men valued these entities" (Campbell & Bunting, 1990, p. 21).

Nightingale had chafed at the limitations and restrictions placed on women, especially "wealthy" women with nothing to do: "What these [women] suffer—even physically—from the want of such work no one can tell. The accumulation of nervous energy, which has had nothing to do during the day, makes them feel every night, when they go to bed, as if they were going mad. . . ." Despite these vivid words, authored by Nightingale (1852/1979) in the fiery polemic "Cassandra," which was used as a rallying cry in many feminist circles, her view of the solution was measured. Her own resolution, painfully arrived at, was to break from her family and actualize her caring mission, that of nurse. One of the many results of this was that a useful occupation for other women to pursue was founded. Although Nightingale approved of this occupation, outside of the home, for other women, certain other occupations—that of doctor, for example—she viewed with hostility, and as inappropriate for women. Why should these women not be nurses or nurse midwives, a far superior calling, in Nightingale's view, than that of a medicine "man"? (Monteiro, 1984).

Welch (1990) terms Nightingale a "Christian feminist" on the eve of her departure to the Crimea. She returned even more skeptical of women. Writing to her close friend Mary Clarke Mohl, she described women that she worked with in the Crimea as being incompetent and incapable of independent thought (Woodham-Smith, 1983; Welch, 1990). According to Palmer (1977), by this time in her life, the concerns of the British people and the demands of service to God took precedence over any concern she had ever had about the rights of women.

In other words, Nightingale, despite the clear freedom in which she lived her own life, nonetheless genderized the nursing role, leaving it rooted in nineteenth-century morality. Nightingale is seen constantly trying to improve the existing order, and to work within that order; she was above all a reformer, seeking to improve the existing order, not to radically change the terrain.

Lady Margaret Rhondda, leading British feminist and wife of Lord Rhondda, the minister of food during World War I, had the following to say about reformers: "[N]ow almost every women's organization recognizes that reformers are far more common than Feminists, that the passion to decide to look after your fellow men, to do good to them in your way, is far more common than the desire to put into everyone's hand the power to look after themselves" (cited in Firestone, 1971). And it is clear that Nightingale

was foremost a reformer. The word *reform* comes from the Latin *re,* meaning "again," and *formare,* meaning "to form": thus, "to form again," "to make better," "to improve or remove faults." Readings from the history of the humanitarian and philanthropic movements of nineteenth-century Britain make clear that it was "reform" that was on the minds of most. A "radical" position calls for a whole new order; a reformist position seeks to make the existing order better, but does not question the status quo.

One of Nightingale's goals, as a reformer, was to create employment for women. In Nightingale's mind, the specific "scientific" activity of nursing—hygiene—was the central element in health care, without which medicine and surgery would be ineffective:

The Life and Death, recovery or invaliding of patients generally depends not on any great and isolated act, but on the unremitting and thorough performance of every minute's practical duty. (Nightingale, 1860/1969)

And this "practical duty" was the work of women. This conception of the proper division of labor resting upon work demands internal to each respective "science," nursing and medicine, obscured the professional inequality. This inequity was heightened by the later successes of medical science. The scientific grounding espoused by Nightingale for nursing was ephemeral at best, as later nineteenth-century discoveries proved much of her analysis wrong, although nonetheless powerful. Much of her strength was in her rhetoric; if not always logically consistent, it certainly was morally resonant (Rosenberg, 1979).

Despite exceptional anomalies, such as women physicians, what Nightingale effectively accomplished was a genderization of the division of labor in health care: male physicians and female nurses. This appears to be a division that Nightingale supported. Because this "natural" division of labor was rooted in the family, women's work outside the home ought to resemble domestic tasks and complement the "male principle" with the "female." Thus, nursing was left on a shifting sand of a soon outmoded "science," the main focus of its authority grounded in an equally shaky moral sphere, also subject to change and devaluation in an increasingly secularized, rationalized, and technological twentieth century.

Nightingale failed to provide institutionalized nursing with an autonomous future, on an equal parity with medicine. She did, however, succeed in providing women's work in the public sphere, establishing for numerous women an identity and source of employment. Although that public identity grew out of women's domestic and nurturing roles in the family, the conditions of a modern society required public as well as private forms of care. It is questionable whether more could have been achieved at that point in time (King, 1988).

If cherished Victorian institutions—the family, the patriarchal state, and God the Father—are examined closely and through the life of a woman such as Nightingale, one can see the power that surges beneath the apparent victimization of women in this society. The subjugation of women can then be seen as a reflexive and defensive response.

A woman, Queen Victoria, presided over the age: "Ironically, Queen Victoria, that panoply of family happiness and stubborn adversary of female independence, could not help but shed her aura upon single women." The queen's early and lengthy widowhood, her "relentlessly spreading figure and commensurately increasing empire, her obstinate longevity which engorged generations of men and the collective shocks of history, lent an epic quality to the lives of solitary women" (Auerbach, 1982, pp. 120–121). Both Nightingale and the queen saw themselves as working through men, yet their lives add new, unexpected, and powerful dimensions to the myth of Victorian womanhood, particularly that of a woman alone and in command (Auerbach, 1982, pp. 120–121).

Nightingale's clearly chosen spinsterhood repudiated the Victorian family. Her unmarried life provides a vision of a powerful life lived on her own terms. This is not the spinsterhood of convention—one to be pitied, one of broken hearts—but a *radically* new image. She is freed from the trivia of family complaints and scorns the feminist collectivity; yet in this seemingly solitary life, she finds union not with one man but with all men, personified by the British soldier.

Lytton Strachey's well-known evocation of Nightingale, iconoclastic and bold, is perhaps closest to the decidedly masculine imagery she selected to describe herself, as evidenced in this imaginary speech to her mother written in 1852:

> Well, my dear, you don't imagine with my "talents," and my "European reputation" and my "beautiful letters" and all that, I'm going to stay dangling around my mother's drawing room all my life! . . . [Y]ou must look upon me as your vagabond son . . . I shan't cost you nearly as much as a son would have done, or had I married. You must consider me married or a son. (Woodham-Smith, 1983, p. 66)

This is the female hero, creating herself, emerging "most vividly in idioms wrested from men who could not have imagined her" (Auerbach, 1982, p. 121).

Did Nightingale fail in her basic undertaking? Was her scope of vision, though broad enough to carry the nursing profession into the twentieth century, not adequate for the new twenty-first century? Was Nightingale able to sever her ties with male politicians and medical men? Has not nursing been sold out time and again to these same two groups? Clearly, she did not wholeheartedly throw her lot in with the early suffragettes. Are these some of the same reasons the nursing profession finds itself in such an intractable position today, as Reverby has suggested? Is the limited vision of some of our early founders still obscuring the contemporary view of the future?

The true legacy Florence Nightingale left is that of her own heroic life—the life of a rebel. Florence Nightingale lived an independent life, one that she had fought for fiercely, on her own terms. According to Auerbach (1982, p. 121), the Victorian spinster lived a psychic life of "'silence, exile, and cunning.' For heroes of both sexes it is in such conditions that myths are born, giving rise to new selves and new lives." It is now up to us, individually and collectively, to imagine and to create this new life. The gauntlet is there, for us to pick up, if we dare.

IDEAS ABOUT NURSING: EXPRESSIONS OF CARING

Every day sanitary knowledge, or the knowledge of nursing, or in other words, of how to put the constitution in such a state as that it will have no disease, or that it can recover from disease, takes a higher place.

—**Florence Nightingale,** *Notes on Nursing* (1860/1969), **Preface**

Evelyn R. Barritt, professor of nursing, suggested that nursing became a science when Nightingale identified her laws of nursing, also referred to as the laws of health, or nature (Barritt, 1973). The remainder of all nursing theory may be viewed as mere branches, and "acorns," all fruit of the roots of Nightingale's ideas. Early writings of Nightingale, compiled in *Notes on Nursing: What It Is and What It Is Not* (1860/1969), provided the earliest systematic perspective for defining nursing. Analysis and application of universal "laws" would promote well-being and relieve the suffering of humanity, according to Nightingale. This was the goal of nursing.

As noted by the caring theorist Madeline Leininger, Nightingale never defined human care or caring in Nightingale's *Notes on Nursing* (1859/1992, p. 31), and she goes on to wonder if Nightingale considered "components of care such as comfort, support, nurturance, and many other care constructs and characteristics and how they would influence the reparative process." Although Nightingale's conceptualizations of nursing, hygiene, the laws of health, and the environment never explicitly identify the construct of caring, an underlying ethos of care and commitment to others echoes in her words, and most importantly resides in her actions and the drama of her life.

Nightingale did not theorize in the way we are accustomed to today. Patricia Winstead-Fry (1993), in a review of the 1992 commemorative edition of Nightingale's *Notes on Nursing* (1859/1992, p. 161), states: "Given that theory is the interrelationship of concepts which form a system of propositions that can be tested and used for predicting practice, Nightingale was not a theorist. None of her major biographers present her as a theorist. She was a consummate politician and health care reformer." Her words and ideas, contextualized in the earlier portion of this chapter, ring differently than those of the other nursing theorists you will study in this book. However, her underlying ideas continue to be relevant, and, some would argue, prescient.

Karen Dennis and Patricia Prescott (1985) note that including Nightingale among the nurse theorists has been a recent development. They make the case that nurses today continue to incorporate in their practice the insight, foresight, and, most important, the clinical acumen of Nightingale's century-old vision of nursing. As part of a larger study, they collected a large base of descriptions from both nurses and physicians describing "good" nursing practice. Over 300 individual interviews were subjected to content analysis; categories were named inductively and validated by four members of the project staff, separately.

Noting no marked differences in the descriptions obtained from either the nurses or physicians, the authors report that despite their independent derivation, the categories that emerged during the study bore a striking resemblance to nursing practice as described by Nightingale: prevention of illness and promotion of health, observation of the sick, and attention to physical environment. Also referred to by Nightingale as the "health of houses," this physical environment included ventilation of both the patient's rooms and the larger environment of the "house"; light, cleanliness, and the taking of food; attention to the interpersonal milieu, which included variety; and not indulging in superficialities with the sick or giving them false encouragement.

The authors note that "the words change but the concepts do not" (Dennis & Prescott, 1985, p. 80).

In keeping with the tradition established by Nightingale, they note that nurses continue to foster an interpersonal milieu that focuses on the person, while manipulating and mediating the environment to "put the patient in the best condition for nature to act upon him" (Nightingale, 1860/1969, p. 133).

Afaf I. Meleis, nurse scholar, does not compare Nightingale to contemporary nurse theorists; nonetheless, she refers to her frequently. Meleis states that it was Nightingale's conceptualization of environment as the focus of nursing activity and her deemphasis of pathology, emphasizing instead the "laws of health" (as yet unknown), that were the earliest differentiation of nursing and medicine. Meleis (1997, pp. 114–116) describes Nightingale's concept of nursing as including "the proper use of fresh air, light, warmth, cleanliness, quiet, and the proper selection and administration of diet, all with the least expense of vital power to the patient. These ideas clearly had evolved from Nightingale's observations and experiences. The art of observation was identified as an important nursing function in the Nightingale model. And this observation was what should form the basis for nursing ideas. Meleis speculates on how differently the theoretical base of nursing might have evolved if we had continued to consider extant nursing practice as a source of ideas.

Pamela Reed and Tamara Zurakowski (1983/1989, p. 33) call the Nightingale model "visionary." They state: "At the core of all theory development activities in nursing today is the tradition of Florence Nightingale." They also suggest four major factors that influenced her model of nursing: religion, science, war, and feminism, all of which are discussed in this chapter.

Margaret Newman, twentieth-century nurse theorist, cites Nightingale in recognizing the need for knowledge specific to nursing. She quotes Nightingale as follows: "I believe . . . that the very elements of nursing are all but unknown . . . are as little understood for the well as for the sick" (Nightingale, cited in Newman, 1972, pp. 449–453). Newman (Nightingale, 1859/1992, p. 44) was to note the following about Nightingale: "Nightingale's views on health, person-environment interaction in relation to health, and the nurse's place in facilitating health set the direction for nursing knowledge development." Newman states that it was Nightingale, as early as 1859, who established the essential parameters of nursing knowledge: nurse, person, environment, and health.

The assumptions in the following section were identified by Victoria Fondriest and Joan Osborne (1994).

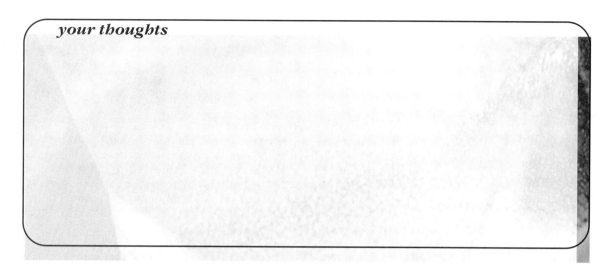

your thoughts

NIGHTINGALE'S ASSUMPTIONS

1. Nursing is separate from medicine.
2. Nurses should be trained.
3. The environment is important to the health of the patient.
4. The disease process is not important to nursing.
5. Nursing should support the environment to assist the patient in healing.
6. Research should be utilized through observation and empirics to define the nursing discipline.
7. Nursing is both an empirical science and an art.
8. Nursing's concern is with the person in the environment.
9. The person is interacting with the environment.
10. Sick and well are governed by the same laws of health.
11. The nurse should be observant and confidential.

The goal of *nursing* as described by Nightingale is assisting the patient in his or her retention of "vital powers" by meeting his or her needs, and thus, putting the patient in the best condition for nature to act upon (Nightingale, 1860/1969). This must not be interpreted as a "passive state," but rather one that reflects the patient's capacity for self-healing facilitated by nurses' ability to create an environment conducive to health. The focus of this nursing activity was the proper use of fresh air, light, warmth, cleanliness, quiet, proper se-

> The goal of nursing is assisting the patient in retention of "vital powers" by meeting his or her needs and putting him or her in the best condition for nature to act upon.

lection and administration of diet, and monitoring the patient's expenditure of energy and observing. This activity was directed toward the environment and the patient.

Health was viewed as an additive process, the result of environmental, physical, and psychological factors, not just the absence of disease. Disease was the reparative process of the body to correct a problem, and could provide an opportunity for spiritual growth. The laws of health, as defined by Nightingale, were those to do with keeping the person, and the population, healthy. This was dependent upon proper environmental control—for example, sanitation. The environment was what the nurse manipulated. It included those physical elements external to the patient. Nightingale isolated five environmental components essential to an individual's health: clean air, pure water, efficient drainage, cleanliness, and light.

The *patient* is at the center of the Nightingale model, which incorporates a holistic view of the person as someone with psychological, intellectual, and spiritual components. This is evidenced in her acknowledgment of the importance of "variety." For example, she wrote of "the degree . . . to which the nerves of the sick suffer from seeing the same walls, the same ceiling, the same surroundings" (Nightingale, 1860/1969). Likewise, her chapter on "chattering hopes and advice" illustrates an astute grasp of human nature and of interpersonal relationships. She remarked upon the spiritual component of disease and illness, she felt they could present an opportunity for spiritual growth. In this, all persons were viewed as equal.

A *nurse* was defined as any woman who had "charge of the personal health of somebody" whether well, as in caring for babies and children, or sick, as an "invalid" (Nightingale, 1860/1969). It was assumed that all women, at one time or another in their lives, would nurse. Thus, all women needed to know the laws of health. Nursing proper, or "sick" nursing, was both an art and a science and required organized, formal education to care for those suffering from disease. Above all, nursing was "service to God in relief of man"; it was a "calling" and "God's work" (Barritt, 1973). Nursing activities served as an "art form" through which spiritual development might occur (Reed & Zurakowski, 1983/1989). All nursing actions were guided by the nurses' *caring,* which was guided by underlying ideas about God.

> **Five environmental factors were essential to health: clean air, pure water, efficient drainage, cleanliness, and light.**

Consistent with this caring base is Nightingale's views on *nursing as an art and a science.* Again, this was a reflection of the marriage, essential to Nightingale's underlying worldview, of science and spirituality. On the surface, these might appear to be odd bedfellows; however, this marriage flows directly from Nightingale's underlying religious and philosophic views, which were operationalized in her nursing practice. Nightingale was an empiricist, valuing the "science" of observation with the intent of use of that knowledge to better the life of humankind. The application of that knowledge required an artist's skill, far greater than that of the painter or sculptor:

> Nursing is an art; and if it is to be made an art, it requires as exclusive a devotion, as hard a preparation, as any painter's or sculptor's work; for what is the having to do with dead canvas or cold marble, compared with having to do with the living body—the Temple of God's spirit? It is one of the Fine Arts; I had almost said, the finest of the Fine Arts. (Florence Nightingale, cited in Donahue, 1985, p. 469)

Nightingale's ideas about nursing health, the environment, and the person were grounded in experience; she regarded one's sense *observations* as the only reliable means of obtaining and verifying knowledge. Theory must be reformulated if inconsistent with empirical evidence. This experiential knowledge was then to be transformed into empirically based generalizations, an inductive process, to arrive at, for example, the laws of health. Regardless

of Nightingale's commitment to empiricism and experiential knowledge, her early education and religious experience also shaped this emerging knowledge (Hektor, 1992).

> **"Nursing is an art . . . It is one of the Fine Arts; I had almost said, the finest of the Fine Arts."**

According to Nightingale's model, nursing contributes to the ability of persons to maintain and restore health directly or indirectly through managing the environment. The person has a key role in his or her own health, and this health is a function of the interaction between person, nurse, and environment. However, neither the person nor the environment is discussed as influencing, in turn, the nurse. Nightingale's education, spiritual development, her time in the Crimea, as well as the role of women in the nineteenth century all affected the development of Nightingale's ideas about nursing (Figure 4-5).

Although it is difficult to describe the interrelationship of the concepts in the Nightingale model, Figure 4-6 is a schema that attempts to delineate this. Note the prominence of "observation" on the outer circle, important to all nursing functions, as well as the interrelationship of the specifics of the in-

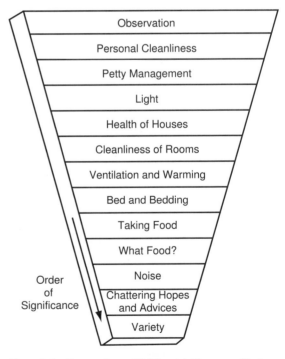

Figure 4–5 *Perspective on Nightingale's 13 canons. Illustration developed by V. Fondriest, RN, BSN and J. Osborne, RN, C BSN in October 1994.*

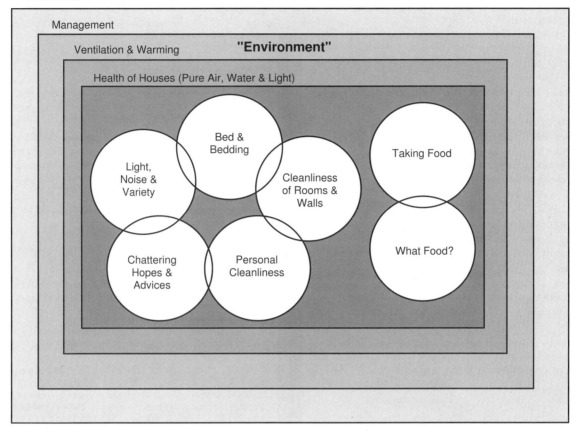

Figure 4–6 *Nightingale's model of nursing and the environment. Illustration developed by V. Fondriest, RN, BSN and J. Osborne, RN, C BSN.*

terventions such as "bed and bedding" and "cleanliness of rooms and walls" that go into making up the "health of houses" (Fondriest & Osborne, 1994).

Summary

NIGHTINGALE'S LEGACY OF CARING

Philip and Beatrice Kalisch (1987, p. 26) describe the popular and glorified images that arose out of the portrayals of Florence Nightingale during and after the Crimean War—that of nurse as self-sacrificing, refined, virginal, an "angel of mercy"—a far less threatening image than one of educated and skilled professional nurses. They attribute nurses' low pay to the perception of nursing as a "calling," a way of life for devoted women with private means, like Florence Nightingale (Kalisch & Kalisch, 1987, p. 20). Well over 100 years later the amount of scholarship on Nightingale provides a more realistic albeit still compelling portrait of a complex and brilliant woman—again, to quote Auerbach (1982) and Strachey (1918), "a demon, a rebel. . . ."

There are various goals to historical inquiry—to analyze, to provide insight into current problems through reflection on the patterns revealed in the past. It may also have descriptive and aesthetic aims: to document and describe anew, and to inspire and refresh. That is the intent of this chapter.

Florence Nightingale's legacy of caring and the activism it implies is carried on in nursing today. There is a resurgence and inclusion of concepts of spirituality in current nursing practice, and a delineation of nursing's caring base that began in essence with the nursing life of Florence Nightingale. Nightingale's caring, as demonstrated in this chapter, extended beyond the individual patient, beyond the individual person. She herself said that the specific business of nursing was the least important of the functions into which she had been forced in the Crimea. Her caring encompassed a broadened sphere—that of the British Army, and indeed the entire British Commonwealth.

The unique aspects of her personality and social position, combined with historical circumstances, laid the groundwork for the evolution of the modern discipline of nursing. Are the challenges and obstacles that we face today any more daunting than what confronted Nightingale when she arrived in the Crimea in 1854? Nursing for Florence Nightingale was what we might call today her "centering force." It allowed her to express her spiritual values as well as enabling her to fulfill her needs for leadership and authority. I am assuming that you are studying nursing because you care about people, because you deeply care about health care. We are challenged, as historian Susan Reverby noted, with the dilemma of how to practice our integral values of caring in a health care system that does not value caring. Let us look again to Florence Nightingale for inspiration, for she remains a role model "par excellence" on the transformation of values of caring into an *activism* that could potentially transform our current health care system into a more humanistic one. Florence Nightingale's legacy of connecting caring with activism can then truly be said to continue.

References

Ackernecht, E. (1982). *A short history of medicine*. Baltimore: Johns Hopkins University Press.

Arnstein, W. (1988). *Britain: Yesterday and today*. Lexington, MA: D.C. Heath & Co.

Auerbach, N. (1982). *Women and the demon: The life of a Victorian myth*. Cambridge, MA: Harvard University Press.

Barritt, E. R. (1973). Florence Nightingale's values and modern nursing education. *Nursing Forum, 12*, 7–47.

Bunting, S., & Campbell, J. (1990). Feminism and nursing: An historical perspective. *Advances in Nursing Science, 12*, 11–24.

Calabria, M., & Macrae, J. (Eds.). (1994). *Suggestions for thought by Florence Nightingale: Selections and commentaries*. Philadelphia: University of Pennsylvania Press.

Cohen, I. B. (1981). Florence Nightingale: The passionate statistician. *Scientific American, 250*(3): 128–137.

Cook, E. T. (1913). *The life of Florence Nightingale* (Vols. 1–2). London: Macmillan.

Dennis, K. E., & Prescott, P. A. (1985). Florence Nightingale: Yesterday, today and tomorrow. *Advances in Nursing Science, 7*(2), 66–81.

Dolan, J. (1971). *The grace of the great lady*. Chicago: Medical Heritage Society.

Donahue, P. (1985). *Nursing: The finest art*. St. Louis: Mosby.

Dossey, B. (1998). Florence Nightingale: A 19th century mystic. *Journal of Holistic Nursing, 16*(2), 111–164.

Erickson, E. (1950). *Childhood and society*. New York: W.W. Norton & Co., Inc.

Erikson, E. (1958). *Young man Luther*. New York: W. W. Norton & Co., Inc.

Erikson, E. (1974). *Dimensions of a new identity*. New York: W. W. Norton & Co., Inc.

Firestone, S. (1971). *The dialectic of sex*. New York: Bantam Books.

Fondriest, V., & Osborne, J. (1994). A theorist before her time? Presentation, NGR 5110, Nursing Theory and Advanced Practice Nursing, School of Nursing, Florida International University, N. Miami, FL.

Goldie, S. (1987). *I have done my duty: Florence Nightingale in the Crimean War, 1854–1856*. Iowa City: University of Iowa Press.

Hektor, L. M. (1984). *Florence Nightingale, 1837–1853: Identity, crisis and resolution*. Unpublished master's thesis. Hunter-Bellevue School of Nursing, New York, NY.

Hektor, L. M. (1992). *Nursing, science, and gender: Florence Nightingale and Martha E. Rogers*. Unpublished doctoral dissertation, University of Miami.

Houghton, W. (1957). *The Victorian frame of mind*. New Haven, CT: Yale University Press.

Huxley, E. (1975). *Florence Nightingale*. New York: G. P. Putnam's Sons.

Kalisch, P. A., & Kalisch, B. J. (1987). *The changing image of the nurse*. Menlo Park, CA: Addison-Wesley.

King, M. G. (1988). Gender: A hidden issue in nursing's professionalizing reform movement. Boston: Boston University School of Nursing. In *Strategies for Theory Development V*, March 10–12.

Macrae, J. (1995). Nightingale's spiritual philosophy and its significance for modern nursing. *Image: Journal of Nursing Scholarship, 27*, 8–10.

Meleis, A. I. (1997). *Theoretical nursing: Development and progress* (3rd ed.). Philadelphia: J. B. Lippincott.

Monteiro, L. (1984). On separate roads: Florence Nightingale and Elizabeth Blackwell. *Signs: Journal of Women in Culture & Society, 9*, 520–533.

Newman, Margaret A. (1972). Nursing's theoretical evolution. *Nursing Outlook, 20*, 449–453.

Nightingale, F. (1852/1979). *Cassandra,* with an introduction by Myra Stark. Westbury, NY: Feminist Press.

Nightingale, F. (1859/1992). *Notes on nursing: Commemorative edition with commentaries by contemporary nursing leaders*. Philadelphia: J. B. Lippincott.

Nightingale, F. (1859). *Notes on nursing: What it is and what it is not*. London: Harrison & Sons.

Nightingale, F. (1860). *Suggestions for thought to searchers after religious truths* (Vols. 2–3). London: George E. Eyre & William Spottiswoode.

Nightingale, F. (1860/1969). *Notes on nursing: What it is and what it is not*. New York: Dover.

Palmer, I. S. (1977). Florence Nightingale: Reformer, reactionary, research. *Nursing Research, 26*, 84–89.

Perkins, J. (1987). *Women and marriage in nineteenth century England.* Chicago: Lyceum Books, Inc.

Quinn, V., & Prest, J. (Eds.). (1981). *Dear Miss Nightingale:A selection of Benjamin Jowett's letters to Florence Nightingale, 1860-1893.* Oxford: Clarendon Press.

Reed, P. G., & Zurakowski, T. L. (1983/1989). Nightingale: A visionary model for nursing. In Fitzpatrick, J., & Whall, A. (Eds.), *Conceptual models of nursing: Analysis and application.* Bowie, MD: Robert J. Brady.

Reverby, S. M. (1987). *Ordered to care:The dilemma of American nursing (1865-1945).* New York: Cambridge University Press.

Rosenberg, C. (1979). *Healing and history.* New York: Science History Publications.

Sattin, A. (Ed.). (1987). *Florence Nightingale's letters from Egypt:A journey on the Nile, 1849-1850.* New York: Weidenfeld & Nicolson.

Shyrock, R. (1959). *The history of nursing.* Philadelphia: W. B. Saunders & Co.

Slater, V. E. (1994). The educational and philosophical influences on Florence Nightingale, an enlightened conductor. *Nursing History Review, 2,* 137-152.

Strachey, L. (1918). *Eminent Victorians:Cardinal Manning, Florence Nightingale, Dr. Arnold, General Gordon.* London: Chatto & Windus.

Summers, A. (1988). *Angels and citizens:British women as military nurses, 1854-1914.* London: Routledge & Kegan Paul.

Swazey, J., & Reed, K. (1978). Louis Pasteur: Science and the application of science. In Swazey, J., & Reed, K. (Eds.), *Today's medicine, tomorrow's science.* U.S. Government Printing Office: DHEW Pub. No. NIH 78-244. Washington, DC: U.S. Government Printing Office.

Vicinus, M. & Nergaard, B. (Eds.). (1990). *Ever yours, Florence Nightingale: Selected letters.* Cambridge, MA: Harvard University Press.

Watson, J. (1992). Commentary. In *Notes on nursing: What it is and what it is not* (pp. 80-85). Commemorative edition. Philadelphia: J. B. Lippincott.

Welch, M. (1986). Nineteenth-century philosophic influences on Nightingale's concept of the person. *Journal of Nursing History, 1*(2), 3-11.

Welch, M. (1990). Florence Nightingale: The social construction of a Victorian feminist. *Western Journal of Nursing Research, 12,* 404-407.

Widerquist, J. G. (1992). The spirituality of Florence Nightingale. *Nursing Research, 41,* 49-55.

Winstead-Fry, P. (1993). Book review: Notes on nursing: What it is and what it is not. Commemorative edition. *Nursing Science Quarterly,* 6(3), 161-162.

Woodham-Smith, C. (1983). *Florence Nightingale.* New York: Atheneum.

Bibliography

Aiken, C. A. (1915). *Lessons from the life of Florence Nightingale.* New York: Lakeside.

Aldis, M. (1914). *Florence Nightingale.* New York: NOPHN.

Andrews, M. R. (1929). *A lost commander.* Garden City, NY: Doubleday.

Baly, M. E. (1986). *Florence Nightingale:The nursing legacy.* New York: Methuen.

Bishop, W. J. (1962). *A bio-bibliography of Florence Nightingale.* London: Dawson's of Pall Mall.

Boyd, N. (1982). *Three Victorian women who changed their world.* New York: Oxford.

Bullough, V., Bullough, B., & Stanton, M. (Eds.). (1990). *Florence Nightingale and her era: A collection of new scholarship.* New York: Garland Publishing.

Cope, Z. (1958). *Florence Nightingale and the doctors.* Philadelphia: J. B. Lippincott.

Cope, Z. (1961). *Six disciples of Florence Nightingale.* New York: Pitman.

Davies, C. (1980). *Rewriting nursing history.* London: Croom Helm.

Donahue, P. (1985). *Nursing:The finest art.* St. Louis, MO: Mosby.

French, Y. (1953). *Six great Englishwomen.* London: H. Hamilton.

Goldsmith, M. L. (1937). *Florence Nightingale:The woman and the legend.* London: Hodder & Stoughton.

Gordon, R. (1979). *The private life of Florence Nightingale.* New York: Atheneum.

Haldale, E. (1931). *Mrs. Gaskell and her friends.* New York: Appleton.

Herbert, R. G. (1981). *Florence Nightingale:Saint, reformer or rebel?* Melbourne: F. L. Krieger.

Nash, R. (1937). *A sketch for the life of Florence Nightingale.* London: Society for Promoting Christian Knowledge.

Newtown, M. E. (1949). *Florence Nightingale's philosophy of life and education.* Unpublished doctoral dissertation, Stanford University, School of Education, Stanford, CA.

Nightingale, F. (1911). *Letters from Miss Florence Nightingale on health visiting in rural districts.* London: King.

Nightingale, F. (1954). *Selected writings.* Compiled by Lucy R. Seymer. New York: Macmillan.

Nightingale, F. (1974). *Letters of Florence Nightingale in the History of Nursing Archive.* Boston: Boston University Press.

Nightingale, F. (1976). *Notes on hospitals.* New York: Gordon.

O'Malley, I. B. (1931). *Life of Florence Nightingale, 1820-1856.* London: Butterworth.

Pollard, E. (1902). *Florence Nightingale:The wounded soldiers' friend.* London: Partridge.

Rosenberg, C. (Ed.). (1989). *Florence Nightingale on hospital reform.* New York: Garland Publishing.

Selanders, L. C. (1993). *Florence Nightingale:An environmental adaptation theory.* Newbury Park, CA: Sage Publications.

Seymer, L. R. (1951). *Florence Nightingale.* New York: Macmillan.

Showalter, E. (1981). Florence Nightingale's feminist complaint: Women, religion, and suggestions for thought. *Signs, 5.*

Smith, F. B. (1982). *Florence Nightingale:Reputation and power.* New York: St. Martin's.

Tooley, S. A. (1905). *The life of Florence Nightingale.* New York: Macmillan.

Woodsey, A. H. (1950). *A century of nursing*. New York: Putnam.

Wren, D. (1949). *They enriched humanity:Adventurers of the 19th century*. London: Skilton.

PERIODICALS

Address given at fiftieth anniversary of founding by Florence Nightingale of first training school for nurses at St. Thomas's Hospital, London, England. *American Journal of Nursing, 11,* 331-361.

Agnew, L. R. (1958). Florence Nightingale: Statistician. *American Journal of Nursing, 58,* 644.

Baly, M. (1986). Shattering the Nightingale myth. *Nursing Times, 82*(24), 16-18.

Baly, M. E. (1969). Florence Nightingale's influence on nursing today. *Nursing Times, 65,* 1-4.

Barker, E. R. (1989). Caregivers as casualties: War experiences and the postwar consequences for both Nightingale-and-Vietnam-era nurses. *Western Journal of Nursing Research, 11,* 628-631.

Bishop, W. J. (1957a). Florence Nightingale bibliography. *International Nursing Review, 4,* 64.

Bishop, W. J. (1957b). Florence Nightingale letters. *American Journal of Nursing, 57,* 607.

Blanchard, J. R. (1939). Florence Nightingale: A study in vocation. *New Zealand Nursing Journal, 32,* 193-197.

Boylen, J. O. (1974). The Florence Nightingale–Mary Stanley controversy: Some unpublished letters. *Medical History, 18*(2), 186-193.

Brow, E. J. (1954). Florence Nightingale and her international influence. *International Nursing Review, 1,* 17-19.

Clayton, R. E. (1974). How men may live and not die in India: Florence Nightingale. *Australian Nurses Journal, 2,* 10-11.

Collins, W. J. (1945). Florence Nightingale and district nursing. *Nursing Mirror, 81,* 74.

Cope, Z. (1960). Florence Nightingale and her nurses. *Nursing Times, 56,* 597.

Dunbar, V. M. (1954). Florence Nightingale's influence on nursing education. *International Nursing Review, 1,* 17-23.

Extracts from letters from the Crimea. (1932). *American Journal of Nursing, 32,* 537-538.

Fink, L. G. (1934). Catholic influences in the life of Florence Nightingale. *Hospital Progress, 15,* 482-489.

Florence Nightingale's letter of advice to Bellevue. (1911). *American Journal of Nursing, 11,* 361-364.

Florence Nightingale's letter. (1932*). Nursing Times, 28,* 699.

Florence Nightingale as a leader in the religious and civic thought of her time. (1936). *Hospitals, 10,* 78-84.

Florence Nightingale bibliography. (1956). *Nursing Research, 5,* 87.

Grier, B., & Grier, M. (1978). Contributions of the passionate statistician (Florence Nightingale). *Research in Nursing and Health, 1*(3), 103-109.

Gropper, E. I. (1990). Florence Nightingale: Nursing's first environmental theorist. *Nursing Forum, 25*(3), 30-33.

Hektor, L. M. (1994). Florence Nightingale and the women's movement. Friend or foe? *Nursing Inquiry, 1*(1), 38-45.

Iveson-Iveson, J. (1983). Nurses in society: A legend in the breaking (Florence Nightingale). *Nursing Mirror, 156*(19), 26-27.

Jones, H. W. (1940). Some unpublished letters of Florence Nightingale. *Bulletin of the History of Medicine, 8,* 1389-1396.

Kerling, N. J. (1976). Letters from Florence Nightingale. *Nursing Mirror, 143*(1), 68.

Konstatinova, M. (1923). In the cradle of nursing. *American Journal of Nursing, 24,* 47-49.

Kopf, E. W. (1978). Florence Nightingale as statistician. *Research in Nursing and Health, 1*(3), 93-102.

Levine, M. E. (1963). Florence Nightingale: The legend that lives. *Nursing Forum, 2,* 24.

Loane, S. F. (1911). Florence Nightingale and district nursing. *American Journal of Nursing, 11,* 383-384.

Mackie, T. T. (1942). Florence Nightingale and tropical and military medicine. *American Journal of Tropical Medicine, 22,* 1-8.

McCarthy, D. O., Ouimet, M. E., & Daun, J. M. (1991). Shades of Florence Nightingale: Potential impact of noise stress on wound healing. *Holistic Nursing Practice, 5*(4), 39-48.

Monteiro, L. (1972). Research into things past: Tracking down one of Miss Nightingale's correspondents. *Nursing Research, 21,* 526-529.

Monteiro, L. A. (1985a). Florence Nightingale on public health nursing. *American Journal of Public Health, 75,* 181-186.

Monteiro, L. A. (1985b). Response in anger: Florence Nightingale on the importance of training for nurses. *Journal of Nursing History, 1*(1), 11-18.

Nagpal, N. (1985). Florence Nightingale: A multifaceted personality. *Nursing Journal of India, 76,* 110-114.

Newton, M. E. (1952). Florence Nightingale's concept of clinical teaching. *Nursing World, 126,* 220-221.

Notting, M. A. (1927). Florence Nightingale as a statistician. *Public Health Nursing, 19,* 207-209.

Noyes, C. D. (1931). Florence Nightingale: Sanitarian and hygienist. *Red Cross Courier, 10,* 41, 42.

Oman, C. (1950). Florence Nightingale as seen by two biographers. *Nursing Mirror, 92,* 30-31.

Palmer, I. S. (1976). Florence Nightingale and the Salisbury incident. *Nursing Research, 25*(5), 370-377.

Palmer, I. S. (1983a). Florence Nightingale: The myth and the reality. *Nursing Outlook, 79,* 40-42.

Palmer, I. S. (1983b). Nightingale revisited. *Nursing Outlook, 31*(4), 229-233.

Parker, P. (1977). Florence Nightingale: First lady of admininstrative nursing. *Supervisor Nurse, 8,* 24-25.

Pearce, E. C. (1954). The influence of Florence Nightingale on the spirit of nursing. *International Nursing Review, 1,* 20-22.

Pope, D. S. (1995). Music, noise and the human voice in the nurse-patient environment. *Image Journal of Nursing Scholarship, 27,* 291-295.

Rajabally, M. (1994). Florence Nightingale's personality: A psychoanalytic profile. *International Journal of Nursing Studies, 31*(3), 269-278.

Richards, L. (1920). Recollections of Florence Nightingale. *American Journal of Nursing, 20,* 649.

Richards, L. (Ed.). (1934). Letters of Florence Nightingale. *Yale Review, 24*, 326-347.

Ross, M. (1954). Miss Nightingale's letters. *American Journal of Nursing, 53*, 593-594.

Scovil, E. R. (1911). Personal recollections of Florence Nightingale. *American Journal of Nursing, 11*, 365-368.

Seymer, L. R. (1951). Florence Nightingale at Kaiserwerth. *American Journal of Nursing, 51,* 424-426.

Seymer, L. R. (1970). Nightingale nursing school: 100 years ago. *American Journal of Nursing, 60*, 658.

Seymer, S. (1979). The writings of Florence Nightingale. *Nursing Journal of India, 70*(5), 121, 128.

Sparacino, P. S. A. (1994). Clinical practice: Florence Nightingale: A CNS role model. *Clinical Nurse Specialist, 8*(2), 64.

Thomas, S. P. (1993). The view from Scutari: A look at contemporary nursing. *Nursing Forum, 28*(2), 19-24.

White, F. S. (1923). At the gate of the temple. *Public Health Nursing, 15*, 279-283.

Whittaker, E., & Oleson, V. L. (1967). Why Florence Nightingale? *American Journal of Nursing, 67*, 2338.

Widerquist, J. G. (1992). The spirituality of Florence Nightingale. *Nursing Research, 41*, 499-555.

Woodham-Smith, Mrs. C. (1947). Florence Nightingale as a child. *Nursing Mirror, 85*, 91-92.

Woodham-Smith, Mrs. C. (1952). Florence Nightingale revealed. *American Journal of Nursing, 52*, 570-572.

Woodham-Smith, Mrs. C. (1954). The greatest Victorian. *Nursing Times, 50*, 737-741.

Yeates, E. L. (1962). The Prince Consort and Florence Nightingale. *Nursing Mirror, 113*, iii-iv.

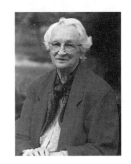

Chapter 5

Hildegard E. Peplau
The Process of Practice-based
Theory Development

Ann R. Peden

INTRODUCING THE THEORIST

Hildegard Peplau was an outstanding leader and pioneer in psychiatric nursing whose career spanned seven decades. A review of the events in her life also serves as an introduction to the history of modern psychiatric nursing. With the publication of *Interpersonal Relations in Nursing* in 1952, Peplau provided a framework for the practice of psychiatric nursing that would result in a paradigm shift in this field of nursing. Prior to this, patients were viewed as objects to be observed. Peplau taught that patients were not objects but subjects, and that we, as psychiatric nurses, must participate with the patients, engaging in the nurse-patient relationship. This was a revolutionary idea. Although *Interpersonal Relations in Nursing* was not well received when it was first published in 1952, it has since been reprinted (1988) and translated into at least six languages.

Hildegard Peplau was born on September 1, 1909, in Reading, Pennsylvania. She described herself as coming from a working-class family. For young women at that time, there were limited career options: nursing, teaching, or becoming a nun. Peplau lacked money for an education that would prepare her to be a teacher. She chose nursing, because as a diploma-school student, she would be paid while working to become a registered nurse. She entered nursing for practical reasons, seeing it as a way to leave home and have an occupation. As she adapted to nursing school, she made the conscious decision that if she were going to be a nurse, then she would be a good one (Peplau, 1998).

As a child, Peplau was a keen observer. She witnessed the influenza epidemic of 1918, and the delirious behaviors of individuals with high fevers. She also saw, daily, individuals who lived in her community who were considered odd or eccentric. As a child she was not allowed to make fun of these individuals and had to be respectful toward them. Their behaviors fascinated her.

In 1931, Peplau graduated from the Pottstown (Pennsylvania) Hospital School of Nursing. During Peplau's basic nursing education, psychiatric nursing was not emphasized. She spent four afternoons a month at Norristown State Hospital. Students were not allowed to speak with physicians; physicians were viewed as important people, and nursing students were the workers. No nursing instructor accompanied the students to Norristown State Hospital; however, Peplau was fortunate to meet Dr. Arthur Noyes, who was a psychiatrist at that hospital. He encouraged students to ask questions. Peplau described Dr. Noyes as a friend to psychiatric nursing, urging nurses to learn a trained technique that would guide them in caring for psychiatric patients. Peplau identified him as an early influence on her nursing career.

Peplau served as the college head nurse and later as executive officer of the Health Service at Bennington College, Vermont. While working there as a nurse, she began taking courses that would lead to a bachelor of arts degree in interpersonal psychology. Dr. Eric Fromm was one of her teachers at Bennington. An experience while working in the Health Service served to pique Peplau's interest in psychiatric nursing. A young student with symptoms of schizophrenia came to the clinic seeking help. Peplau did not know what to do for her. The student left Bennington to receive treatment and returned to complete her education later. The successful recovery of this young woman was a positive experience for Peplau.

Bennington offered its students eight-week field experiences during the winter. Peplau spent one of these experiences at Bellevue, at that time the best psychiatric program available. While at Bellevue, Peplau attended lectures given for the medical staff and worked on the psychiatric wards. Peplau spent another field experience at Chestnut Lodge in Rockville, Maryland. This experience was probably the most influential in the development of Peplau's ideas about interpersonal theory and nursing. While at Chestnut Lodge, she received weekly supervision from Freida Fromm Reichmann. She also was introduced to the work of Harry Stack Sullivan which was an important introduction to theory development in psychiatric nursing. Additionally, she spent field experiences with Dr. David Levy, a leading child psychiatrist of that time, and did private duty nursing with psychiatric patients who were confined to their homes. These experiences fueled Peplau's interest in psychiatric nursing (Peplau, 1998).

Upon graduation from Bennington, Peplau joined the Army Nurse Corps. She was assigned to the School of Military Neuropsychiatry in England. This experience introduced her to the psychiatric problems of soldiers at war and allowed her to work with many great psychiatrists, including the Menningers. After the war, Peplau attended Columbia University on the GI Bill and earned her master's in psychiatric-mental health nursing.

In 1946, the Mental Health Act was passed. It identified four disciplines that would receive federal support for education. During the first few years after this act was passed, schools with programs in psychiatric nursing could not spend all the money allotted. There were, at that time, few programs that offered master's degrees, fewer teachers who could teach in these programs, and a limited number of students with bachelor's of science in nursing degrees who were eligible. Psychiatric nursing was "ripe" for a leader to emerge.

After her graduation in 1948, Peplau was invited to remain at Columbia and teach in their master's program. She immediately searched the library for books to use with students, but she found very few. At that time, the psychiatric nurse was viewed as a companion to patients, someone who would play games and take walks but talk about nothing substantial. In fact, nurses were instructed not to talk to patients about their problems, thoughts, or feelings. Peplau began teaching at Columbia, knowing that she wanted to change the education and practice of psychiatric nursing. There was no direction for what to include in graduate nursing programs. She took educational experiences from psychiatry and psychology and adapted them to nursing education. Peplau described this as a time of "innovation or nothing." Peplau's innovation in nursing education was criticized by her colleagues.

Her goal was to prepare nurse psychotherapists, referring to this training as "talking to patients" (Peplau, 1960, 1962). She arranged clinical experiences for her students at Brooklyn State Hospital, the only hospital in the New York City area that would take them. At the hospital, students were assigned to back wards, working with the most chronic and severely ill patients. Each student met twice weekly with the same patient, for a session lasting one hour. According to Peplau, the nurses resisted this practice tremendously and thought this was an awful thing to do (Peplau, 1998). Using carbon paper, verbatim notes were taken during the session. Students then met individually with Peplau to go over the interaction in detail. Through this process, both Peplau and her students began to learn what was helpful and what was harmful in the interaction.

Peplau struggled daily to keep her students working at this clinical site. She and her students were challenged not to make waves or risk losing this experience at Brooklyn State. Although they were assigned to the most severely ill patients, Peplau and her students met few licensed personnel—only untrained attendants. As patients showed improvement as a result of the interactions with Peplau and her students, the untrained staff behaved in ways that seemed to indicate that they wanted patients to stay sick. This was Peplau's first introduction to illness-maintaining behaviors that were common in state hospitals. As she reported, "The pathology of the patients we worked with was so blatant, we couldn't miss it" (Peplau, cited in Hatherleigh, 1998).

In 1955, Peplau left Columbia to teach at Rutgers, where she began the Clinical Nurse Specialist program in psychiatric-mental health nursing. The students were prepared as nurse psychotherapists, developing expertise in individual, group, and family therapies. Peplau required of her students "unflinching self-scrutiny," examining their own verbal and nonverbal communication and its effects on the nurse-patient relationship. Students were encouraged to ask, "What message am I sending?"

In 1956, Peplau began spending her summers touring the country, offering week-long clinical workshops in state hospitals. This activity was instrumental in teaching interpersonal theory and the importance of the nurse-patient relationship to psychiatric nurses. The workshops also provided a forum from which Peplau could promote advanced education for psychiatric nurses. Her belief that psychiatric nurses must have advanced degrees encouraged large numbers of psychiatric nurses to seek master's degrees and eventual certification as psychiatric-mental health clinical specialists.

During her career as a nursing educator, a total of 100 students had the opportunity to study with Peplau. These students have become leaders in psychiatric nursing. Many have gone on to earn doctoral degrees, becoming psychoanalysts, writing prolifically in the field of psychiatric nursing, and entering and influencing the academic world. Their influence has resulted in the integration of the nurse-patient relationship and the concept of anxiety into the culture of nursing. In 1974, Peplau retired from Rutgers. This allowed her more time to devote to the larger profession of nursing. Throughout her career, Peplau actively contributed to the American Nurses' Association (ANA) by serving on various committees and task forces. Peplau lived in New York City and later New Jersey; this close proximity to ANA and National League for Nursing (NLN) headquarters enabled her to participate in policy making and influence nursing practices (Sills, 1998). She served as chairperson of the ANA Division of Psychiatric Mental Health Nursing and was a member of the ANA Congress on Nursing Practice. As a member of this congress, Peplau argued for the certification of specialists in nursing. She is the only person who has been both the executive director and president of ANA. Peplau served on the ANA committee that wrote the Social Policy Statement. For the first time in nursing's history, nursing had a phenomenological focus—human responses.

Peplau held 11 honorary degrees. In 1994, she was inducted into the American Academy of Nursing's Living Legends Hall of Fame. She was named one of the 50 great Americans by *Marquis Who's Who* in 1995. In 1997, Peplau received the Christiane Reiman Prize, nursing's most prestigious award. In 1998, she was inducted into the ANA Hall of Fame.

Internationally, Peplau was an advisor to the World Health Organization (WHO); she was a member of their First Nursing Advisory Committee and contributed to WHO's first paper on psychiatric nursing. She served as a consultant to the Pan-American Health Association, and served two terms on the International Council of Nurses' Board of Directors. Even after her retirement, she continued to mentor nurses in many countries.

Peplau entered the field of psychiatric nursing at a time when there were no role models. She described herself as never having a mentor, although she mentored countless students and nurses herself. As she was developing as a psychiatric nurse and leader, Peplau learned more from the many psychiatrists she worked with than from nurses. Grayce Sills, colleague and long-time friend of Peplau, wrote, "[T]he persistent theme is that of a woman of uncommon intellect, socialized outside the 1940s model of nursing in the United States, who developed a paradigm of professionalism. She then brought, in a half century of commitment, a model of professionalism that has permeated every aspect of her long and distinguished career. It is a legacy that will survive and continue to serve the profession well into the 21st century" (Sills, 1998, p. 171).

Hildegard Peplau died in March 1999 at her home in Sherman Oaks, California.

THE EXPERIENCE OF A THIRD-GENERATION PEPLAU STUDENT

In 1987, I began doctoral study at the University of Alabama at Birmingham. At that time, Dr. Elizabeth Morrison was assigned as my faculty advisor and chaired my dissertation committee. Dr. Morrison is one of the 100 students who studied directly with Peplau and is a Peplau scholar. Peplau described her as "a professor's delight: intelligent, responsible, responsive, career-oriented and always cheerful . . . she has taken her own career and further professional development seriously and has contributed greatly to the advancement of the profession" (Peplau, personal communication, September 16, 1998). After Dr. Morrison's graduation from Rutgers, she maintained a relationship with Peplau and has tested Peplau's theory in practice (Morrison, 1992; Morrison, Shealy, Kowalski, LaMont, & Range, 1996).

While beginning work on my dissertation, I began to read the writings of Peplau more carefully. Like most psychiatric nurses, I applied her interpersonal theory in my clinical practice. I had actually been taught interventions developed by Peplau as an undergraduate nursing student in psychiatric nursing. However, like many nurses educated before the 1980s, I was not told that a theorist named Peplau was guiding my practice. This I discovered after graduating from my baccalaureate program, when I began to read Peplau's work, especially her writings on anxiety and hallucinations (Peplau, 1952, 1962). In the course of reading her work with the "eye" of a doctoral student, I discovered her paper on theory development that had been presented at the first Nursing Theory Conference in 1969. In that paper, Peplau (1989a) described the process of practice-based theory development. Reading this work was very exciting. In the paper, Peplau described a methodology for developing theory in practice. This will be described more completely later in this chapter.

As my dissertation proposal developed, Dr. Morrison encouraged me to send it to Peplau for her to read. This idea made me extremely anxious, but Dr. Morrison persisted. She had talked to Peplau and Peplau said that she would be glad to read my proposal. This began a correspondence with Peplau that continued for years, until her death in 1999. She enriched my professional life and I am honored that she was interested in what I thought and what I was doing. When considering the link between Peplau, Elizabeth Morrison, and me, I consider myself a third-generation student of Peplau. From the beginning of her research career, Peplau provided guidance, direction, and feedback—answering many questions, sharing resources, and providing contacts with other psychiatric nurse researchers. She shared her knowledge and expertise with countless numbers of psychiatric nurses. In fact, this has been a hallmark of her professional life—sharing, developing, and responding to nurses as they sought knowledge. Psychiatric nursing has benefited from the leadership of this scholar who was always ahead of her time—a pioneer who led the way in nursing.

PEPLAU'S PROCESS OF PRACTICE-BASED THEORY DEVELOPMENT

In 1969, at the first Nursing Theory Conference, Hildegard Peplau proposed a research methodology to guide "development of knowledge from observations in nursing situations" (Peplau, 1989a, p. 22).

Peplau asserted that nursing was an applied science and that nurses used established knowledge for beneficial purposes. According to Peplau (1988, p. 12), nurses not only "use the knowledge that 'producing scientists' publish," but they, in practice, create the context whereby this knowledge is transformed into nursing knowledge, linking nursing processes with nursing practice (Reed, 1996). Peplau urged nurses to use nursing situations as a source of observations from which unique nursing concepts could be derived. Practice provided the context for initiating and testing nursing theory. To direct nurses in the development of practice-based theory, Peplau (1989a) proposed a three-step process that would assist in this pursuit.

> Peplau urged nurses to use nursing situations as a source of observations from which unique nursing concepts could be derived.

Theory development begins with observations made in practice. In the first step, the nurse observes a phenomenon, which is then named, categorized, or classified. The nurse relies on an already existing body of knowledge from which to derive the name of the concept or phenomenon. By relying on existing literature to assist in naming the concept, further information about the concept is gained. Included in this step are the continuing clinical observations of the nurse who seeks regularities in the phenomenon. Peplau (1952) identified several methods of observation, including participant observation, spectator observation, and interviewer and random observation. Participant observation, in which the nurse observes while participating, yields the most valuable clinical knowledge. This includes the recording of observations of both self and other in order to analyze the interpersonal process. Peplau identified the participant observer as one of the characteristic roles of the professional nurse (Peplau, 1989b). Validation of the nurse's observations, either with other professionals or with patients, is encouraged, in order to decrease observer bias (Peplau, 1989c). A nurse enters clinical situations with "theoretical understanding, personal bias, and previously acquired nursing knowledge" (Reed, 1996, p. 31).

In the second step of the process, the nurse sorts and classifies information about the phenomenon. Decoding, subdividing data, categorizing data, identifying layers of meaning at different levels of abstraction, and applying a conceptual framework to explain the phenomenon may occur as a means of interpreting observations (Peplau, 1989b). At that time, a structure for obtaining more information about the phenomenon emerges. Further observation or interviewing leads to a clearer, more explicit description of the phenomenon or concept. The nurse works to identify all of the behaviors associated with the concept. Included in this step is the collection of information about patterns or processes that accompany the phenomenon.

Using Peplau's process, clinical data are collected via observation and interview. Verbatim recordings of interactions with patients are examined for regularities. The nurse, as the interviewer, assists the patient in providing a thorough description of the concept or process. Peplau (1989d) offered interview techniques that encouraged description, for example: "Describe one time that you were . . ."; "Describe one example . . ."; "Say more about that . . ."; and "Fill in the details about that experience" (Peplau, 1989d, pp. 221–222). Only by thorough description of the

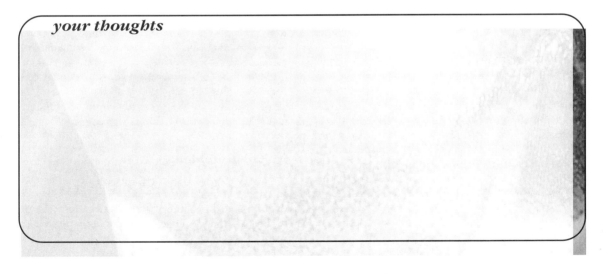

your thoughts

concept or process can the nurse assure that all of the behaviors associated with the process are identified.

The last step of the process leads to the development of interventions. Peplau viewed nursing interventions as those that "assisted patients in gaining interpersonal and intellectual competencies evolved through the nurse-patient relationship" (O'Toole & Welt, 1989, p. 351). Useful interventions are derived and tested (Peplau, 1989c).

Peplau used this process to study clinical phenomena. Both she and her students collected verbatim recordings of interactions with patients. These recordings were examined for regularities. Similar-looking data were then transcribed onto 3-by-5-inch index cards, which were then sorted, classified, and counted. As early as 1948, Peplau's students at Teachers College (Columbia University) were asked to make carbon copies of their interactions with patients. Peplau studied these and noticed that the students could not talk in a friendly way until the patients had said "I need you" or "I like you." Her analysis of similar nurse-patient interactions led to her theory of anxiety and subsequently to nursing interventions to decrease anxiety (O'Toole & Welt, 1989).

PEPLAU'S PRACTICE-BASED PROCESS AND A PROGRAM OF RESEARCH

Peplau's process of practice-based theory development has directed a program of research in the area of depression in women (Peden, 1998). Beginning with the identification of a clinical phenomenon, women recovering from depression, and culminating in the testing of an intervention to reduce negative thinking in depressed women, Peplau's process of practice-based theory development has provided direction and structure for four studies.

The treatment of depression had been studied extensively. However, lacking in the literature were women's accounts of recovering from depression. A thorough description of the process of recovering in women with depression was not reflected in the literature. The identification of a clinical phenomenon and a review of available information related to that phenomenon were the first step in Peplau's process.

In the second step, a descriptive, exploratory study (Peden, 1993) was conducted. Seven women who were recovering from depression were interviewed and a process of recovering was described. Peplau assisted in the design of the semistructured interview guide (personal communication, December 14, 1990). Verbatim transcripts of the audiotaped interviews were analyzed. The process of recovering in women who were depressed was initiated by a crisis or "turning point" experience. It continued with professional support and the support of friends and family. Recovering, according to the participants, required determination, work over time,

> Peplau's process provided direction and structure for four studies of women recovering from depression, concluding with testing a nursing intervention.

and a series of successes that enhanced self-esteem and maintained balance. The process was dynamic, occurring in a nonserial order, with back-and-forth movement among the categories and phases. It was internal and ongoing. This study raised many questions and provided further direction for study. While participating in the interviews, the women shared strategies or techniques that facilitated recovering (Peden, 1994). These included cognitive skills, positive self-talk, and use of affirmations. They also identified negative thinking as the most difficult symptom to overcome.

Follow-up Study

Continuing in step 2 of the process, a follow-up study (Peden, 1996) was conducted a year later, to describe further the process of recovering in women who had been depressed. No new phases of the recovering process were identified. Interventions that assisted patients in recovering instilled hope, were psychoeducational in nature, included cognitive interventions that change thinking styles, and provided for individualized treatment.

Peden's study (1996) concluded with the realization that more information was needed on the symptom of negative thinking. To understand a phenomenon, one must analyze its etiology, its cause, its meaning, and any clues to successful intervention (Peplau, 1989c). At the suggestion of Peplau (personal communication, January 16, 1993), work began, returning to the first step of the process, to gather more information about the symptom of negative thinking.

Negative Thinking

A qualitative study (Peden, 2000) was designed to describe the nature or inherent quality of negative thoughts, their content or subject matter, and the origins of the negative thoughts experienced by women with major depression. The participants also shared strategies they used to manage the negative thoughts. The sample consisted of six women with a diagnosis of major depression who were experiencing or had experienced negative thoughts and were willing to talk about the experiences. The women participated in a series of six group interviews, the purpose of which was to elicit negative views/thoughts held by the group participants. The group interviews were conducted weekly, for 6 consecutive weeks. Each interview lasted 1 hour. A semi-structured interview guide, developed in consultation with Peplau (personal communication, January 16, 1993), was used to facilitate the interviews. The group interviews focused on the women's life experiences, views of self and significant others, lifestyles, and past experiences. Descriptions of negative thoughts held by the women were sought.

Verbatim transcripts were examined for regularities (Peplau, 1989b). A coding guide was developed. Codes were derived from available literature and based on recommendations from Peplau (personal communication, January 16, 1993); other codes that emerged from the initial review of the data. Codes included negative thinking related to self, negative thinking related to significant others, interactions with significant others, and developing view of self. After coding the data, recurring themes were sought (Peplau, 1989a).

For the six women who participated in the study, the negative thoughts had their origins in childhood. Common childhood experiences included suppression of emotion, restrictive parenting, learning to be passive, lack of praise or compliments, high parental expectations, stifled communication, and lack of emotional support. The negative thoughts focused primarily on self, being different, disappointing self and others, not being perfect, and always failing. The women described their self-talk as constant, negative, and demeaning. They identified various means of managing the negative thoughts. Once again, the use of affirmations, positive self-talk, and learning to change thinking were identified as reducing negative thinking. Steps 1 and 2 of the process of practice-based theory development had provided direction for moving into the third step, design of an intervention.

Testing an Intervention

A 6-week group intervention was designed specifically to incorporate cognitive-behavioral techniques to assist in reducing negative thinking in depressed women. As described earlier, thought stopping and positive self-talk (or affirmations) were identified as key strategies in reducing negative thoughts. The intervention was designed using specific content from Gordon and Tobin's (1991) *Insight* program, *The De-*

pression Workbook (Copeland, 1992), and the investigator's own clinical experiences with depressed women. Affirmations, direct actions, thought stopping, and information on distorted thinking styles were introduced to the group members. Depressed women benefit from group treatment (Gordon & Tobin, 1991; Van Survellan & Dull, 1981). Group sessions allow contact with peers with similar problems, reduce isolation, promote change, and are cost-effective. Guided by Peplau's (1952) Theory of Interpersonal Nursing, the introduction of cognitive-behavioral techniques did not occur until the second group session. The focus of the first week was on enhancing the development of the nurse-patient relationship to decrease anxiety, increase trust and security within the group, and lay the foundation for the intervention.

To pilot-test the intervention, 13 women with a diagnosis of major depression were randomly assigned either to a control or to an experimental group. All subjects were under psychiatric care in an outpatient clinic and receiving antidepressant medication. The experimental group ($n = 5$) participated in the 6-week cognitive-behavioral group intervention for 1 hour per week. The control group ($n = 8$) continued with routine psychiatric care.

Pre- and post-test measures were collected on depression using the Beck Depression Inventory (Beck, Ward, Mendelson, Mock, & Erbaugh, 1961) and negative thinking using the Crandall Cognitions Inventory (Crandall & Chambless, 1986) and the Automatic Thoughts Questionnaire (Hollon & Kendall, 1980). Feedback from the five participants in the experimental group indicated that the intervention was beneficial. There were significant decreases from pretest to post-test in the experimental group in negative thoughts ($p < .05$) and depressive symptoms ($p < .05$) and an increase in self-esteem ($p < .05$). The reduction in depressive symptoms in both groups was expected. However, for the experimental group, the Beck Depression Inventory (BDI) mean scores decreased from 22 (moderate to severe depression) to 7 (normal), a reduction of 15 points from pre- to post-test. For the control group, the Beck scores decreased from 18 (moderate depression) to 11 (mild depression), a reduction of 7 points. Although the sample size was small, the intervention had a significant positive effect on depression.

Testing the Intervention with At-Risk Women

Upon recommendation of Peplau (personal communication, January 16, 1993), the intervention was

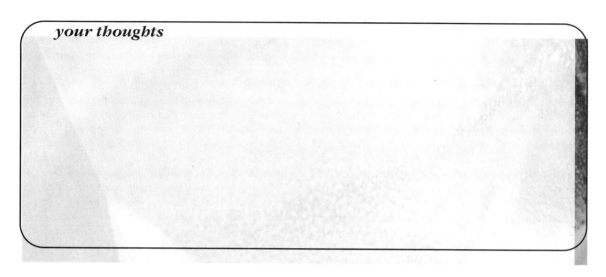

tested on at-risk college women to determine if it had preventive effects (Peden, Hall, Rayens, & Beebe, 2000). A randomized controlled prevention trial was conducted to test the efficacy of a cognitive-behavioral group intervention in reducing negative thinking and depressive symptoms and enhancing self-esteem in a sample of 92 college women ages 18 to 24. Depression risk status was determined by scores on the Center for Epidemiologic Studies—Depression Scale (CES-D) (Radloff, 1977) and the BDI (Beck and coworkers, 1961).

As they were enrolled, the participants were randomly assigned to either the control or experimental groups. Those participants assigned to the experimental group participated in the 6-week cognitive-behavioral group intervention. Data on self-esteem, depressive symptoms, and negative thinking were collected from both groups 1 month after the intervention and at 6-month follow-up sessions to assess the interventions' long-term effects. Currently, 18-month follow-up data are being collected.

Based on the preliminary findings of this study, the intervention did have a positive effect on depressive symptoms, negative thinking, and self-esteem in a group of at-risk college women. Reducing negative thinking in at-risk individuals may decrease the risk for depression. At this point, plans are underway to test the intervention with other at-risk groups to continue to gather support for its preventive effects.

PEPLAU FOR THE FUTURE

Study of Peplau's work is very timely. She proposed, in 1969, using practice as the basis for theory development. At that time this was a radical idea. Now the trend is to return to practice for knowledge develop-

ment. Peplau used clinical situations to derive theories inductively that were then tested in clinical practice. She also applied existing social science theories to nursing phenomena, combining induction (observation and classification) with deduction (the application of known concepts and processes to data). This provided a creative, nonlinear approach to the formation of ideas.

She also proposed the linkage of qualitative and quantitative methods. Using her methodology, the nurse would begin with an in-depth look at a phenomenon, which would evolve into a quantitative study testing an intervention directed at the phenomenon. These ideas, proposed during the positivist period of nursing, were highly revolutionary. It is unlikely that Peplau's contemporaries would have embraced her process of practice-based theory development. In fact, the debates related to knowledge development in nursing and the accompanying quantitative/qualitative rift did not occur until the 1980s. However, as nursing has come to recognize practice knowledge as one of the ways of knowing, researchers may return to Peplau's ideas offered at the first Nursing Theory Conference (Peplau, 1969) for direction.

> Peplau's theory keeps pace with postmodern influences, reinforcing nurses' awareness of the knowledge-rich context of practice, at the level of the patient.

Peplau's theory is very timely today, keeping pace with the postmodern influences that have reinforced nurses' awareness of the knowledge-rich context of practice, at the level of the patient. A study of Peplau's work introduces you to a woman whose ideas were ahead of her time. These ideas have arrived!

Summary

Peplau's process of practice-based theory development came at a time in nursing when grand theories were being developed and theoretical nursing was highly valued. These theories are now being criticized as too broad and too remote from nursing to be applied. The trend now is to return to practice for knowledge development. Peplau, always ahead of her time, provided an "approach to knowledge development through the scholarship of practice; nursing knowledge is developed in practice as well as for practice" (Reed, 1996, p. 29). Peplau used observations in clinical situations as the basis for hypotheses and interventions that were then tested in clinical practice. She also applied existing theories from the social sciences to nursing phenomena:

> The process of combining induction (observation and classification) with deduction (the application of known concepts and processes to data) provides a creative nonlinear approach to the formation of ideas, one that uses the data of practice, as well as extant theories as the basis of those formulations. (O'Toole & Welt, 1989, p. 355)

Peplau's methodology also linked qualitative and quantitative methods. After a qualitative, in-depth look at a phenomenon, a quantitative study would be developed to test an intervention directed at the phenomenon. Peplau's ideas and approach to nursing were highly revolutionary at the time; few of her contemporaries openly embraced her process of practice-based theory development. It was not until the 1980s that nursing scholars debated approaches to knowledge development in nursing and a rift developed between advocates of quantitative versus qualitative approaches. However, as nursing has come to recognize practice knowledge as one of the ways of knowing, researchers may return to the ideas Peplau offered at the first Nursing Theory Conference (Peplau, 1989a) for direction:

> Peplau's theory has kept pace with post modern influences that have reinforced nurses' awareness of the knowledge-laden context of practice, at the level of the patient." (Reed, 1996, p. 30)

The use of Peplau's process of practice-based theory development as a research methodology has provided the structure for developing my program of research in the area of depression in women. The identification of a clinical problem and an in-depth look at its etiology, patterns, and processes directed the design and testing of an intervention. As interventions were tested and supported in clinical research, the findings were reported to support the growing body of psychiatric nursing knowledge. Peplau's Theory of Interpersonal Nursing and her mentorship have been invaluable to me in developing each phase of my research program.

References

Beck, A. T., Ward, C. H., Mendelson, M., Mock, L., & Erbaugh, J. (1961). An inventory for measuring depression. *Archives of General Psychiatry, 4*, 561–571.

Copeland, M. E. (1992). *The Depression Workbook.* Oakland, CA: New Harbinger.

Crandell, C. J., & Chambless, D. L. (1986). The validation of an inventory for measuring depressive thoughts: The Crandell Cognitions Inventory. *Behavioral Research and Theory, 24*, 402–411.

Gordon, V., & Tobin, M. (1991). *Insight: A cognitive enhancement program for women.* Available from Verona Gordon, University of Minnesota, Minneapolis.

Hollon, S. D., & Kendall, P. C. (1980). Cognitive self-statements in depression: Development of an automatic thoughts questionnaire. *Cognitive Theory and Research, 4*, 383–395.

Morrison, E. G. (1992). Inpatient practice: An integrated framework. *Journal of Psychosocial Nursing and Mental Health Services, 30*(1), 26–29.

Morrison, E. G., Shealy, A. H., Kowalski, C., LaMont, J., & Range, B. A. (1996). Work roles of staff nurses in psychiatric settings. *Nursing Science Quarterly, 9*, 17–21.

O'Toole, A., & Welt, S. R. (1989). *Interpersonal theory in nursing practice: Selected works of Hildegarde Peplau.* New York: Springer.

Peden, A. (1993). Recovering in depressed women: Research with Peplau's theory. *Nursing Science Quarterly, 6*(3), 140–146.

Peden, A. R. (1994). Up from depression: Strategies used by women recovering from depression. *Journal of Psychiatric and Mental Health Nursing, 2*, 77–84.

Peden, A. R. (1996). Recovering from depression: A one-year follow-up. *Journal of Psychiatric and Mental Health Nursing, 3*, 289–295.

Peden, A. R. (1998). The evolution of an intervention: The use of Peplau's process of practice-based theory development. *Journal of Psychiatric and Mental Health Nursing, 5*(3), 173–178.

Peden, A. R. (2000). Negative thoughts of depressed women. *Journal of the American Psychiatric Nurses Association, 6*, in press.

Peden, A. R., Hall, L. A., Rayens, M. K., & Beebe, L. L. (2000). Negative thinking mediates the effect of self-esteem on depressive symptoms in college women. *Nursing Research, 50*, in press.

Peplau, H. E. (1952). *Interpersonal relations in nursing*. New York: G. P. Putnam's Sons. (English edition reissued as a paperback in 1988 by Macmillan Education Ltd., London.)

Peplau, H. E. (1960). Talking with patients. *American Journal of Nursing, 60*, 964–967.

Peplau, H. E. (1962). The crux of psychiatric nursing. *American Journal of Nursing, 62*, 50–54.

Peplau, H. E. (1988). The art and science of nursing: Similarities, differences and relations. *Nursing Science Quarterly, 1*, 8–15.

Peplau, H. E. (1989a). Theory: The professional dimension. In O'Toole, A., & Welt, S. R. (Eds.), *Interpersonal theory in nursing practice: Selected works of Hildegard Peplau* (pp. 21–30). New York: Springer.

Peplau, H. E. (1989b). Interpersonal relations: The purpose and characteristics of professional nursing. In O'Toole, A., & Welt, S. R. (Eds.), *Interpersonal theory in nursing practice: Selected works of Hildegard Peplau* (pp. 42–55). New York: Springer.

Peplau, H. E. (1989c). Interpretation of clinical observations. In O'Toole, A., & Welt, S. R. (Eds.), *Interpersonal theory in nursing practice: Selected works of Hildegard Peplau* (pp. 149–163). New York: Springer.

Peplau, H. E. (1989d). Investigative counseling. In O'Toole, A., & Welt, S. R. (Eds.), *Interpersonal theory in nursing practice: Selected works of Hildegard Peplau* (pp. 205–229). New York: Springer.

Peplau, H. E. (1998). *Life of an angel: Interview with Hildegard Peplau (1998)*. Hatherleigh Co. Audiotape available from the American Psychiatric Nurses Association. www.apna.org/items.htm

Radloff, L. S. (1977). The CES-D Scale: A self-report depression scale for research in the general population. *Applied Psychological Measurement, 1*, 385–401.

Reed, P. G. (1996). Transforming practice knowledge into nursing knowledge: A revisionist analysis of Peplau. *Image, 28*, 29–33.

Sills, G. (1998). Peplau and professionalism: The emergence of the paradigm of professionalization. *Journal of Psychiatric and Mental Health Nursing, 5*(3), 167–172.

Van Survellan, G. M., & Dull, L. V. (1981). Group psychotherapy for depressed women: A model. *Journal of Psychosocial Nursing, 19*, 25–31.

Bibliography

Armstrong, M., & Kelly, A. (1993). Enhancing staff nurses' interpersonal skills: Theory to practice. *Clinical Nurse Specialist, 7*(6), 313–317.

Armstrong, M., & Kelly, A. (1995). More than the sum of their parts: Martha Rogers and Hildegard Peplau. *Archives of Psychiatric Nursing, 9*(1), 40–44.

Barker, P. (1993). The Peplau legacy: Hildegard Peplau. *Nursing Times, 89*(11), 48–51.

Barker, P. (1998). The future of the Theory of Interpersonal Relations: A personal reflection on Peplau's legacy. *Journal of Psychiatric and Mental Health Nursing, 5*(3), 213–220.

Beeber, L. S. (1998). Treating depression through the nurse-client relationship. *Nursing Clinics of North America, 33*, 153–172.

Beeber, L. S., & Bourbonniere, M. (1998). The concept of interpersonal pattern in Peplau's Theory of Nursing. *Journal of Psychiatric and Mental Health Nursing, 5*(3), 187–192.

Beeber, L. S., & Caldwell, C. L. (1996). Pattern integrations in young depressed women: Parts I–II. *Archives of Psychiatric Nursing, 10*, 151–164.

Burd, S. F. (1963). The development of an operational definition using the process of learning as a guide. In S. F. Burd & A. Marshall (Eds.), *Some clinical approaches to psychiatric nursing*. New York: Macmillan.

Burton, G. (1958). Personal, impersonal, and interpersonal relations. Cited in S. A. Smoyak & S. Rouslin (Eds.) (1982), *A collection of classics in psychiatric nursing literature*. Thorofare, NJ: Charles B. Slack.

Buswell, C. (1997). A model approach to care of a patient with alcohol problems. *Nursing Times, 93*, 34–35.

Chambers, M. (1998). Interpersonal mental health nursing: Research issues and challenges. *Journal of Psychiatric and Mental Health Nursing, 5*(3), 203–212.

Comley, A. (1994). A comparative analysis of Orem's self-care model and Peplau's interpersonal theory. *Journal of Advanced Nursing, 20*(4), 755–760.

Dennis, S. (1996). Implementing a nursing model for ward-based students. *Nursing Standard, 11*, 33–35.

Doncliff, B. (1994). Putting Peplau to work. *Nursing New Zealand, 2*(1), 20–22.

Feely, M. (1997). Using Peplau's theory in nurse-patient relations. *International Nursing Review, 44*, 115–120.

Field, W. E., Jr. (Ed.). (1979). *The psychotherapy of Hildegard E. Peplau*. New Braunfels, TX: PSF Publications.

Forchuk, C. (1993). *Hildegard E. Peplau: Interpersonal Nursing*. Newbury Park, CA: Sage.

Forchuk, C. (1994). The orientation phase of the nurse-client relationship: Testing Peplau's theory. *Journal of Advanced Nursing, 20*(3), 532–537.

Forchuk, C., & Dorsay, J. (1995). Hildegard Peplau meets family systems nursing: Innovation in theory-based practice. *Journal of Advanced Nursing, 21*(1), 110–115.

Forchuk, C., Jewell, J., Schofield, R., Sircelj, M., & Valledor, T. (1998). From hospital to community: Bridging therapeutic relationships. *Journal of Psychiatric and Mental Health Nursing, 5*(3), 197–202.

Forchuk, C., Westwell, J., Martin, A., Azzapardi, W. B., Kosterewa-Tolman, D., & Hux, M. (1998). Factors influencing movement of chronic psychiatric patients from the orientation to the working phase of the nurse-client relationship on an inpatient unit. *Perspectives in Psychiatric Care, 34*, 36–44.

Fowler, J. (1994). A welcome focus on a key relationship: Using Peplau's model in palliative care. *Professional Nurse, 10*(3), 194–197.

Fowler, J. (1995). Taking theory into practice: Using Peplau's model in the care of patients. *Professional Nurse, 10*(4), 226–230.

Garrett, A., Manuel, D., & Vincent, C. (1976). Stressful experiences identified by student nurses. *Journal of Nursing Education, 15*(6), 9-21.

Gregg, D. E. (1978). Hildegard E. Peplau: Her contributions. *Perspective in Psychiatric Care, 16*(3), 118-121.

Hall, K. (1994). Peplau's model of nursing: Caring for a man with AIDS. *British Journal of Nursing, 3*(8), 418-422.

Hays, D. (1961). Teaching a concept of anxiety. *Nursing Research, 10*(2), 108-113.

Hofling, C. K., & Leininger, M. M. (1960). Basic psychiatric concepts in nursing. Cited in Smoyak, S. A., & Rouslin, S. (Eds.) (1982), *A collection of classics in psychiatric nursing literature*. Thorofare, NJ: Charles B. Slack.

Iveson, J. (1982). A two-way process . . . theories in nursing practice . . . Peplau's nursing model. *Nursing Mirror, 155*(18), 52.

Jewell, J. A., & Sullivan, E. A. (1996). Application of nursing theories in health education. *Journal of the American Psychiatric Nurses Association, 2*, 79-85.

Jones, A. (1995). Utilizing Peplau's psychodynamic theory for stroke patient care. *Journal of Clinical Nursing, 4*(1), 49-54.

Jones, A. (1996). The value of Peplau's theory for mental health nursing. *British Journal of Nursing, 5*, 877-881.

Keda, A. (1970). From Henderson to Orlando to Wiedenbach: Thoughts on completion of translation of basic principles of clinical nursing. *Comprehensive Nursing Quarterly, 5*(1), 85-94.

Kelley, S. J. (1996). "It's just me, my family, and my nurse . . . oh, yeah, and Nintendo: Hildegard Peplau's day with kids with cancer. *Journal of the American Psychiatric Nurses Association, 2*, 11-14.

LaMonica, E. (1981). Construct validity of an empathy instrument. *Research in Nursing and Health, 4*, 389-400.

Lego, S. (1980). The one-to-one nurse-patient relationship. *Perspectives in Psychiatric Care, 18*(2), 67-89. (Reprinted from *Psychiatric nursing 1946-1974: A report on the state of the art,* American Journal of Nursing Co.)

Lego, S. (1998). The application of Peplau's theory to group psychotherapy. *Journal of Psychiatric and Mental Health Nursing, 5*(3), 193-196.

Marshall, J. (1963). Dr. Peplau's strong medicine for psychiatric nurses. *Smith, Kline & French Reporter, 7*, 11-14.

McCarter, P. (1980). New statement defines scope of practice: Discussion with Dr. Lane and Dr. Peplau. *American Nurse, 12*(4), 1, 8, 24.

Methven, D., & Schlotfeldt, R. M. (1962). The social interaction inventory. *Nursing Research, 11*(2), 83-88.

Muff, J. (1996). Images of life on the verge of death: Dream and drawing of people with AIDS. *Perspectives in Psychiatric Care, 32*, 10-22.

Nursing Theories Conference Group. J. B. George, Chairperson. (1980). *Nursing theories: The base for professional nursing practice* (pp. 73-89). Englewood Cliffs, NJ: Prentice-Hall.

Olson, T. (1996). Fundamental and special: The dilemma of psychiatric-mental health nursing. *Archives of Psychiatric Nursing, 10*, 3-15.

Orlando, I. (1961). The dynamic nurse-patient relationship. Cited by Smoyak, S. A., & Rouslin, S. (Eds.) (1982), *A collection of classics in psychiatric nursing literature*. Thorofare, NJ: Charles B. Slack.

Osborne, O. (1984). Intellectual traditions in psychiatric nursing. *Journal of Psychosocial Nursing, 22*(1), 27-32.

Peplau, H. E. (1964). *Basic principles of patient counseling* (2nd ed.). Philadelphia: Smith, Kline, & French Laboratories.

Price, B. (1998). Explorations in body image care: Peplau and practice knowledge. *Journal of Psychiatric and Mental Health Nursing, 5*(3), 179-186.

Reynolds, W. J. (1997). Peplau's theory in practice. *Nursing Science Quarterly, 10*, 168-170.

Sills, G. M. (1977). Research in the field of psychiatric nursing, 1952-1977. *Nursing Research, 28*(3), 201-207.

Sills, G. M. (1978). Hildegard E. Peplau: Leader, practitioner, academician, scholar, and theorist. *Perspectives in Psychiatric Care, 16*(3), 122-128.

Slevin, E. (1996). Interpreting problematic behavior in people with learning disabilities. *British Journal of Nursing, 5*, 610-612, 625-627.

Smoyak, S. A., & Rouslin, S. (Eds.). (1982). *A collection of classics in psychiatric nursing literature*. Thorofare, NJ: Charles B. Slack.

Spring, F. E., & Turk, H. (1962, Fall). A therapeutic behavior scale. *Nursing Research, 11*(4), 214-218.

Thelander, B. L. (1997). The psychotherapy of Hildegard Peplau in the treatment of people with serious mental illness. *Perspectives in Psychiatric Care, 33*, 24-32.

Thomas, M. D., Baker, J. M., & Estes, N. J. (1970). Anger: A tool for developing self-awareness. *American Journal of Nursing, 70*(12), 2586-2590.

Topf, M., & Dambacher, B. (1979). Predominant source of interpersonal influence in relationships between psychiatric patients and nursing staff. *Research in Nursing and Health, 2*(1), 35-43.

Usher, K. J., & Arthur, D. (1997). Nurses and neuroleptic medication: Applying theory to a working relationship with clients and their families. *Journal of Psychiatric & Mental Health Nursing, 4*, 117-123.

Yamashita, M. (1997). Family caregiving: Application of Newman's and Peplau's theories. *Journal of Psychiatric & Mental Health Nursing, 4*, 401-405.

OTHER SOURCES

Arnold, W., & Nieswiadomy, R. (1993). Peplau's theory with an emphasis on anxiety. In S. M. Ziegler (Ed.), *Theory-directed nursing practice*. New York: Springer.

Forchuk, C. (1993). *Hildegard E. Peplau: Interpersonal nursing theory*. Newbury Park, CA: Sage.

BOOK CHAPTERS

Peplau, H. E. (1969). Theory: The professional dimension. In C. Norris (Ed.), *Proceedings of the first nursing theory conference* (March 21-28). Kansas

City: University of Kansas Medical Center, Department of Nursing Education.

Peplau, H. E. (1987). Nursing science: A historical perspective. In R. Parse (Ed.), *Nursing science: Major paradigms, theories, critiques*. Philadelphia: W. B. Saunders.

JOURNAL ARTICLES

Peplau, H. E. (1951). Toward new concepts in nursing and nursing education. *American Journal of Nursing, 52*(12), 722-724.

Peplau, H. E. (1952). The psychiatric nurses' family group. *American Journal of Nursing, 52*(12), 1475-1477.

Peplau, H. E. (1953). The nursing team in psychiatric facilities. *Nursing Outlook, 1*(2), 90-92.

Peplau, H. E. (1953). Themes in nursing situations: Power. *American Journal of Nursing, 52*(10), 1221-1223.

Peplau, H. E. (1953). Themes in nursing situations: Safety. *American Journal of Nursing, 53*(11), 1343-1346.

Peplau, H. E. (1955). Loneliness. *American Journal of Nursing, 55*(12), 1476-1481.

Peplau, H. E. (1956). Present day trends in psychiatric nursing. *Neuropsychiatry, 111*(4), 190-204.

Peplau, H. E. (1956). An undergraduate program in psychiatric nursing. *Nursing Outlook, 4*, 400-410.

Peplau, H. E. (1957). What is experiential teaching? *American Journal of Nursing, 57*(7), 884-886.

Peplau, H. E. (1958). Educating the nurse to function in psychiatric services. In *Nursing Personnel for Mental Health Programs* (pp. 37-42). Atlanta: Southern Regional Educational Board.

Peplau, H. E. (1960). Anxiety in the mother-infant relationship. *Nursing World, 134*(5), 33-34.

Peplau, H. E. (1960, March). A personal responsibility: A discussion of anxiety in mental health. *Rutgers Alumni Monthly*, pp. 14-16.

Peplau, H. E. (1963). Interpersonal relations and the process of adaptations. *Nursing Science, 1*(4), 272-279.

Peplau, H. E. (1964). Psychiatric nursing skills and the general hospital patient. *Nursing Forum, 3*(2), 28-37.

Peplau, H. E. (1965). The heart of nursing: Interpersonal relations. *Canadian Nurse, 61*(4), 273-275.

Peplau, H. E. (1965). Specialization in professional nursing. *Nursing Science, 3*(4), 268-287.

Peplau, H. E. (1966). Trends in nursing and nursing education. *NJSNA News Letter, 22*(3), 17-27.

Peplau, H. E. (1967). Interpersonal relations and the work of the industrial nurse. *Industrial Nurse Journal, 15*(10), 7-12.

Peplau, H. E. (1967). The work of psychiatric nurses. *Psychiatric Opinion, 4*(1), 5-11.

Peplau, H. E. (1968). Psychotherapeutic strategies. *Perspectives in Psychiatric Care, 6*(6), 264-289.

Peplau, H. E. (1969). Professional closeness as a special kind of involvement with a patient, client, or family group. *Nursing Forum, 8*(4), 342-360.

Peplau, H. E. (1970). Professional closeness as a special kind of involvement with a patient, client or family group. *Comprehensive Nurse Quarterly, 5*(3), 66-81.

Peplau, H. E. (1971). Communication in crisis intervention. *Psychiatric Forum, 2*, 1-7.

Peplau, H. E. (1972). The independence of nursing. *Imprint, 9*, 11.

Peplau, H. E. (1972). The nurse's role in health care delivery systems. *Pelican News, 28*, 12-14.

Peplau, H. E. (1974). Creativity and commitment in nursing. *Image: Journal of Nursing Scholarship, 6*, 3-5.

Peplau, H. E. (1974). Is health care a right? Affirmative response. *Image: Journal of Nursing Scholarship, 7*, 4-10.

Peplau, H. E. (1974). Talking with patients. *Comprehensive Nursing Quarterly, 9*(3), 30-39.

Peplau, H. E. (1975). Interview with Dr. Peplau: Future of nursing. *Japanese Journal of Nursing, 39*(10), 1046-1050.

Peplau, H. E. (1975). An open letter to a new graduate. *Nursing Digest, 3*, 36-37.

Peplau, H. E. (1977). The changing view of nursing. *International Nursing Review, 24*, 43-45.

Peplau, H. E. (1978). Psychiatric nursing: Role of nurses and psychiatric nurses. *International Nursing Review, 25*, 41-47.

Peplau, H. E. (1980). The psychiatric nurses: Accountable? To whom? For what? *Perspectives in Psychiatric Care, 18*, 128-134.

Peplau, H. E. (1982). Some reflections on earlier days in psychiatric nursing. *Journal of Psychosocial Nursing Mental Health Services, 20*, 17-24.

Peplau, H. E. (1987). American Nurses' Association social policy statement: Part I. *Archives of Psychiatric Nursing, 1*(5), 301-307.

Peplau, H. E. (1987). Tomorrow's world. *Nursing Times, 83*, 29-33.

Peplau, H. E. (1989). Future direction in psychiatric nursing from the perspective of history. *Journal of Psychosocial Nursing, 27*(2), 18-28.

Peplau, H. E. (1992). Interpersonal relations: A theoretical framework for application in nursing practice. *Nursing Science Quarterly, 5*(1), 13-18.

Peplau, H. E. (1995). Hildegard Peplau in a conversation with Mark Welch, Part I. *Nursing Inquiry, 2*(1), 53-56.

Peplau, H. E. (1995). Hildegard Peplau in a conversation with Mark Welch, Part II. *Nursing Inquiry, 2*(2), 115-116.

Peplau, H. E. (1996). Commentary. *Archives of Psychiatry Nursing, 10*(1), 14-15.

Peplau, H. E. (1996). Encounters along a career line. *Journal of the American Psychiatric Nurses Association, 2*, 36.

Peplau, H. E. (1997). The ins and outs of psychiatric-mental health nursing and the American Nurses' Association. *Journal of the American Psychiatric Nurses Association, 3*, 10-16.

Peplau, H. E. (1997). Peplau's theory of interpersonal relations. *Nursing Science Quarterly, 10*, 162-167.

Peplau, H. E. (1997). Is health care a right? *Image, 29*, 220-224.

INTERVIEWS

Peplau, H. E. (1985). Help the public maintain mental health. *Nursing Success Today, 2*(5), 30-34.

Peplau, H. E. (1985). The power of the dissociative state. *Journal of Psychosocial Nursing, 23*(8), 31-33.

CHAPTERS AND PAMPHLETS

Peplau, H. E. (1956). *The yearbook of modern nursing*. New York: G. P. Putnam's Sons.

Peplau, H. E. (1959). Principles of psychiatric nursing. In *American Handbook of Psychiatry* (Vol. 2). New York: Basic Books.

Peplau, H. E. (1962). Will automation change the nurse, nursing, or both? *Technical innovations in health care: Nursing implications* (Pamphlet 5). New York: American Nurses' Association.

Peplau, H. E. (1963). Counseling in nursing practice. In Harms, E., & Schreiber, P. (Eds.), *Handbook of counseling techniques*. New York: Pergamon.

Peplau, H. E. (1967). Psychiatric nursing. In Freedman, A. M., & Kaplan, A. I. (Eds.), *Comprehensive textbook of psychiatry*. New York: Williams & Wilkins.

Peplau, H. E. (1968). Operational definitions and nursing practice. In Zderad, L. T., & Belcher, H. C.

(Eds.), *Developing behavioral concepts in nursing*. Atlanta: Southern Regional Education Board.

Peplau, H. E. (1969). Pattern perpetuation in schizophrenia. In D. Sankar (Ed.), *Schizophrenia: Current concepts and research*. Hicksville, NY: PJD Publications.

Peplau, H. E. (1992). Notes on Nightingale. In F. Nightingale (1859/1992), *Notes on nursing: What it is, and what it is not*. Philadelphia: J. B. Lippincott.

Peplau, H. E. (1995). Another look at schizophrenia from a nursing standpoint. In *Psychiatric Nursing 1946 to 1994: A report on the state of the art*. St. Louis: Mosby.

Peplau, H. E. (1995). Preface. In *Psychiatric nursing 1946 to 1994: A report on the state of the art*. St. Louis: Mosby.

THESES

Peplau, H. E. (1953). *An exploration of some process elements which restrict or facilitate instructor-student interaction in a classroom, Type B*. Doctoral Project, Teachers College, Columbia University, New York.

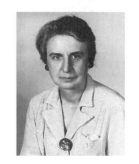

Chapter 6

Ernestine Wiedenbach
Clinical Nursing: A Helping Art

Theresa Gesse and Marcia Dombro

INTRODUCING THE THEORIST

The focus of this chapter is a review of the theoretical work of Ernestine Wiedenbach. A complete acknowledgment of her work, however, must include something about this extraordinary person who lived the philosophy that was the basis of her nursing theory.

Wiedenbach was born in 1900 in Germany to an American mother and a German father who migrated to the United States when Ernestine was a child. The affluent family supported the idea of a college education for their daughter and she graduated with a bachelor of arts degree from Wellesley College in 1922. Her later interest in a nursing career was reluctantly accepted by her family. Pursuing nursing in this era was atypical for someone who came from a family of gentility.

Her independent characteristics overruled her parents' reluctance and she enrolled in a hospital school of nursing. Early in her studies there, her advocacy for quality nursing education and her leadership role with her classmates resulted in dismissal from the school. Through the intervention of friends and faculty, including that of Adelaide Nutting, who realized her potential, she was admitted to Johns Hopkins School of Nursing and graduated in 1925 (Nickel, Gesse, & MacLaren, 1992.)

Wiedenbach had many interests and held a variety of professional positions. Because of her interest in education, she began taking graduate courses part-time at Columbia University. She was also involved with the New York State Nurses' Association and with various nursing committees. After completing a master of arts in 1934, she became a professional writer for the *American Journal of Nursing* (AJN).

This position brought new opportunities to experience many different facets of nursing and to meet national leaders in both nursing and health care. Her tenure in the AJN office included the years during World War II, when she played a critical role in the recruitment of nursing students and military nurses.

After the war, she returned to clinical practice and to her love of maternal-child nursing. At age 45, she began her studies in nurse-midwifery. At the Maternity Center in New York City, her personal mentors included such pioneers as Hazel Corbin and Hattie Hemschemeyer.

In 1952, Wiedenbach joined the faculty of Yale University School of Nursing where her roles as practitioner, teacher, author, and theorist would be consolidated. She retired from Yale in 1966 as an associate professor emeritus and subsequently held part-time positions at California State University and the University of Florida. She eventually moved to a Miami, Florida, retirement village with her college roommate and lifelong friend, Caroline Falls.

In 1972, Marcia Dombro, who was active in Miami's childbirth education movement, heard that Wiedenbach was living nearby. She telephoned and requested Wiedenbach's participation in a childbirth education conference being held at Florida International University (FIU). Wiedenbach graciously accepted and invited Dombro to her house for tea to discuss it further.

Following this contact and the childbirth education conference, Wiedenbach and Falls became involved in developing and teaching a university course on communication in nursing. Her pattern of intellectual productivity continued with the publication of another book: *Communication: Key to Effective Nursing* (Wiedenbach & Falls, 1978).

Wiedenbach's love for interaction with students persisted even after her mobility decreased. She and Caroline Falls continued to give informal seminars in their home for Professor Theresa Gesse and the University of Miami nurse-midwifery students. They enjoyed discussing the past, present, and future of nursing and nurse-midwifery and she always reminded students and faculty of the need for clarity of purpose, based on reality.

This rekindling of ties to the nursing education community did not deter Wiedenbach from being an advocate for the residents of the retirement village. She was an activist in promoting change in policies and practices related to nutrition and creative activities for the many talented residents now in their late stages of life. She was adamant about improvement of the quality of life and level of independence for those who lived in the village, where she continued to apply her prescriptive theory of nursing in everyday living. She even continued to use her gift for writing to transcribe books for the blind, including a Lamaze childbirth manual, which she prepared on her Braille typewriter. Wiedenbach continued to be productive and maintain a central purpose as long as she was able.

In 1992, events began to occur that profoundly affected Wiedenbach's remaining years. During this period, her friend Caroline Falls died of heart failure, and Hurricane Andrew destroyed the retirement village, causing a temporary relocation into unfamiliar surroundings. Susan Nickel, who had become a personal friend, searched for Wiedenbach after the storm and found her in an area nursing home. Wiedenbach was much in need of the caring that she herself had promoted so strongly in nursing. Wiedenbach stayed at Ms. Nickel's home for several months until the retirement village was restored.

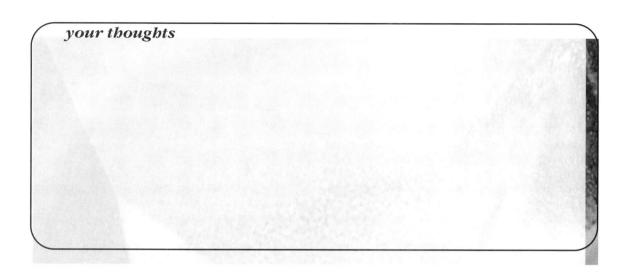
your thoughts

Until the end of her life, Wiedenbach continued to maintain the independent spirit that originally fueled her productivity and creativity. In April 1998, Wiedenbach died at age 98.

THE EVOLUTION OF WIEDENBACH'S PRESCRIPTIVE THEORY

Fellow Yale University faculty members William Dickoff and Patricia James were acknowledged by Wiedenbach for noting her early theory conceptualization and for their continuing guidance in its development. They were professors and theorists in Yale's Department of Philosophy who conducted seminars for the School of Nursing faculty on philosophical constructs, theory development, and research. It was through this association that Wiedenbach initially sought their feedback on her work, which they determined was a prescriptive theory. In Wiedenbach's words, "I had written the first book, Dickoff, James and Wiedenbach (1968), *Family Centered Maternity Nursing,* and Bill and Pat read it. We were discussing it and they said, 'You know, it's interesting. You've really followed pretty much the pattern of a prescriptive theory.' They said, 'Yes, you have the agent, you have the recipient.' "

Ida Orlando was a fellow faculty member at Yale. According to Wiedenbach, she was interested in the dynamics of interaction and was anxious to have a clinical area where she could put her theories to practice. Wiedenbach encouraged Orlando: "By all means, go ahead, do it right here on the maternity service. . . . [We] used to talk a great deal about purpose. This was one of the things that startled me when I was teaching students. I would ask them, . . . 'What's your purpose in nursing?' They would look blank and they would just say, 'It's just to take care of people . . . of those who need care.' That's not a real purpose in nursing. It is your commitment which specifies what you want to accomplish through your actions. So I had in my book, 'the *purpose,*' and talked about 'the *agent,*' which is the nurse [and] 'the *recipient,*' who would be the mother or the family" (Nickel, 1981b, videotaped interview).

> Theory is an abstract phenomenon that lies dormant in the mind until it is "given expression either through action and/or through words."

Another colleague at Yale was Virginia Henderson, who, along with Wiedenbach and Orlando, made unique contributions to nursing theory. Orlando was the youngest of the three, by more than 25 years. They frequently discussed their shared belief in the integration of mind, body, and spirit (Nickel, 1981a, videotaped interview).

THE PRESCRIPTIVE THEORY

The following are excerpts from Wiedenbach's personal papers, in which she explained the essence of her prescriptive theory. In an unpublished paper presented at Duke University on May 8, 1970 (Wiedenbach, 1970, p. 1), she prefaced her presentation with impressions about the topic title she had been given. She stated, "I take issue with the concept implied in your topic for inquiry, namely *Application of*

Theory to Nursing Practice. It suggests to me that theory is something apart from practice—and that it must be developed and then applied—like one might a poultice—to nursing practice."

She then defined *theory* as an abstract phenomenon that lies dormant in the mind until it is "given expression either through action and/or through words" (Wiedenbach, 1970, p. 1). She continued, "[P]ractice is a concrete phenomenon, characterized primarily by action. And when that action is goal-directed, as nursing practice may be said to be, then practice immediately becomes theory-based. Theory thus would seem to be inextricably interlocked with practice. . . . To say that theory may be applied to practice suggests, furthermore, that practice precedes theory (we practice first and then formulate a theory for our practice). Actually I think it is the other way around. Theory of some sort precedes practice" (Wiedenbach, 1970, p. 1).

Wiedenbach's explanation of her prescriptive theory follows: "Account must be taken of the motivating factors that influence the nurse not only in doing what she does but also in doing it the way she does it with the realities that exist in the situation in which she is functioning." Such account is incorporated in a prescriptive theory (Wiedenbach, 1970, p. 2).

Three ingredients essential to a prescriptive theory are:

1. The nurse's *central purpose* in nursing. It constitutes the nurse's professional commitment.
2. The *prescription.* It indicates the broad general action that the nurse deems appropriate to fulfillment of her central purpose.
3. The *realities.* They are the aspects of the immediate situations that influence the results the nurse achieves through what she does (Wiedenbach, 1970, p. 3).

During the presentation, Wiedenbach referred to her article in the *American Journal of Nursing* (1963) and her book, *Meeting the Realities in Clinical Teaching* (1969), in which she presented her concept of prescriptive theory. However, during this presentation, she expressed the need at this time to elaborate further on these concepts to her audience. The following is her explanation of the components of the theory and their interrelationships: "It defines the quality [the nurse] desires to bring about or sustain in her patient's condition, attitude, or situation, and specifies what she recognizes to be her social responsibility in caring for him. It is the outcome that ideally she consistently *strives* to obtain through her nursing action" (Wiedenbach, 1970, p. 3).

She emphasizes that the nurse's central purpose is grounded in her philosophy, "those beliefs and values that shape her attitude toward life, toward fellow human beings and toward herself." The three concepts that epitomize the essence of a philosophy are:

1. Reverence for the gift of life.
2. Respect for the dignity, autonomy, worth, and individuality of each human being.
3. Resolution to act dynamically in relation to one's beliefs. (Wiedenbach, 1970, p. 4)

She took the position that one must explore each of these, "since the beliefs on which a philosophy is founded, determine the validity of the concept. If the concepts have meaning for the nurse and she can subscribe to them, that will serve her as valuable guides for making choices and decisions." For example, the second concept—respect for the dignity, autonomy, worth and individuality of each human being—when I explored it for the beliefs on which I think it is founded, revealed, among others, the following four beliefs:

1. Each human being is endowed with unique potential to develop—within himself—resources that enable him to maintain and sustain himself.
2. The human being basically strives toward self-direction and relative independence, and desires not only to make best use of his capabilities and potentialities, but to fulfill his responsibilities as well.
3. The human being needs positive social interaction in order to make best use of his capabilities and realize his self-worth.
4. Whatever the individual does, represents his best judgment at the moment of doing it. (Wiedenbach, 1970, p. 4)

Wiedenbach felt that her beliefs guided her thinking "when trying to formulate a statement of purpose that I can regard as my central purpose in nursing." She went on to say, "Because you may want to know what it is, I'll state it. It is to motivate the individual and/or facilitate his efforts to overcome the obstacles that may now as well as later, interfere with his ability to respond capably to the demands made of him by the realities in his situation" (Wiedenbach, 1970, p. 4).

She emphasized that this was her own central purpose in nursing, and that "others—each of you, for instance, may hold different beliefs and thus you may see your overall commitment in nursing somewhat differently from the way I see mine." She was equally emphatic that it is a personal "central purpose *in* nursing rather than the central purpose *of*

> **To formulate one's central purpose in nursing is a soul-searching experience.**

nursing" (Wiedenbach, 1970 [emphasis added]). She further stated: "To formulate one's central purpose in nursing is a soul-searching experience. Has each of you, I wonder, undergone it, and are you willing and ready to present your central purpose in nursing for examination and discussion when appropriate?" (Wiedenbach, 1970, p. 5).

In her elaboration of the second component, "prescription," Wiedenbach explained that it "specifies both the nature of the action that will most likely lead to fulfillment of the nurse's central purpose in nursing, and the thinking process that determines it." She categories nursing as a practice that is discipline- and goal-directed: "[P]resumably, the nurse has thought through the kind of results she wants to obtain from what she does, gears her action to obtaining them and accepts accountability not only for what she does but for the outcome of her acts as well. Nursing action, thus, is a deliberate action" (Wiedenbach, 1970, p. 5).

It is in the explanation of "deliberate action" that Wiedenbach illustrates the linkage of these components with the concepts of her philosophy. She delineates three kinds of deliberate action:

1. Mutually understood and agreed upon
2. Patient-directed
3. Nurse-directed

Each of these three may have a very different effect on the patient—a fact that the nurse needs to recognize *before* she acts. ". . . The kind of action she will resort to, depends, I think, on her clarity about her central purpose in nursing, and consequently on the way she may view the patient at any particular moment that she is caring for him" (Wiedenbach, 1970, p. 6).

Wiedenbach then presented an example of a nurse's bed-bath assignment to illustrate her point. Note the incorporation of her philosophical concepts:

> Her action may be considered to be *mutually-understood and agreed-upon,* if it reflects that she respects the patient's dignity, worth, autonomy and individuality, and she makes sure that [the patient] is psychologically receptive to her giving him the bath before she starts the procedure. This kind of action suggests that the nurse's central purpose in nursing is to facilitate the patient's effort to respond capably to the bed-bath what she desires to give him.

> The effect of this kind of action on the patient will, in all probability, be positive. He presumably understands that she is about to do or is doing and is in accord with her efforts and action. (Wiedenbach, 1970, p. 6)

Using the same example, she explains "patient-directed" as assisting according to the patient's needs and directions:

> This kind of action implies that the nurse's central purpose in nursing is to be accessible to the patient to give whatever help he indicates he wants in relation to his bed-bath. Thus she supports what she assumes to be his desire for independence. (Wiedenbach, 1970, p. 6)

She explains "nurse-directed" action in the bed-bath example as follows:

> [T]he nurse respects the patient's dignity and worth, but not particularly his individuality and autonomy. She gives him the bath without consulting him about it, and thus implies that she, the nurse, knows best what the patient needs. For this kind of action, the nurse's central purpose would seem to be to do for the patient (or with him) what she thinks he needs to have done for or with him.

> Prescription thus represents a directive to the nurse for effecting the kind of results she desires. It is inextricably tied to her central purpose in nursing. Consequently, once she has formulated her central purpose and has accepted it as her commitment she not only has established the prescription for *her* nursing, but is ready to implement it within the realities of the clinical situation. (Wiedenbach, 1970, p. 7)

Wiedenbach professed that there are "realities" in nursing practice that are "physical, physiological, emotional and spiritual that are at play in a situation in which nursing action occurs at any given moment" (Wiedenbach, 1970, p. 7). She describes these as follows:

The Agent, who is the nurse or her delegate, and who supplies the propelling force for any nursing action that may be taken.

The Recipient, the patient, who receives the agent's action or in whose behalf the action is taken

The Framework, which comprises all the extraneous factors and facilities in the situation that affect the nurse's ability to obtain the kind of results she wants to obtain, through her nursing.

The Goal, which represents the end to be attained through the activity which the nurse plans or undertakes in behalf of the patient. And—

The Means, which comprise the activities and devices through which the nurse is enabled to attain her goal. (Wiedenbach, 1970 p. 7)

Wiedenbach expressed in her presentation the need to elaborate on features of the realities because of their strong influence on effective nursing practice.

She described the nurse as the *agent* who supplies the "propelling force for the overt actions that determine the effectiveness of her practice" (Wiedenbach, 1970, p. 8). She emphasized the responsibility of the nurse,

> . . . not only for clarifying her central purpose in nursing and her prescription for fulfilling it, but also for recognizing the responsibilities that are hers by virtue of her resolve to fulfill her central purpose and implement her prescription. (Wiedenbach, 1970, p. 8)

Four responsibilities of the agent (nurse) that she considered to be outstanding are:

1. To reconcile her assumptions about the realities in the clinical situation with her central purpose in nursing. (This presumes not only that she has clarified her central purpose in nursing for herself, but that she respects the need to validate her assumptions before acting on them!)
2. To specify the objectives of her practice in terms of behavioral outcomes that are realistically attainable.
3. To practice nursing in accordance with her objectives.
4. To engage in related activities which contribute to her self-realization as to the improvement of nursing practice (p. 8).

The patient is viewed as the *recipient* of the nurse's ministrations in a vulnerable position. She explains that this is so because the patient subjects himself to another's care. There is a risk of losing one's individuality, dignity, worth, and autonomy. However, according to Wiedenbach, the patient has

> . . . one unassailable resource that he can use as a secret weapon! It is his sensitivity—his feelings. [By the use of it] he can defeat or frustrate those responsible for his care, by thwarting their efforts to obtain the results they desire from their efforts and ministrations. (Wiedenbach, 1970, p. 9)

Wiedenbach used an enema procedure as an example of this. The success of the procedure was directly related to the patient's (recipient's) cooperation in receiving and holding the enema fluid. Because of a lack of sensitivity about the patient's feelings of autonomy, the nurse's efforts were thwarted. "The patient's feelings, thus, were a powerful mechanism in his defense" (Wiedenbach, 1970, p. 9).

The next reality defined is the *framework*:

> In nursing practice, the framework constitutes a complex of factors which, though [intangible] as a whole, have, nevertheless, potential for limiting or expanding the scope of the nurse's ability to function as she would like to function at any given time. It derives from a combination of extraneous elements and circumstances which imagined or real are present or are introduced into every nursing situation. By their existence, they share the course of events. In addition, they influence not only the care with which the nurse is able to achieve desired results from her nursing, but also the ease with which the patient is able to benefit from the nurse's ministrations. (p. 10)

The arrival of fresh linen or the unexpected absence of a nursing staff member are two of many examples Wiedenbach cited as factors that could "shape the course of events" (Wiedenbach, 1970, p. 10). She views the framework as

> . . . a conglomerate that may include objects, existing or missing, policies, setting, atmosphere, time of day, humans and happenings that may be current, past and recalled, or anticipated. Depending on its makeup, it may promote, complicate, facilitate, alter, impair or impede the nurse's ability to function effectively in her practice.

She pointed out that not only must the nurse recognize that a "framework" always exists to be reckoned with, but also, the patient must be aware of it and "we must strive to enable our patient to cope with it capably as well" (Wiedenbach, 1970, p. 11).

The fourth aspect of the realities is the *goal*. She describes "goal" as the end to be attained through whatever the nurse undertakes in her practice. She states: "In the context of a prescriptive theory, goal is included in any statement of purpose." She uses the example of an individual's "capability" as a specified goal in any given situation that the nurse might strive toward. However, in the context of realities, the goal "specifies the particular result which the nurse desires to achieve through the particular activity she plans or initiates" (p. 11). One example she gives is that of relieving a patient of discomfort when carrying out a procedure. She believes that "stipulation of an activity's goal gives focus to the nurse's action, implies her reason for taking it and paves the way for its effective realization" (p. 11).

She emphasizes that one cannot reach a goal simply by articulating it. She cites three necessary and distinct steps. These are:

1. Goal in intent specifies the attitude that the nurse believes the patient must manifest in order to be able to benefit from her ministrations. It is an attitude, consequently that she needs to foster or engender consciously, as part of her effort to attain her activity's goal. Goal in intent derives mainly from the nurse's central purpose in nursing. If her purpose, for instance, is to have the patient benefit from her ministrations, her goal in intent will most likely be inducement of a receptive attitude toward them, on the patient's part. If, on the other hand, her purpose is to have the patient become independent of her ministrations, her goal in intent might be inducement of an assertive attitude on her patient's part. (Wiedenbach 1970, p. 12)

2. Goal in application specifies the kind of framework that the nurse believes is essential to achievement of the goal she has set for the activity she plans to undertake. I think it could be called a supportive framework [environment]—which means that the nurse has available to her, appropriate equipment with which to carry out the activity; that the physical environment is adjusted to the patient's tolerance and the nurse's ease in functioning; and that the human elements consisting not only of professionals but also of nonprofessionals who may also include the patient's family, are accepting of the nurse's plan to engage in a particular activity in the patient's behalf. (p. 12)

She explains that goal in application is often taken for granted but "needs to be recognized and respected not only as an integral part of the nurse's practice, but as one that is crucial to her obtaining the kind of results she desires from what she does" (p. 12).

3. Goal in execution specifies the relationship that the nurse desires to maintain between the realities and her activity while she is actually carrying out the activity. I would designate it as a *symbiotic* relationship. (p. 13)

Wiedenbach elaborates on goal in execution in reference to the nurse's characteristics: Attainment of the goal calls for *vigilance, sensitivity,* and *wisdom* on

the part of the nurse, all the while that she is engaging in the activity; vigilance for signs of resistance in the patient toward the activity; and sensitivity to untoward changes in the framework or in herself that could prevent attainment of the activity's goal and wisdom in dealing objectively and kindly with what she is aware of in the situation so that the patient's ability to benefit from the activity may be supported, restored, or enhanced (Wiedenbach, 1970, p. 13).

Wiedenbach reiterated the importance of these three goals in action to effective nursing. Although their significance may not always be recognized, "when the nurse makes their attainment a conscious part of her nursing, she is taking a major step toward obtaining desired results in her practice" (p. 13).

The last of the realities is described as the means. These are:

> The expedients that the nurse uses to achieve the objectives of her practice. They include the whole gamut of skills, knowledge, techniques, procedures and devices that the nurse may use to *identify* her patient's experienced need for help[,] [a]dminister the help he needs, or validate that the help she gave was indeed helpful. (Wiedenbach, 1970, p. 13)

Although Wiedenbach (1970) views the means as

> . . . indispensable resources the nurse relies on, their value for the patient depends largely on the way the nurse uses them. It is the nurse's *way* of giving a treatment, for example, that enables the patient to benefit from it, not just the fact that he is given a treatment. And it is her *way* of expressing her concern, not just the fact that she is present or speaks that enables him to reveal his fears. The nurse's way of using the means available to her to achieve the results she desires, in her practice, is an *individual* matter, determined to a large degree, by her central purpose in nursing and the prescription she regards as appropriate to its fulfillment. (p. 13)

Wiedenbach summarized her presentation to the audience at Duke University (1970) by stating that:

> This then is my concept of a prescriptive theory of nursing. Its components are, first of all, a *central purpose* that suggests the nurse's reason for being—the mission she believes is hers to accomplish. Second, a *prescription* that suggests the action she deems appropriate to the accomplishment of her mission. And third, the *realities*, which, by their pervasiveness, challenge the nurse's ingenuity and creativity

as she endeavors to fulfill her central purpose in nursing through her practice.

Like all theory, a prescriptive theory, too, is a system of conceptualizations invented for some purpose. The relationship to practice is close and inseparable. Its *value* manifests itself when each nurse probes the depths of her value system and beliefs, makes them explicit, uses them as the basis of *her* theory of nursing practice, and reflects them in everything she does. (p. 14)

WIEDENBACH'S THEORY AND CLINICAL PRACTICE

Wiedenbach consistently emphasized "purpose" and "patient" in her many writings and presentations about her perspective of nursing practice. She stated: "The practice of clinical nursing is goal directed, deliberately carried out and patient centered" (Wiedenbach, 1964, p. 23). Figure 6–1 represents a spherical model she created in 1962 that depicts the "experiencing individual" as the central focus. The published version of the model appeared two years later in her text *Clinical Nursing: A Helping Art* (Wiedenbach, 1964). In a presentation entitled "A Concept of Dynamic Nursing" at a conference in Pittsburgh, Pennsylvania (Wiedenbach, 1962, p. 7), she described the model as follows:

> In its broadest sense, Practice of Dynamic Nursing may be envisioned as a set of concentric circles, with the experiencing individual in the circle at its core. Direct service, with its three components, identification of the individual's experienced need for help, ministra-

tion of help needed and validation that the help provided fulfilled its purpose, fills the circle adjacent to the core. The next circle holds the essential concomitants of direct service: coordination, i.e., charting, recording, reporting, and conferring; consultation, i.e., conferencing, and seeking help or advice; and collaboration, i.e., giving assistance or cooperation with members of other professional or nonprofessional groups concerned with the individual's welfare. The content of the fourth circle represents activities which are essential to

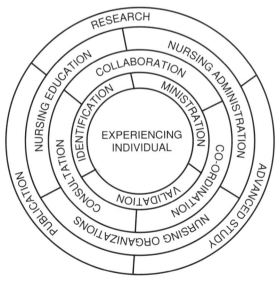

Figure 6–1 *Professional nursing practice focus and components. Reprinted with permission from the Wiedenbach Reading Room (1962), Yale University School of Nursing.*

the ultimate well-being of the experiencing individual, but only indirectly related to him; nursing education, nursing administration and nursing organizations. The outermost circle comprises research in nursing, publication and advanced study, the key ways to progress in every area of practice.

In this same presentation, Wiedenbach shared schematic drawings of the elements of the second sphere (circle), identification, ministration, and validation. These are presented here in Figures 6-2, 6-3, and 6-4. These also were later edited and published in *Clinical Nursing: A Helping Art* (Wiedenbach, 1964).

She explained the elements of the second sphere to her presentation audience (Wiedenbach, 1962, p. 9) in the following way:

Implicit in identification is the individualization of the individual and what he is experiencing. This calls for awareness of how the individual differs in appearance, manner, and behavior, from any other individual, and from the nurse's expectation of him. It calls for recognition too, that the individual's perception of his condition or situation grows out of *his* background of experiences and understandings, which may be called his frame-of-reference; while the nurse's perception of it is in relation to *her* background of experiences and understandings, that is, her frame-of-reference. Activity in this unit of Practice (identification) is directed toward ascertaining 1) whether the individual is experiencing discomfort or incapability; 2) the cause of the discomfort or incapability he may be experiencing; 3) the need required to restore comfort or capability; and 4) whether the need represents a need-for-help, one, in other words which the individual is unable to meet himself, unaided.

The unit Ministration involves providing the help which is needed. Underlying it, is the assumption that the individual must be accepting of any applied resource, be it a bit of advice, a recommendation, or a comfort or therapeutic measure, if he is to derive maximum benefit from it. Application of resource, thus, is dependent first of all, on selection of one which is appropriate to the need which has been identified, and second, on its acceptability to the individual. In this unit of Practice, i.e., Ministration-of-Help-Needed, the full range of resources to which the nurse has access may come into play, and the greater her stock

of resources, the greater her potential for effective service. Included in such range would be her own beliefs, values, knowledge, skills and know-how; those of others whom she knows or of whom she has heard, i.e., members of other professions or the laity; and those represented by facilities of the community and beyond.

Validation has as its goal, evidence that, as a result of the help that was provided, the individual is experiencing improvement in his feeling of comfort and capability in relation to his immediate situation. Such improvement may be measured by the individual's verbal and non-verbal behavior, on the assumption that he will respond behaviorally, to how he is currently experiencing his situation. Implicit in this unit are 1) clarification of the meaning to the individual, of his behavior; and 2) classification of his meaning according to the nurse's concept of comfort and capability in the context of the individual's situation. Essentially, this means that to validate the effectiveness of Practice, how the individual is experiencing his immediate situation must be consistent with the nurse's expectation of the outcome of her ministration.

Wiedenbach's clinical application of her prescriptive theory was always evident in her logical clinical examples. They often related to general basic nursing procedures, but more so with maternity nursing practice. In discussing the practice and process of nursing, she stated:

The focus of Practice is the experiencing individual, i.e., the individual for whom the nurse is caring, and the way he and only he perceived his condition or situation. For example, a mother had a red vaginal discharge on her first postpartum day. The doctor had recognized it as lochi, a normal concomitant of the phenomenon of involution, and had left an order for her to be up and move about. Instead of trying to get up, the mother remained, immobile in her bed. The nurse who wanted to help her out of bed expressed surprise at the mother's unwilling to do so, when she seemed to be progressing so well. The mother explained that she had a red discharge, and this to her was evidence of onset of hemorrhage. This terrified her and made her afraid to move. Her sister, she added, had hemorrhaged and almost lost her life the day after she had her baby two years ago. The nurse expressed her

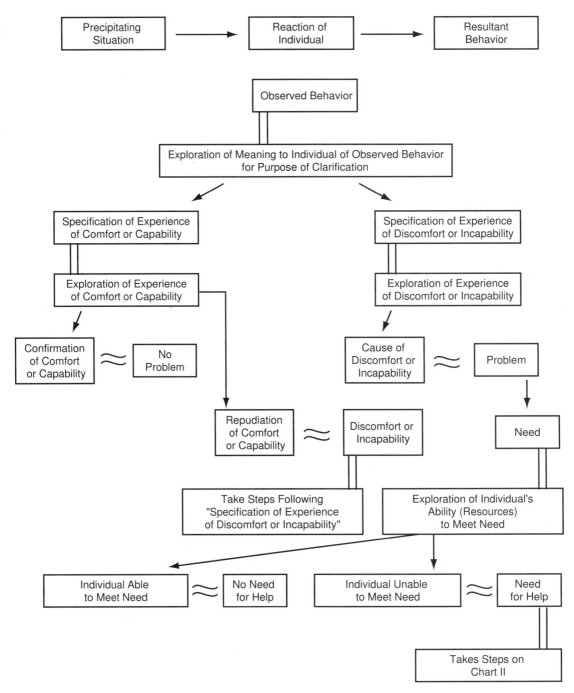

Figure 6–2 *Identifying an experienced need for help. Reprinted with permission from the Wiedenbach Reading Room (1962), Yale University School of Nursing.*

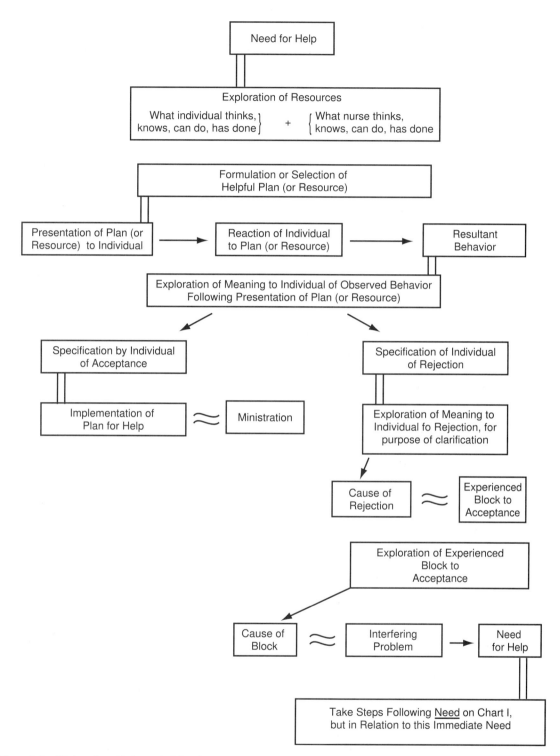

Figure 6–3 *Ministration of help needed. Reprinted with permission from the Wiedenbach Reading Room (1962), Yale University School of Nursing.*

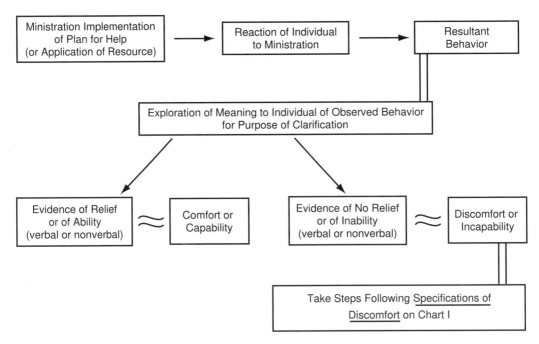

Figure 6–4 *Validation that need for help was met. Reprinted with permission from the Wiedenbach Reading Room (1962), Yale University School of Nursing.*

understanding of the mother's fear, but then encouraged her to compare her current experience with that of her sister. When the mother tried to do this, she recognized gross differences, and accepted the nurse's explanation of the origin of the discharge. The mother then voiced her relief, and validated it by getting out of bed without further encouragement. (Wiedenbach, 1962, pp. 6–7)

In another example, she recalled an experience as a student:

> . . . assigned to a multiparous woman in early labor. With each mild contraction, the woman would clutch the student's hand and scream, "Nurse, don't leave me!" After observing this behavior for some time, Wiedenbach asked the woman why she was acting so frightened. The woman replied that she overheard the physician tell a nurse that she would "dilate" that night and the woman interpreted this as "die late" that night. Wiedenbach told the historian that this incident revealed to her how little a woman may

> **The practice of clinical nursing is goal directed, deliberately carried out and patient centered.**

know about the process of childbirth and how carefully one must explain things to them. She believes that this experience impressed upon her the importance of always understanding the meaning of a patient's behavior. (Nickle, Gessey, & MacLaren, 1992, p. 162)

Critics of Wiedenbach's work have indicated that utilization of her practice theory is limited to the responsive patient. A graduate student chose Wiedenbach's concepts to demonstrate the use of identification, ministration, and validation in providing care for a newborn infant in intensive care (Miller, 1985). She believes that Wiedenbach's prescriptive theory is adaptable to a nonresponsive patient as well, and presented the following example.

Miller described identification as a need for "observation, understanding, cause, help needed," which she translated into signs and symptoms of respiratory distress. She called this a "physiological perception" and "a need-for-help." Ministration was interpreted as the nurse's response to the infant's hypoxic state by taking appropriate measures. Validation was achieved by the infant's positive response to the ministration (Miller, 1985, pp. 10–11). This situation has merit for a linking of most of the concepts of Wiedenbach's prescriptive theory in the care of this ill newborn.

McKenna (1997) has observed that Wiedenbach's theory emerged from a strong clinical practice association. He cites Orlando and Travelbee as well as Wiedenbach, all of whom, while giving or observing nursing care, used grounded theory methods of data collection, that is, case studies, interviews, and observations. Wiedenbach, Orlando, and Travelbee analyzed likenesses and differences of the data and then developed concepts and linkages. McKenna called this a "practice-theory strategy" (McKenna, 1997).

> Wiedenbach addressed this in her thinking about "theory" as being an abstract phenomenon. It develops within the mind but derives from reality and influences action. It is the outgrowth of an intellectual process set in motion by observations. From them, ideas are generated. Then, by means of the intellect, the ideas—we'll call them concepts—may be consciously brought into meaningful relationship with one another for such purposes as to identify or isolate factors, to characterize or classify them, to predict effect from cause, or to prescribe a course of action by which to obtain desired results. When such a relationship is articulated, a theory has been formulated. (McKenna, 1997, p. 1057)

However, Wiedenbach considered nursing a "practical phenomenon" that involved action. She believed that this was necessary to understand the theory that underlies the "nurse's way of nursing." This involved "knowing what the nurse wanted to accomplish, how she went about accomplishing it, and in what context she did what she did" (Wiedenbach, 1970, p. 1058). This, then, is the foundation of the central purpose, prescription, and realities of the prescriptive theory in clinical practice.

WIEDENBACH'S THEORY AND CLINICAL TEACHING

There is a uniqueness in Wiedenbach's prescriptive theory in that it is so adaptable to nursing education as well as to clinical practice. She logically related the concepts of the three main components of her theory to education in a practice discipline. In her text, *Meeting the Realities in Clinical Teaching* (Wiedenbach, 1969), she defined the components as:

> Purpose—to motivate the student and/or facilitate her efforts to overcome the obstacles that now—or may later—interfere with her ability to gain the knowledge, insights, and skill she

needs [as the agent] who is responsible, as the propelling force, for student learning. (p. 9).

> Prescription—Factors that, when combined, give direction to the instructor's action as well as the thinking process that hopefully will lead to the results desired. (p. 11)

Realities—The factors are listed here, that influence teaching and learning. These are:

1. The agent—the instructor who is responsible, as the propelling force, for student learning.
2. The recipient—the student, who is presumed to want specific knowledge, skills, abilities and understanding that will enable her to assume professional responsibilities.
3. The framework—the complex factors (such as time of day, people present, atmospheric conditions, activities going on, et cetera) that limit or expand the scope of the instructors and students' abilities to function.
4. The goal—the end to be attained
   a. goal-in-intent—the attitude of the student
   b. goal-in-application—the kind of framework essential for successful learning.
   c. goal-in-execution—the student's realization of her potential for learning.
5. The means—the sum and substance of the teaching program. (Wiedenbach, 1969, pp. 21–156)

Wiedenbach believed very strongly in the need to develop one's own philosophy, as well as central purpose, and expected each student to do so. She felt that the clinical instructor's basic philosophy of nursing would influence her attitude toward the student and could serve as a frame of reference for decision making (Nickel, 1981a). She taught as well as practiced from the framework of her prescriptive theory and therefore presented a consistency for students in both classroom and clinical activities.

Encouraging students to think was very important to Wiedenbach and made its appearance in many ways. She distributed a list of eight "Student Responsibilities" (expected behaviors) to her students. The list included being friendly, helpful, neat, prompt, and seeking help when needed, but the last on the list was "THINK!"

She instituted a "Summary of Thinking" as a means of evaluation of students. In composition, students were encouraged to identify what they had learned by their experiences, not only in terms of skills, but also "factors which affected his/her ability to gain them. The 'Summary of Thinking' reconstructed the students' activities in terms of purpose and outcomes" (Nickel, 1981a, p. 75).

A letter from Wiedenbach dated May 27, 1958, to a student gave the following suggestions regarding her thesis:

1. Organize the study in terms of the stated purpose.
2. Give a clear statement of the hypothesis.
3. Present the collected data in tables.
4. Make your analysis from the tables.
5. Draw your conclusions and state them succinctly. (Nickel, 1981, p. 76)

The emphasis on individual responsibility and reflection was clear in a presentation Wiedenbach gave, in which she stated, "How much better it would be, wouldn't you agree . . . if each nurse would think through, deliberately, the theory that she would like her practice to reflect. Only by making it explicit for herself, I believe, can she harmonize her practice with her theory, and give it the constancy, consistency, and the spiritual meaning that nursing, in its finest connotation, implies" (Wiedenbach, 1970, pp. 14–15).

Summary

The central purpose of this chapter has been to share rather than critique or analyze Wiedenbach's work. It is a privilege to have access to her personally verbalized thoughts and explanations of her prescriptive theory. Through audio- and videotapes acquired by Nickel, and other personal materials she reviewed and reported on in her thesis, in addition to the authors' personal contacts and recollections, it has been possible to bring about an account of Wiedenbach's work that summarizes but cannot equal the theorist's own writing.

Her philosophy continues to be reflected in today's focus on "humanism" and on "transculturalism" in nursing literature, practice, and education, as well as in health care in general. Her focus on the "respect for dignity, worth, autonomy, and individuality" became a part of the philosophy of the American College of Nurse-Midwives in 1961 and has remained a hallmark of nurse-midwifery practice.

In 1983, social scientist Donald Schon wrote a text on the need for reflection when carrying out one's professional service. He presented his analysis of what he called "reflective-in-action." He noted that most professions practice technical rationality, that is, problem solving by applying specialized scientific knowledge in a routinized manner. He believed that rather than a standard application of knowledge, one must reflect on action taken or to be taken and also recognize the individual differences of those receiving services. Thus, such reflection leads to inquiry and ultimately to new theories and new knowledge. Davies (1995, p. 167) noted the "disjuncture between theory and practice" that plagues nursing education. She instituted "reflective activities" for her students in their clinical practice in an effort to address this problem. Of many findings reported, two of particular consequence were that the students began to accept more responsibility for their learning and identifying their own learning needs, and they began to view the client as the central focus. In their

your thoughts

reflection, they began to expand in terms of their thinking and nursing action (Davies, 1995).

The introduction of prescriptive theory in nursing by Dickoff, James, and Wiedenbach (1968) more than 30 years ago was evolutionary for nursing theory. However, it was never taken seriously because nurse theorists focused on middle-range theories that were believed necessary for nursing to be accepted as a scientific discipline. (Lenz, Supp, Gift, and associates, 1995; Ruland & Moore, 1998). Today, there is renewed interest in the work of Wiedenbach and the concepts she promoted. Perhaps it is a matter of going back to our roots to grasp the essence of nursing too often swallowed by technology and impersonal care and driven by economics; or perhaps it is the recognition, finally, that Wiedenbach's early efforts to link theory, practice, and research had merit. She herself recognized that she "never systematically validated her theory or published such results" (Nickel, Gesse, & MacLaren, 1992, p. 166). The challenge to do so is ours. In Wiedenbach's own words:

> May each of you spark nurses in and of the future, to make theory a conscious part of their practice. The opportunity you have to do this is exciting! And it is rewarding, for, by helping nurses to uncover the theory that underlies their practice, you are paving the way for them to render a finer quality of service to the patient, and to gain a deepened sense of fulfillment for themselves. (Wiedenbach, 1970, p. 15)

References

Davies, E. (1995). Reflective practice: Focus for caring. *Journal of Nursing Education, 34*(167).
Dickoff, J., James, P., & Wiedenbach, E. (1968). Theory in a practice discipline. *Nursing Research, 14*(5).
Lenz, E., Supp., F., Gift, A., Pugh, L., & Milligan, R. (1995). Collaborative development of middle range nursing theories: Toward a theory of unpleasant symptoms. *Advances in Nursing Science, 17*(1).
McKenna, H. (1997). *Nursing theories and models.* London: Routledge.
Miller, C. (1985). *Nursing theory.* Unpublished paper, Barry University, Miami, FL.
Nickel, S. (1981a). *A historical nursing review: The life and career contributions of Ernestine Wiedenbach.* Unpublished thesis, University of Miami.
Nickel, S. (1981b). Audio-visual taped interview with Ernestine Wiedenbach. Tape 1, October 20, 1980; Tape 2, February 2, 1981; Tape 3, May 22, 1981. Copy in University of Miami School of Nursing Archives, Coral Gables, FL.
Nickel, S., Gesse, T., & MacLaren, A. (1992). Her professional legacy. *Journal of Nurse Midwifery, 3*(161).
Ruland, C., & Moore, S. (1998). Theory construction based on standards of care: Proposed theory of the peaceful end of life. *Nursing Outlook, 46*(169).
Wiedenbach, E. (1962). *A concept of dynamic nursing: Philosophy, purpose, practice and process.* Paper presented at the Conference on Maternal and Child Nursing, Pittsburgh, PA. Archives, Yale University School of Nursing, New Haven, CT.
Wiedenbach, E. (1963). The helping art of nursing. *American Journal of Nursing, 63*(11).
Wiedenbach, E. (1964). *Clinical nursing: A helping art.* New York: Springer.
Wiedenbach, E. (1969). *Meeting the realities in clinical teaching.* New York: Springer.
Wiedenbach, E. (1970). *A systematic inquiry: Application of theory to nursing practice.* Paper presented at Duke University, Durham, NC (author's personal files).
Wiedenbach, E., & Falls, C. (1978). *Communication: Key to effective nursing.* New York: Tiresias Press.

Bibliography

BOOKS

Schon, D. (1983). *The reflective practitioner.* New York: Basic Books.
Wiedenbach, E. (1958/1967). *Family centered maternity nursing* (2nd ed. rev.). New York: Putnam.
Wiedenbach, E. (1972/1977). Maternity nursing today. In *The nursing process in maternity nursing* (2nd ed. rev). New York: McGraw Hill Publishing.

JOURNAL ARTICLES

Wiedenbach, E. (1940, January). Toward educating 130 million people—A history of the Nursing Information Bureau. *American Journal of Nursing, 40,* 13–18.
Wiedenbach, E. (1942, November). Overcoming mental barriers—A true story. *American Journal of Nursing, 42,* 1247–1252.
Wiedenbach, E. (1949, August). Childbirth as mothers say they like it. *Public Health Nursing, 51,* 417–426.
Wiedenbach, E. (1960, May). Nurse-midwifery . . . Purpose, practice and opportunity. *Nursing Outlook, 8,* 256–259.
Wiedenbach, E. (1962, Summer). Contributions of murse-midwifery to maternity care today. *Bulletin of the American College of Nurse Midwives, 8.*
Wiedenbach, E. (1965, December). Family nurse practitioner for maternal and child care. *Nursing Outlook, 13.*
Wiedenbach, E. (1968, June). Nurse's role in family planning. *Nursing Clinics of North America, 3*(6), 355–365.
Wiedenbach, E. (1968, May). Genetics and the nurse. *Bulletin of the American College of Nurse-Midwifery, 13*(5), 8–13.
Wiedenbach, E. (1970, May). Nurses' wisdom in nursing theory. *American Journal of Nursing, 70,* 1057–1062.
Wiedenbach, E., Dickoff, J., & James, P. (1968, September–October). Theory in a practice dis-

cipline. Part 1. *Nursing Research 17*(5), 415–437.

Wiedenbach, E., Dickoff, J., & James, P. (1968, November–December). Theory in a practice discipline. Part II. *Nursing Research 17*(6), 545–554.

Wiedenbach, E., & Thomas, H. (1954, September). Support during labor. *Journal of the American Medical Association, 156*(9), 3–10.

UNPUBLISHED MANUSCRIPTS

Wiedenbach, E. (1961). *Growth and development of the nurse-midwifery program at Yale.* Unpublished manuscript, Yale University School of Nursing.

Wiedenbach, E. (1962). Professional nursing practice—focus and components. Unpublished manuscript, Yale University School of Nursing, New Haven, CT.

Wiedenbach, E. (1963). *Suggested statement of philosophy.* Unpublished manuscript, Yale University School of Nursing, New Haven, CT.

Wiedenbach, E. (1965). *Qualities and competencies students are expected to acquire.* Unpublished manuscript, Yale University School of Nursing, New Haven, CT.

Wiedenbach, E. (1965). *Emergency maternal and newborn care.* Paper presented to the Connecticut State Council on Civil Defense Nursing, December 2, 1965. Yale University School of Nursing, New Haven, CT.

Wiedenbach, E. (1965). *Interpretation of elements in evaluation functional ability.* Unpublished manuscript, Yale University School of Nursing, New Haven, CT.

Wiedenbach, E. (1966, January 26). *Functions of the professional nurse and the impact of nursing education.* Paper presented at the South Ohio League for Nursing, Cincinnati, OH.

Wiedenbach, E. (1969, October 27). *The meaning of theory to clinical practice.* Paper presented at the University of Colorado School of Nursing, Denver, CO.

UNPUBLISHED RECORDING

Wiedenbach, E. (1981). Audiovisual taped interview with Ernestine Wiedenbach. February 14, 1981. University of Miami School of Nursing Archives, Coral Gables, FL.

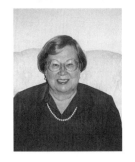

Chapter 7

Dorothy Johnson Behavioral System Model for Nursing

- ❖ Introducing the Theorist
- ❖ The Johnson Behavioral System Model
- ❖ Major Concepts of the Model
- ❖ Role of the Model in Nursing Practice, Administration, Research, and Education
- ❖ Summary
- ❖ References

Bonnie Holaday

INTRODUCING THE THEORIST

The "grand theorists" discussed in this book are all different from one another, yet most of them agree to attach enormous importance to the idea of frameworks that give meaning and significance to phenomena of interest to nursing. Dorothy Johnson's earliest publications pertained to what knowledge base nurses needed for nursing care (Johnson, 1959, 1961). Throughout her career, Johnson stressed that nursing had a unique independent contribution to health care that was distinct from "delegated medical care." Johnson was one of the first "grand theorists" to present her views as a conceptual model at Vanderbilt University in 1968. Her model was the first to provide both a guide to understanding and a guide to action. These two ideas—understanding seen first as a holistic, behavioral system process mediated by a complex framework and second as an active process of encounter and response—are central to the work of other theorists who followed her lead and developed conceptual models for nursing practice.

Dorothy Johnson was born on August 21, 1919, in Savannah, Georgia. She received her associate of arts degree from Armstrong Junior College in Savannah, Georgia, in 1938 and her bachelor of science in nursing degree from Vanderbilt University in 1942. She practiced briefly as a staff nurse at the Chatham-Savannah Health Council before attending Harvard University, where she received her master of public health (MPH) in 1948. She began her academic career at Vanderbilt University School of Nursing. A call from Lulu Hassenpplug, dean of the School of Nursing, enticed her to go to the University of California at Los Angeles (UCLA) in 1949. She served there as an assistant, associate, and professor of pediatric nursing until her retirement in 1978. She moved to Key Largo and later to New Smyrna Beach and continued her interest in "systems" as a shell collector.

During her academic career Dorothy Johnson addressed issues related to nursing practice, nursing education, and nursing science. While she was a pediatric nursing advisor at the Christian Medical College School of Nursing in Vellare, South India, she wrote a series of clinical articles for the *Nursing Journal of India* (Johnson, 1956, 1957). She worked with the California Nurses' Association, National League for Nursing, and American Nurses' Association to examine the role of the clinical nurse specialist, the scope of nursing practice, and the need for nursing research. She also completed a Public Health Service–funded research project ("Crying as a Physiologic State in the Newborn Infant") in 1963 (Johnson & Smith, 1963). The foundations of her model and her beliefs about nursing are clearly evident in these early publications. Dorothy Johnson's body of published work includes more than 30 articles, 4 books, and numerous proceedings, reports, and abstracts.

Ms. Johnson received many awards, including the Founders Medal from Vanderbilt University (1942), the Faculty Award from UCLA graduate students (1975), the Lulu Hassenplug Distinguished Achievement Award from the California Nurses' Association (1977), the Vanderbilt University School of Nursing Award for Excellence in Nursing (1981), and induction as an honorary fellow in the American Academy of Nursing (1997). She enjoyed activities with the Class of '42 and took great pride in the career achievements of her former students. Dorothy Johnson, RN, MPH, FAAN passed away in February 1999.

THE JOHNSON BEHAVIORAL SYSTEM MODEL
Paradigmatic Origins

Johnson has noted that her theory evolved from philosophical ideas, theory and research, her clinical background, and many years of thought, discussions, and writing (Johnson, 1968). She cited a number of sources for her theory. From Florence Nightingale came the belief that nursing's concern is a focus on the person rather than the disease. Systems theorists (Buckley, 1968; Chin, 1961; Parsons & Shils, 1951; Rapoport, 1968; and Von Bertalanffy, 1968) were all sources for her model. Johnson's background as a pediatric nurse is also evident in the development of her model. In her papers, Johnson cited developmental literature to support the validity of a behavioral system model (Ainsworth, 1964; Crandal, 1963; Gerwirtz, 1972; Kagan, 1964; and Sears, Maccoby, & Levin, 1954). Johnson also noted that a number of her subsystems had biological underpinnings.

Johnson's theory and her related writings reflect her knowledge about both development and general systems theories. I think her model demonstrates a marvelous fitting together of theory and concepts from both areas. The combination of nursing, development, and general systems introduces into the rhetoric about nursing theory development some of the specifics

> Johnson's model incorporates five principles of system thinking: wholeness and order, stabilization, reorganization, hierarchic interaction, and dialectical contradiction.

that make it possible to test hypotheses and conduct critical experiments. I will conclude this section with a discussion of some aspects of my own thinking about Johnson's use of development and systems in the Johnson Behavioral System Model (JBSM).

Johnson's model incorporates five core principles of system thinking: wholeness and order, stabilization, reorganization, hierarchic interaction, and dialectical contradiction. Each of these general systems principles has analogs in developmental theories that Johnson used to verify the validity of her model (Johnson, 1980, 1990). Wholeness and order provide the basis for continuity and identity, stabilization for development, reorganization for growth and/or change, hierarchic interaction for discontinuity, and dialectical contradiction for motivation. Johnson conceptualized a person as an open system with organized, interrelated, and interdependent subsystems. By virtue of subsystem interaction and independence, the whole of the human organism (system) is greater than the sum of its parts (subsystems). Wholes and their parts create a system with dual constraints: Neither has continuity and identity without the other.

The overall representation of the model can also be viewed as a behavioral system within an environment. The behavioral system and the environment are linked by interactions and transactions. We define the person (behavioral system) as being comprised of subsystems and the environment as being comprised of physical, interpersonal (e.g., father, friend, mother, sibling), and sociocultural (e.g., rules and mores of home, school, country, and other cultural contexts) components that supply the sustenal imperatives (Grubbs, 1980; Holaday, 1997; Johnson, 1990; Meleis, 1991).

The developmental analogy of wholeness and order is continuity and identity. Given the behavioral systems potential for plasticity, a basic feature of the system is that both continuity and change can exist across the life span. The presence of or potentiality for at least some plasticity means that the key way of casting the issue of continuity is not a matter of deciding what exists for a given process or function of a subsystem. Instead, the issue should be cast in terms of determining patterns of interactions among levels of the behavioral system that may promote continuity for a particular subsystem at a given point in time. Johnson's work infers that continuity is in the relationship of the parts rather than in their individuality. Johnson (1990) noted that at the psychological level, attachment (affiliative) and dependency are examples of important specific behaviors that change over time while the representation (meaning) may remain the same. Johnson (1990, p. 28) stated: "[D]evelopmentally, dependence behavior in the socially optimum case evolves from almost total dependence on others to a greater degree of dependence on self, with a certain amount of interdependence essential to the survival of social groups." In terms of behavioral system balance, this pattern of dependence to independence may be repeated as the behavioral system engages in new situations during the course of a lifetime.

Stabilization or behavioral system balance is another core principle of the JBSM. Dynamic systems respond to contextual changes by either a homeostatic or homeorhetic process. Systems have a set point (like a thermostat) that they try to maintain by altering internal conditions to compensate for changes in external conditions. Human thermoregulation is an example of a homeostatic process that is primarily biological but is also behavioral (turning on the heater). Narcissism or the use of attribution of ability or effort are behavioral homeostatic processes we use to interpret activities so they are consistent with our mental organization.

From a behavioral system perspective, homeorhesis is a more important stabilizing process than is homeostatis. In homeorhesis the system stabilizes around a trajectory rather than a set point. A toddler placed in a body cast may show motor lags when the cast is removed but soon shows age-appropriate motor skills. An adult newly diagnosed with asthma who does not receive proper education until a year after diagnosis can successfully incorporate the material into her daily activities. These are examples of homeorhetic processes or self-righting tendencies that can occur over time.

What we as nurses observe as development or adaptation of the behavioral system is a product of stabilization. When a person is ill or threatened with illness, he or she is subject to biopsychosocial perturbations. The nurse, according to Johnson (1980, 1990), acts as the external regulator, and monitors patient response and looks for successful adaptation to occur. If behavioral system balance returns, there is no need for intervention, and if not, the nurse intervenes to help the patient restore behavioral system balance. It is hoped that the patient matures and with additional hospitalizations the previous patterns of response have been assimilated and there are few disturbances.

Adaptive reorganization occurs when the behavioral system encounters new experiences in the environment that cannot be balanced by existing system mechanisms. Adaptation is defined as change that permits the behavioral system to maintain its set

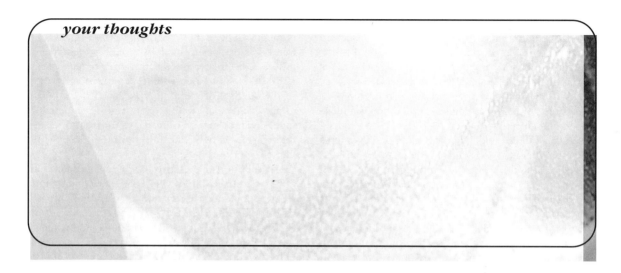

points best in new situations. To the extent that the behavioral system cannot assimilate the new conditions with existing regulatory mechanisms, accommodation must occur either as a new relationship between subsystems or by the establishment of a higher order or different cognitive schema (set, choice). The nurse acts to provide conditions or resources essential to help the accommodation process, may impose regulatory or control mechanisms to stimulate or reinforce certain behaviors, or may attempt to repair structural components (Johnson, 1980).

The difference between stabilization and reorganization is that the latter involves change or evolution. A behavioral system is embedded in an environment, but it is capable of operating independently of environmental constraints through the process of adaptation. The diagnosis of a chronic illness, the birth of a child, or the development of a healthy lifestyle regimen to prevent problems in later years are all examples where accommodation not only promotes behavioral system balance but also involves a developmental process that results in the establishment of a higher order or more complex behavioral system.

Each behavioral system exists in a context of hierarchical relationships and environmental relationships. From the perspective of general systems theory, a behavioral system that has the properties of wholeness and order, stabilization and reorganization will also demonstrate a hierarchic structure (Buckley, 1968). Hierarchies, or a pattern of relying on particular subsystems, lead to a degree of stability. A disruption or failure will not destroy the whole system but leads instead to a decomposition to the next level of stability.

The judgement that a discontinuity has occurred is typically based on a lack of correlation between assessments at two points of time. One's lifestyle (or one's usual set, choice, and action) prior to surgery is not a good fit postoperatively. These discontinuities can provide opportunities for reorganization and development.

The last core principle is the motivational force for behavioral change. Johnson (1980) described these as drives and noted that these responses are developed and modified over time through maturation, experience, and learning. I have also discussed stabilization and reorganization as reactions to environmental changes. A person's activities in the environment lead to knowledge and development. However, by acting on the world, each person is constantly changing it and his or her goals, and therefore changing what he or she needs to know. The number of environmental domains that the person is responding to include the biological, psychological, cultural, familial, social, and physical setting. The person needs to resolve (maintain behavioral system balance of) a cascade of contradictions between goals related to physical status, social roles, and cognitive status when faced with illness or the threat of illness. Nurses' interventions during these periods can make a significant difference in the lives of the persons involved. Behavioral system balance is restored and a new level of development is attained.

In summary, I believe Johnson's pragmatic origins included general systems theory as well as dominant themes from developmental theory. This has given the model some unique features that are absent in other models. One may analyze the patient's response in terms of behavioral system balance, and, from a developmental perspective, ask, Where did

> The client is seen as a collection of behavioral subsystems that interrelate to form the behavioral system. There are eight subsystems, along with their goals and functions.

this come from and where is it going? The developmental component necessitates that we identify and understand the processes of stabilization and sources of disturbances that lead to reorganization. These need to be evaluated by age, gender, and culture. The combination of systems theory and development identifies "nursing's unique social mission and our special realm of original responsibility in patient care" (Johnson, 1990, p. 32).

MAJOR CONCEPTS OF THE MODEL

Person

Johnson conceptualized a nursing client as a behavioral system. The behavioral system is orderly, repetitive, systematic, and organized with interrelated and interdependent biological and behavioral subsystems. The client is seen as a collection of behavioral subsystems that interrelate to form the behavioral system. The system may be defined as "those complex, overt actions or responses to a variety of stimuli present in the surrounding environment that are purposeful and functional" (Auger, 1976, p. 22). These ways of behaving form an organized and integrated functional unit that determines and limits the interaction between the person and environment, and establishes the relationship of the person to the objects, events, and situations in the environment. Johnson (1980, p. 209) considered such "behavior to be orderly, purposeful and predictable; that is, it is functionally efficient and effective most of the time, and is sufficiently stable and recurrent to be amenable to description and exploration."

The parts of the behavioral system are called *subsystems*. They carry out specialized tasks or functions needed to maintain the integrity of the whole behavioral system and manage its relationship to the environment. Each of these subsystems has a set of behavioral responses that is developed and modified through motivation, experience, and learning.

Johnson identified seven subsystems. However, in my operationalization of the model, as in Grubbs (1980), I have included eight subsystems. These eight subsystems and their goals and functions are described in Table 7–1. Johnson noted that these subsystems are found cross-culturally and across a broad range of the phylogenetic scale. She also noted the significance of social and cultural factors involved in the development of the subsystems. She did not consider the seven subsystems as complete, because "the ultimate group of response systems to be identified in the behavioral system will undoubtedly change as research reveals new subsystems or indicated changes in the structure, functions, or behavioral groupings in the original set" (Johnson, 1980, p. 214).

Each subsystem has functions that serve to meet the conceptual goal. Functional behaviors are those activities carried out to meet these goals. These behaviors may vary with each individual, depending on the person's age, sex, motives, cultural values, social norms, and self-concepts. In order for the subsystem goals to be accomplished, behavioral system structural components must meet functional requirements of the behavioral system.

Each subsystem is composed of at least four structural components that interact in a specific pattern. These parts are goal, set, choice, and action. The goal of a subsystem is defined as the desired result or consequence of the behavior. The basis for the goal is a universal drive whose existence can be supported by scientific research. In general, the drive of each subsystem is the same for all people, but there are variations among individuals (and within individuals over time) in the specific objects or events that are drive-fulfilling, in the value placed on goal attainment, and in drive strength. With drives as the impetus for the behavior, goals can be identified and are considered universal.

Behavioral set is a predisposition to act in a certain way in a given situation. The behavioral set represents a relatively stable and habitual behavioral pattern of responses to particular drives or stimuli. It is learned behavior and is influenced by knowledge, attitudes, and beliefs. Set contains two components: perseveration and preparation. Perseveratory set refers to consistent tendency to react to certain stimuli with the same pattern of behavior. The preparatory set is contingent upon the function of the perseveratory set. The preparatory set functions to establish priorities for attending or not attending to various stimuli.

The conceptual set is a component that I have added to the model (Holaday, 1982). The conceptual set is a process of ordering that serves as the mediating link between stimuli from the preparatory and perseveratory sets. Here attitudes, beliefs, information, and knowledge are examined before a choice is made. There are three levels of processing—an inadequate conceptual set, a developing conceptual set, and a sophisticated conceptual set.

TABLE 7-1	*The Subsystems of Behavior* *	
Achievement Subsystem		
Goal	Mastery or control of self or the environment	
Function	To set appropriate goals	
	To direct behaviors toward achieving a desired goal	
	To perceive recognition from others	
	To differentiate between immediate goals and long-term goals	
	To interpret feedback (input received) to evaluate the achievement of goals	
Affiliative Subsystem		
Goal	To relate or belong to someone or something other than oneself; to achieve intimacy and inclusion	
Function	To form cooperative and interdependent role relationships within human social systems	
	To develop and use interpersonal skills to achieve intimacy and inclusion	
	To share	
	To be related to another in a definite way	
	To use narcissistic feelings in an appropriate way	
Aggressive/Protective Subsystem		
Goal	To protect self or others from real or imagined threatening objects, persons, or ideas, to achieve self-protection and self-assertion	
Function	To recognize biological, environmental, or health systems that are potential threats to self or others	
	To mobilize resources to respond to challenges identified as threats	
	To use resources or feedback mechanisms to alter biological, environmental, or health input or human responses in order to diminish threats to self or others	
	To protect one's achievement goals	
	To protect one's beliefs	
	To protect one's identify or self-concept	
Dependency Subsystem		
Goal	To obtain focused attention, approval, nurturance, and physical assistance; to maintain the environmental resources needed for assistance; to gain trust and reliance	
Function	To obtain approval, reassurance about self	
	To make others aware of self	
	To induce others to care for physical needs	
	To evolve from a state of total dependence on others to a state of increased dependence on the self	
	To recognize and accept situations requiring reversal of self-dependence (dependence upon others)	
	To focus on another or oneself in relation to social, psychological, and cultural needs and desires	

TABLE 7-1	*Continued*

Eliminative Subsystem

Goal	To expel biological wastes; to externalize the internal biological environment
Function	To recognize and interpret input from the biological system that signals readiness for waste excretion
	To maintain physiological homeostasis through excretion
	To adjust to alterations in biological capabilities related to waste excretion while maintaining a sense of control over waste excretion
	To relieve feelings of tension in the self
	To express one's feelings, emotions, and ideas verbally or nonverbally

Ingestive Subsystem

Goal	To take in needed resources from the environment to maintain the integrity of the organism or to achieve a state of pleasure; to internalize the external environment
Function	To sustain life through nutritive intake
	To alter ineffective patterns of nutritive intake
	To relieve pain or other psychophysiological subsystems
	To obtain knowledge or information useful to the self
	To obtain physical and/or emotional pleasure from intake of nutritive or nonnutritive substances

Restorative Subsystem

Goal	To relieve fatigue and/or achieve a state of equilibrium by reestablishing or replenishing the energy distribution among the other subsystems; to redistribute energy
Function	To maintain and/or return to physiological homeostasis
	To produce relaxation of the self system

Sexual Subsystem

Goal	To procreate, to gratify or attract; to fulfill expectations associated with one's sex; to care for others and to be cared about by them
Function	To develop a self-concept or self-identity based on gender
	To project an image of oneself as a sexual being
	To recognize and interpret biological system input related to sexual gratification and/or procreation
	To establish meaningful relationships in which sexual gratification and/or procreation may be obtained

Source: Based on J. Grubbs (1980). An interpretation of the Johnson behavioral system model. In J. P. Riehl & C. Roy (Eds.), *Conceptual models for nursing practice* (2nd ed., pp. 217–254). New York: Appleton-Century-Crofts; D. E. Johnson (1980). The behavioral system model for nursing. In J. P. Riehl & C. Roy (Eds.), *Conceptual models for nursing practice* (2nd ed., pp. 207–216). New York: Appleton-Century-Crofts; D. Wilks (1987). *Operationalization of the JBSM.* Unpublished paper. University of California, San Francisco; and B. Holaday (1972). *Operationalization of the JBSM.* Unpublished paper. University of California, Los Angeles.

The third and fourth components of each subsystem are choice and action. Choice refers to the individual's repertoire of alternative behaviors in a situation that will best meet the goal and attain the desired outcome. The larger the behavioral repertoire of alternative behaviors in a situation, the more adaptable is the individual. The fourth structural component of each subsystem is the observable action of the individual. The concern is with the efficiency and effectiveness of the behavior in goal attainment. Actions are any observable responses to stimuli.

For the eight subsystems to develop and maintain stability, each must have a constant supply of functional requirements (sustenal imperatives). The notion of functional requirements of the behavioral system remains one of the cloudiest, and empirically, one of the most debatable concepts of this model. The concept of functional requirements tends to be confined to conditions of survival of the system, and it includes biological as well as psychosocial needs. The problems are related to establishing the types of functional requirements (universal versus highly specific), and finding procedures for validating the assumptions of these requirements. It also suggests a classification of the various states or processes on the basis of some principle and perhaps the establishment of a hierarchy among them. The Johnson model proposes that, for the behavior to be maintained, it must be protected, nurtured, and stimulated: It requires protection, from noxious stimuli that threaten the survival of the behavioral system; nurturance, which provides adequate input to sustain behavior; and stimulation, which contributes to continued growth of the behavior and counteracts stagnation. A deficiency in any or all of these functional requirements threatens the behavioral system as a whole, or the effective functioning of the particular subsystem with which it is directly involved.

In summary, the behavioral system is a complex of observable features and actions of a person that describe his interaction with the environment. It is an integrative response system that adaptively relates to various stimuli and communicates the status of internal processes to the surrounding environment. Therefore, even though each of the subsystems has a specialized function, the system as a whole depends on an integrated performance of these subsystems.

Environment

Johnson referred to the internal and external environment of the system. She also referred to the interaction between the person and the environment and to the objects, events, and situations in the environment. She also noted that there are forces in the environment that impinge on the person and to which the person adjusts. Thus, the environment consists of all elements that are not a part of the individual's behavioral system but influence the system and can serve as a source of sustenal imperatives. Some of these elements can be manipulated by the nurse to achieve health (behavioral system balance or stability) for the patient. Johnson provided no other specific definition of the environment, nor did she identify what she considered internal versus external environment. But much can be inferred from her writings, and system theory also provides additional insights into the environment component of the model. For those who choose to use this model, I encourage you to continue to define this domain.

I view the external environment as people, objects, and phenomena that can potentially permeate

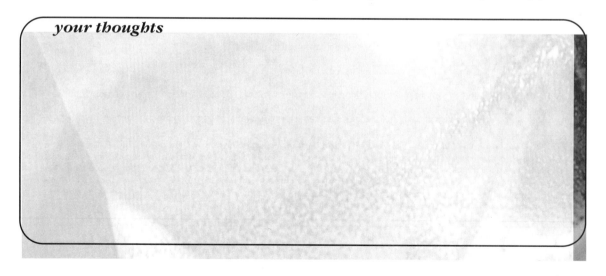

your thoughts

the boundary of the behavioral system. This external stimulus forms an organized or meaningful pattern that elicits a response from the individual. The behavioral system attempts to maintain equilibrium in response to environmental factors by assimilating and accommodating to the forces that impinge upon it. Areas of external environment of interest to nurses include the physical settings, people, objects, phenomena, and psychosocial-cultural attributes of an environment.

No definition of "internal environment" was provided in Johnson's published material. However, she provided detailed information about the internal structure and how it functions. She also noted that "[i]llness or other sudden internal or external environmental change is most frequently responsible for system malfunction" (Johnson, 1980, p. 212). I focus my attention on internal regulatory mechanisms. Therefore, I view such factors as physiology, temperament, ego, age, and related developmental capacities, attitudes, and self-concept as general regulators that may be viewed as a class of internalized intervening variables that influence set, choice, and action. They are key areas for nursing assessment. For example, a nurse attempting to respond to the needs of an acutely ill hospitalized 6-year-old would need to know something about the developmental capacities of a 6-year-old, and about self-concept and ego development, to understand the child's behavior.

Health

Johnson viewed health as efficient and effective functioning of the system, and as behavioral system balance and stability. Behavioral system balance and stability are demonstrated by observed behavior that is purposeful, orderly, and predictable. Such behavior is maintained when it is efficient and effective in managing the person's relationship to the environment.

Behavior changes when efficiency and effectiveness are no longer evident, or when a more optimal level of functioning is perceived. Individuals are said to achieve efficient and effective behavioral functioning when their behavior is commensurate with social demands, when they are able to modify their behavior in ways that support biologic imperatives, when they are able to benefit to the fullest extent during illness from the physician's knowledge and skill, and when their behavior does not reveal unnecessary trauma as a consequence of illness (Johnson 1980, p. 207).

Behavior system imbalance and instability are not described explicitly, but can be inferred from the following statement to be a malfunction of the behavioral system:

> The subsystems and the system as a whole tend to be self-maintaining and self-perpetuating so long as conditions in the internal and external environment of the system remain orderly and predictable, the conditions and resources necessary to their functional requirements are met, and the interrelationships among the subsystems are harmonious. If these conditions are not met, malfunction becomes apparent in behavior that is in part disorganized, erratic, and dysfunctional. Illness or other sudden internal or external environmental change is most frequently responsible for such malfunctions. (Johnson 1980, p. 212)

Thus, it can be inferred that behavioral system imbalance and instability are equated with illness. However, as Meleis (1991) has pointed out, we must consider that illness may be separate from behavioral system functioning. Johnson also referred to physical and social health, but did not specifically define wellness. Just as the inference about illness may be made, it may be inferred that wellness is behavioral system balance and stability, as well as efficient and effective behavioral functioning.

> Nursing is viewed as a service that is complementary to medicine and other health professions, but which makes distinctive contributions to the health and well-being of people.

Nursing and Nursing Therapeutics

Nursing is viewed as "a service that is complementary to that of medicine and other health professions, but which makes its own distinctive contribution to the health and well-being of people." Johnson (1980, p. 207) distinguished nursing from medicine by noting that nursing views the patient as a behavioral system, and medicine views the patient as a biological system. In her view, the specific goal of nursing action is "to restore, maintain, or attain behavioral system balance and stability at the highest possible level for the individual" (Johnson, 1980, p. 214). This goal may be expanded to include helping the person achieve an optimal level of balance and functioning when this is possible and desired.

The goal of action of the system is behavioral system balance. For the nurse, the area of concern is a behavioral system threatened by the loss of order and predictability through illness or the threat of illness. The goal of action of the nurses is to maintain or restore the individual's behavioral system balance and stability, or to help the individual achieve a more optimal level of balance and functioning.

Johnson did not specify the steps of the nursing process, but clearly identified the role of the nurse as an external regulatory force. She also identified questions to be asked when analyzing system functioning, and provided diagnostic classifications to delineate disturbances and guidelines for interventions.

Johnson (1980) expected the nurse to base judgements about behavioral system balance and stability on knowledge and an explicit value system. One important point she made about the value system is that "given that the person has been provided with an adequate understanding of the potential for and means to obtain a more optimal level of behavioral functioning than is evident at the present time, the final judgement of the desired level of functioning is the right of the individual" (Johnson, 1980, p. 215).

The source of difficulty arises from structural and functional stresses. Structural and functional problems develop when the system is unable to meet its own functional requirements. As a result of the inability to meet functional requirements, structural impairments may take place. In addition, functional stress may be found as a result of structural damage or from the dysfunctional consequences of the behavior. Other problems develop when the system's control and regulatory mechanisms fail to develop or become defective.

The model differentiates four diagnostic classifications to delineate these disturbances. A disorder originating within any one subsystem is classified as either an insufficiency, which exists when a subsystem is not functioning or developed to its fullest capacity due to inadequacy of functional requirements, or as a discrepancy, which exists when a behavior does not meet the intended conceptual goal. Disorders found between more than one subsystem are classified either as an incompatibility, which exists when the behaviors of two or more subsystems in the same situation conflict with each other to the detriment of the individual, or as dominance, which exists when the behavior of one subsystem is used more than any other, regardless of the situation or to the detriment of the other subsystems. This is also an area where Johnson believed additional diagnostic classifications would be developed. Nursing therapeutics deal with these three areas.

The next critical element is the nature of the interventions the nurse would use to respond to the behavioral system imbalance. The first step is a thorough assessment to find the source of the difficulty or the origin of the problem. There are at least three types of interventions that the nurse can use to bring about change. The nurse may attempt to repair damaged structural units by altering the individual's set and choice. The second would be for the nurse to temporarily impose regulatory and control measures. The nurse acts outside the patient environment to provide the conditions, resources, and controls necessary to restore behavioral system balance. The nurse also acts within and upon the external environment and the internal interactions of the subsystem to create change and restore stability. The third, and most common, treatment modality is to supply or to help the client find his or her own supplies of essential functional requirements. The nurse may provide nurturance (resources and conditions necessary for survival and growth, train the client to cope with new stimuli, encourage effective behaviors), stimulation (provision of stimuli that brings forth new behaviors or increases behaviors, motivation for a particular behavior, and that provides opportunities for appropriate behaviors), and protection (safeguarding from noxious stimuli, defending from unnecessary threats, coping with a threat on the individual's behalf). The nurse and the client negotiate the treatment plan.

ROLE OF THE MODEL IN NURSING PRACTICE, ADMINISTRATION, RESEARCH, AND EDUCATION

Fundamental to any professional discipline is the development of a scientific body of knowledge that can be used to guide its practice. The Johnson Behavioral System Model (JBSM) has served as a means for identifying, labeling, and classifying phenomena important to the discipline of nursing. The JBSM model has been used by nurses since the early 1970s and has demonstrated its ability to provide a medium for theoretical growth; provide organization for nurses' thinking, observations, and interpretations of what was observed; provide a systematic structure and rationale for activities; provide direction to the search for relevant research questions; provide solutions for patient care problems; and, finally, provide criteria to determine if a problem had been solved. Rather than provide a cursory overview of many articles, I have reviewed the work of nurses who have used the JBSM to guide a program of study over time.

Research

Stevenson and Woods (1986, p. 6) state: "Nursing science is the domain of knowledge concerned with the adaptation of individuals and groups to actual or potential health problems, the environments that influence health in humans and the therapeutic interventions that promote health and affect the consequences of illness." This position focuses efforts in nursing science on the expansion of knowledge about clients' health problems and nursing therapeutics. Nurse researchers have demonstrated the usefulness of Johnson's model in a clinical practice in a variety of ways. The majority of the research focuses on clients' functioning in terms of maintaining or restoring behavioral system balance, understanding the system and/or subsystems by focusing on the basic sciences, or focusing on the nurse as an agent of action who uses the JBSM to gather diagnostic data or provide care that influences behavioral system balance.

Dr. Anayis Derdiarian's program of research involves both the client and the nurse as agents of action. Derdiarian's early research tested an instrument designed to measure and describe, using the JBSM perspective, the perceived behavioral changes of cancer patients (Derdiarian, 1983; Derdiarian & Forsythe, 1983). The research was based on Johnson's premise that illness is a noxious stimulus that affects the balance of the behavioral system. The results demonstrated by the instrument possessed content validity, strong internal consistency, and thus strong reliability. A later study (Derdiarian, 1988) explained the effects of the variables of age, site, and stage of cancer on "set" behaviors of the eight behavioral subsystems of the Johnson model. The study also served to further validate her instrument.

These studies were important for two reasons. First, Derdiarian examined the impact of three moderator variables on set behavior. The scores and subscores from her instrument were used to summarize commonalities and not a specific behavior. Thus, the measure can be taken as an indicator of the construct of "behavioral set." The construct was defined by a network of relations that were tied to observables and were therefore empirically testable. Thus, this validation study linked a particular measure, the Derdiarian Behavioral System Model (DBSM), to the more general theoretical construct, "behavioral set," that was embedded in the more comprehensive theoretical network of the JBSM.

The results indicated significant differences in some mean factor scores in the subsystems among the groups stratified by age, site of cancer, and stage of cancer. Therefore, this study extended the development of the "nomological network" (Cronbach & Meehl, 1955) of the Johnson model. It provided evidence that the measure exhibited, at least in part,

the network of relations derived from the theory of the construct. It also elaborated the nomological network by increasing the definiteness of the components of the model (e.g., connections between the moderator variables, behavioral set, and subsystem behaviors). The linking of instrument behaviors to a more general attribute provided not only an evidential basis for interpreting the process underlying the instrument scores, but also a basis for inferring researchable implications of the scores from the broader network of the construct's meaning. A further test of the instrument (Derdiarian & Schobel, 1990) indicated a rank order among the subsystems' response frequency counts as well as among their importance values. Derdiarian also found that changes in the aggressive/protective subsystem made both direct and indirect effects on changes in other subsystems (Derdiarian, 1990).

Derdiarian also examined the nurse as an action agent within the practice domain. She focused on the nurses' assessment of the patient using the DBSM and the effect of using this instrument on the quality of care (Derdiarian, 1990, 1991). This approach expanded the view of nursing knowledge from exclusively client-based to knowledge about the context and practice of nursing that is model-based. The results of these studies found a significant increase in patient and nurse satisfaction when the DBSM was used. Derdiarian also found that a model-based valid and reliable instrument could improve the comprehensiveness and the quality of assessment data, the method of assessment, and the quality of nursing diagnosis, interventions, and outcomes.

Derdiarian's body of work reflects the complexity of nursing's knowledge as well as the strategic problem-solving capabilities of the JBSM. Her article (Derdiarian, 1991) demonstrated the clear relationship between Johnson's theory and nursing practice.

My program of research has examined normal and atypical patterns of behavior of children with a chronic illness and the behavior of their parents, and the interrelationship between the children and the environment. My goal was to determine the causes of instability within and between subsystems (e.g., breakdown in internal regulatory or control mechanisms), and to identify the source of problems in behavioral system balance.

My first study (Holaday, 1974) compared the achievement behavior of chronically ill and healthy children. The study showed that chronically ill children differed in attributional tendencies when compared with healthy children, and that the response patterns differed within the chronically ill group when compared to certain dimensions (e.g., gender,

age at diagnosis). Males and children diagnosed at birth attributed both success and failure to the presence or absence of ability and little to effort. This is a pattern found in children with low achievement needs. The results indicated behavioral system imbalance and focused my attention on interventions directed toward set, choice, and action.

The next series of studies used the concept of "behavioral set" and examined how mothers and their chronically ill infants interacted (Holaday, 1981, 1982, 1987). Patterns of maternal response provided information related to the setting of the "set goal" or behavioral set, that is, the degree of proximity and speed of maternal response. Mothers with chronically ill infants rarely did not respond to a cry indicating a narrow behavioral set. Further analysis of the data led to the identification of a new structural component of the model-conceptual set. A person's conceptual set was defined as an organized cluster of cognitive units that were used to interpret the content information from the preparatory and preservatory sets. A conceptual set may differ both in the number of cognitive units involved and in the degree of organization exhibited. Thus, the various cognitive units that make up a conceptual set may vary in complexity depending on the situation. Three levels of conceptual set have been identified, ranging from a very simple to a complex "set" with a high degree of connectedness between multiple perspectives (Holaday, 1982). Thus, the conceptual set functions as an information collection and processing unit. Examining a person's set, choice, and conceptual set offered a way to examine issues of individual cognitive patterns and its impact on behavioral system balance.

The most recent study (Holaday, Turner-Henson, & Swan, 1997) drew from the knowledge gained from previous studies. This study viewed the JBSM as holistic, in that it assumed that all part processes—biological, physical, psychological, and sociocultural—are interrelated; developmental, in that it assumed that development proceeds from a relative lack of differentiation toward a goal of differentiation and hierarchic integration of organismic functioning; and system-oriented, in that a unit of analysis was the person in the environment where the physical and/or biological (e.g., health), psychological, interpersonal, and sociocultural levels of organization of the person are operative and interrelated with the physical, interpersonal, and sociocultural levels of organization in the environment. Our results indicate that it was possible to determine the impact of a lack of functional requirements on a child's actions, to identify behavioral system imbalance and the need for specific types of nursing intervention.

The goal of my program of research has been to describe the relations both among and within the subsystems that make up the integrated whole as well as to identify the type of nursing interventions that restore behavioral system balance. The process of clinical assessment to attain such information is described elsewhere (Holaday, 1997). The program of research is linked to systems as well as developmental aspects of the JBSM. The research problems were selected with the systems-based assumption that a disturbance in any part of the behavioral system or the environment that supplies sustenal imperatives would impact the system as a whole. Moreover, with respect to development, we are touching on a set of conditions that has developmental relevance, namely the functioning of the person under stressful (e.g., diagnosis and management of a chronic illness) versus more optimal conditions of functioning. Changes in the person, in the environment, or in the relations between them can cause behavioral system imbalance, which may, in turn, depending on the nursing interventions, make for developmental progression (change). Thus, my approach has been to use the complementarity of explication (description) and causal explanation (condition under which cause-effect relations occur) rather than being restricted to one approach.

Other nurse researchers have demonstrated the utility of Johnson's model for clinical practice. Wilke, Lovejoy, Dodd, and Tesler (1988) used the JBSM to examine cancer pain control behaviors. Their findings supported the assumption that aggressive/protective subsystem behaviors are developed and modified over time. Lovejoy (1983) found that leukemic children were affected by their perceptions of family behavioral disturbances. Lewis and Randell (1990) used the JBSM to identify the most common nursing diagnoses of hospitalized geopsychiatric patients. They found that 30% were related to the achievement subsystem. They also found that the JBSM was more specific than NANDA (North American Nursing Diagnosis Association) diagnoses, which demonstrated considerable overlap. Poster, Dee, and Randell (1997) found the JBSM was an effective framework to use to evaluate patient outcomes. All of these studies have tested the JBSM and have increased nursing's body of knowledge.

Education

Johnson's model was used as the basis for undergraduate education at the UCLA School of Nursing. The curriculum was developed by the faculty; however, no published material is available that describes this process. Texts by Wu (1973) and Auger (1976) extended Johnson's model and provided some idea of the content of that curriculum. Later, in the 1980s, Harris (1986) described the use of Johnson's theory as a framework for UCLA's curriculum. The Universities of Hawaii, Alaska, and Colorado also used the JBSM as a basis for their undergraduate curricula.

Loveland-Cherry and Wilkerson (1983) analyzed Johnson's model and concluded that the model could be used to develop a curriculum. The primary focus of the program would be the study of the person as a behavioral system. The student would need a background in systems theory and the biological, psychological, and sociological sciences.

Nursing Practice and Administration

Johnson has influenced nursing practice because she enabled nurses to make statements about the links between nursing input and health outcomes for clients. The model has been useful in practice because it identifies an end product (behavioral system balance), which is the goal of nursing. Nursing's specific objective is to maintain or restore the person's behavioral system balance and stability, or to help the person achieve a more optimum level of functioning. The model provides a means for identifying the source of the problem in the system. Nursing is seen as the external regulatory force that acts to restore balance (Johnson, 1980).

> Nursing's objective is to maintain or restore the person's behavioral system balance and stability, or help the person achieve a more optimum level of functioning.

One of the best examples of the use of the model in practice has been at the University of California, Los Angeles, Neuropsychiatric Hospital (UCLA—NPI). Auger and Dee (1983) designed a patient classification system using the JBSM. Each subsystem of behavior was operationalized in terms of critical adaptive and maladaptive behaviors. The behavioral statements were designed to be measurable, relevant to the clinical setting, observable, and specific to the subsystem. The use of the model has had a major impact on all phases of the nursing process, including a more systematic assessment process, identification of patient strengths as well as problem areas, and an objective means for evaluating the quality of nursing care (Dee & Auger, 1983).

The early works of Dee and Auger lead to further refinement in the patient classification system. Behavioral indices for each subsystem have been further operationalized in terms of critical adaptive and maladaptive behaviors. Behavioral data is gathered to determine the effectiveness of each subsystem (Dee & Randell, 1989; Dee, 1990). Based on behavioral data, each subsystem is assigned a behavioral category score ranging from 1 to 4 (1 = effective; 2 = inconsistently effective; 3 = ineffective; and 4 = severely ineffective). In addition, data is gathered to determine the degree to which the internal and external environments protect, nurture, and/or stimulate the behavioral subsystems. The diagnostic process is based on the degree of effectiveness or on the effectiveness of each behavioral subsystem. An overall behavioral category score is determined for the entire behavioral system ranging from 1 to 4 (1 = health, 2 = potential for health deviation; 3 = illness; and 4 = critical illness). Priorities are established and mutual goal-setting is conducted between patient/family and nurse (Dee & Randell, 1989). Nursing

TABLE 7–2　Nursing Staffing Budget Unit: 2–South

Shift	Actual No. Patients	Levels of Nursing Interventions				# Stf	Patient Hours	—Total Cost—			—Cost per Patient—		
		I	II	III	IV			Budget	Actual	Var	Budget	Actual	Var
N	12.3	1.5	7.1	3.5	0.1	2.49	1.65	181734	154156	27578	40.2	35.2	5.0
D	12.0	1.2	7.3	3.4	0.2	4.24	2.91	358208	338014	20194	79.1	79.6	−0.4
E	12.2	1.2	7.3	3.6	0.1	3.82	2.55	183008	270855	−87847	40.4	61.9	−21.5
	Totals					10.55	7.11	722950	763025	−40075	159.7	176.7	−16.9

Source: V. Dee & B. Randell (1989). *NPH Patient Classification System: A theory-based nursing practice model for staffing.* Paper presented at the UCLA Neuropsychiatric Institute and Hospital.

interventions are ranked according to frequency, intensity, and nature of nursing contract. Predicted outcomes and short-term goals are measured to determine whether increased behavioral effectiveness was achieved.

The scores serve as an acuity rating system and provide a basis for allocating resources. Resources are allocated based on the assigned levels of nursing intervention, and resource needs are calculated based on the total number of patients assigned according to levels of nursing interventions and the hours of nursing care associated with each of the levels (Dee & Randell, 1989) (see Table 7–2). The development of this system has provided nursing administration with the ability to identify the levels of staff needed to provided care (licensed vocational nurse versus registered nurse), bill patients for actual nursing care services, and identify nursing services that are absolutely necessary in times of budgetary restraint. Recent research has demonstrated the importance of a model-based nursing database in medical records (Poster, Dee, & Randell, 1997) and the effectiveness of using a model to identify the characteristics of a large hospital's managed behavioral health population in relation to observed nursing care needs, level of patient functioning on admission and discharge, and length of stay (Dee, Van Servellen, & Brecht, 1998).

The work of Vivien Dee and her colleagues has demonstrated the validity and usefulness of the JBSM as a basis for clinical practice within a health care setting. From the findings of their work, it is clear that the JBSM established a systematic framework for patient assessment and nursing interventions, provided a common frame of reference for all practitioners in the clinical setting, provided a framework for the integration of staff knowledge about the clients, and promoted continuity in the delivery of care. These findings should be generalizable to a variety of clinical settings.

Summary

The Johnson Behavioral System Model captures the richness and complexity of nursing. While the perspective presented here is embedded in the past, there remains the potentiality for the further development of the theory, as well as the uncovering and shaping of significant research problems that have both theoretical and practical value. There are a variety of problem areas worthy of investigation that are suggested by the JBSM assumptions and from previous studies. Some examples include examining the levels of integration (biological, psychological, and sociocultural) within and between the subsystems. For example, a study could examine the way a person deals with the transition from health to illness with the onset of asthma. There is concern with the relations between one's biological system (e.g., unstable, problems breathing), one's psychological self (e.g., achievement goals, need for assistance, self-concept), self in relation to the physical environment (e.g., allergens, being away from home), and transactions related to the sociocultural context (e.g., attitudes and values about the sick). The study of transitions (e.g., the onset of puberty, menopause, death of a spouse, onset of acute illness) also represents a treasury of open problems for research with the JBSM. Findings obtained from these studies will provide not only an opportunity to revise and advance the theoretical conceptualization of the JBSM but also information about nursing interventions. The JBSM approach leads us to seek common organizational parameters in every scientific explanation and does so using a shared language about nursing and nursing care.

References

Ainsworth, M. (1964). Patterns of attachment behavior shown by the infant in interactions with mother. *Merrill-Palmer Quarterly, 10,* 51–58.

Auger, J. (1976). *Behavioral systems and nursing.* Englewood Cliffs, NJ: Prentice-Hall.

Auger, J., & Dee, V. (1983). A patient classification system based on the Behavioral Systems Model of Nursing: Part 1. *Journal of Nursing Administration, 13*(4), 38–43.

Buckley, W. (Ed.). (1968). *Modern systems research for the behavioral scientist.* Chicago: Aldine.

Chin, R. (1961). The utility of system models and developmental models for practitioners. In Benne, K., Bennis, W., & Chin, R. (Eds.), *The planning of change.* New York: Holt.

Crandal, V. (1963). Achievement. In Stevenson, H. W. (Ed.), *Child psychology.* Chicago: University of Chicago Press.

Cronbach, L. J., & Meehl, P. (1955). Construct validity in psychological tests. *Psychological Bulletin, 52,* 281–301.

Dee, V. (1990). Implementation of the Johnson Model: One hospital's experience. In Parker, M. (Ed.), *Nursing Theories in Practice* (pp. 33–63). New York: National League for Nursing.

Dee, V., & Auger, J. (1983). A patient classification system based on the Behavioral System Model of Nursing: Part 2. *Journal of Nursing Administration, 13*(5), 18–23.

Dee, V., & Randell, B. P. (1989). *NPH patient classification system: A theory based nursing practice model for staffing.* Paper presented at the UCLA Neuropsychiatric Institute and Hospital, Los Angeles, CA.

Dee, V., Van Servellen, G., & Brecht, M. (1998). Managed behavioral health care patients and their nursing care problems, level of functioning and impairment on discharge. *Journal of the American Psychiatric Nurses Association, 4*(2), 57-66.

Derdiarian, A. K. (1983). An instrument for theory and research development using the behavioral systems model for nursing: The cancer patient. *Nursing Research, 32,* 196-201.

Derdiarian, A. K. (1988). Sensitivity of the Derdiarian Behavioral Systems Model Instrument to age, site and type of cancer: A preliminary validation study. *Scholarly Inquiring for Nursing Practice, 2,* 103-121.

Derdiarian, A. K. (1990). The relationships among the subsystems of Johnson's Behavioral System model. *Image, 22,* 219-225.

Derdiarian, A. (1991). Effects of using a nursing model-based instrument on the quality of nursing care. *Nursing Administration Quarterly, 15*(3), 1-16.

Derdiarian, A. K., & Forsythe, A. B. (1983). An instrument for theory and research development using the behavioral systems model for nursing: The cancer patient. Part II. *Nursing Research, 3,* 260-266.

Derdiarian, A. K., & Schobel, D. (1990). Comprehensive assessment of AIDS patients using the behavioral systems model for nursing practice instrument. *Journal of Advanced Nursing, 15,* 436-446.

Gerwitz, J. (Ed.). (1972). *Attachment and dependency.* Englewood Cliffs, NJ: Prentice-Hall.

Grubbs, J. (1980). An interpretation of the Johnson behavioral system model. In Riehl, J. P., & Roy, C. (Eds.), *Conceptual models for nursing practice* (pp. 217-254). New York: Appleton-Century-Crofts.

Harris, R. B. (1986). Introduction of a conceptual model into a fundamental baccalaureate course. *Journal of Nursing Education, 25,* 66-69.

Holaday, B. (1972). Unpublished operationalization of the Johnson Model. University of California, Los Angeles.

Holaday, B. (1974). Achievement behavior in chronically ill children. *Nursing Research, 23,* 25-30.

Holaday, B. (1981). Maternal response to their chronically ill infants' attachment behavior of crying. *Nursing Research, 30,* 343-348.

Holaday, B. (1982). Maternal conceptual set development: Identifying patterns of maternal response to chronically ill infant crying. *Maternal Child Nursing Journal, 11,* 47-59.

Holaday, B. (1987). Patterns of interaction between mothers and their chronically ill infants. *Maternal Child Nursing Journal, 16,* 29-45.

Holaday, B. (1997). Johnson's behavioral system model in nursing practice. In M. Alligood & A. Marriner-Tomey (Eds.), *Nursing theory: Utilization and application* (pp. 49-70). St. Louis: Mosby-Year Book.

Holaday, B., Turner-Henson, A., & Swan, J. (1997). The Johnson Behavioral System Model: Explaining activities of chronically ill children. In Hinton-Walker, P., & Newman, B. (Eds.), *Blueprint for use of nursing models: Education, research, practice, and administration* (pp. 33-63). New York: National League for Nursing.

Johnson, D. E. (1956). A story of three children. *The Nursing Journal of India, XLVII*(9), 313-322.

Johnson, D. E. (1957). Nursing care of the ill child. *The Nursing Journal of India, XLVIII*(1), 12-14.

Johnson, D. E. (1959). The nature and science of nursing. *Nursing Outlook, 7,* 291-294.

Johnson, D. E. (1961). The significance of nursing care. *American Journal of Nursing, 61,* 63-66.

Johnson, D. E. (1968). *One conceptual model of nursing.* Unpublished lecture. Vanderbilt University.

Johnson, D. E. (1980). The behavioral system model for nursing. In J. P. Riehl C. Roy (Eds.), *Conceptual models for nursing practice* (2nd ed., pp. 207-216). New York: Appleton-Century-Crofts.

Johnson, D. E. (1990). The Behavioral System Model for Nursing. In Parker, M. E. (Ed.), *Nursing theories in practice* (pp. 23-32). New York: National League for Nursing.

Johnson, D. E., & Smith, M. M. (1963). *Crying as a physiologic state in the newborn infant.* Unpublished research report, PHS Grant NV-00055-01 (formerly GS-9768).

Kagan, J. (1964). Acquisition and significance of sex role identity. In Hoffman, R., & Hoffman, G. (Eds.), *Review of child development research.* New York: Russell Sage Foundation.

Lewis, C., & Randell, R. B. (1990). Alteration in self-care: An instance of ineffective coping in the geriatric patient. In Carroll-Johnson, R. M. (Ed.), *Classification of nursing diagnosis: proceedings of the 9th conference.* Philadelphia: J. B. Lippincott.

Lovejoy, N. (1983). The leukemic child's perceptions of family behaviors. *Oncology Nursing Forum, 10*(4), 20-25.

Loveland-Cherry, C., & Wilkerson, S. (1983). Dorothy Johnson's behavioral system model. In Fitzpatrick, J., & Whall, A. (Eds.), *Conceptual models of nursing: Analysis and application.* Bowie, MD: Robert J. Brady.

Meleis, A. I. (1991). *Theoretical nursing: Development and progress.* Philadelphia: J. B. Lippincott.

Parsons, T., & Shils, E. A. (Eds.). (1951). *Toward a general theory of action: Theoretical foundations for the social sciences.* New York: Harper & Row.

Poster, E. C., Dee, V., & Randell, B. P. (1997). The Johnson Behavioral Systems Model as a framework for patient outcome evaluation. *Journal of the American Psychiatric Nurses Association, 3*(3), 73-80.

Rapoport, A. (1968). Forward to modern systems research for the behavior scientist. In Buckley, W. (Ed.), *Modern systems research for the behavioral scientist.* Chicago: Aldine.

Sears, R., Maccoby, E., & Levin, H. (1954). *Patterns child rearing.* White Plains, NY: Row & Peterson.

Stevenson, J. S., & Woods, N. F. (1986). Nursing science and contemporary science: Emerging paradigms. In *Setting the agenda for year 2000: Knowledge development in nursing* (pp. 6-20). Kansas City, MO: American Academy of Nursing.

Von Bertalanffy, L. (1968). *General systems theory: Foundations, development, application.* New York: George Braziller.

Wilkie, D. (1987). Unpublished operationalization of the Johnson model. University of California, San Francisco.

Wilkie, D., Lovejoy, N., Dodd, M., & Tesler, M. (1988). Cancer pain control behavior: Description and correlation with pain intensity. *Oncology Nursing Forum, 15,* 723–731.

Wu, R. (1973). *Behavior and Illness.* Englewood Cliffs, NJ: Prentice-Hall.

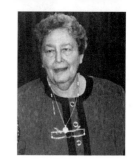

Chapter 8

Myra Levine
Conservation Model:
A Model for the Future

Karen Moore Schaefer

Nursing is human interaction.... Nursing knowledge, thoroughly grounded in modern scientific concepts, allows for a sensitive and productive relationship between the nurse and the individual entrusted to her care. In the care of the sick, this has always been true, but never before has there been available to the nurse so rich and demanding a body of knowledge to use in the patient's behalf

—**Myra Levine (1973, p. 1)**

INTRODUCING THE THEORIST

Myra Levine has been called a Renaissance woman—highly principled, remarkable, and committed to what happens to the quality of life of patients. She was a daughter, sister, wife, mother, friend, educator, administrator, student of humanities, scholar, enabler, and confidante. She was amazingly intelligent, opinionated, quick to respond, loving, caring, trustworthy, and global in her vision of nursing. She was committed to her Jewish faith; she planted a tree in Israel in memory of my father. What a precious gift she was! "In the Talmudic tradition of her ancestors, she was a forthright spokesperson for social justice and the inherent dignity of the human person as a child of God" (Mid-Year Convocation, 1992). She lives on in my heart, as I hope she will in yours, as you learn about her and the model she unknowingly created to develop nursing knowledge.

Myra was born in Chicago and raised with a sister and brother with whom she shared a close, loving relationship (Levine, 1988b). She was also very fond of her father, who was a hardware man. He was often ill and frequently hospitalized with gastrointestinal problems. She thinks that this might have been why she had such a great interest in nursing. Myra's mother was a strong woman who kept the home filled with love and warmth. She was very supportive of Myra's choice to be a nurse. "[My mother] probably knew as much about nursing as I did," (Levine, 1988b) because she was devoted to caring for her father when he was ill.

Myra completed most of her education in Chicago schools. She went to elementary and high school in the "windy city." She started undergraduate work at the University of Chicago, but after 2 years she left the university and had to consider other options. She claimed that she originally wanted to be a physician but she was discouraged from pursuing this career because she was a woman and Jewish. In her last year of high school she had an emergency appendectomy and "fell in love" with nursing. When she could

no longer afford the University of Chicago, she chose to attend Cook County School of Nursing.

Being in nursing school was a new experience for her; she called it a "great adventure" (Levine, 1988b). She had never before been away from home. At Cook County she had a room all to herself with a desk, a bed, and a chair. Before this time in her life she had always shared a room with her sister. She received her diploma from Cook County in 1944. She later received her bachelor of science degree from the University of Chicago in 1949 and her master of science in nursing from Wayne State University in 1962.

Myra married Edwin Levine in 1944. They had three children. Their first son, Benjamin, died 3 days after birth. Bill and Pat were born several years later. Myra talked of the difficulty of living with the loss of her child, Benoni, but soon found that even this sad event became a blessing to her (Levine, 1988b). She said of her children: "Bearing, nurturing, and growing with children creates parent as person. My children—all three—created me" (Levine, 1988b, p. 223).

Education was always Myra's primary interest, although she had clinical experience in the operating room and in oncology nursing. She was a civilian nurse at the Gardiner General Hospital, director of nursing at Drexel Home in Chicago, clinical instructor at Bryan Memorial Hospital in Lincoln, Nebraska, and administrative supervisor at University of Chicago Clinics and Henry Ford Hospital in Michigan. She was chairperson of clinical nursing at Cook County School of Nursing and a faculty member at Loyola University, Rush University, and University of Illinois. She was a visiting professor at Tel Aviv University in Israel and Recanti School of Nursing at Ben Gurion University of the Negev in Beer Sheeva, Israel. She was professor emeritus in Medical Surgical Nursing, University of Chicago, a charter fellow of the American Association of Nurses (FAAN), and a member of Sigma Theta Tau, from which she received the Elizabeth Russell Belford Award as distinguished educator. She received an honorary doctorate from Loyola University in 1992. Dr. Jacqueline Fawcett, Jane Benson Pond, and I were thrilled to share this momentous event with her. This is when I first met her and learned that she loved pizza as much as I did. I also learned that her hugs were "warm fuzzies."

Myra passed away on March 20, 1996. It was comforting to know that many of her friends were able to spend time with her in her final days. This was a sad day for all those who loved her, especially her family and friends.

INTRODUCTION TO THE FOUNDATIONS FOR CLINICAL NURSING

F. A. Davis Company published the first edition of Myra Levine's textbook, *Introduction to Clinical Nursing*, in 1969, and the second and last edition in 1973. In discussing the first edition of her book, Levine (1969a, p. 39) said: "I decided against using 'holistic' in favor of 'organismic,' largely because the term 'holistic' had been appropriated by pseudoscientists endowing it with the mythology of transcendentalism. I used 'holism' in the second edition in 1973 because I realized it was too important to be abandoned to the mystics. I believed that it was the proper description of the way the internal environment and the external environment were joined in the real world." In the introduction to the second edition, she wrote (Levine, 1973, p. vii):

> There is something very final about a printed page, and yet books do have a life all their own. They gather life from the use to which they are put, and when they succeed in communicating among many individuals in many places, then their intent is most truly served. The most remarkable fact about the first edition of this book has been the exchange of interests that has resulted from the willingness with which its readers and users have communicated with its author.

This passage suggests that Levine's original book (1969) provided a model to teach medical surgical nursing and created a dialogue among colleagues about the plan itself. The text has continued to create dialogue about the art and science of nursing with ongoing research serving as a testament to its value.

Myra's original reason for writing the book was to find a way to teach the foundations of nursing that would be focused on nursing and organized in such a way that nursing students would learn the skill as well as the rationale for the skill. She felt that too often the focus was on skill and not on the reasons why the skill is performed. She felt that nursing research was generally ignored. Her intent was to bring practice and research together to establish nursing as an applied science. The book was used as a beginning nursing text by by Myra and many of her colleagues.

The first chapter of her text was entitled the "Introduction to Patient Centered Nursing Care," a model of care delivery that is now acclaimed to be the answer to cost-effective delivery of health-care services today. She believed that patient-centered care was "individualized nursing care" (Levine, 1973, p. 23). She was truly visionary. She discussed the theory of causation, a unified theory of health and disease, the meaning of the conservation principles, the hospital as environment, and patient-centered intervention. The nursing care chapters in her text focus on nursing care of the patient with:

1. failure of the nervous system,
2. failure of the integration resulting from hormonal imbalance,
3. disturbance of homeostasis: fluid and electrolyte imbalance,
4. disturbance of homeostasis: nutritional needs,

your thoughts

5. disturbance of homeostasis: systemic oxygen needs,
6. disturbance of homeostasis: cellular oxygen needs,
7. disease arising from aberrant cellular growth,
8. inflammatory problems, and
9. holistic response.

Her way of organizing the material was a shift from teaching nursing based on the disease model. Her final chapter on the holistic response represented a major shift away from disease to the systems way of thinking. Informed by other disciplines, she discusses the integrated system, the interaction of systems creating the sense of well-being, energy exchange at the organism level as well as the cellular level, perception of self, the affect of space on self-perception, and the circadian rhythm.

As Myra wrote her book, major changes took place in the curriculum at Cook County Hospital (Levine, 1988b). She and her colleagues began to focus on the importance of nursing research, and taught perception, sleep, distance (space), and periodicity as a factor in health and disease.

THE CONSERVATION MODEL INFORMED BY THE ADJUNCTIVE SCIENCES

Levine used the inductive method to develop her model. She "borrowed" information from other disciplines while retaining the basic structure of nursing in the model (Levine 1988a). As she continued to write about her model, she integrated information from other sciences and increasingly cited personal experiences as evidence of the validity of her work. The following is a list of the influences in the development of her philosophy of nursing and the conservation model.

1. Myra Levine credited Florence Nightingale (1859) with the importance of observation to the process of nursing. Observation is a guardian activity (Levine, 1992). Levine indicated that Nightingale provided great attention to energy conservation and recognized the need for structural integrity. Levine relates Nightingale's discussion of social integrity to Nightingale's concern for sanitation, which she says implies an interaction between the person and the environment.
2. Irene Beland was Myra's teacher and thesis advisor. Beland influenced her thinking about nursing as a compassionate art and rigid intellectual

pursuit (Levine, 1988b). Levine also credited Beland (1971) for the theory of specific causation and multiple factors.
3. Feynman (1965) provided support for Myra's position that conservation was a natural law, arguing that the development of theory cannot deny the importance of natural law (Levine, 1973).
4. Bernard (1957) is recognized for his contribution in the identification of the interdependence of bodily functions (Levine, 1973).
5. Levine (1973) emphasized the dynamic nature of the internal milieu, using Waddington's (1968) term "homeophoresis."
6. Use of Bates's (1967) formulation of the external environment as having three levels of factors—perceptual, operational, and conceptual—challenging the integrity of the individual, helped to emphasize the complexity of the environment.
7. The description of illness is based on Wolf's (1961) description of disease as adaptation to noxious environmental forces.
8. Selye's (1956) definition of "stress" is included in Levine's (1989c, p. 30) description of her organismic stress response as "being recorded over time and . . . influenced by the accumulated experience of the individual."
9. The perceptual organismic response incorporates Gibson's (1966) work on perception as a mediator of behavior. His identification of the five perceptual systems, including hearing, sight, touch, taste, and smell, contributed to the development of the perceptual response.
10. The notion that individuals seek to defend their personhood is grounded in Goldstein's (1963) explanation of the soldiers who, despite brain injury, sought to cling to some semblance of self-awareness.
11. Dubos's (1965) discussion of the adaptability of the organism helped support Levine's explanation that adaptation occurs within a range of responses.
12. Levine's personal experiences influenced her thinking in several ways. When hospitalized, "the experience of wholeness is universally acknowledged," she said (Levine, 1996, p. 39).

THE COMPOSITION OF THE CONSERVATION MODEL

As an organizing framework for nursing practice, the goal of the Conservation Model is to promote adaptation and maintain wholeness using the principles of conservation. The model guides the nurse to focus on the influences and responses at the organismic level. The nurse accomplishes the goals of the model through the conservation of energy, structure, and personal and social integrity (Levine, 1967). Interventions are provided in order to improve the patient's condition (therapeutic) or to promote comfort (supportive) when change in the patient's condition is not possible. The outcomes of the interventions are assessed through the organismic response.

Although Levine identified two concepts critical to the use of her model—adaptation and wholeness—conservation is fundamental to the outcomes expected when the model is used. Conservation is therefore handled as the third major concept of the model.

Adaptation is the process of change, and conservation is the outcome of adaptation. Adaptation is the process whereby the patient maintains integrity within the realities of the environment (Levine, 1966, 1989a). Adaptation is achieved through the "frugal, economic, contained, and controlled use of environmental resources by the individual in his or her best interest" (Levine, 1991, p. 5). In her view:

> The environmental "fit" that underscores successful adaptation suggests that every species has fixed patterns of response uniquely designed to ensure success in essential life activities, demonstrating that adaptation is both historical and specific. However, tremendous opportunities for individual accommodations are locked into the gene structure of each species; every individual is one of a kind.

Every individual has a unique range of adaptive responses. These responses will vary based on heredity, age, gender, or challenges of an illness experience. For example, the response to weakness of the cardiac muscle is an increased heart rate, dilation of the ventricle, and thickening of the myocardial muscle. While the responses are the same, the timing and the manifestation of the organismic response (e.g., pulse rate) will be unique for each individual.

Redundancy, history, and specificity characterize adaptation. These characteristics are "rooted in history and awaiting the specific circumstances to which they respond" (Levine, 1991, p. 6). The genetic structure develops over time and provides the foundation for these responses. Specificity, while sharing traits with a species, has individual potential that creates a variety of adaptation outcomes. For example, diabetes has a genetic component, which explains the fundamental decrease in sugar metabolism. However, the organismic responses vary (renal perfusion, blood vessel integrity), for example, based on genetic alterations, age, gender, and therapeutic management techniques.

Redundancy represents the fail-safe options available to the individual to ensure continued adaptation. Levine (1991) believed that health is dependent on the ability to select from redundant options. She hypothesized that aging may be the result of the failure of redundant systems. If this is the case, then survival is dependent on redundant options, which are often challenged and limited by illness, disease, and aging. When the compensatory response to cardiac disease is no longer able to maintain an adequate blood flow to vital organs during activity, survival becomes increasingly difficult. Adaptation represents the accommodation between the internal and external environments.

Conservation is the product of adaptation and is a common principle underlying many of the basic sciences. Conservation is critical to understanding an essential element of human life:

> Implicit in the knowledge of conservation is the fact of wholeness, integrity, unity—all of the structures that are being conserved . . . conservation of the integrity of the person is essential to ensuring health and providing the strength to confront disability . . . the importance of conservation in the treatment of illness is precisely focused on the reclamation of wholeness, of health . . . Every nursing act is dedicated to the conservation, or "keeping together," of the wholeness of the individual. (Levine, 1991, p. 3)

Individuals are continuously defending their wholeness to keep together the life system. Individuals defend themselves in constant interaction with their environment, choosing the most economic, frugal, and energy-sparing options that safeguard their integrity. Conservation seeks to achieve a balance of energy supply and demand that is within the unique biological capabilities of the individual (Schaefer, 1991a).

Maintaining the proper balance involves the nursing intervention coupled with the patient's participation to assure the activities are within the safe limits of the patient's ability to participate. Although energy cannot be directly observed, the consequences

> The nursing practice goal of the Conservation Model is to promote adaptation and maintain wholeness using principles of conservation.

of energy exchanges are predictable, recognizable, and manageable (Levine, 1973; 1991).

Wholeness is based on Erikson's (1964, p. 63) description of wholeness as an open system: "Wholeness emphasizes a sound, organic, progressive mutuality between diversified functions and parts within an entirety, the boundaries of which are open and fluid." Levine (1973, p. 11) stated that "the unceasing interaction of the individual organism with its environment does represent an 'open and fluid' system, and a condition of health, wholeness, exists when the interaction or constant adaptations to the environment, permit ease—the assurance of integrity . . . in all the dimensions of life." This continuous dynamic, open interaction between the internal and external environment provides the basis for holistic thought, the view of the individual as whole.

Using the model in practice requires that the nurse understand the commonplaces (Barnum, 1994) of health, person, environment, and nursing.

Health and disease are patterns of adaptive change. From a social perspective, health is the ability to function in social roles. Health is culturally determined: "[I]t is not an entity, but rather a definition imparted by the ethos and beliefs of the groups to which the individual belongs" (personal communication, February 21, 1995). Health is an individual response that may change over time in response to new situations, new life challenges, aging; or social, political, economic, and spiritual factors. Health is implied to mean unity and integrity. The goal of nursing is to promote health. Levine (1991, p. 4) clarified what she meant by health as:

> . . . the avenue of return to the daily activities compromised by ill health. It is not only the insult or the injury that is repaired but the person himself or herself. . . . It is not merely the healing of an afflicted part. It is rather a return to self hood, where the encroachment of the disability can be set aside entirely, and the individual is free to pursue once more his or her own interests without constraint.

In all of life challenges, individuals will constantly attempt to attain, retain, maintain, or protect their integrity (health, wholeness, and unity).

The *person* is "a holistic being who is sentient, thinking, future-oriented, and past-aware." The whole-

> Conservation is the product of adaptation and is critical to understanding human life.

ness (integrity) of the individual demands that the "individual life has meaning only in the context of social life" (Levine, 1973, p. 17). The person responds to change in an integrated, sequential, yet singular fashion while in constant interaction with the environment. Levine (1996, p. 40) defined "the person" as a spiritual being, quoting Genesis 1:27: "And God created man in his own image, in the image of God created He him. Male and female created He them. . . . Sanctity of life is manifested in everyone. The holiness of life itself [testifies] to its spiritual reality." "Person" can be an individual, a family, or a community.

The *environment* completes the wholeness of the individual. The individual has both an internal and external environment. The internal environment combines the physiological and pathophysiological aspects of the individual and is constantly challenged by the external environment.

The external environment includes those factors that impinge on and challenge the individual. The environment as described by Levine (1973) was adapted from the three levels of environment identified by Bates (1967). The perceptual environment includes aspects of the world that individuals are able to seize or interpret through the senses. The individual "seeks, selects, and tests information from the environment in the context of his [her] definition of himself [herself], and so defends his [her] safety, his [her] identity, and in a larger sense, his [her] purpose" (Levine, 1971, p. 262). The operational environment includes factors that may physically affect individuals but are not directly perceived by them such as radiation, microorganisms, and pollution. The conceptual environment includes the cultural patterns characterized by spiritual existence and mediated by language, thought, and history. Factors that affect behavior—such as norms, values, and beliefs—are also part of the conceptual environment.

Nursing is "human interaction" (Levine, 1973, p. 1). "The nurse enters into a partnership of human experience where sharing moments in time—some trivial, some dramatic—leaves its mark forever on each patient" (Levine, 1977, p. 845). The goal of nursing is to promote adaptation and maintain wholeness (health). The goal is accomplished through the use of the conservation principles: energy, structure, personal, and social.

Energy conservation is dependent on the free exchange of energy with the internal and external environment to maintain the balance of energy supply and demand. Conservation of structural integrity is dependent on an intact defense system (immune system) that supports heal-ing and repair to pre-serve the structure and function of the whole being.

The conservation of personal integrity ac-knowledges the individ-ual as one who strives for recognition, respect, self-awareness, humanness, self-hood, and self-deter-mination. The conservation of social integrity recog-nizes the individual as a social being who functions in a society that helps to establish boundaries of the self. The value of the individual is recognized, but it is also recognized that the individual resides within a family, a community, a religious group, an ethnic group, a political system, and a nation (Levine, 1973).

The outcome of nursing involves the assessment of organismic responses. The nurse is responsible for [responding to a request for health care] and for rec-ognizing altered health and the patient's organismic response to altered health. An organismic response is a change in behavior or change in the level of func-tioning during an attempt to adapt to the environ-ment. The organismic responses are intended to maintain the patient's integrity. The levels of organis-mic response include (Levine, 1973):

1. *Response to fear (flight/fight response).* This is the most primitive response. It is the physiologi-cal and behavioral readiness to respond to a sud-den and unexpected environmental change; it is an instantaneous response to real or imagined threat.
2. *Inflammatory response.* This is the second level of response intended to provide for structural in-tegrity and the promotion of healing. Both are de-fenses against noxious stimuli and the initiation of healing.
3. *Response to stress.* This is the third level of re-sponse, which is developed over time and influ-enced by each stressful experience encountered by the patient. If the experience is prolonged, the stress can lead to damage to the systems.
4. *Perceptual response.* This is the fourth level of re-sponse. It involves gathering information for the environment and converting it to a meaningful experience.

The organismic responses are redundant in the sense that they coexist. The four responses help individuals

protect and maintain their integrity. They are inte-grated by their cognitive abilities, wealth of previous experiences, ability to define relationships, and the strength of their adaptive abilities.

Nurses use the scientific process and creative abil-ities to provide nursing care to the patient (Schaefer, 1997). The nursing process incorporates these abili-ties, thereby improving the care of the patient (Table 8–1).

PHILOSOPHICAL NOTES

Assumptions

1. The person is viewed as a holistic being: "The experience of wholeness is the foundation of all human enterprises" (Levine, 1991, p. 3).
2. Human beings respond in a singular yet inte-grated fashion.
3. Each individual responds wholly and completely to every alteration in his or her life pattern.
4. Individuals cannot be understood out of the context of their environment.
5. "Ultimately, decisions for nursing care are based on the unique behavior of the individual patient. . . . A theory of nursing must recognize the importance of unique detail of care for a sin-gle patient within an empiric framework which successfully describes the requirements of all pa-tients" (Levine, 1973, p. 6).
6. "Patient centered care means individualized nursing care. It is predicated on the reality of common experience: every man is a unique individual, and as such requires a unique constellation of skills, techniques, and ideas designed specially for him" (Levine, 1973, p. 23).
7. "Every self sustaining system monitors its own behavior by conserving the use of resource re-quired to define its unique identity" (Levine, 1991, p. 4).
8. The nurse is responsible for recognizing the state of altered health and the patient's organis-mic response to altered health.
9. Nursing is a unique contributor to patient care (Levine, 1988a).
10. The patient is in an altered state of health (Levine, 1973). A patient is one who seeks health care because of a desire to remain healthy or identifies a known or possible risk behavior.
11. A guardian angel activity assumes that the nurse accepts responsibility and shows concern based

TABLE 8-1	Use of the Nursing Process According to Levine	
Process	**Application of the Process**	
Assessment Collection of provocative facts through observation and interview of challenges to the internal and external environments.	The nurse observes the patient for organismic responses to illness, reads medical reports, evaluates results of diagnostic studies, and talks with patients and their families (support persons) about their needs for assistance. The nurse assesses for physiological and pathophysiological challenges to the internal environment and the factors in the perceptual, operational, and conceptual levels of the external environment that challenge the individual.	
Trophicognosis* Nursing diagnosis that gives the provocative facts meaning.	The nurse arranges the provocative facts in a way that they provide meaning to the patient's predicament. A judgement is the trophicognosis.**	
Hypotheses Direct the nursing interventions with the goal of maintaining wholeness and promoting adaptation.	Nurses seek validation of the patients' problems with the patients or support persons. The nurses then propose hypotheses about the problems and the solutions, such as: Eight glasses of water a day will improve bowel evacuation. These become the plan of care.	
Interventions Test the hypotheses.	Nurses use hypotheses to direct care. The nurse tests proposed hypotheses. Interventions are designed based on the conservation principles: conservation of energy, structural integrity, person integrity, and social integrity. Interventions are not imposed, but are determined to be mutually acceptable. The expectation is that this approach will maintain wholeness and promote adaptation.	
Evaluation Observation of organismic response to interventions.	The outcome of hypothesis testing is evaluated by assessing for organismic response that means the hypotheses are supported or not supported. Consequences of care are either therapeutic or supportive: therapeutics measures improve the sense of well-being; supportive measures provide comfort when the downward course of illness cannot be influenced. If the hypotheses are not supported, the plan is revised and new hypotheses are proposed.	

*The novice nurse may use the conservation principles at this point to assist with the organization of the provocative facts. The expert nurse integrates this into the environmental assessments.

**Trophicognosis is a nursing care judgement arrived at through the use of the scientific process (Levine, 1965). The scientific process is used to make observations and select relevant data to form hypothetical statements about the patients' predicaments (Schaefer, 1991).

Source: Table 6–1, "Levine's Nursing Process Using Critical Thinking." In M. R. Alligood & A. Marriner-Tomey (Eds.). (1997). *Nursing theory: Utilization and application.* St. Louis: Mosby. Revised and used with permission of Mosby.

on knowledge that makes it possible to decide on the patient's behalf and in his [or her] best interest (Levine, 1973).

Values

1. All nursing actions are moral actions.
2. Two moral imperatives are the sanctity of life and the relief of suffering.
3. Ethical behavior "is the day-to-day expression of one's commitment to other persons and the ways in which human beings relate to one another in their daily interactions" (Levine, 1977, p. 846).

4. A fully informed individual should make decisions regarding life and death in advance of the situations. These decisions are not the role of the health care providers or families (Levine, 1989b).
5. Judgments by nurses or doctors about quality of life are inappropriate and should not be used as a basis for the allocation of care (Levine, 1989b).
6. "Persons who require the intensive interventions of critical care units enter with a contract of trust. To respect trust . . . is a moral responsibility" (Levine, 1988b, p. 88).

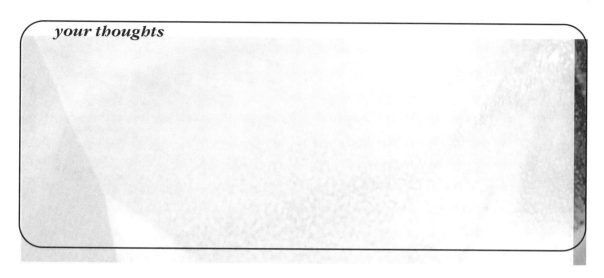

your thoughts

THE MODEL'S FIT WITH PRACTICE

The universality of the model is supported by the use of the model in a variety of situations and patients' conditions across the life span. A growing body of research is providing the support for the development of scientific knowledge related to the model.

Use of the Conservation Model in Practice

The model has been used to guide patient care in settings such as critical care (Brunner, 1985; Langer, 1990; Littrell & Schumann, 1989; Lynn-McHale & Smith, 1991; Tribotti, 1990), acute care (Foreman, 1989, 1991, 1996; Molchany, 1992; Schaefer, 1991a; Schaefer & Shober-Potylycki, 1993; Schaefer, Swavely, Rothenberger, 1996), emergency room (Pond & Taney, 1991), primary care (Pond, 1991), operating room (Crawford-Gamble, 1986), long-term/extended care (Cox, 1991), homeless (Pond, 1997), and the community (Dow & Mest, 1997; Pond, 1991).

This model has been used with a variety of patients across the life span, including the neonate (Tribotti, 1990), infant (Newport, 1984; Savage & Culbert, 1989), young child (Dever, 1991), pregnant woman (Roberts, Fleming, & Yeates-Giese, 1991), young adult (Pasco & Halupa, 1991), long-term ventilator patient (Higgins, 1998), and older adult and elderly patients (Cox, 1991; Foreman, 1991, 1996; Hirschfeld, 1976), including the frail elderly patient. (M. Happ, personal communication, January 31, 1995; Roberts, Brittin, Cook, & deClifford, 1994).

The model has been used as a framework for wound care (Cooper, 1990), managing respiratory illness (Dow & Mest, 1997; Roberts, Brittin, Cook, & deClifford, 1994), managing sleep in the patient with a myocardial infarction (Littrell & Schumann, 1989), developing nursing diagnoses (MacLean, 1989; Taylor, 1989), practicing enterostomal therapy (Neswick, 1997), assessing for changes in bladder function in posthysterectomy women (O'Laughlin, 1986); for developing plans of care for women with chronic illness (Schaefer, 1997), care of intravenous sites (Dibble, Bostrom-Ezrati, & Rizzuto, 1991), and skin care (Burd et al., 1994); for developing day room admission (Clark, Fraaza, Schroeder, & Maddens, 1995); and for care of patients undergoing treatment for cancer (Webb, 1993). Universities and colleges are considering continued and new use of the model as the framework for undergraduate (Grindley & Paradowski, 1991) and graduate programs (Schaefer, 1991b). Current work on the model is in process in the areas of community health. The following is a brief summary of beginning clarification of the model's use in community-based care.

The Conservation Model as a Model for Community-based Care— A Modification of the Model

The principles of community health nursing that are fundamental to community-based care can be practiced in any setting. This particular discussion focuses on community-based care using Levine's Conservation Model to provide a foundation for the future of nursing practice and dispel the myth that the model is inappropriate for the community.

The focus of health in the community is based on the assumption that community-based care is informed often by the one-to-one care provided to individuals. Using Levine's Conservation Model, community was initially defined as "a group of people living

your thoughts

together within a larger society, sharing common characteristics, interests, and location" (*National League for Nursing Self Study Report,* 1978). Clark (1992) provides examples of the use of the conservation principles with the individual, family, and community as a testament to the model's flexibility/ universality.

The approach to community begins with the collection of facts and a thorough assessment (provocative facts). The internal environment assessment directs the nurse to examine the patterns of health and disease among the people of the community and their use of programs available to promote a healthy community. The assessment of the external environment directs the nurse to examine the perceptual, operational, and conceptual levels of the environment in which the people live. The perceptual environment incorporates those factors that are processed by the senses. On a community basis these factors might include an assessment of:

1. how the media affect the health of the people,
2. how the quality of the air influences health patterns and housing development,
3. the availability of nutritious and affordable foods throughout the community,
4. noise pollution, and
5. relationships among the subcultures of the community.

The operational environment would encourage a more detailed assessment of the factors in the environment that affect the health of the individual but are not perceived by the people. These might include assessment for the use of toxins in industry, disposal of waste products, consideration for expo-

sure to radiation from electrical lines, and examination of buildings for asbestos and radon.

The conceptual environment will focus the assessment on the ethnic and cultural patterns in the community. An assessment of types of houses of worship and health-care settings might be included. In this area, the effect of the communities external to the one being assessed would be addressed in order to determine factors that may influence the function of the target community.

The novice nurse will benefit from using the conservation principles to guide continued assessment to assure a thorough understanding of the community. When considering energy conservation, areas to assess might include:

1. hours of employment
2. water supply
3. community budget

An assessment of structural integrity might include:

1. city planning
2. availability of resources
3. transportation
4. public services

Assessment of personal integrity might include:

1. community identity
2. mission of the government
3. political environment

Assessment of the social integrity might include:

1. recreation
2. social services

See Table 8-2, Levine's Conservation Model—Nursing Process in the Community.

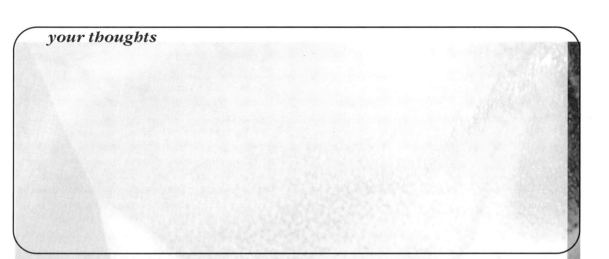

your thoughts

Process	Application of the Process
TABLE 8-2	*Levine's Conservation Model–Nursing Process in the Community*
Assessment Collection of provocative facts through observation and interview.	The nurse uses observation, review of census data, statistics, data from community member interviews, etc. to collect provocative facts about the community. Use of wind shield assessments or other formally developed community assessments are helpful in the collection of data.
Trophicognosis Community Diagnosis.	The nurse organizes that data in such a way as to provide meaning. A judgement or trophicognosis is made.
Hypothesis Directs the nurse to provide interventions that will promote adaptation and maintain wholeness of the community.	In discussion with the members of the community the nurse validates her judgements about the communities predicament. The nurse then proposes hypotheses about the problems and solutions, such as: Providing shelter to abused women will reduce the morbidity associated with continuous uninterrupted abuse.
Interventions Test the hypotheses.	Nurses use the hypotheses to direct the plan of care for the community. The nurse tests the proposed hypotheses to try to remedy the predicament. The nurses select the most appropriate solutions with the help of the community members. Interventions are based on the conservation principles of energy, structural integrity, personal integrity, and social integrity. The shelter for abused women provides for structural integrity of the community while preserving the energy, personal and social integrity of the women who choose shelter.
Evaluation Observation of organismic response to interventions.	The outcome of hypothesis testing is evaluated by assessing for organismic response. For example, an expected outcome of shelters for abused women might be a reduction in emergency visits for injury resulting from suspected abuse or an increase in the number of women who are able to remove themselves from an abusive relationship.

Source: Table 6–1, "Levine's Nursing Process Using Critical Thinking." In M. R. Alligood & A. Marriner-Tomey (Eds.). (1997). *Nursing theory: Utilization and application.* St. Louis: Mosby. Revised and used with permission of Mosby.

RESEARCH BASED ON THE CONSERVATION MODEL

"Nurses are constantly testing what they propose will work in their practice based on what they know" (Schaefer, 1991a, p. 45). This continuous testing expands what is known about practice and offers new insights to improve the practice of nursing. Levine (1973) maintained that research is critical to the development of a scientifically sound body of knowledge for nursing. She felt that the conservation principles offer an approach to nursing that is scientific, research-oriented, and universal in practice. She said that the "focus of research should be on the maintenance of wholeness and the interface between the internal and external environments of the person (Levine, 1978). For the purpose of discovery, and contrary to the notion of wholeness, Levine supported the testing of variables that represent a single integrity. For example, Lane and Winslow (1987) focused on energy conservation, whereas Roberts, Fleming, and (Yeates) Giese (1991) focused on energy conservation and structural integrity. To be true to the model, investigators can explain their findings within the framework and consider how the findings support the goal of promoting adaptation and maintaining wholeness.

Because the model supports understanding and description, both qualitative and quantitative approaches are appropriate to develop the model and theories derived from the model. The qualitative approach helps to explain how the patient experiences the challenges to their internal and external environments. The quantitative approach helps to test the relationships between the variables, and, in some cases, provides for the testing of causal models. These predictive models help clinicians alter the environments to promote adaptation and maintain wholeness.

Combining qualitative and quantitative (triangulation) approaches to the study concepts using Levine's model helps to preserve the art and the science of nursing. Interactions with patients are both predictive and creative. Qualitative research helps to provide a way for the nurses to share the creative aspects of their work in a way that they can be shared again and again. Qualitative data help to explain the quantitative data and provide a more holistic perspective regarding the data experience.

Several investigators have contributed significant research to the support and expansion of the Conservation Model as a model for nursing practice. Theories developed from the model will provide propositions from which hypotheses can be developed and tested. Following is a summary of the conclusions of research using the Conservation Model as a framework.

1. Responding to involuntary urges was as efficient as, and resulted in less perineal damage than, sustained breath holding during the second stage of labor (Yeates & Roberts, 1984). There were no differences in the mean duration of the second stage of labor between the two groups.
2. Interventions that are employed as a course of routine rather than based on individual needs actually increase the physiological burden of healing following birth and act as a significant threat to the psychological adjustments of the postpartum period (Fleming, 1988).
3. Conservation of energy can be maintained by placing the infant skin to skin on the mother's chest, covered with a warm blanket (Newport, 1984).
4. Ludington (1990) found that simple skin-to-skin contact was effective in reducing activity and state-related energy expenditure in the newborn of 34 to 36 weeks' gestation.
5. An initial study of patients with rheumatoid arthritis who engaged in a balance of physical activity and rest increased their activity more than patients in the control group. Rest served as a restorative measure.
6. There is no significant difference in energy expenditure between basin, tub, or shower bathing 5 to 17 days postmyocardial infarction (Winslow, Lane, & Gaffney, 1985). The differences that did exist were related more to subject variability than the type of bathing. The experimental group had significantly lower oxygen consumption than did the control group.
7. There are no significant differences in oxygen consumption when comparing unoccupied and occupied bed making, but it was significantly higher than when at rest. Heart rate differed significantly between rest and unoccupied bed making. The researchers concluded that the findings provide no basis for restricting either bed-making technique (Lane & Winslow, 1987).
8. Generally the use of water beds for preterm infants produces a soothing effect and reduces activity. However, the expected reduction in heart rate as a measure of energy cost does not occur. The use of heart rate as a measure of energy use needs further investigation. The high variability among and within subjects raises questions about the value of heart rate as a measure of energy cost.

9. Age, arterial pressure on bypass, and body temperature on the first and third postoperative days best predicts delirious patients (Foreman, 1989). Acutely confused patients were differentiated best from those not confused by 10 variables representing all four conservation principles.

10. Foreman (1996) is in the process of analyzing measures of cognition and psychophysiological variables associated with delirium in the elderly. The four conservation principles provided the basis for the selection of variables. The results, as of 1996, supported the conclusion through confirmatory factor analysis that the model explained 87.3% of the variance in cognition. The results also support that the Conservation Model of Nursing is a framework with which to examine complex clinical phenomena, and for deriving effective plans of care for preventing and treating delirium in this vulnerable population.

11. Higgens (1998) found that fatigue was present in ventilator patients 100% of the time, and that fatigue and depression were significantly correlated. Despite the fact that sleep disturbances were present and nutrition was compromised, there were no significant relationships with fatigue.

12. Boomerang pillows used to provide comfort are safe for individuals who are healthy and do not have respiratory problems (Roberts, Brittin, Cook, & deClifford, 1994). The use of the pillows does not interfere with energy conservation. A secondary finding was that vital capacity was significantly lower in the semi-Fowler's position than in a straight chair.

13. After 10 minutes on boomerang pillows, frail elderly patients experienced a significant reduction in vital capacity (Roberts, Brittin, & deClifford, 1995). Boomerang pillows interfere with energy conservation in women whose respiratory capacity is compromised by age.

14. Schaefer's (1991b; Schaefer & Shober-Potylycki, 1993) research supports the finding that the experience of fatigue in congestive heart failure is an experience that affects one's whole sense of being.

Winslow (personal communication, October 14, 1993) indicated that an important outcome of her studies of bathing and toileting was that hospitalized patients had a significantly lower oxygen consumption during these activities than did healthy subjects. Patients moved more slowly and deliberately than did the healthy subjects. Consistent with Levine's (1973, p. 7) notion that we "reduce activity to that which is absolutely necessary," patients seem to reduce activity on their own to promote healing. Levine (1989, p. 332) later stated that:

> The conservation of energy is clearly evident in the very sick, whose lethargy, withdrawal, and self-concern are manifested while, in its wisdom, the body is spending its energy resource on the processes of healing.

Many of the studies using the Conservation Model as the basis for the investigation are single studies or the beginning research program development. There is no replication and little consistency in how the variables are measured. The results of the studies are therefore not sufficient to change nursing practice but they do cluster in two areas that with continued study could have a major influence on how nurses practice.

In general, the studies support that energy can be conserved with nursing interventions and can be measured through the assessment of organismic responses. Patients inherently conserve their own energy when confronted with environmental challenges. The second important finding is that attention to the conservation principles explains the organismic response of confusion (delirium) better than does any single principle alone. This supports the assumption that using the conservation principles to guide interventions will promote adaptation and maintain wholeness.

> Three major concepts of Levine's model are critical to health-care delivery of the future: adaptation, wholism, and conservation.

Investigators are encouraged to continue their excellent work with Levine's model. New investigators are encouraged to consider the Conservation Model as a basis for study and to test the propositions developed from the theories discussed later in this chapter. It is only with continued research that a scientific basis for nursing will be developed.

THE CONSERVATION MODEL IN THE TWENTY-FIRST CENTURY

Nurses of the future will continue to build on the basic principles of nursing established by Florence Nightingale (1859). Nightingale was a visionary woman who knew that nurses should be prepared professionals in institutions of higher education. Myra Levine continued in this tradition and focused a great deal of her professional career on preparing advanced practice nurses as clinical nurse specialists.

Nurses of the future will be leaders in health care. Their leadership will increasingly provide direction for care in community settings and less in acute care settings. The skills and knowledge required of these nurses will include:

1. an understanding of the predicaments associated with health promotion, health restoration, health maintenance, and illness prevention;
2. a working knowledge of health care and information systems, marketing and financial management, strategic planning, and program development and evaluation;
3. the ability to practice as professionals in a variety of settings, and to direct and manage personnel;
4. the ability to assess the value of and provide complementary therapies to appropriate patients; and
5. the ability to make contributions to the understanding and the maintenance of quality care delivery systems through program evaluation and research to support evidence based practice.

Levine's Conservation Model and the theories developed from the model provide a basis for the future of professional nursing. The model includes a method for assessment; identification of problems; development of a hypothesis about the problem; the identification, selection, and application of an intervention; and an evaluation of the response. The interventions are provided based on the assumption that if the intervention attends to the conservation of energy, structural, social, and personal integrities, the patient will return to wholeness (health). Health is a goal for individuals, families, communities, and populations at large. From a global perspective, "health for all" is an appropriate metaphor. Wholeness is universally understood. The model includes three major concepts that are critical to understanding the healthcare delivery systems of the future: adaptation, wholism (health), and conservation (balance of energy supply and demand within the capabilities of the patient [organization, community, and universe]).

The Conservation Model provides the conceptual basis for the development of three theories: the Theory of Conservation, the Theory of Redundancy, and the Theory of Therapeutic Intention. About theory, Levine said:

1. "The serious study of any discipline requires a theoretical baseline which gives it substance and meaning" (Levine, 1969a, p. xi).
2. "The essential science concepts develop the rationale [for nursing actions], using ideas from all areas of knowledge that contribute to the development of the nursing process in the specific area of the model" (cited in Fawcett, 1995, p. 136).
3. Nursing theory should define the boundaries of nursing.
4. "Nursing theory is too important an enterprise to be undertaken without the strictest rules of scientific discovery and explanation. . . . It is the researcher who should challenge the cherished ideas and find the data that will support or refute the theorist's claims. The practitioner must provide the ultimate test of relevance to the theorist's work. Unless the theory can be interpreted by the nurse who reaches the patient wherever nursing is practiced, theory will remain a questionable entity . . . theory should teach nurses what they are" (Levine, 1988a, pp. 20–21).
5. It is essential that concepts that are shared from other disciplines are accurately reproduced and used appropriately (Levine, 1996). The sharing of concepts from other disciplines has enhanced nursing scholarship and provided nurses with the knowledge and skills to provide holistic care.
6. "At every level where theory is taught . . . the content of courses in nursing theory ought to excite what Brunner (1985) called the effective surprise, where the combination of recognition and discovery adds new dimensions to nursing practice" (Levine, 1995, p. 12).
7. "[I]t is imperative that there be a variety [of nursing theories]—for there is no global theory of nursing that fits every situation" (Levine, 1995, p. 13).
8. "Not everything that is accepted as theory now can—nor should—survive, but 'serious intellectual inquiry' will create new theories, and nursing can only prosper when it does" (Levine, 1995, p. 14).

In summary, Levine proposed that nursing theory is an adjunctive science, provides for the development of the intellectual component of nursing essential for understanding the why of nursing actions, is tested through use by practitioners, is not universal in the sense that there is no one global theory of nursing that will fit all situations, and should be refined and further developed by new researchers. She noted that some theories might be time limited and new theories would be developed. Levine's work continues to encourage the intellectual pursuits of "her" students. We learn and grow as we continue to review and reinterpret her work in preparation for the future of nursing.

Alligood (1997) first made the Theory of Conservation explicit. The Theory of Conservation is rooted in the concept of conservation and is based on the assumption that all nursing actions are conservation principles (Levine, 1973, p. 13). Conservation is natural law that is fundamental to many basic sciences. The purpose of conservation is "to keep together." "To keep together means to maintain a proper balance between active nursing interventions coupled with patient participation on the one hand and the safe limits of the patients' abilities to participate on the other." The Theory of Conservation is based on the universal principle of conservation, which provides the foundation for the conservation principles in the model. Conservation assures wholeness, integrity, and unity.

The conservation principles form the major propositions (Levine, 1973, pp. 444, 446, and 13):

1. The individual is always within an environment milieu, and the consequences of his awareness of his environment persistently influence his behavior at any given moment.
2. The individual protects and defends himself within his environment by gaining all the information he can about it.
3. The nurse participates actively in every patient's environment, and much of what she does supports his adaptations as he struggles in the predicament of illness.
4. Even in the presence of disease, the organism responds wholly to the environment interaction in which it is involved, and considerable element of nursing care is devoted to restoring the symmetry of response—symmetry that is essential to the well-being of the organism (Levine, 1969b, p. 98).

The Theory of Therapeutic Intention was developed with the intent of providing a way to organize nursing interventions out of the biological realities that nurses had to confront (Fawcett, 1995). The biological realities faced by nurses include areas of concern that focus on living organisms; their structure, form, function, behavior, growth, and development; and relationships to their environment and organisms like and unlike themselves. Given the biological realities of health, illness, and disease, nurses are organizing interventions across the life span, in a variety of settings, and based on the principles drawn from nursing and other disciplines (epidemiology, psychology, sociology, theology, etc.). The Theory of Therapeutic Intention is directly related to the biological realities. Therefore, the guiding assumptions for this theory are:

1. Conservation is the outcome of adaptation.
2. Change associated with therapeutic intervention results in adaptation.
3. The proper application of conservation (conservation principles) results in the restoration of health.
4. Activities directed toward the preservation of health include health promotion, surveillance, illness prevention, and follow-up activities.

According to Fawcett, Levine (cited in Fawcett, 1995) identified the following goals of the Theory of Therapeutic Intention:

1. Facilitate integrated healing and optimal restoration of structure and function [by supporting and enhancing] the natural response to disease. This goal can be reached if the nurse caring for a patient with burns changes dressing as ordered, provides medication to reduce the pain associated with treatment, offers complementary pain-reducing techniques, listens carefully to the concerns the patient may have regarding self related to scarring from the burns, refers to appropriate counseling, and works closely with the family or support persons to maintain connections for the patient.
2. Provide support for a failing autoregulatory portion of the integrated system (e.g., medical/surgical treatments).
3. Restore individual integrity and well-being (e.g., work with children with ADHD—attention deficit hyperactivity disorder).
4. Provide supportive measures to assure comfort and promote human concern when therapeutic measures are not possible (e.g., care of the dying).
5. Balance a toxic risk against the threat of disease (e.g., nurses who facilitate immunization).
6. Manipulate diet and activity to correct metabolic imbalances and to stimulate physiological processes (e.g., care of the anorexic young woman).
7. Reinforce or antagonize usual response to create a therapeutic change (e.g., enhance pain relief with music therapy).

The expected outcome of therapeutic intentions would be a therapeutic response measured by the organismic change (e.g., adaptation resulting in conservation).

The Theory of Redundancy is grounded in the concept of adaptation. Change is the process of adaptation and conservation is the outcome of adaptation. The Theory of Redundancy assumes that there are fail-safe options available in the physiological, anatomical, and psychological responses of individuals that are employed in the development of patient care. The body has more than one way for its function to be accomplished. It involves a series of adaptive responses (cascade of integrated responses—simultaneous, not separate) available when the stability of the organism is challenged (Schaefer, 1991b). The selection of an option rests with the knowledge of the health-care provider in consultation with the patient. When redundant choices are lost, survival becomes difficult and ultimately fails for lack of fail-safe options—either those that the patient possesses (e.g., two lungs) or those that can be employed on his or her behalf (e.g., medications or a pacemaker) (Levine, 1991).

Summary

Levine's notion of the environment as complex provides an excellent basis for continuing to develop an improved understanding of the environment. Studying the interactions between the external and the internal environment will provide for a better understanding of adaptation. This focus will provide for additional information about the challenges in the external environment and how they change over time. It is important that we understand the changes that occur and how the person who adapted before now changes the adaptive response in order to maintain balance or integrity. This adaptive response will inform the organismic response. With an improved repertoire of organismic responses we can test how to predict these responses, hence assure that the responses that are adaptive will occur. This is said with the understanding that nurses recognize when the goal is to maintain comfort only (e.g., supportive interventions).

Moving to a more global perspective, the environment as defined according to Levine (1973) provides nurses with the opportunity to enhance their understanding of it and to provide interventions for communities that suffer from environmental disasters. An assessment of the internal environment's response to the challenge of the external environment (e.g., destruction from hurricanes) will identify the altered health status of the community and the community needs immediately. An assessment of the external environment will provide an understanding of the changes occurring due to the assault on the internal environment and a more detailed assessment of the perceptive, organismic, and conceptual levels of the environmental challenges. There is no question that this approach to describing, defining, and planning for environmental challenges will identify (1) the

perceptual challenges, (2) the organismic challenges that may not be immediately known to the residents (e.g., pollution of air and water), and (3) the conceptual issues that increase the nurses' awareness of the social, political, and economic impact on the predicament. This provides the nurses with the opportunity to develop a political agenda and perhaps design public policy that might improve interventions in the context of a disaster. The Conservation Model has the components needed to provide nurses with a global perspective of the environment.

Future practitioners and researchers are encouraged to continue to focus on studies that will develop and enhance the model as well as the theories of conservation, therapeutic intention, and redundancy. Schaefer (1991a, p. 223) expressed excitement about the development of the Theory of Therapeutic Intention because, "[n]ot only will the nurse have a repertoire of tested interventions, given that a theory provides specific information about care delivery, but [the nurse] also . . . should have information about the expected responses. With this in mind, the theory provides the direction for quality [improvement] activities and measure of cost effectiveness." Nurses are encouraged to test interventions guided by the propositions of the theory to define further the boundaries of nursing practice.

Development of the theories of conservation and redundancy is also encouraged. It is suggested that the natural law of conservation be thoroughly examined in all disciplines with attention to the implications for nursing practice. A brief search revealed that many studies address the issue of conservation without the use of the Conservation Model as a foundation. It is possible that the completed studies will provide parameters for the issue of conservation in nursing and substantiate its significance to a Theory of Conservation for nursing.

Two areas appropriate to the Theory of Redundancy are important to nursing practice and warrant further investigation: the importance of choice in the management of an individual's health and the significance of availability of fail-safe options. Although there is evidence that patients benefit from a feedback system, compensatory systems, and two kidneys, lungs, and eyes, the value of this knowledge for the practice of nursing must be carefully investigated. This theory will benefit all health-care providers and perhaps provide a foundation for collaborative practice (e.g., consider the context in which kidney transplantation takes place). As more choices become available for patients, development of this theory becomes imperative. To enhance the development of knowledge, scientists may want to consider an integrated theory that considers the principles associated with redundancy and moral theory. Levine's perspective on ethical and moral care has been made explicit (Levine, 1977, 1982a, 1982b, 1989b, 1989c, 1989d).

Levine's (1968a, 1968b, 1973) discussion of the person includes recognition that the person is defined to a certain degree based on the boundaries defined by Hall (1966) as personal space. Levine rejected the notion that energy can be manipulated and transferred from one human to another as in therapeutic touch. Yet a person is affected by the presence of another relative to his or her personal space boundaries. Admittedly some of this is defined based on cultural ethos, yet what is it about the "bubble" that results in a specific organismic response? It may be that the energy involved in the interaction is not clearly defined. Scientists are challenged to examine this. Levine encouraged creativity such as therapeutic touch but rejected activities that are not scientifically sound.

And finally, the practice of nurses and advanced practice nurses is changing rapidly to keep up with the current speed of health-care system changes. Levine's Conservation Model provides an approach that educates good nurses and provides a foundation for their practice, whatever the role or the setting. Nurse practitioners, case managers, program planners, nurse midwives, nurse anesthetists, and nurse entrepreneurs are encouraged to test the model as a basis for improving and guiding their practice. Whatever the results, they should publish them to assure the continued development of the art and science of nursing. Myra will applaud their efforts.

Theory is the poetry of science. The poet's words are familiar each standing alone, but brought together they sing, they astonish, they teach. The theorist offers a fresh vision, familiar concepts brought together in bold, new designs . . . the theorist and poet seek excitement in the sudden insights that make ordinary experience extraordinary, but theory caught in the intellectual exercises of the academy becomes alive only when it is made a true instrument of persuasion. (Levine, 1995, p. 14)

References

Alligood, M. R. (1997). Models and theories: Critical thinking structures. In Alligood, M. R., & Marriner-Tomey, A. (Eds.), *Nursing theory: Utilization and application* (pp. 31–45). St. Louis: Mosby.

Barnum, B. J. S. (1994). *Nursing theory:Analysis, application, evaluation* (4th ed.). Philadelphia: J. B. Lippincott.

Bates, M. (1967). A naturalist at large. *Natural History, 76,* 8–16.

Beland, I. (1971). *Clinical nursing:Pathophysiological and psychological implications* (2nd ed.). New York: Dover.

Bernard, C. (1957). *An introduction to the study of experimental medicine.* New York: Dover.

Bruner, J. (1979). *On knowing:Essays for the left hand.* New York: Argenaemun.

Brunner, M. (1985). A conceptual approach to critical care nursing using Levine's model. *Focus on Critical Care, 12*(2), 39–44.

Burd, C., Olson, B., Langemo, D., Hunter, S., Hanson, D., Osowki, K. F., & Sauvage, T. (1994). Skin care strategies in a skilled nursing home. *Journal of Gerontological Nursing, 20*(11), 28–34.

Clark, L. R., Fraaza, V., Schroeder, S., & Maddens, M. E. (1995). Alternative nursing environments: Do they affect hospital outcomes. *Journal of Gerontological Nursing, 21*(11), 32–38.

Clark, M. J. (1992). *Nursing in the community.* Norwalk, CT: Appleton & Lange.

Cooper, D. H. (1990). Optimizing wound healing: A practice within nursing's domain. *Nursing Clinics of North America, 25*(1), 165–180.

Cox, R. A. Sr. (1991). A tradition of caring: Use of Levine's model in long-term care. In Schaefer, K. M., & Pond, J. B. (Eds.), *The conservation model:A framework for nursing practice* (pp. 179–197). Philadelphia: F. A. Davis.

Crawford-Gamble, P. E. (1986). An application of Levine's conceptual model. *Perioperative Nursing Quarterly, 2*(1), 64–70.

Dever, M. (1991). Care of children. In Schaefer, K. M., & Pond, J. B. (Eds.), *The conservation model:A framework for nursing practice* (pp. 71–83). Philadelphia: F. A. Davis.

Dibble, S. L., Bostrom-Ezerati, J., & Ruzzuto, C. (1991). Clinical predictors of intravenous site symptoms. *Research in Nursing & Health, 14,* 413–420.

Dow, J. S., & Mest, C. G. (1997). Psychosocial interventions for patients with chronic obstructive pulmonary disease. *Home-Healthcare-Nurse, 15*(6), 414–420.

Dubos, R. (1965). *Man adapting.* New Haven: Yale University Press.

Erickson, E. H. (1964). *Insight and responsibility.* New York: W. W. Norton & Co.

Fawcett, J. (1995). *Conceptual models of nursing* (3rd ed.). Philadelphia: F. A. Davis.

Feynman, R. (1965). *The character of physical law.* Cambridge, MA: MIT Press.

Fleming, N. (1988). Comparison of women with different perineal conditions after childbirth. *Dissertation Abstracts International, 48,* 2924B. Microfilm No. 8728762.

Foreman, M. D. (1989). Confusion in the hospitalized elderly: Incidence, onset, and associated factors. *Research in Nursing & Health, 12*(1), 21–29.

Foreman, M. D. (1991). Conserving cognitive integrity of the hospitalized elderly. In Schaefer, K. M., & Pond, J. B. (Eds.), *The conservation model:A frame-*

work for nursing practice (pp. 133-150). Philadelphia: F. A. Davis.

Foreman, M. D. (1996). The evolution of delirium. Abstract. Midwest Nursing Research Society. Kansas City, MO.

Gibson, J. E. (1966). The senses considered as perceptual systems. Boston: Houghton Mifflin.

Goldstein, K. (1963). The organism. Boston: Beacon Press.

Grindley, J., & Paradowski, M. B. (1991). Developing an undergraduate program using Levine's model. In Schaefer, K. M., & Pond, J. B. (Eds.), The conservation model: A framework for nursing practice (pp. 199-208). Philadelphia: F. A. Davis.

Hall, E. (1966). The hidden dimension. Garden City, NY: Doubleday.

Happ, M. B., Williams, C. C., Strumpf, N. E., & Burger, S. G. (1996). Individualized care for frail elderly: Theory and Practice, Journal of Gerontological Nursing, 22(3), 7-14.

Higgins, P. A. (1998). Patients' perception of fatigue while undergoing long-term mechanical ventilation: Incidence and associated factors. Heart and Lung: Journal of Acute and Critical Care, 27(3), 177-183.

Hirschfeld, M. H. (1976). The cognitively impaired older adult. American Journal of Nursing, 76, 1981-1984.

Lane, L. D., & Winslow, E. H. (1987). Oxygen consumption, cardiovascular response, and perceived exertion in healthy adults during rest, occupied bedmaking, and unoccupied bedmaking activity. Cardiovascular Nursing, 23(6), 31-36.

Langer, V. S. (1990). Minimal handling protocol for the intensive care nursery. Neonatal Network, 9(3), 23-27.

Levine, M. E. (1965). Trophicognosis: An alternative to nursing diagnosis. ANA Regional Clinical Conferences, 2, 55-70.

Levine, M. E. (1966). Adaptation and assessment: A rationale for nursing intervention. American Journal of Nursing, 66, 2450-2453.

Levine, M. E. (1967). The four conservation principles of nursing. Nursing Forum, 6, 45-59.

Levine, M. E. (1968a). Knock before entering personal space bubbles (Part I). Chart, 65(1), 58-62.

Levine, M. E. (1968b). Knock before entering personal space bubbles (Part II). Chart, 65(2), 82-84.

Levine, M. E. (1969a). Introduction to clinical nursing. Philadelphia: F. A. Davis.

Levine, M. E. (1969b). The pursuit of wholeness. American Journal of Nursing, 69, 93-98.

Levine, M. E. (1971). Holistic nursing. Nursing Clinics of North America, 6(2), 253-263.

Levine, M. E. (1973). Introduction to clinical nursing (2nd ed.). Philadelphia: F. A. Davis.

Levine, M. E. (1977). Nursing ethics and the ethical nurse. American Journal of Nursing, 77(5), 845-849.

Levine, M. E. (1978). Cancer chemotherapy: A nursing model. Nursing Clinics of North American, 13(2), 271-280.

Levine, M. E. (1982a). Bioethics of cancer nursing. Rehabilitation Nursing 7, 27-31, 41.

Levine, M. E. (1982b). The bioethics of cancer nursing. Journal of Enterostomal Therapy, 9, 11-13.

Levine, M. E. (1988a). Antecedents from adjunctive disciplines: Creation of nursing theory. Nursing Science Quarterly, 1(1), 16-21.

Levine, M. E. (1988b). Myra Levine. In T. M. Schoor & A. Zimmerman (Eds.), Making choices, taking chances: Nurse leaders tell their stories (pp. 215-228). St. Louis: C. V. Mosby.

Levine, M. E. (1989a). The conservation model: Twenty years later. In J. P. Riehl-Sisca (Ed.), Conceptual models for nursing practice (pp. 325-337). Norwalk, CT: Appleton & Lange.

Levine, M. E. (1989b). Ration or rescue: The elderly in critical care. Critical Care Nursing, 12(1), 82-89.

Levine, M. E. (1989c). The ethics of nursing rhetoric. Image: Journal of Nursing Scholarship, 21(1), 4-5.

Levine, M. E. (1989d). Beyond dilemma. Seminars in Oncology Nursing, 5, 124-128.

Levine, M. E. (1991). The conservation model: A model for health. In Schaefer, K. M., & Pond, J. B. (Eds.), The conservation model: A framework for nursing practice (pp. 1-11). Philadelphia: F. A. Davis.

Levine, M. E. (1992). Nightingale redux. In B. S. Barnum (Ed.), Nightingale's notes on nursing. Philadelphia: J. B. Lippincott.

Levine, M.E. (1995). The rhetoric of nursing theory. Image: Journal of Nursing Scholarship, 27(2), 11-14.

Levine, M. E. (1996). The conservation principles: A retrospective. Nursing Science Quarterly, 9(1), 38-41.

Littrell, K., & Schumann, L. (1989). Promoting sleep for the patient with a myocardial infarction. Critical Care Nurse, 9(3), 44-49.

Ludington, S. M. (1990). Energy conservation during skin-to-skin contact between premature infants and their mothers. Heart & Lung, 19(5), 445-451.

Lynn-McHale, D. J., & Smith, A. (1991). Comprehensive assessment of families of the critically ill. In Leske, J. S. (Ed.), AACN clinical issues in critical care nursing (pp. 195-209). Philadelphia: J. B. Lippincott.

MacLean, S. L. (1989). Activity intolerance: Cues for diagnosis. In Carroll-Johnson, R. M. (Ed.), Classification proceedings of the Eighth Annual Conference of North American Nursing Diagnosis Association (pp. 320-327). Philadelphia: J. B. Lippincott.

Mid-Year Convocation: Loyola University, Chicago. The Conferring of Honorary Degrees by R. C. Baumhart. Candidate for the degree of Doctor of Humane Letters, 1992, p. 6.

Molchany, C. A. (1992). Ventricular septal and free wall rupture complicating acute MI. Journal of Cardiovascular Nursing, 6(4), 38-45.

National League for Nursing Self Study Report. (1978). Allentown College of St. Francis de Sales, Department of Nursing.

Neswick, R. S. (1997). Myra E. Levine: A theoretical basis for ET nursing. Professional Practice, 24(1), 6-9.

Newport, M. A. (1984). Conserving thermal energy and social integrity in the newborn. Western Journal of Nursing Research, 6(2), 175-197.

Nightingale, F. (1859). Notes on nursing: What it is, and what it is not. London: Harrison & Sons.

O'Laughlin, K. M. (1986). Change in bladder function in the woman undergoing radical hysterectomy for cervical cancer. Journal of Obstetric, Gynecologic and Neonatal Nursing, 15(5), 380-385.

Section II *Evolution of Nursing Theory: Essential Influences*

Pasco, A., & Halupa, D. (1991). Chronic pain management. In Schaefer, K. M., & Pond, J. B. (Eds.), *The conservation model: A framework for nursing practice* (pp. 101–117). Philadelphia: F. A. Davis.

Pond, J. B. (1991). Ambulatory care of the homeless. In Schaefer, K. M., & Pond, J. B. (Eds.), *The conservation model: A framework for nursing practice* (pp. 167–178). Philadelphia: F. A. Davis.

Pond, J. B., & Taney, S. G. (1991). Emergency care in a large university emergency department. In Schaefer, K. M., & Pond, J. B. (Eds.), *The conservation model: A framework for nursing practice* (pp. 151–166). Philadelphia: F. A. Davis.

Roberts, J. E., Fleming, N., & (Yeates) Giese, D. (1991). Perineal integrity. In Schaefer, K. M., & Pond, J. B. (Eds.), *The conservation model: A framework for nursing practice* (pp. 61–70). Philadelphia: F. A. Davis.

Roberts, K. L., Brittin, M., Cook, M., & deClifford, J. (1994). Boomerang pillows and respiratory capacity. *Clinical Nursing Research, 3*(2), 157–165.

Roberts, K. L., Brittin, M., & deClifford, J. (1995). Boomerang pillows and respiratory capacity in frail elderly women. *Clinical Nursing Research, 4*(4), 465–471.

Savage, T. A., & Culbert, C. (1989). Early interventions: The unique role of nursing. *Journal of Pediatric Nursing, 4*(5), 339–345.

Schaefer, K. M. (1991a). Levine's conservation principles and research. In Schaefer, K. M., & Pond, J. B. (Eds.), *The conservation model: A framework for nursing practice* (pp. 45–59). Philadelphia: F. A. Davis.

Schaefer, K. M. (1991b). Care of the patient with congestive heart failure. In Schaefer, K. M., & Pond, J. B. (Eds.), *The conservation model: A framework for nursing practice* (pp. 119–132). Philadelphia: F. A. Davis.

Schaefer, K. M. (1997). Levine's conservation model: Use of the model in practice. In Alligood, M. R., & Marriner-Tomey, A. (Eds.), *Nursing theories: Utilization and practice* (89–107), St. Louis: Mosby.

Schaefer, K. M., & Pond, J. B. (1994). Levine's conservation model as a guide to nursing practice. *Nursing Science Quarterly, 7*(2), 53–54.

Schaefer, K. M., & Shober-Potylycki, M. J. (1993). Fatigue associated with congestive heart failure: Use of Levine's Conservation Model. *Journal of Advanced Nursing, 18,* 260–268.

Schaefer, K. M., Swavely, D., Rothenberger, C., Hess, S., & Willistin, D. (1996). Sleep disturbances post coronary artery bypass surgery. *Progress in Cardiovascular Nursing, 11*(1), 5–14.

Schaefer, K. M. et al. (1998). Myra Estrin Levine: The Conservation Model. In Tomey, A. M., & Alligood, M. R. (Eds.), *Nursing theorists and their work* (4th ed., pp. 195–206). St. Louis: Mosby.

Selye, H. (1956). *The stress of life.* New York: McGraw-Hill.

Taylor, J. W. (1989). Levine's conservation principles: Using the model for nursing diagnosis in a neurological setting. In Riehl-Sisca, J. P. (Ed.), *Conceptual models for nursing practice* (3rd ed., pp. 349–358). Norwalk, CT: Appleton & Lange.

Tribotti, S. (1990). Admission to the neonatal intensive care unit: Reducing the risks. *Neonatal Network, 8*(4), 17–22.

Waddington, C. H. (Ed.). (1968). *Towards a theoretical biology: I. Prolegomena.* Chicago: Aldine.

Webb, H. (1993). Holistic care following palliative Hartmann's procedure. *British Journal of Nursing, 2*(2), 128–132.

Winslow, E. H., Lane, L. D., & Gaffney, F. A. (1985). Oxygen consumption and cardiovascular response in patients and normal adults during in-bed and out-of-bed toileting. *Journal of Cardiac Rehabilitation, 4,* 348–354.

Wolf, S. (1961). Disease as a way of life: Neural integration in systemic pathology. *Perspectives on Biological Medicine, 5,* 288–303.

Yeates, D. A., & Roberts, J. E. (1984). A comparison of two bearing-down techniques during the second stage of labor. *Journal of Nurse Midwifery, 29,* 3–11.

Bibliography

Bunting, S. M. (1988). The concept of perception in selected nursing theories. *Nursing Science Quarterly, 1*(4), 39–44.

Fawcett, J., Tulman, L., & Samarel, N. (1995). Enhancing function in life transitions and serious illness. *Advanced Practice Nursing, 1*(3), 50–57.

Fawcett, J., Brophy, S. F., Rather, M. L., & Ross, J. (1997). Commentary about Levine's *On Creativity in Nursing. Image: Journal of Nursing Scholarship, 29*(3), 218–219.

Flaskerud, J. H., & Halloran, E. J. (1980). Areas of agreement in nursing theory development. *Advances in Nursing Sciences, 3*(1), 1–17.

Frauman, A. C., & Rasch, R. T. R. (1995, Winter). Myra Levine, At last a clear voice of reason [Letter to the editor]. *Image: Journal of Nursing Scholarship, 27,* 262.

Griffith-Kenney, J. W., & Christensen, P. (1986). *Nursing process: Application of theories, frameworks, and models* (pp. 6, 24–25), St. Louis: Mosby.

Hall, K. V. (1979). Current trends in the use of conceptual frameworks in nursing education. *Journal of Nursing Education. 18*(4), 26–29.

Leonard, M. K. (1990). Myra Estrin Levine. In George, J. B. (Ed.), *Nursing theories: The base for professional nursing practice* (pp. 181–192). Englewood Cliffs, N.J: Prentice-Hall.

Levine, M. E. (1963). Florence Nightingale: The legend that lives. *Nursing Forum, 2*(4), 24–35.

Levine, M. E. (1964). Not to startle, though the way were deep. *Nursing Science, 2*(4), 58–67.

Levine, M. E. (1964). There need be no anonymity. *First, 18*(9), 4.

Levine, M. E. (1965a). The professional nurse and graduate education. *Nursing Science, 3,* 206–214.

Levine, M. E. (1965). Trophicognosis: An alternative to nursing diagnosis, *ANA Regional Clinical Conferences, 2,* 55–70.

Levine, M. E. (1967a). Medicine-nursing dialogue belongs at patient's bedside. *Chart, 64*(5), 136–137.

Levine, M. E. (1967b). This I believe about patient-centered care. *Nursing Outlook, 15,* 53–55.

Levine, M. E. (1967c). For lack of love alone. *Accent, 39*(7), 179–202.

Levine, M. E. (1968). The pharmacist in the clinical setting: A nurse's viewpoint. *American of Hospital Pharmacy, 25*(4), 168-171.

Levine, M. E. (1969a). Nursing in the 21st century. *National Student Association.*

Levine, M. E. (1969b). Constructive student power. *Chart, 66*(2), 42FF.

Levine, M. E. (1969c). Small hospital—Big nursing (Part I). *Chart, 66,* 265-269.

Levine, M. E. (1969d). Small hospital—Big nursing (Part II). *Chart, 66,* 310-315.

Levine, M. E. (1970a). Dilemma. *ANA Clinical Conferences,* 338-342.

Levine, M. E. (1970b). Symposium on a drug compendium: View of a nursing educator. *Drug Information Bulletin,* 133-135.

Levine, M. E. (1970c). Breaking through the medications mystique. Published simultaneously in *American Journal of Nursing, 70*(4), 799-803; and *American Journal of Hospital Pharmacy, 27*(4), 294-299.

Levine, M. E. (1971a). Consider the implications for nursing in the use of physician's assistant. *Hospital Topics, 49,* 60-63.

Levine, M. E. (1971b). The time has come to speak of health care. *AORN Journal, 13,* 37-43.

Levine, M. E. (1971c). *Renewal for nursing.* Philadelphia: F. A. Davis.

Levine, M. E. (1971d). Nursing grand rounds: Congestive heart failure. *Nursing '72, 2,* 18-23.

Levine, M. E. (1972a). Nursing educators—An alienating elite? *Chart, 69*(2), 56-61.

Levine, M. E. (1972b). Nursing grand rounds: Complicated care of CVA. *Nursing '72, 2*(3), 3-34.

Levine, M. E. (1972c). Nursing grand rounds: Insulin reactions in a brittle diabetic. *Nursing '72, 2*(5), 6-11.

Levine, M. E. (1972d). Issues in rehabilitation: The quadriplegic adolescent. *Nursing '72, 2,* 6.

Levine, M. E. (1972e). Nursing grand rounds: Severe trauma. *Nursing '72, 2*(9), 33-38.

Levine, M. E. (1972). Benoni. *American Journal of Nursing, 12*(3), 466-468.

Levine, M. E. (1973a). A letter from Myra. *Chart, 70*(9). (Also in *Israel Nurses' Journal,* December 1973, in English and Hebrew.)

Levine, M. E. (1973b). On creativity in nursing. *Image: Journal of Nursing Scholarship, 3*(3), 15-19.

Levine, M. E. (1974). The pharmacist's clinical role in interdisciplinary care: A nurse's viewpoint. *Hospital Formulary Management, 9,* 47.

Levine, M. E. (1975). On creativity in nursing. *Nursing Digest, 3,* 38-40.

Levine, M. E. (1976). On the nursing ethic and the negative command. *Proceedings of the Intensive Conference, Faculty of the University of Illinois Medical Center.* Philadelphia, PA: Society for Health and Human Values.

Levine, M. E. (1977a). History of nursing in Illinois. *Proceedings of the Bicentennial Workshop of the University of Illinois College of Nursing.* Chicago, IL: University of Illinois Press.

Levine, M. E. (1977b). Primary nursing: Generalist and specialist education. *Proceedings of the American Academy of Nursing,* Kansas City, MO: American Nurses Association.

Levine, M. E. (1978a). Kapklvoo and nursing, too (editorial). *Research in Nursing and Health, 1*(2), 51.

Levine, M. E. (1978b). Does continuing education improve practice? *Hospitals, 52*(21), 138-140.

Levine, M. E. (1979). Knowledge base required by generalized and specialized nursing practice. *ANA Publication* (G-127), 57-69.

Levine, M. E. (1980). The ethics of computer technology in health care. *Nursing Forum, 19*(2), 193-198.

Levine, M. E. (1984a). A conceptual model for nursing: The four conservation principles. *Proceedings from Allentown College of St. Francis de Sales.*

Levine, M. E. (1984b). *Myra Levine.* Paper presented at the Nurse Theorist Conference, Edmonton, Alberta, Canada (cassette recording).

Levine, M. E. (1985a). What's right about rights? In Carmi, A., & Schneider, S., (Eds.), *Proceedings of the First International Congress of Nursing Law and Ethics.* Berlin: Springer Verlag.

Levine, M. E. (1985b). [Review of the book *Magic Bullets*]. *Oncology Nursing Forum, 12,* pp. 101-102.

Levine, M. E. (1985c, August) *Myra Levine.* Paper presented at the conference on Nursing Theory in Action, Edmonton, Alberta, Canada. (Cassette recording).

Levine, M. E. (1988). What does the future hold for nursing? 25th Anniversary Address, 18th District. *Illinois Nurses Association Newsletter, XXIV*(6), 1-4.

Levine, M. E. (1990). Conservation and integrity. In M. Parker (Ed.), *Nursing theories in practice* (pp. 189-201). New York: National League for Nursing.

Levine, M. E. (1994). Some further thought on nursing rhetoric. In J. F. Kilkuchi & H. Simmons (Eds.), *Developing a philosophy of nursing* (pp. 104-109). Thousand Oaks, CA: Sage.

Levine, M. E. (1995a). The rhetoric of nursing theory. *Image: Journal of Nursing Scholarship, 27*(1), 11-14.

Levine, M. E. (1995b, Winter). Myra Levine responds [Letter to the editor]. *Image: Journal of Nursing Scholarship, 27,* 262.

Levine, M. E. (1996). On humanities in nursing. *Canadian Journal of Nursing Research, 27*(2), 19-23.

Levine, E. B., & Levine, M. E. (1965). Hippocrates, father of nursing, too? *American Journal of Nursing, 65*(12), 86-88.

Martsolf, D. S., & Mickley, J. R. (1998). The concept of spirituality in nursing theories: Differing worldviews and extent focus. *Journal of Advanced Nursing, 27,* 294-303.

Melies, A. I. (1985). Myra Levine. In Meleis, A. I. (Ed.), *Theoretical nursing: Development and progress* (pp. 275-283). Philadelphia: F. A. Davis.

Newman, M. A. (1995, Winter). Margaret Newman and the rhetoric of nursing theory [Letter to the editor]. *Image: Journal of Nursing Scholarship, 27,* 262-262.

The nursing theorists: Portraits of excellence: Myra Levine. (1988). Oakland: Studio III [videotape]. (Available from Fuld Video Project, 370 Hawthorne Avenue, Oakland, CA 94609)

Peiper, B. A. (1983). Levine's nursing model. In J. J. Fitzpatrick & A. L. Whall (Eds.), *Conceptual models of nursing: Analysis and application* (pp. 101-115). New York: National League for Nursing.

Pond, J. B. (1990). Application of Levine's Conservation Model to nursing the homeless. In M. E. Parker (Ed.), *Nursing theories in practice* (pp. 203-215). New York: National League for Nursing.

Pond, J. B. (1996, May). Nursing mourns the loss of two great leaders. *The Nursing Spectrum,* Greater Philadelphia/Tri-State edition, *5*(8), 10-11.

Schaefer, K. M. (1991). Developing a graduate program in nursing: Integrating Levine's philosophy. In Schaefer, K. M., & Pond, J. B. (Eds.), *The Conservation Model: A framework for nursing practice* (pp. 209-218). Philadelphia: F. A. Davis.

Schaefer, K. M. (1996). Levine's Conservation Model: Caring for women with chronic illness. In Hinton,

P. H., & Neuman, B. (Eds.), *Blueprint for use of nursing models: Education, research, practice, and adminstration* (pp. 187-227). New York: National League for Nursing.

Schaefer, K. M., & Pond, J. B. (1990). Effects of waterbed flotation on indicators of energy expenditure in preterm infants. *Nursing Research, 39*(5), 293.

Schaefer, K. M., & Pond, J. B. (Eds) (1991). *The conservation model: A framework for nursing practice.* Philadelphia: F. A. Davis.

Servellen, G. M. V. (1982). The concept of individualized nursing practice. *Nursing & Health Care, 3,* 482-485.

Tompkins, E. S. (1980). Effect of restricted mobility and dominance on perceived duration. *Nursing Research, 29*(6), 333-338.

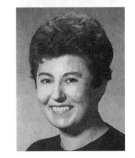

Chapter 9

Ida Jean Orlando (Pelletier)
The Dynamic Nurse-Patient
Relationship

- ❖ Introducing the Theorist
- ❖ A Conversation with the Theorist
- ❖ Assumptions of the Theory
- ❖ Major Theoretical Concepts
- ❖ Relevance of the Theory for Nursing Practice
- ❖ Applicability in Today's Health-Care System
- ❖ Summary
- ❖ References

Maude R. Rittman

INTRODUCING THE THEORIST

Nursing is responsive to individuals who suffer or anticipate a sense of helplessness; it is focused on the process of care in an immediate experience; it is concerned with providing direct assistance to individuals in whatever setting they are found for the purpose of avoiding, relieving, diminishing or curing the individual's sense of helplessness.

—**Ida Jean Orlando (1972)**

The above quotation summarizes Ida Jean Orlando's theoretical contributions in defining what nursing is and what constitutes effective nursing practice. Her theory, dubbed the "dynamic nurse-patient relationship," has also been called a "theory of effective nursing practice" (George, 1990; Mariner-Tomey, 1994; Schmieding, 1993) and will be reviewed from the perspective of its application in clinical practice. Before applying a theory, whether for practice, research, or education, the user needs to know the origins of the theory, as well as the underlying assumptions or beliefs embedded in the theory, and assess its adequacy and appropriateness for the context in which it will be used. Following a discussion of these points, an exploration of the applicability of Orlando's work to clinical practice in today's nursing environment is presented.

Although the focus of this chapter is on application of Orlando's theory to practice, the theory has been used to guide nursing research. Probably the most extensive review of Orlando's theory was written by Norma Jean Schmieding (1993). Orlando directed me to Schmieding's book and other published materials. Orlando stated that Schmieding's work most accurately describes her theory. In her book, entitled *Ida Jean Orlando: A Nursing Process Theory,* Schmieding summarizes the research that was completed shortly after Orlando's theory was published, including her own research applying the theory to nursing administration.

Ida Jean Orlando was born August 12, 1926, in New York. She received a diploma in nursing from the New York Medical College, Lower Fifth Avenue Hospital, School of Nursing, New York, in 1947, and a bachelor of science degree in public health nursing from St. John's University in Brooklyn, New York, in 1951. Orlando completed her master's degree at Teachers College, Columbia University, in New York in 1954, with emphasis on education and psychiatric-mental health nursing. Her master's degree was completed during the era when nurse leaders were concerned about defining nursing as a profession and separating nursing functions from the traditional role of physicians' handmaid.

In understanding the evolution of Orlando's theoretical developments, it is interesting to note that her early education is firmly grounded in clinical practice. Her background experiences culminated in an interest in and focus on the nurse-patient relationship. Her studies at Teachers College contributed a strong educational perspective with which she approached the study of nursing practice. Schmieding attributes Orlando's focus on the role of past experiences influencing the meaning of present experiences to her graduate education. She studied with Professor L. Thomas Hopkins, who was teaching education courses at Columbia University (Schmieding, 1993).

> Orlando's theory is research-based, using naturalistic inquiry methods.

Early in her nursing career, Orlando worked briefly in clinical practice in obstetrics, medicine, surgery, and emergency room nursing. Following her master's degree in 1954, she went to Yale University, where she completed research upon which she developed her theory. Her research blended her previous experience and interests in nursing practice, psychiatric-mental health nursing, and nursing education. After completing her research and publishing her first book in 1961, Orlando moved to Massachusetts, where she worked at McLean Hospital as a clinical nursing consultant. During the 1960s and early 1970s, she tested the applicability of her theory and taught her theory to nurses. Later she was an assistant director of nursing for education and research at the Metropolitan State Hospital in Waltham, Massachusetts. She has also been nationally and internationally recognized as a consultant and speaker on nursing and health care issues. Her last public presentation was probably on the issue of independence of nursing practice, an issue about which she continues to feel strongly.

Orlando's theory is research-based, evolving out of a study funded by the National Institute of Mental Health to improve the education of nurses. Specifically, the study was aimed at improving the education of nurses on psychiatric-mental health concepts and probably at least partially accounts for the strong emphasis on interpersonal relationships. Orlando was one of the earliest qualitative nurse researchers. She used an inductive method to obtain her data using naturalistic inquiry methods. The definitive text of Orlando's theory is *The Dynamic Nurse-Patient Relationship: Function, Process, and Principles,* which was first published in 1961 and remained out of print until 1990, when it was reissued by the National League for Nursing. The book, dedicated to her students, is a report of findings from a study to identify factors that promoted or inhibited the integration of mental health principles in nursing educational programs.

Qualitative methods of participant observations and interviews were used to collect data over a 3-year period on experiences of nursing faculty, nurses, students, and patients. Data were analyzed to identify the content of instruction, the teaching process, and the learning environment important in shaping students' professional development. It is not surprising that the dynamic nurse-patient relationship theory has it roots in psychiatric-mental health nursing, clinical practice, and education. Orlando's theory was originally developed to provide professional nurses with a theory of effective nursing practice with a focus on the patient's experience with illness and what is required from the nurse to meet the needs of the patient. The theory reflects Orlando's strong belief in the nurse-patient relationship, meeting the needs of patients as they perceive them, and the power of communication in clinical practice.

Over the next 10 years, Orlando continued to develop her theory while she was a clinical nursing consultant at McLean Hospital in Belmont, Massachusetts. In this position, she continued to study interactions between patients and nurses. Using her theory as a framework for nursing practice at McLean Hospital, she developed a training program for nurses and reorganized the nursing service around her theory. She also received federal funding to evaluate the training program. She published findings from this phase of her work in her second book, *The Discipline and Teaching of Nursing Process: An Evaluative Study* (1972).

A CONVERSATION WITH THE THEORIST

In October 1998, I contacted Ida Jean Orlando. She agreed to talk with me about her theory but warned me that her health would not allow her to talk very long (she was 72 years old). We made an appointment and talked for about 20 minutes a few weeks later about her life and her work. I was thrilled to be able to speak directly with one of the early nurse theorists and felt a sense of awe in being able to talk with a nurse who had made a significant contribution to the nursing profession before I had even entered college. I immediately felt a sense of respect and admiration for her and for all of the early theorists in nursing as I reflected on their work and contributions to the nursing profession.

My impression of Orlando was that she still holds very strong beliefs about nursing and what nursing is. She emphasized in our talk about nursing that today's nurses need to reconnect with the patient, to learn about what the patient perceives his or her needs to be, and to address those needs. She vividly described her own recent experiences with the health-care system that were both positive and negative. She attributed the difference to the quality of care provided by the nurse who assisted her. She spoke eloquently about the need today for nurses to serve as advocates for patients, and stay focused on what is valued and needed by the patient. She stated that if nurses do not ensure that patients get what they need, there is no one else who will help guide them through the system. When I asked her to tell me about significant life experiences that might have influenced her in developing her theory, she quipped, "Who knows? I don't, and I am not sure it is so important." She went on to explain that when she became a nurse, she tried to make sense out of what it meant to be a nurse and realized that, as a profession, nursing needed to define itself and its unique contribution in

> Nurses must stay connected to patients and assure that patients get what they need. There is no one else who will help guide them through the system.

health care and to patients. The quest for answering these questions is what influenced Orlando and shaped her career in nursing.

I asked her if there were any misconceptions about her or her work that she would like to address. She stated that some authors have presented a misconception about the origins of her work by saying that Hildegard Peplau influenced her thinking. She said that this was absolutely incorrect: Although Orlando and Peplau were of the same generation of theorists, Orlando's work was not influenced by Peplau's thinking. It seemed important to her to set the record straight. She told me how she came to know Peplau. She and Peplau became acquainted while she was at Yale and Peplau consulted with her while she was at McLean Hospital. Peplau made a presentation at McLean Hospital while Orlando was working as a clinical nurse consultant there. Orlando stated that she enjoyed knowing Peplau and that they had similar interests. Peplau authored her theory of interpersonal relationships in nursing in 1952. Peplau and Orlando enjoyed a collegial relationship for several years.

Orlando stressed the need for nurses to stay connected to patients and to advocate to make sure that

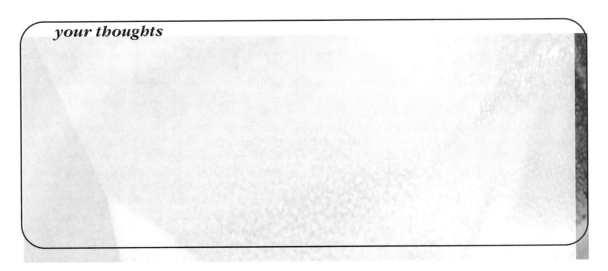

your thoughts

patients receive what they need from the health-care system in order to recover. She expressed concern about nurse practitioners, because she said many of them practice in a manner that is closer to physician practice than it is to nursing practice. For example, she said that she did not support the idea of nurses ordering medications—she believed that ordering medications should be the responsibility of physicians. Nonetheless, she went on to describe the wonderful assistance she and her husband received from a nurse practitioner who, according to her, functioned in an independent role. She stated that the nurses who are her heroes are the nurses in Appalachia, who sometimes deliver care on horseback and must function independently. She strongly believed that nurses should "take care of the patients and think for themselves."

We also talked about the role of nursing theory today. She laughed about the interest in "all this theory stuff" and stated that "students must hate having to learn all these theories." Orlando said that educators should let nursing students take care of patients and that it is only in engaging in practice that one can learn how to be a nurse. As she talked, I realized that many of the issues important in her era are still with us today and remain largely unresolved. Nurses continue to define and redefine nursing as a profession, and the many issues involved in the overlap between medicine and nursing are still important.

ASSUMPTIONS OF THE THEORY

Defining the assumptions, or "givens," inherent in a theory is important in order to develop an understanding of the theory. Underlying assumptions can also influence a decision regarding the appropriate-

ness of using the theory in a particular clinical setting. Orlando's theory reflects her belief that nursing practice should be based on the needs of the patient. Hence, communication with the patient was foundational to understanding the needs and providing effective nursing care. The essence of her theory is its focus on the patient and his or her needs and the communicative interface between the nurse and the patient. The following assumptions are identified in her writings:

1. The nursing process includes identifying the needs of patients, the response of the nurse, and nursing actions. The nursing process described by Orlando is not the linear nursing process model taught today in nursing education but is more reflexive and circular, occurring during encounters with patients.

2. Understanding the meaning of the patient's behavior is influenced by the nurse's perceptions, thoughts, and feelings requiring deliberative responses. Orlando argued that this deliberative process can be taught in educational programs and nursing students can learn to use it in patient care situations.

3. Patients experience distress when they cannot cope with their needs.

4. The nurse must take the initiative in helping the patient express the meaning of behavior to ascertain distress. The basis for nursing action is determined by the distress experienced by the patient.

> Nursing is an interpersonal process aimed at assisting patients when they are experiencing distress. It is a deliberative process that can be learned.

Section II *Evolution of Nursing Theory: Essential Influences*

5. Direct and indirect observations of patient behavior can be used to determine its meaning, and thus provide knowledge about the patient in planning nursing care.
6. Interactions with patients are unique, complex, and dynamic processes.
7. Professional nurses function in an independent role separate from physicians and others.

MAJOR THEORETICAL CONCEPTS

The major concepts included in Orlando's theory are person, needs, perceptions, thoughts, and feelings of the nurse, and deliberative action. The four major theoretical concepts in nursing are client (or patient), nursing action, environment, and health (Kim, 1983). Orlando's theory addresses all but environment, and the concept of health is implicit in the theory. The domain of environment includes the physical, social, and symbolic environment of the patient and is an essential concept for holistic nursing practice.

RELEVANCE OF THE THEORY FOR NURSING PRACTICE

Meleis (1985) stated that to be useful in practice, a theory has to be evaluated in terms of its goals. In addition to goals of the theory, and in order to judge the practical value of Orlando's theory, I will use four criteria recommended by Glaser and Strauss regarding evaluating theory: whether it fits, its understandability, whether it is sufficiently general, and whether it provides at least partial control over situations that it addresses (Glaser, 1967). Each of these criteria is discussed below.

Goals

Orlando conceptualized nursing practice as an interactive process focused on the patient's needs and/or responses to the environment. She defined *nursing* as a deliberative interaction process that is learned and includes the patients' needs, the nurse's reactions, and the nursing interventions to assist the patient. In Orlando's view, the major goal of nursing as an interpersonal process is to assist patients when they are experiencing distress.

Fit

According to Glaser (1967), a theory must closely fit the area in which it will be used. The strength of Orlando's theory is that it was developed inductively from the study of nursing practice. This grounding in the clinical world is evident in its emphasis on recognizing the patient's needs, on the nurse-patient relationship as the vehicle for achieving the goals of nursing practice, and on the nursing process. The theory was developed prior to the high technology that we take for granted in today's health-care settings. Information that influences the assessment of patient needs comes from a variety of sources. The patient is one source but not the only source of information.

Understandability

Glaser's second criterion (1967) is that the theory must be readily understood. Understandability is a hallmark of this theory because Orlando used words that are common to the practice of nursing and that are easy to comprehend.

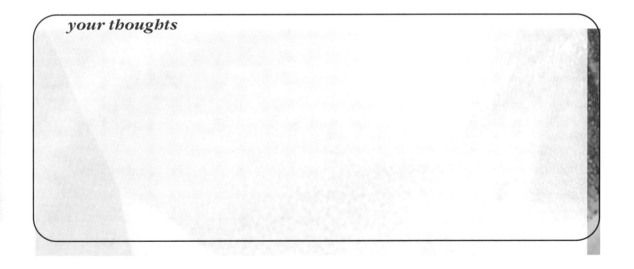

your thoughts

Sufficiently General

Third, the theory must be sufficiently general in order to be applicable to multiple and diverse situations. The applicability of Orlando's theory to multiple and diverse nursing care situations is strong in that almost all nursing practice situations depend on nurse-patient relationships to some extent. However, in complex health-care settings, the theory is an important aspect of the nursing situation but does not sufficiently address all of the functions and responsibilities that nurses encounter in their work. In this sense, Orlando's theory is sufficient for understanding the interactions between nurses and patients but fails to address other important areas of practice.

Control

The last criterion (Glaser, 1967), is that theory should provide at least partial control over situations as they change over time. Orlando's theory is a general approach to nursing interactions and interpersonal relationships with patients and is not focused on a particular patient population. Hence, control over specific clinical situations is weak.

APPLICABILITY IN TODAY'S HEALTH-CARE SYSTEM

The health-care system as we know it today is vastly different from the health-care system that existed during Ida Jean Orlando's era. Today we are faced with health-care systems that are largely operating in an economic paradigm, in which costs are driving the way hospitals and health maintenance organizations (HMOs) do business. Emphasis today is on outcomes that demonstrate cost reductions or cost-effectiveness. Price squeezing has led to altered staffing patterns. Nurses are expected to deliver nursing care to patients who are "short stay" with fewer and fewer resources. In today's context, every contact with a patient has to contribute to improved outcomes.

As hospitals move into the periphery of the health-care scene, more care is provided in the home or at other sites. Little concern is focused on nurse-patient relationships. Even as health-care systems strive to improve "customer service," the connection between nurse-patient relationships and satisfied customers seems to be glossed over. Health-care administrators are looking to the business community to improve efficiency of operations and are losing sight of the purpose of the industry: to provide care.

As a nurse-scientist in a clinical setting, I have considered the usefulness of Orlando's theory in today's practice setting. Almost 40 years have passed since this theory was developed from the study of clinical nursing practice. It was before the era of intensive care units, life-sustaining technologies, electronic monitoring, and many aspects of modern nursing as we know it today. With all of the benefits that modern technology and modern health care bring—and there are many—we need to pause and ask the question, What is at risk in health care today? I believe the answer to that question leads us to reconsider the value of Orlando's theory in nursing and the critical link between meaningful relationships and the preservation of humankind—a risk with high stakes.

Summary

The most important contribution of Orlando's nursing theory is what it says about the values underpinning our profession. Inherent in this theory is a strong value that what transpires between the patient and the nurse is of the highest value. Orlando's theory reveals and bears witness to the essence of nursing as a practice discipline. I believe the true worth of Orlando's theory of nursing is that it clearly states what nursing is or should be. Regardless of the changes in the health-care system, the human transaction between the nurse and the patient in any setting that nurses have ever practiced holds the greatest value, not only for nursing but for society at large. Orlando's theory can serve as a philosophy as well as a theory, because it is the foundation upon which our profession has been built.

References

George, J. B. (1990). *Nursing theories: The base for professional nursing practice* (3rd ed.). Norwalk, CT: Appleton & Lange.

Glaser, B. G., & Strauss, A. L. (1967). *The discovery of grounded theory.* Chicago: Aldine Publishing Co.

Kim, H. S. (1983). *The nature of theoretical thinking in nursing.* Norwalk, CT: Appleton-Century-Crofts.

Mariner-Tomey, A. (1994). *Nursing theorists and their work* (3rd ed.). St. Louis: Mosby.

Meleis, A. I. (1985). *Theoretical nursing: Development and progress.* Philadelphia: J. B. Lippincott.

Orlando, I. J. (1961/1990). *The dynamic nurse-patient relationship: Functions, process, and principles.* New York: National League for Nursing. (reprinted from 1961 edition, New York: G. P. Putnam's Sons).

Orlando, I. J. (1972). *The discipline and teaching of nursing process: An evaluative study.* New York: G. P. Putnam's Sons.

Schmieding, N. J. (1993). *Ida Jean Orlando: A nursing process theory.* Newbury Park, CA: Sage.

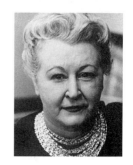

Chapter *10*

Lydia Hall
The Care, Core,
and Cure Model

Theris A. Touhy and Nettie Birnbach

INTRODUCING THE THEORIST

Lydia Hall and her conceptual model of nursing will be described in this chapter, along with her work at the Loeb Center for Nursing and Rehabilitation, the implications of her work for practice and research, and, finally, our views about how Hall might reflect on the future of nursing in the twenty-first century. Our purpose in writing this chapter is to share the story of Lydia Hall's life and her contribution to professional nursing rather than to critique a nursing theory.

Visionary, risk-taker, and consummate professional, Lydia Hall touched all who knew her in a special way. She inspired commitment and dedication through her unique conceptual framework for nursing practice that viewed professional nursing as the key to the care and rehabilitation of patients.

A 1927 graduate of the York Hospital School of Nursing in Pennsylvania, Hall held various nursing positions during the early years of her career. In the mid-1930s she enrolled at Teachers College, Columbia University, where she earned a bachelor of science degree in 1937, and a master of arts degree in 1942. She worked with the Visiting Nurse Service of New York from 1941 to 1947 and was a member of the nursing faculty at Fordham Hospital School of Nursing from 1947 to 1950. Hall was subsequently appointed to a faculty position at Teachers College, where she developed and implemented a program in nursing consultation and joined a community of nurse leaders. At the same time, she was involved in research activities for the U.S. Health Service. Active in nursing's professional organizations, Hall also provided volunteer service to the New York City Board of Education, Youth Aid, and other community associations (Birnbach, 1988).

Hall's most significant contribution was to nursing practice in the form of the model she designed and put into place in the Loeb Center for Nursing and Rehabilitation at Montefiore Medical Center in New York. Opened in 1963, the Loeb Center was the culmination of 5 years of planning and construction under Hall's direction. The circumstances that brought Hall and the Loeb Center together date back to 1947, when Dr. Martin Cherkasky was named director of the new hospital-based home care division of Montefiore Medical Center in Bronx, New York. At that time, Hall was employed by the Visiting Nurse Service at its Bronx office and had frequent contact with the Montefiore home care program. Hall and Cherkasky shared congruent philosophies regarding health care and the delivery of quality service, which served as the foundation for a long-standing professional relationship (Birnbach, 1988).

In 1950, Cherkasky was appointed director of the Montefiore Medical Center. During the early years of his tenure existing traditional convalescent homes fell into disfavor. Convalescent treatment was undergoing rapid change due largely to medical advances, new pharmaceuticals, and technological discoveries. One of the homes that closed as a result of the emerging trends was the Solomon and Betty Loeb Memorial Home in Westchester County, New York. Cherkasky and Hall collaborated in convincing the board of the Loeb Home to join with Montefiore in founding the Loeb Center for Nursing and Rehabilitation. Using the proceeds realized from the sale of the Loeb Home, plans for construction of the Loeb Center proceeded over a 5-year period, from 1957 to

your thoughts

1962. Although the Loeb Center was, and still is, an integral part of the Montefiore physical complex, it was separately administered, with its own board of trustees that interrelated with the Montefiore board.

Under Hall's direction, patients for the Loeb Center were selected by nurses based on their potential for rehabilitation. Qualified professional nurses provided direct care to patients and coordinated needed services. Hall frequently described the center as "a halfway house on the road home," where the nurse worked with the patients as active participants in achieving desired outcomes (Hall, 1963a, p. 2). Over time, the effectiveness of Hall's practice model was validated by the significant decline in the number of readmissions among former Loeb patients as compared with those who received other types of posthospital care ("Montefiore cuts," 1966).

In 1967, Hall received the Teachers College Nursing Alumni Award for Distinguished Achievement in Nursing Practice. She shared her innovative ideas about the practice of nursing with numerous audiences around the country and contributed articles to nursing journals. In those articles, she referred to nurses using feminine pronouns. Because gender-neutral language was not yet an accepted style, and women comprised 96 percent of the nursing workforce, the feminine pronoun was used almost exclusively.

Hall died of heart disease on February 27, 1969, at Queens Hospital in New York. In 1984, she was inducted into the American Nurses' Association Hall of Fame. Following Hall's death, her legacy was kept alive at the Loeb Center, until 1984, under the capable leadership of her friend and colleague Genrose Alfano.

Remembered by her colleagues for her passion for nursing, her flamboyant personality, and the excitement she generated, Hall was indeed a force for change. At a time when task-oriented team nursing was the preferred practice model in most institutions, she implemented a professional patient-centered framework whereby patients received a standard of care unequaled anywhere else. At the Loeb Center, Lydia Hall created an environment in which nurses were empowered, in which patients' needs were met through a continuum of care, and in which, according to Genrose Alfano, "nursing was raised to a high therapeutic level" (personal communication, January 27, 1999).

HISTORICAL BACKGROUND

During the 1950s and 1960s, the health-care milieu in which Lydia Hall functioned was undergoing tremendous change. As previously stated, the type of nursing home model then in use failed to meet expectations, and care of the elderly was a growing problem. Increasing recognition that the elder population was in the greatest need of health-care insurance generated years of debate among legislators, the medical profession, and the public. Finally, in 1965, Medicare legislation was enacted that provided hospital, nursing home, and home care for those citizens age 65 and over. Medicaid was established to provide health-care services for the medically indigent irrespective of age. These programs provided a source of revenue for the nation's hospitals and, as public confidence in hospitals grew, there was concomitant growth in the need for more hospitals. Subsequent congressional legislation provided for construction of new facilities, which, in turn, created more opportunities for the employment of nurses. Undoubtedly, all of these factors were relevant to Hall as she proceeded to implement her vision.

With respect to nursing, the 1960s witnessed the growth of specialization, the movement toward preparation of nurse practitioners and clinical nurse specialists, and the emergence of new practice fields such as industrial nursing. Although most nurses worked in hospitals at that time, a beginning trend to community-based practice was evolving. In regard to nursing education, the advent of degree-granting, 2-year programs in community colleges proved to be an attractive alternative to the apprenticeship model—hospital-based, diploma school education—through which most nurses had previously been prepared. And, with publication of the American Nurses' Association's position statement on educational preparation in 1965, baccalaureate education was receiving renewed recognition as the preferred method for preparing professional nurses. The correlation between higher education and professional practice seems to agree with Hall's ideas and probably elicited her support. Her model of nursing at the Loeb Center clearly required nurses to be educated, professional, and caring. Its success depended upon the ability of the nurses to relate to each patient with sensitivity and understanding. Hall was clear in her vision of the registered professional nurse as the appropriate person to fulfill that role.

Scholars and practitioners today continue to grapple with questions about how to define nursing and to demonstrate the unique contribution of professional nursing to the health and well-being of people. Lydia Hall's belief that the public deserves and can benefit from professional nursing care was not only articulated in her theory of nursing but also demonstrated in practice at the Loeb Center under her guidance. Hall stated (1963c, p. 805):

> The program at the Loeb Center was designed to alleviate some of the growing problems which face our health-conscious public today: the complex and long-term nature of illnesses besetting all age groups; the high cost of services utilized in overcoming these illnesses; the negative reactions of the public and the health professions to patient care offered by institutions; and the confusion among all groups about the definition of nursing, its organization for service, and the kind of educational preparation it requires.

These questions and concerns are as relevant today as they were when Hall articulated her ideas over 30 years ago. Perhaps they are even more relevant now, as we face a rapidly increasing older population with needs for long-term care and an era of cost containment that often limits access to professional care and services.

> Hall believed that in spite of successes in keeping people alive, there was failure in helping them live fully with chronic pathology.

VISION OF NURSING

Lydia Hall would not have considered herself a nurse-theorist. She did not set out to develop a theory of nursing but rather to offer a view of professional nursing. Wiggins (1980, p. 10) reflected on the status of nursing theory during this time and stated: "[T]he excitement of the possibility of development by nurses of nursing theories was in its barest beginnings." Hall's observations of hospital care at the time led her to articulate her beliefs about the value of professional nursing to patient welfare. She observed that care was fragmented; patients often felt depersonalized; and patients, physicians, and nurses were voicing concern about the lack and/or poor quality of nursing care. She reflected that in the early part of the twentieth century, a person came to the hospital for care. In the 1950s and 1960s, the focus changed, and a person came to the hospital for cure. However, the health problems of the time were long-term in nature and often not subject to cure. It was Hall's belief that in spite of successes in keeping people alive, there was a failure in helping patients live fully with chronic pathology. After the biological crisis was stabilized, Hall believed that care should be the primary

focus and that nurses were the most qualified to provide the type of care that would enable patients to achieve their maximum potential. In fact, she questioned why medicine would want the leadership and suggested that the patient with a long-term illness would come to nursing (Hall, 1965).

Hall described the two phases of medical care that she saw existing in hospitals at the time. The first phase is when the patient is in biological crisis with a need for intensive medicine. Phase 2 begins when the acute crisis is stabilized and the patient is in need of a different form of medicine. Hall labeled this as "follow-up"—evaluative medicine—and felt that it is at this point that professional nursing is most important. She criticized the practice of turning over the patient's care to practical nurses and aides at this point while the professional nurse attended to new admissions in the biological crisis phase. Hall (1969, p. 87) stated:

> Now when the patient reaches the point where we know he is going to live, he might be interested in learning how to live better before he leaves the hospital. But the one nurse who could teach him, the one nurse who has the background to make this a truly learning situation, is now busy with the new patients in a state of biological crisis. She rarely sees those other patients who have survived this period, unless there is something investigative or potentially paining to do! The patients in the second stage of hospitalization are given over to straight comforters, the practical nurses and aides. No teaching is available and the patient doesn't change a bit. No wonder so many people keep coming back for readmission. They've never had the invitation nor the opportunity to learn from this experience. So I say, if that's the way it is, take [the patient] from the medical center at this point in his follow-up evaluative medical care period and transfer him to the Loeb Center, where nurturing will be his chief therapy and medicine will become an ancillary one.

Hall also opposed the concept of team nursing, which was being implemented in many acute care settings at the time. According to Hall (1958), team nursing viewed nursing as a set of functions, ranging from simple to complex. Simple functions were considered those in which few factors were taken into consideration before making a nursing judgement. The tasks or activities of nursing were divided among nursing personnel, simply or complexly educated, with the highest educated leading the nursing team.

Hall believed that the concept of team nursing was detrimental to nursing and reduced nursing to a vocation or trade. Hall (1958, p. 1) stated: "There is nothing simple about patients who are complex human beings, or a nurse who is also complex and who finds herself involved in the complexities of disease and health processes in a complex helping relationship." Hall was convinced that patient outcomes are improved when direct care is provided by the professional nurse.

CARE, CORE, AND CURE

Hall enumerated three aspects of the person as patient: the person, the body, and the disease. These aspects were envisioned as overlapping circles that influence each other. Hall stated:

> Everyone in the health professions either neglects or takes into consideration any or all of these, but each profession, to be a profession, must have an exclusive area of expertness with which it practices, creates new practices, new theories and introduces newcomers to its practice. (Hall, 1965, p. 4)

She believed that medicine's responsibility was the area of pathology and treatment. The area of person, which, according to Hall, has been sadly neglected, belongs to a number of professions, including psychiatry, social work, and the ministry, among others. She saw nursing's expertise as the area of body as body, and also as influenced by the other two areas.

Hall clearly stated that the focus of nursing is the provision of intimate bodily care. She reflected that the public has long recognized this as belonging exclusively to nursing (Hall, 1958, 1964, 1965). Being expert in the area of body involved more than simply knowing how to provide intimate bodily care. To be expert, the nurse must know how to modify the care depending on the pathology and treatment while considering the unique needs and personality of the patient.

> **Nursing is required when persons are not able to provide intimate bodily care for themselves. The nursing intent of this care is to comfort.**

Based on her view of the person as patient, Hall conceptualized nursing as having three aspects, and delineated the area that is the specific domain of nursing, as well as those areas that are shared with other professions (Hall, 1955, 1958, 1964, 1965) (Figure 10–1). Hall believed that this model reflected

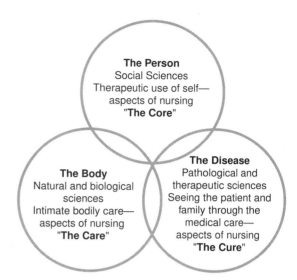

Figure 10–1   *Care, core, and cure model. From Hall, L. (1964, Feb.). Nursing: What is it?* The Canadian Nurse, *60 (2), 151. Reproduced with permission from* The Canadian Nurse.

the nature of nursing as a professional interpersonal process. She visualized each of the three overlapping circles as an "aspect of the nursing process related to the patient, to the supporting sciences and to the underlying philosophical dynamics" (Hall, 1958, p. 1). The circles overlap and change in size as the patient progresses through a medical crisis to the rehabilitative phase of the illness. In the acute care phase, the cure circle is the largest. During the evaluation and follow-up phase, the care circle is predominant. Hall's framework for nursing has been described as the "Care, Core, and Cure Model" (Chinn & Jacobs, 1987; Marriner-Tomey, Peskoe, & Gumm, 1989; Stevens-Barnum, 1990).

Care

Hall suggested that the part of nursing that is concerned with intimate bodily care (e.g., bathing, feeding, toileting, positioning, moving, dressing, undressing, and maintaining a healthful environment) belongs exclusively to nursing. Nursing is required when people are not able to undertake these activities for themselves. This aspect provided the opportunity for closeness and required seeing the process as an interpersonal relationship (Hall, 1958). Hall labeled this aspect "care," and identified knowledge in the natural and biological sciences as foundational to practice. The intent of bodily care is to comfort the patient. Through this comforting, the person of the patient, as well as his or her body, responds to the physical care. Hall cautioned against viewing intimate bodily care as a task that can be performed by anyone when she stated:

> To make the distinction between a trade and a profession, let me say that the laying on of hands to wash around a body is an activity, it is a trade; but if you look behind the activity for the rationale and intent, look beyond it for the opportunities that the activity opens up for something more enriching in growth, learning and healing production on the part of the patient—you have got a profession. Our intent when we lay hands on the patient in bodily care is to comfort. While the patient is being comforted, he feels close to the comforting one. At this time his person talks out and acts out those things that concern him—good, bad and indifferent. If nothing more is done with these, what the patient gets is ventilation or catharsis, if you will. This may bring relief of anxiety and tension but not necessarily learning. If the individual who is in the comforting role has in her preparation all of the sciences whose principles she can offer a teaching-learning experience around his concerns, the ones that are most effective in teaching and learning, then the comforter proceeds to something beyond—to what I call "nurturer"—someone who fosters learning, someone who fosters growing up emotionally, someone who even fosters healing. (Hall, 1969, p. 86)

> Cure is an aspect of nursing that is shared with medicine. The nurse may assume medical functions, or help the patient with these through comforting and nurturing.

Cure

The second aspect of the nursing process is shared with medicine and is labeled the "cure." During this aspect, the nurturing process may be modified as this aspect overlaps it. Hall (1958) comments on the two ways that this medical aspect of nursing may be viewed. It may be viewed as the nurse assisting the doctor by assuming medical tasks or functions. The other view of this aspect of nursing is to see the nurse helping the patient through his or her medical, surgical, and rehabilitative care in the role of comforter and nurturer. Hall felt that the nursing profession was assuming more and more of the medical aspects of care while at the same time giving away the nurturing process of nursing to less well-prepared persons. Hall stated:

> Interestingly enough, physicians do not have practical doctors. They don't need them . . . they have nurses. Interesting, too, is the fact that most nurses show by their delegation of nurturing to others, that they prefer being second class doctors to being first class nurses. This is the prerogative of any nurse. If she feels better in this role, why not? One good reason why not for more and more nurses is that with this increasing trend, patients receive from professional nurses second class doctoring; and from practical nurses, second class nursing. Some nurses would like the public to get first class nursing. Seeing the patient through [his or her] medical care without giving up the nurturing will keep the unique opportunity that personal closeness provides to further [the] patient's growth and rehabilitation. (Hall, 1958, p. 3)

> The nurse who knows self can love and trust the patient enough to work *with* him professionally, rather than *for* him technically, or *at* him vocationally.

Core

The third area that nursing shares with all of the helping professions is that of using relationships for therapeutic effect—the core. This area emphasizes the social, emotional, spiritual, and intellectual needs of the patient in relation to family, institution, community, and the world (Hall, 1955, 1958, 1965). Knowledges foundational to the core were based on the social sciences and therapeutic use of self. Through the closeness offered by the provision of intimate bodily care, the patient will feel comfortable enough to explore with the nurse "who he is, where he is, where he wants to go and will take or refuse help in getting there—the patient will make amazingly more rapid progress toward recovery and rehabilitation" (Hall, 1958, p. 3). Hall believed that through this process, the patient would emerge as a whole person.

Knowledge and skills important for the nurse to be able to use self therapeutically include knowing self and learning interpersonal skills. The goals of the interpersonal process are to help patients to understand themselves as they participate in problem focusing and problem solving. Hall discussed the importance of nursing with the patient as opposed to nursing at, to, or for the patient. Hall reflected on the value of the therapeutic use of self by the professional nurse when she stated:

> The nurse who knows self by the same token can love and trust the patient enough to work *with* him professionally, rather than *for* him technically, or *at* him vocationally. Her goals cease being tied up with "where can I throw my nursing stuff around," or "how can I explain my nursing stuff to get the patient to do what we want him to do," or "how can I understand my patient so that I can handle him better." Instead her goals are linked up with "what is the problem?" and "how can I help the patient understand himself?" as he participates in problem facing and solving. In this way, the nurse recognizes that the power to heal lies in the patient and not in the nurse unless she is healing herself. She takes satisfaction and pride in her ability to help the patient tap this source of power in his continuous growth and development. She becomes comfortable working cooperatively and consistently with members of other professions, as she meshes her contributions with theirs in a concerted program of care and rehabilitation. (Hall, 1958, p. 5)

Hall believed that the role of professional nursing was enacted through the provision of *care* that facilitates the interpersonal process and invited the patient to learn to get at the *core* of his difficulties while seeing him through the *cure* that is possible. Through the professional nursing process, the patient has the opportunity of making the illness a learning experience from which he may emerge even healthier than before his illness (Hall, 1965).

THE LOEB CENTER FOR NURSING AND REHABILITATION

Lydia Hall was able to actualize her vision of nursing through the creation of the Loeb Center for Nursing and Rehabilitation at Montefiore Medical Center. The major orientation of the center was rehabilitation and subsequent discharge to home or to a long-term care institution if further care was needed. Doctors referred patients to the center and a professional nurse made admission decisions. Criteria for admission were based on the patient's need for rehabilitation nursing. What made the Loeb Center uniquely different was the model of professional nursing that was implemented under Lydia Hall's guidance. The guiding philosophy of the center was Hall's belief that during the rehabilitation phase of an illness ex-

perience, professional nurses were the best prepared to foster the rehabilitation process, decrease complications and recurrences, and promote health and prevent new illnesses. She saw this being accomplished by the special and unique way nurses work with patients in a close interpersonal process with the goal of fostering learning, growth, and healing. At the Loeb Center, nursing was the chief therapy, with medicine and the other disciplines ancillary to nursing. A new model of organization of nursing services was implemented and studied at the center. Hall stated:

> Within this proposed organization of services, the chief therapeutic agent for the patient's rehabilitation and progress will be the special and unique way the nurse will work with the individual patient. She will be involved not only in direct bedside care but she will also be the instrument to bring the rehabilitation service of the Center to the patient. Specialists in related therapies will be available on staff as resource persons and as consultants. (Hall, 1963b, p. 4)

Nursing was in charge of the total health program for the patient and responsible for integrating all aspects of care. Only registered professional nurses were hired. The 80-bed unit was staffed with 44 professional nurses employed around the clock. Professional nurses gave direct patient care and teaching and were responsible for eight patients and their families. Senior staff nurses were available on each ward as resources and mentors for staff nurses. For every two professional nurses there was one nonprofessional worker called a "messenger-attendant." The messenger-attendants did not provide hands-on care to the patients. Instead, they performed such tasks as getting linen and supplies, thus freeing the nurse to nurse the patient (Hall, 1969). Additionally, there were four ward secretaries. Morning and evening shifts were staffed at the same ratio. Night-shift staffing was less; however, Hall (1965, p. 2) noted that there were "enough nurses at night to make rounds every hour and to nurse those patients who are awake around the concerns that may be keeping them awake." In most institutions of that time, the number of nurses was decreased during the

> The chief focus of the patient's rehabilitation at the Loeb Center was the special and unique way the nurse worked with each patient. Patients participated in all care decisions.

evening and night shifts because it was felt that larger numbers of nurses were needed during the day to get the work done. Hall took exception to the idea that nursing service was organized around work to be done rather than the needs of the patients.

The patient was the center of care at Loeb and participated actively in all care decisions. Families were free to visit at any hour of the day or night. Rather than strict adherence to institutional routines and schedules, patients at the Loeb Center were encouraged to maintain their own usual patterns of daily activities, thus promoting independence and an easier transition to home. There was no chart section labeled "Doctor's Orders." Hall believed that to order a patient to do something violated the right of the patient to participate in his or her treatment plan. Instead, nurses shared the treatment plan with the patient and helped him or her to discuss his or her concerns and become an active learner in the rehabilitation process. Additionally, there were no doctor's progress notes or nursing notes. Instead, all charting was done on a form entitled "Patient's Progress Notes." These notes included the patient's reaction to care, his concerns and feelings, his understanding of the problems, the goals he has identified, and how he sees his progress toward those goals. Hall believed that what was important to record was the patient's progress, not the duties of the nurse or the progress of the physician. Patients were also encouraged to keep their own notes to share with their caregivers.

Referring back to Hall's care, core, and cure model, the care circle enlarges at Loeb. The cure circle becomes smaller, and the core circle becomes very large. It was Hall's belief that the nurse reached the patient's person through the closeness of inti-

mate bodily care and comfort. The interpersonal process established by the professional nurse during the provision of care was the basis for rehabilitation and learning on the part of the patient. Alfano (1982, p. 213) noted that "Hall's process for nursing care was based upon a theory that incorporated the teachings of Harry Stack Sullivan, Carl Rogers, and John Dewey." Nurses were taught to use a nondirective counseling approach that emphasized use of a reflective process. Within this process, it was important for nurses to learn to know and care for self so that they could use the self therapeutically in relationship with the patient (Hall, 1965, 1969). Hall reflected:

> If the nurse is a teacher, she will concern herself with the facilitation of the patient's verbal expressions and will reflect these so that the patient can hear what he says. Through this process, he will come to grips with himself and his problems, in which case, he will learn rapidly, i.e. he will change his behavior from sickness to "wellness." (Hall, 1958, p. 4)

Lydia Hall directed the Loeb Center from 1963 until her death in 1969. Genrose Alfano succeeded her in the position of director until 1984. At this time, the Loeb Center became licensed to operate as a nursing home, providing both subacute and long-term care (Griffiths, 1997b). The philosophy, structure, and organization of services established under Hall, and continued under the direction of Genrose Alfano, changed considerably in response to changes in health-care regulation and financing. Hall and others have provided detailed desciptions of the planning and design of the original Loeb Center, its daily operations, and the nursing work that was done from 1963 to 1984 (Alfano, 1964, 1969, 1982;

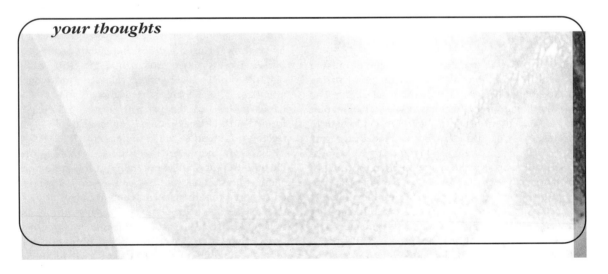

your thoughts

Bowar, 1971; Bowar-Ferres, 1975; Englert, 1971; Hall, 1963a, 1963b; Henderson, 1964; Isler, 1964; Pearson, 1984).

IMPLICATIONS FOR NURSING PRACTICE

The stories and case studies written by nurses who worked at Loeb provide the best testimony of the implications for nursing practice at the time (Alfano, 1971; Bowar, 1971; Bowar-Ferres, 1975; Englert, 1971). Griffiths and Wilson-Barnett (1998, p. 1185) noted: "The series of case studies from staff at the Loeb illustrate their understanding of this practice and describe a shift in the culture of care both between nurses and patient and within the nursing management structure." Alfano (1964) discussed the nursing milieu, including the orientation, education, mentoring, and expectations of the nurses at the Loeb Center. Before hiring, the philosophy of nursing and the concept of professional practice were discussed with the applicant. Alfano stated: "If she agrees to try the nondirective approach and the reflective method of communication, and if she's willing to exercise all her nursing skills and to reach for a high level of clinical practice, then we're ready to join forces" (1964, p. 84). Nurses were given support in learning and developing their professional practice. Administration worked with nurses in the same manner in which they expected nurses to work with patients, emphasizing growth of self. Bowar (1971, p. 301) described the role of senior resource nurse as enabling growth through a teaching-learning process grounded in caring and respect for the "integrity of each nurse as a person."

Staff conferences were held at least twice weekly as forums to discuss concerns, problems, or questions. A collaborative practice model between physicians and nurses evolved and the shared knowlege of the two professions led to more effective team planning (Isler, 1964). The nursing stories published by nurses who worked at Loeb describe nursing situations that demonstrate the effect of professional nursing on patient outcomes. Additionally, they reflect the satisfaction derived from practicing in a truly professional role (Alfano, 1971; Bowar, 1971; Bowar-Ferres, 1975; Englert, 1971). Alfano stated: "The successful implementation of the professional nursing role at Loeb was associated with an institutional philosophy of nursing autonomy and with considerable authority afforded clinical nurses in their practice" (Alfano, 1982, p. 226). The model of professional nursing practice developed at Loeb has been compared to primary nursing (Griffiths & Wilson-Barnett, 1998).

Questions arise about why the concept of the Loeb Center was not replicated in other facilities. Alfano (1982) identified several deterrents to replication of the model. Foremost among these was her belief that many people were not convinced that it was essential for professional nurses to provide direct patient care. Additionally, she postulated that others did not share the definition of the term "professional nursing practice" that was espoused by Hall. She noted that "those who have tried to replicate the program, but have employed nonprofessional or less-skilled persons, have not produced the same results" (Alfano, 1982, p. 226). Other factors included economic incentives that favored keeping the patient in an acute care bed, and the difficulties encountered in maintaining a population of short-term rehabilitation patients in the extended care unit. Pearson (1984, p. 54) suggested that the philosophy of the center may have been "threatening to established hierarchies and power relationships." Alfano (1982, p. 226) speculated that the Loeb Center may have been an "idea ahead of its time" and that dissatisfaction with nursing homes, the nation's excess hospital bed capacities, and an increasing emphasis on rehabilitation might contribute to replication of the Loeb model in the future.

> Research findings suggested that patients at the Loeb Center achieved better outcomes at less overall cost. These findings are consistent with recent research.

Interestingly, the Loeb model was the prototype for the development of several Nursing-Led In-Patient Units (NLIUs) in the United Kingdom. Two British nurses, Peter Griffiths and Alan Pearson, both traveled to the Loeb Center in preparation for the development of NLIUs in the United Kingdom. Both have done extensive writing in the literature describing the units and are involved in active outcome research. In a comprehensive review of the literature, Griffiths and Wilson-Barnett (1998) identify several nursing-led in-patient units, including Loeb; describe their structure; and discuss the research that was conducted to evaluate the centers. The operational definition of nursing-led in-patient units derived from this study includes the following characteristics:

1. in-patient environment offering active treatment;
2. case mix based on nursing need;

3. nurse leadership of the multidisciplinary clinical team;
4. nursing is conceptualized as the predominant active therapy; and
5. nurses have authority to admit and discharge patients. (Griffiths & Wilson-Barnett, 1998, p. 1185)

Unencumbered at the present time by the financial constraints of the American health-care system, the potential for the further development of nursing-led in-patient centers in the United Kingdom seems promising. However, Griffiths (1997b) suggested that future development of NLIUs in the United Kingdom may soon be influenced by financial constraints similar to those in the United States.

IMPLICATIONS FOR NURSING RESEARCH

In addition to case study research by nurses who worked at Loeb, an 18-month follow-up study of the outcomes of care was funded by the Department of Health, Education and Welfare. Alfano (1982) presents a detailed description of the study. The purpose of the longitudinal study was to compare selected outcomes of two groups of patients exposed to different nursing environments (the Loeb program and a control group). Outcomes examined were cost of hospital stay, hospital readmissions, nursing home admissions, mortality, and return to work and social activities. Overall, findings suggested that the Loeb group achieved better outcomes at less overall cost.

The findings of several other studies in nurse-led units lend further support to the benefit of the structure to patient outcomes, including prevention of complications (Daly, Phelps, & Rudy, 1991; Griffiths, 1996; Griffiths & Wilson-Barnett, 1998; Rudy, Daly, Douglas, Montenegro, Song, & Dyer, 1995). There is a critical need for research examining the effect of professional nursing care on patient outcomes in all settings. In a recent study involving 506 hospitals in 10 states, Kovner and Gergen (1998) reported that patients who have surgery done in hospitals with fewer registered nurses per patient run a higher risk of developing avoidable complications following their operation. There was a strong inverse relationship between registered nurse staffing and adverse patient events. Patients in hospitals with fewer full-time registered nurses per in-patient day had a greater incidence of urinary tract infections, pneumonia, thrombosis, pulmonary congestion, and other lung-related problems following major surgery. The authors suggested that these complications can be prevented by hands-on nursing practices and that this

should be considered when developing strategies to reduce costs. Griffiths (1996) suggested the need for further research and cautioned that although clinical outcomes are important, it is equally important to study the processes of care in these units. In doing so, we will begin to understand the resources and methods of nursing care necessary to ensure positive patient outcomes.

Summary

Currently, nurses practice in a health-care environment driven by financial gain, where quality is sacrificed and the patient is lost in a world of mismanaged care. More than ever, these alarming trends indicate a need to return to the basic premise of Hall's philosophy—patient-centered, therapeutic care. According to Griffiths (1997a), however, the Loeb Center presently reflects little resemblance to its former image. It now provides part subacute and part long-term care and, in fact, appears remarkably like the kind of system that Hall was trying to alter. Nursing is bogged down in a morass of paperwork, and the enthusiasm generated by the Hall model is no longer evident.

How would Lydia Hall react to these conditions, and what response might we expect if she spoke with us today? We believe she would be appalled by the diminished presence of professional nurses in health-care facilities and the impediments confronting those who remain. She would encourage us to explore new ways to provide needed nursing care within an existing chaotic climate. She would lead us in challenging the status quo and speak of the necessity for nursing leaders to have a clear vision of nursing practice as well as a willingness to advocate for nursing irrespective of external forces seeking to undermine the profession.

She would foster scientific inquiry that addresses outcomes of care and validates the impact of professional nursing, particularly in long-term care settings. She would agree that the improvement of care to elders in nursing homes is a significant ethical issue for society and that nurses, the largest group of providers of care to elders in nursing homes, play a vital role in the improvement of care. She would call upon us to develop professional models of care and demonstrate the positive outcomes for the health and well-being of elders. She would challenge the widely held belief that provision of care to this population consists only of bed and body care that can be effectively delivered by nonprofessional staff.

She would applaud the movement toward advanced nursing practice but would probably envision it as a means for highly educated nurses to use their expertise more effectively in providing direct patient care outside the hospital. She would encourage advanced practice nurses to continue to develop knowledge related to the discipline of nursing and the unique contribution of nursing to the health of people. And she would identify community nursing organizations as an opportunity for nurses to coordinate and deliver continuity of care in the ambulatory setting and in the home.

Finally, she would urge nurses to recapture the aspects of nursing practice that have been relinquished to others—those nurturing aspects that, according to Hall (1963a), provide the opportunity for nurses to establish therapeutic, humanistic relationships with patients and make it possible for them to work together toward recovery.

References

Alfano, G. (1964). Administration means working with nurses. *American Journal of Nursing, 64,* 83-86.

Alfano, G. (1969). The Loeb Center for Nursing and Rehabilitation. *Nursing Clinics of North America, 4,* 487-493.

Alfano, G. (1971). Healing or caretaking—which will it be? *Nursing Clinics of North America, 6,* 273-280.

Alfano, G. (1982). In Aiken, L. (Ed.), *Nursing in the 1980's* (pp. 211-228). Philadelphia: J. B. Lippincott.

Birnbach, N. (1988). Lydia Eloise Hall, 1906-1969. In Bullough, V. L., Church, O. M., & Stein, A. P. (Eds.), *American Nursing: A biographical dictionary* (pp. 161-163). New York: Garland Publishing.

Bowar, S. (1971). Enabling professional practice through leadership skills. *Nursing Clinics of North America, 6,* 293-301.

Bowar-Ferres, S. (1975). Loeb Center and its philosophy of nursing. *American Journal of Nursing, 75,* 810-815.

Bullough, V. L., Church, O. M., & Stein, A. P. (Eds.). (1988). *American Nursing: A biographical dictionary.* New York: Garland Publishing.

Chinn, P. L., & Jacobs, M. K. (1987). *Theory and nursing.* St. Louis: Mosby.

Daly, B. J., Phelps, C., & Rudy, E. B. (1991). A nurse-managed special care unit. *Journal of Nursing Administration, 21,* 31-38.

Englert, B. (1971). How a staff nurse perceives her role at Loeb Center. *Nursing Clinics of North America, 6* (2), 281-292.

Griffiths, P. (1996). Clinical outcomes for nurse-led in-patient care. *Nursing Times, 92,* 40-43.

Griffiths, P. (1997a). In search of the pioneers of nurse-led care. *Nursing Times, 93,* 46-48.

Griffiths, P. (1997b). In search of therapeutic nursing: Subacute care. *Nursing Times, 93,* 54-55.

Griffiths, P., & Wilson-Barnett, J. (1998). The effectiveness of "nursing beds": A review of the literature. *Journal of Advanced Nursing, 27,* 1184-1192.

Hall, L. E. (1955). *Quality of nursing care.* Manuscript of an address before a meeting of the Department of Baccalaureate and Higher Degree Programs of the New Jersey League for Nursing, February 7, 1955, at Seton Hall University, Newark, New Jersey. Montefiore Medical Center Archives, Bronx, New York.

Hall, L. E. (1958). *Nursing: What is it?* Manuscript. Montefiore Medical Center Archives, Bronx, New York.

Hall, L. E. (1963a, March). *Summary of project report: Loeb Center for Nursing and Rehabilitation.* Unpublished report. Montefiore Medical Center Archives, Bronx, New York.

Hall, L. E. (1963b, June). *Summary of project report: Loeb Center for Nursing and Rehabilitation.* Unpublished report. Montefiore Medical Center Archives, Bronx, New York.

Hall, L. E. (1963c). A Center for Nursing. *Nursing Outlook, 11,* 805-806.

Hall, L. E. (1964). Nursing—what is it? *Canadian Nurse, 60,* 150-154.

Hall, L. E. (1965). *Another view of nursing care and quality.* Address delivered at Catholic University, Washington, D.C. Unpublished report. Montefiore Medical Center Archives, Bronx, New York.

Hall, L. E. (1969). The Loeb Center for Nursing and Rehabilitation, Montefiore Hospital and Medical Center, Bronx, New York. *International Journal of Nursing Studies, 6,* 81-97.

Henderson, C. (1964). Can nursing care hasten recovery? *American Journal of Nursing, 64,* 80-83.

Isler, C. (June, 1964). New concept in nursing therapy: Care as the patient improves. *RN,* 58-70.

Kovner, C., & Gergen, P. (1998). The relationship between nurse staffing level and adverse events following surgery in acute care hospitals. *Image: Journal of Nursing Scholarship, 30,* 315-321.

Marriner-Tomey, A., Peskoe, K., & Gumm, S. (1989). Lydia E. Hall Core, Care, and Cure Model. In Marriner-Tomey, A. M. (Ed.), *Nursing theorists and their work* (pp. 109-117). St. Louis: Mosby.

Montefiore cuts readmissions 80%. (1966, February 23). *The New York Times.*

Obituaries—Lydia E. Hall. (1969). *American Journal of Nursing, 69,* 830.

Pearson, A. (1984, July 18). A centre for nursing. *Nursing Times,* 53-54.

Rudy, E. B., Daly, B. J., Douglas, S., Montenegro, H. D., Song, R., & Dyer, M. A. (1995). Patient outcomes for the chronically critically ill: Special care unit versus intensive care unit. *Nursing Research, 44,* 324-331.

Stevens-Barnum, B. J. (1990). *Nursing theory analysis, application, evaluation* (3rd ed.). Glenview, IL: Scott, Foresman/Little Brown.

Wiggins, L. R. (1980). Lydia Hall's place in the development of nursing theory. *Image, 12,* 10-12.

Bibliography

Hall, L. E. (1955). Quality of nursing care. *Public Health News (New Jersey State Department of Health), 36,* 212-215.

Hall, L. E. (1960). *Report of a work conference on nursing in long-term chronic disease and aging.* National League for Nursing as a League Exchange #50. New York: National League for Nursing.

Hall, L. E. (1963, June). *Report of Loeb Center for Nursing and Rehabilitation project report* (pp. 1515–1562). Congressional Record Hearings before the Special Subcommittee on Intermediate Care of the Committee on Veterans' Affairs. Washington, DC.

Hall, L. E. (1965). Nursing—what is it? In Baumgarten (Ed.), *Concepts of nursing home administration.* New York: Macmillan.

Hall, L. E. (1966). Another view of nursing care and quality. In Straub, M. K. (Ed.), *Continuity of patient care: The role of nursing.* Washington, DC: Catholic University of America Press.

Levenson, D. (1984). *Montefiore—the hospital as social instrument.* New York: Farrar, Straus & Giroux.

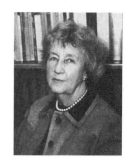

Chapter *11*

Virginia Avenel Henderson
Definition of Nursing

Shirley Countryman Gordon

INTRODUCING THE THEORIST

Virginia Avenel Henderson presented her definition of the nature of nursing in a era when few nurses had ventured into describing the complex phenomena of modern nursing. Henderson wrote about nursing the way she lived it: focusing on what nurses do, how nurses function, and on nursing's unique role in health care. Her works are beautifully written in jargon-free, everyday language. However, Henderson refused to have her definition of nursing endowed as a theory or concept (Smith, 1998). She believed that so-called nursing theories did not make a direct impact on the quality of nursing care delivered to real patients (Smith, 1998).

Virginia Henderson is often referred to as the twentieth-century Florence Nightingale (Halloran, 1991). Her search for a definition of nursing ultimately influenced the practice and education of nursing around the world. Her pioneer work in the area of identifying and structuring nursing knowledge has provided the foundation for nursing scholarship for generations to come.

PERSONAL BACKGROUND

Virginia Avenel Henderson was born in Kansas City, Missouri, on November 30, 1897. She was the fifth of eight children born to Lucy Abott Henderson and Daniel B. Henderson. The family relocated to Virginia in 1901 when her father, an attorney, took a position representing Native-Americans before the government in Washington, D.C.

Henderson's early education was received at home and at a school for boys run by her uncle, Charles Abott. With two of her brothers serving in the armed forces during World War I and in anticipation of a critical shortage of nurses, Virginia Henderson entered the Army School of Nursing at Walter Reed Army Hospital. It was there that she began to question the regimentalization of patient care and the concept of nursing as ancillary to medicine (Henderson, 1991). She described her introduction to nursing as a "series of almost unrelated procedures, beginning with an unoccupied bed and progressing to aspiration of body cavities" (Henderson, 1991, p. 9). It was also at Walter Reed Army Hospital that she met Annie W. Goodrich, the dean of the School of Nursing. Henderson admired Goodrich's intellectual abilities and stated: "Whenever she visited our unit, she lifted our sights above techniques and routine" (Henderson, 1991, p. 11). Henderson credited Goodrich with inspiring her with the "ethical significance of nursing" (Henderson, 1991, p. 10).

Henderson learned to serve in an atmosphere where nurses felt indebted to their patients. During her training, there was a war going on. As a member of society, she considered it a privilege to care for sick and wounded soldiers (Henderson, 1960). This experience forever influenced her ethical understanding of nursing and her appreciation of the importance and complexity of the nurse-patient relationship. She continued to explore the nature of nursing as her student experiences exposed her to different ways of being in relationship with patients and their families.

A pediatric experience as a student at Boston Floating Hospital introduced Henderson to patient-centered care. In this setting nurses were assigned to patients instead of tasks, and, in contrast with the atmosphere of Walter Reed Army Hospital, warm nurse-patient relationships were encouraged. Nurses in this setting were able to come to know the children but were unfamiliar with their parents or home environments (Henderson, 1991).

Following a summer spent with the Henry Street Visiting Nurse Agency in New York City, Henderson began to appreciate the importance of getting to know the patients and their environments. She enjoyed the less formal approach to patient care and become skeptical of the ability of hospital regimes to successfully alter patient's unhealthy ways of living upon returning home (Henderson, 1991).

Based on her experience at Henry Street, Henderson became a visiting nurse after earning her diploma in 1921. Responding to a need for nursing instructors, she left nursing in homes to take a teaching position at Norfolk Protestant Hospital School of Nursing in Norfolk, Virginia. After 5 years of what Henderson (1966) referred to as "learning through teaching," she went back to school to gain more knowledge and to clarify her ideas about the nature of nursing.

THE SEARCH FOR A PERSONAL DEFINITION OF NURSING

Henderson entered Teachers College at Columbia University, earning her baccalaureate degree in 1932 and her master's degree in 1934. She continued at Teachers College as an instructor and associate professor of nursing for the next 20 years.

While at Teachers College, Henderson studied with several people who were influential in clarifying her thoughts about nursing and in developing an analytical approach to patient care. She credits Caroline Stackpole for her understanding of the principle of physiological balance and Edward Thorndike for providing her with a framework focusing on the fundamental needs of humans in which routine nursing activities could be designed and evaluated (Henderson, 1966). Henderson saw the ideas she had been formulating implemented in the rehabilitation work of Dr. George Deaver. She stated: "Nothing made my concept of nursing more concrete that the demonstrations and writings of these rehabilitation experts with their insistence on individualized programs and constant evaluation of the patient's needs and his progress towards the goal of independence" (Henderson, 1966, p. 17).

While working on the 1955 revision of the *Textbook of the Principles and Practice of Nursing,* Henderson focused on the need to be clear about the function of nurses. She opened chapter 1 with the following question: What is nursing and what is the function of the nurse? (Harmer & Henderson, 1955, p. 1) Henderson believed this question was fundamental to anyone choosing to pursue the study and practice of nursing.

> **What is the unique function of the nurse?**

Her often-quoted definition of nursing first appeared in the fifth edition of *Textbook of the Principles and Practice of Nursing* (Harmer & Henderson, 1955, p. 4):

> Nursing is primarily assisting the individual (sick or well) in the performance of those activities contributing to health or its recovery (or to a peaceful death), that he would perform unaided if he had the necessary strength, will, or knowledge. It is likewise the unique contribu-

tion of nursing to help people be independent of such assistance as soon as possible.

Similar definitions later appeared in *Basic Principles of Nursing Care* (Henderson, 1960), *The Nature of Nursing* (Henderson, 1966), and *Principles and Practice of Nursing,* sixth edition (Henderson & Nite, 1978). The subsequent definitions of nursing contain minor wording changes, but the essence of Henderson's definition of nursing has remained consistent with her earliest definition.

In presenting her definition of nursing, Henderson hoped to encourage others to develop their own working concept of nursing and nursing's unique function in society. She believed the definitions of the day were too general and failed to differentiate nurses from other members of the health team. From experience she knew that the functions of health-team members at times overlapped but believed in recognizing the unique function of each member. This knowing led her to consider the following questions: "What *is nursing* that is not also medicine, physical therapy, social work, etc.? And, What is *the unique function of the nurse?*" (Harmer & Henderson, 1955, p. 4). Based on the definition identified above, Henderson described the unique function of the nurse as follows:

> To assist the individual (sick or well) in the performance of those activities contributing to health or its recovery (or to a peaceful death), that he would perform unaided if he had the necessary strength, will, or knowledge. It is likewise her function to help the individual gain independence as rapidly as possible. (Harmer & Henderson, 1955, p. 4)

your thoughts

In addition to declaring nursing functions as unique, Henderson's definition provides a rationale for legitimate nursing activities. Nursing activities are to be performed when an individual lacks part or all of the necessary strength, will, or knowledge to reach the goal of recovery, independence, or peaceful death.

One of Henderson's many contributions to nursing was the introduction of the term "basic nursing care." She identified 14 components that encompassed basic nursing care (Henderson, 1966, pp. 16–17):

1. breathe normally
2. eat and drink adequately
3. eliminate body wastes
4. move and maintain desirable postures
5. sleep and rest
6. select suitable clothes—dress and undress
7. maintain body temperature within normal range by adjusting clothing and modifying the environment
8. keep the body clean and well groomed and protect the integument
9. avoid dangers in the environment and avoid injuring others
10. communicate with others in expressing emotions, needs, fears, or opinions
11. worship according to one's faith
12. work in such a way that there is a sense of accomplishment
13. play or participate in various forms of recreation
14. learn, discover, or satisfy the curiosity that leads to normal development and health and use the available health facilities.

The 14 components reflect needs pertaining to personal hygiene and healthful living, including helping the patient carry out the physician's therapeutic plan (Henderson, 1960, 1966). The focus is on helping individual patients perform patterns of daily living and health-related activities. "The definition of nursing and the fourteen components together outline the functions the nurse can initiate and control" (Furukawa & Howe, 1995, p. 72). They also provide the boundaries for nursing. Patients are returned to independence or health when they are able to perform the 14 components unaided. Henderson (1960) eloquently describes the basic nursing care components in her publication, *Basic Principles of Nursing Care.*

INFLUENCE ON INTERNATIONAL NURSING

Based on the success of *Textbook of the Principles and Practice of Nursing* (fifth edition), Henderson was asked by the International Council of Nurses (ICN) to prepare a short essay that could be used as a guide for nursing in any part of the world. Despite Henderson's belief that it was difficult to promote a universal definition of nursing, *Basic Principles of Nursing Care* (Henderson, 1960) became an international sensation. To date, it has been published in 29 languages and is referred to as the twentieth-century equivalent of Florence Nightingale's *Notes on Nursing.* Henderson continued to question the usefulness of a universal definition of nursing. As recently as 1991, she stated: "Perhaps we should accept the conclusion that it [nursing] depends on the resources of the country involved and the needs of the people it serves" (Henderson, 1991, p. 8). After visiting countries worldwide, she concluded that nursing varied from country to country and that rigorous attempts to define it have been unsuccessful, leaving the "nature of nursing" largely an unanswered question (Henderson, 1991).

> Henderson's definition of nursing called for the nurse to be an expert in basic nursing and to be an independent practitioner.

INFLUENCE ON NURSING EDUCATION

Henderson used the term "nurse" to "refer to a man or woman with a minimum general education represented by graduation from high school, having been prepared for nursing in a recognized basic program of from two and a half to three years" (Harmer & Henderson, 1955, p. 9). Her definition of nursing, which called for the nurse to be an expert in basic nursing care and to be an independent practitioner, required a move from training to education in order to promote nurses knowing the "why" of their practice over adhering to memorized rules (Henderson, 1966).

Henderson outlined basic programs of nursing that included the study of biological and physical sciences, social sciences, medical sciences, and the nursing arts (Harmer & Henderson, 1955). For Henderson, knowledge of the biological and physical sciences was necessary in order for the nurse to understand body functions and to distinguish normal activity from subnormal or pathological activity (Harmer & Henderson, 1955). For this purpose, she recommended study of scientific principles in the areas of biology, chemistry, physics, physiology, and pathology. Without knowing the scientific principles underlying their practice, Henderson believed nurses would be limited in their ability to offer patients help in making healthful decisions and in developing practices or assisting others in developing practices leading to good health (Harmer & Henderson, 1955).

Study in the social sciences was intended to provide the nurse with a better understanding of herself and therefore her patients. In addition, Henderson believed that the nurse must have knowledge of personality development and of the beliefs and customs of different groups in order to assess individual needs accurately (Harmer & Henderson, 1955).

Henderson referred to the following as the "medical sciences": all that is known about the cause; the signs and symptoms; and the occurrence, prevention, treatment, and probable outcome of disease (Harmer & Henderson, 1955). She believed knowledge of the medical sciences was necessary for the nurse to cooperate effectively with the physician's therapeutic plan for the patient.

The nursing arts were described by Henderson as the application of knowledge of the sciences and development of skills related to nursing activities (Harmer & Henderson, 1955). She stated: "It may be that knowledge of the general with application to the specific is central to artistic performances in all arts—including the art of nursing" (Henderson, 1966, p. 62).

In addition to recommendations about curricular content, Henderson had thoughts on the sequencing of learning experiences, tools to facilitate learning, and evaluation of nursing practice. She believed basic programs of nursing should begin with learning the "fundamentals of nursing care" and progress through a sequence of increasingly complex experiences involving mildly ill adults; medical and surgical services; and maternity, pediatrics, and mental health divisions while working beside an older nurse (Harmer & Henderson, 1955). She believed that working with an older nurse enabled the student to develop the ability to "size up" or analyze a nursing situation. For Henderson, this analysis began with an assessment of patient health needs and culminated in a developed plan of care.

Henderson's 1955 revision of Harmer's *Textbook of the Principles and Practice of Nursing* included a chapter on the plan of care for the patient. She placed the responsibility for studying the patient and planning his or her nursing care on the individual nurse assigned to the patient or on the nurse team leader. Henderson stated: "In order to meet the person's health needs it is necessary to know him and his family, and this can only be accomplished by being with them and studying them" (Harmer & Henderson, 1955, p. 3). Studying the patient involved an analysis of factors influencing nursing care that included having knowledge of the patient's age, sex, race, nationality, and religion, along with an estimate of the patient's native intelligence, previous experiences, occupation, and economic status. The nurse also required information about the physician's diagnosis and plan of therapy. Henderson referred to the collection of information about the patient as a "case study" (Harmer & Henderson, 1955). Without the preparation of a case study, Henderson believed that the nurse could not analyze individual needs of the patient required to develop an effective plan of care. She believed that failure to prepare an adequate patient case study would result in a routine pattern of care.

Virginia Henderson also believed in evaluating the quality of basic nursing care provided to patients. She was interested in developing tools that would assist instructors, students, and graduate nurses to evaluate the quality of their care continually. Birnbach (1998, p. 45) recalled Henderson discussing the following three questions that nurses could use to determine how patients perceived their quality of care: What did I do that helped you? What did I do that didn't help you? and What did I not think of that might have helped you?

INFLUENCE ON PRACTICE

Henderson's definition of nursing has had a lasting influence on the way nursing is practiced around the globe. She was one of the first nurses to articulate that nursing had a unique function that made a valuable contribution to the health care of individuals. In writing reflections on the nature of nursing, Henderson (1966) states that her concept of nursing implies universally available health care and a partnership relationship between doctors, nurses, and other healthcare workers.

Based on the assumption that nursing has a unique function, Henderson believed that nursing independently initiates and controls activities related to basic nursing care. Relating the conceptualization of basic care components with the unique functions of nursing provided the initial groundwork for introducing the concept of independent nursing practice. In her 1966 publication, *The Nature of Nursing,* Henderson stated: "It is my contention that the nurse is, and

> Henderson has been heralded as the greatest advocate for nursing libraries worldwide.

should be legally, an independent practitioner and able to make independent judgments as long as he, or she, is not diagnosing, prescribing treatment for disease, or making a prognosis, for these are the physician's functions" (Henderson, 1966, p. 22).

Furthermore, Henderson believed that functions pertaining to the care of patients could be categorized as nursing and non-nursing. She believed that limiting nursing activities to "nursing care" was a useful method of conserving professional nurse power (Harmer & Henderson, 1955). She defined functions that are not a service to the person (mind and body) as non-nursing functions (Harmer & Henderson, 1955). For Henderson, examples of non-nursing functions included ordering supplies, cleaning and sterilizing equipment, and serving food (Harmer & Henderson, 1955).

At the same time, Henderson was not in favor of the practice of assigning patients to lesser trained workers on the basis of level of complexity. For Henderson, "all 'nursing care' . . . is essentially complex because it involves constant adaptation of procedures to the needs of the individual" (Harmer & Henderson, 1955, p. 9).

As the authority on basic nursing care, Henderson believed the nurse has the responsibility to assess the needs of the individual patient, help individuals meet their health needs, and/or provide an environment in which the individual can perform activities unaided. It is the nurse's role, according to Henderson, "to 'get inside the patient's skin' and supplement his strength, will or knowledge according to his needs" (Harmer & Henderson, 1955, p. 5). Conceptualizing the nurse as a substitute for the patient's lack of necessary will, strength, or knowledge to attain good health and to complete or make the patient whole, highlights the complexity and uniqueness of nursing.

INFLUENCE ON LIBRARY RESEARCH AND DEVELOPMENT

Henderson has been heralded as the greatest advocate for nursing libraries worldwide. Following the completion of her revised text in 1955, Henderson moved to Yale University. It was here that she began what would become a distinguished career in library science research.

Of all her contributions to nursing, Virginia Henderson's work on the identification and control of nursing literature is perhaps her greatest. In the 1950s there was an increasing interest on the part of the profession to establish a research basis for the practice of nursing. It was also recognized that the body of nursing knowledge was unstructured and therefore inaccessible to practicing nurses and educators. Henderson encouraged nurses to become active in the work of classifying the nursing literature.

Virginia Henderson and Leo W. Simmons, an anthropologist at Yale University, were asked to make a survey of existing nursing research (Simmons & Henderson, 1964). Working on a grant awarded to Yale University, Henderson went to 30 states to determine what nursing research had been done there, what individuals knew about, and what studies they would do if they had the necessary resources (Henderson, 1991). The results of the survey indicated that awareness of nursing research was limited and that nurse researchers were conducting studies from the perspective of the social sciences (Henderson, 1991).

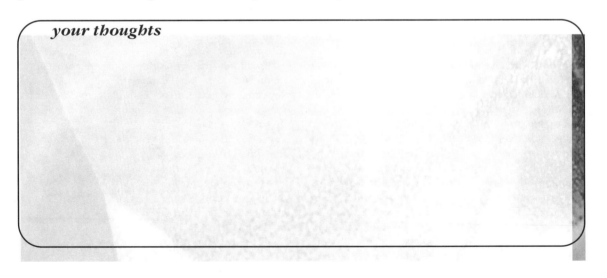

your thoughts

Florence Wald, dean of Yale University School of Nursing, recognized the value of the bibliography developed from the survey and pursued a grant from the U.S. Public Health Service to publish the bibliography. An advisory committee and what would become the Interagency Council on Library Resources for Nursing were formed to support the project. At its completion, the 11-year project was published by J. B. Lippincott Company as the four-volume annotated index to the analytical and historical literature on nursing from 1900 through 1959, known as the Nursing Studies Index (NSI).

The success of the NSI and the efforts of the Interagency Council on Library Resources for Nursing led to the creation of the International Nursing Index (INI) in 1966. The INI is published collaboratively by the *American Journal of Nursing* and the National Library of Medicine and continues to be a major scholastic resource in nursing. The INI includes articles selected from nursing and non-nursing journals, publications of organizations and agencies, nursing books published, and nursing dissertations. In an effort to help nurses use the index more easily, the nursing thesaurus was revised to include commonly used nursing terms as cross-references to the Medical Subject Headings in 1968.

Virginia Henderson remained a strong advocate for nursing resource development throughout her lifetime. In 1990, the Sigma Theta Tau International Library was named in her honor. Henderson insisted that if the library were to bear her name, the electronic networking system would have to advance the work of staff nurses by providing them with current, jargon-free information wherever they were based (McBride, 1997).

Summary

Virginia Henderson's life was devoted to the promotion of nursing and nursing care. Embodied in her writings is a deep sense of obligation to serve others. Henderson's definition of nursing and the 14 basic nursing care components have been widely read and frequently used in guiding the direct nursing care of real patients around the world. Her conceptualizations have empowered others to see nursing from a new perspective and continue to ask questions about the nature of nursing. She has influenced curriculum development and inspired nurses to be clinical scholars by promoting the accessibility and importance of research in day-to-day practice. Miss Henderson's lifetime achievements have provided essential stepping stones in the recognition of nursing as a scientific discipline and profession. But more important, she served by sharing the beauty of nursing with the world.

> I think the beauty of medicine and nursing is the combination of your heart, your head and your hands and where you separate them, you diminish them, diminish the service. (McBride, 1997)

References

Birnbach, N. (1998). Three questions. In Hermann, E. K. (Ed.), *Virginia Avenel Henderson: Signature for nursing.* Indianapolis: Center Nursing Press.

Furukawa, C. Y., & Howe, J. K. (1995). Virginia Henderson. In George, J. B. (Ed.), *Nursing theories: The base for professional nursing practice* (4th ed.). Norwalk, CT: Appleton & Lange.

Halloran, E. (1991). Virginia Henderson. [On-line]. Available: http://www.son.washington.edu/news 1.html.

Harmer, B., & Henderson, V. A. (1955). *Textbook of the principles and practice of nursing.* New York: Macmillan.

Henderson, V. A. (1960). *Basic Principles of nursing care.* Geneva: International Council of Nurses.

Henderson, V. A. (1966). *The nature of nursing.* New York: The National League for Nursing Press.

Henderson, V. A. (1991). *The nature of nursing: Reflections after 25 years.* New York: The National League for Nursing Press.

Henderson, V. A. & Nite, G. (1978). *Principles and practices of nursing* (6th ed.). New York: Macmillan.

McBride, A. B. (Narrator). (1997). Celebrating Virginia Henderson. (Video). (Available from Center for Nursing Press, 550 West North Street, Indianapolis, IN 46202.)

Simmons, L. W., & Henderson, V. A. (1964). *Nursing research: A survey and assessment.* New York: Appleton & Lange.

Smith, J. P. (1998). In my opinion. In Hermann, E. K. (Ed.), *Virginia Avenel Henderson: Signature for nursing.* Indianapolis: Center Nursing Press.

Chapter *12*

Josephine Paterson
and Loretta Zderad
Humanistic Nursing Theory
with Clinical Applications*

- ❖ Introducing the Theorists
- ❖ Humanistic Nursing Theory
- ❖ Clinical Applications of Humanistic Nursing Theory
- ❖ References

Susan Kleiman

*Reprinted with permission of the National League for Nursing, New York.

INTRODUCING THE THEORISTS

While I was struggling to write about Humanistic Nursing Theory, I received a phone call from a registered nurse from the Midwest. She was a graduate student taking her first course in nursing theory and had chosen the Theory of Humanistic Nursing as the topic of her term paper. She was being discouraged by her instructor and dissuaded by some other academic nursing professionals that she had contacted. The reasons given ranged from lack of clarity of the theory, to not enough mention in the literature about clinical or research applications, to the assertion that Humanistic Nursing Theory is a theory that has "had its day." I have heard these criticisms before, both personally and related by other students. The purpose of this section is to clarify these and other relevant issues. The applications presented in the next section are directed toward enhancing the understanding of the practical applications of Humanistic Nursing Theory.

As for Humanistic Nursing Theory having had its day, I still believe that it was before its time and it is only recently, in an atmosphere of theory-based nursing, that it is being received and understood in its full range of meaning. Why now?, you may ask, as this student did. I truly believe that it is related to the changing worldview. There is an increasing acceptance of a worldview that does not embrace the reductionist mind-set as the touchstone of explanatory power. More and more there is an awareness of interrelatedness or, in terms of Humanistic Nursing Theory, the "all-at-once" quality of existence. It includes a temporal component that provides a space-time immediacy to the phenomenon in the "here and now." According to this view, patients and nurses bring all that they are, "all at once," as they engage in a dialogue that is the "essence" of nursing. It is a theory that does not reduce either the patient or the nurse to needs, pathology, or culture. It is an inclusive theory that provides a method for managing the complexities that are the reality of "being in the world." At the same time, it offers a means of prioritizing and focusing, which allows for growth and enrichment. I will show how Humanistic Nursing Theory provides an umbrella; in other words, that it is a meta-theory, under which other nursing theories are subsumed and can be explained.

Questions that students of Humanistic Nursing Theory ask are not only related to the concepts and the application of the theory itself. There are also important questions about how we might use this newly found awareness and understanding of the "essential characteristics of nursing" to enhance nursing as a profession.

Martin Buber (1965, p. 71) has eloquently said that humans have a basic need to be confirmed by others of their kind: "[S]ecretly and bashfully [they] watch for a 'Yes' which allows [them] to be." In Humanistic Nursing Theory we experience that "yes" as we encounter outward expression of that which we have inwardly known. We are uplifted by the "poiesis," the bringing forth and bursting open of the blossom of possibilities that this brings (Heidegger, 1977, p. 10).

The Theorists

Who are the theorists who authored Humanistic Nursing Theory? Dr. Josephine Paterson is originally from the East Coast and Dr. Loretta Zderad is from the Midwest. Each attended different diploma schools of nursing and different undergraduate pro-

your thoughts

grams, both receiving their bachelor's degree in nursing education. In their graduate work, Dr. Zderad majored in psychiatric nursing at the Catholic University of America and Dr. Paterson in public health nursing at Johns Hopkins University. They met in the mid-1950s, when they both worked at Catholic University. Their task was to create a new program that would encompass the community health component and the psychiatric component of the graduate program. That started a process of collaboration and dialogue and friendship that has lasted for over 35 years.

Dr. Zderad earned her doctorate in philosophy from Georgetown University and Dr. Paterson earned her doctor of nursing science degree from Boston University. Dr. Zderad's dissertation was on empathy and Dr. Paterson's was on comfort. They shared and developed their concepts, approaches, and experiences of "existential phenomenology," which evolved into the formal Theory of Humanistic Nursing. They incorporated these into their work as educators and shared them across the country in seminars and workshops on Humanistic Nursing Theory. This theory may be considered a prototype for some of the more recent experiential-based nursing theories (Benner, 1984; Parse, 1981; Watson, 1988).

My first contact with Humanistic Nursing Theory was when I was a graduate student in psychiatric mental health nursing. Josephine Paterson's name was given to me as a possible preceptor for my clinical placement. At that time, Dr. Paterson was working as a psychotherapist at the Veterans Hospital in Northport, Long Island, in the Mental Hygiene Clinic and was also adjunct associate professor at Adelphi University. Loretta Zderad was at that time the associate chief of nursing service for education at the same Veterans Hospital.

Dr. Paterson and Dr. Zderad came to the Veterans Administration (VA) Hospital in Northport in 1971. They were hired for their original positions as nursologists by a forward-thinking administrator who recognized the need for staff support during a period of change in the VA system. The position of nursologist involved a three-pronged approach to the improvement of patient care through clinical practice, education, and research. These functions were integrated within the framework of humanistic nursing. They worked with the nurses at Northport in this manner from 1971 until 1978. At that time they assumed the positions they held when I met them.

My initial interview with Dr. Paterson went well and she agreed to work with me over the next 2 years. Perhaps she had an attraction to the "all at onceness" of my multidimensional life. At that time, I was working full time, a graduate student, a wife, a mother, and a homemaker. I am eternally grateful to her for those sunrise hours of supervision before I went off to work. The following week I had the privilege of meeting Loretta Zderad.

When I first met Dr. Paterson and Dr. Zderad, I had no awareness of Humanistic Nursing Theory. During our discussions, however, it became apparent that we shared an interest in certain writers. For example, we spoke about Martin Buber and the "I and Thou" concept and "dialogue" as the process of intersubjective relating. We also spoke about Rollo May (1995) and his work on creativity. At some point Dr. Paterson casually mentioned that I might be interested in reading a book that she and Dr. Zderad had written. She indicated that the book referenced these writers as well as some existentialists such as Marcel, Desan, and Popper. The book was *Humanistic Nursing* (1988). The following 2 years brought me a world of enrichment. For Dr. Paterson and Dr. Zderad the next 2 years culminated in their retirement and relocation to the South. I, on the other hand, continue the work that they started, as a fellow theorist, and as a friend and colleague in nursing.

Since their retirement, Dr. Zderad and Dr. Paterson refer inquiries about Humanistic Nursing Theory to me. The reasons for this honor I have been told are that they believe I have "a real grasp of what the theory is about." They also appreciate how alive it is in my everyday practice of nursing. It has given me the opportunity to speak individually to students or to present and discuss the theory with groups of nurses. At these times I am aware of the disappointment that nurses feel in not being able to have more direct access to the theorists themselves. I feel privileged to have had a professional and a personal relationship in which I have been able to dialogue with Dr. Paterson and Dr. Zderad about Humanistic Nursing Theory. With this privilege I also experience a responsibility to share what that dialogue has offered me. I do, however, have concerns when they refer people to me that I represent Humanistic Nursing Theory accurately and adequately.

My call to Dr. Paterson and Dr. Zderad for validation of my representation of their theory in discourse and in writing has been responded to with confirmation that I have done what they had hoped nurses would do. That is, I have taken Humanistic Nursing Theory and made it my own, expanded it, and articulated it to others. And so while I may use a different style, and in our world scholars at times may differ, I am confident based on their validation that the core concepts of the theory have not been distorted. Perhaps my particular contribution is that I have taken the basic theoretical concepts of Humanistic Nursing Theory that were originally articulated and conceptualized through the shared experiences of nurses, and shown how nurses can use those concepts to expand and enrich themselves, their patients, nursing, and health care in general. Dr. Paterson and Dr. Zderad's response to my call was that it was now our theory. "Our theory" to me means a theory in progress, to be owned, expanded upon, and hopefully articulated by all those nurses who embrace it as their own.

HUMANISTIC NURSING THEORY

Humanistic Nursing Theory is multidimensional. It speaks to the essences of nursing and embraces the dynamics of being, becoming, and change. It is an interactive theory of nursing that provides a methodology for reflective articulation of nursing essences. It is also a theory that provides a methodological bridge between theory and practice by providing a broad guide for nursing "dialogue" in a myriad of settings.

Nursing as seen through Humanistic Nursing Theory is the ability to struggle with another through "peak experiences related to health and suffering in which the participants in the nursing situation are and become in accordance with their human potential" (Paterson & Zderad, 1976, p. 7). The struggle is shared through a dialogue between the participants. This mandate to share "struggles with" is what allows for each to "become" in relationship with the other. In nursing, the purpose of this dialogue, or intersubjective relating, according to Josephine Paterson and Loretta Zderad, is, "[n]urturing the well-being and more-being of persons in need" (p. 4). Humanistic Nursing Theory is grounded in existentialism and emphasizes the lived experience of nursing. One of the existential themes that it builds on is the affirmation of being and becoming of both the patient and the nurse through the choices they make and the intersubjective relationships they engage in. This dynamic is expressed as nursing's concern with the struggle toward self-actualizing potential or "more-being."

> Nursing is nurturing the well-being and more-being of persons. It is the ability to enter into nursing situations and to struggle with another in his or her experiences of health and suffering toward his or her self-actualizing potential.

The new adventurer in humanistic nursing theory may at first find some of these terms and phrases awkward. When I spoke to a colleague of the "moreness" and of "relating all-at-once," she remarked, "Oh, oh, you're beginning to sound just like them," meaning Dr. Paterson and Dr. Zderad. What was of note to her has become natural to me. It is reflective of my grasp of nursing as an ever-changing process. Think of your nursing experiences, whatever the contexts may be. Are these experiences of static settings? Or is there a pervasive sense of activity associated with them? Just as nursing in actual practice is never inert, so Humanistic Nursing Theory is in its essence dynamic. I reflect with a smile on Josephine Paterson's description of humanistic nursing: "Our 'here and now' stage of humanistic nursing practice theory development at times is experienced as an all-at-once octopus at a discotheque, stimulation personified gyrating in many colors" (1977, p. 4). It is a bonus when a theory not only can be useful but also can be fun.

While this approach to theory may seem somewhat lighthearted, it addresses the need to feel comfortable with theory. Theory, like research, is not just for those in ivory towers. Theory and research are a part of every nurse and all that is nursing. If we look at theory through R. D. Lang's eyes as "an articulated vision of experience" (Zderad, 1978, p. 4), we can see that in one sense by looking at our own experience of nursing, as proposed in Humanistic Nursing Theory, we all become theorists. I do not use the term "comfortable with" in the generic sense, but rather in the humanistic nursing sense. Comfort in this view is that which allows persons to be all that they can be in particular lived situations. Theory should offer nurses comfort in their everyday nursing. In other words, theory should offer nurses assistance to be all that they can be in their particular lived nursing situations.

If I were asked to succinctly conceptualize humanistic nursing theory, I would have to say, "call and response." These three words encapsulate for me the core themes of this quite elegant and very profound theory. In what follows, you will come to understand that through this paradigm, Josephine Paterson and Loretta Zderad have presented a vision of nursing that withstands variation in practice settings and the changing patterns of nursing over time.

According to Humanistic Nursing Theory, there is a call from a person, a family, a community, or from humanity for help with some health-related issue. A nurse, a group of nurses, or the community of nurses hearing and recognizing that call responds in a manner that is intended to help the caller with the health-related need. What happens during this dialogue, the "and" in the "call-and-response," the "between," is nursing.

In their book *Humanistic Nursing* (1976), Drs. Paterson and Zderad share with other nurses their method for exploring the "between," again emphasizing that it is the "between" that they conceive of as nursing. The method is phenomenological inquiry (Paterson & Zderad, 1976 p. 72). Engaging in phenomenological inquiry sensitizes the inquiring nurse to the excitement, fear, and uncertainty of approaching the nursing situation openly. Through a spirit of receptivity, a readiness for surprise, and the courage to experience the unknown, there is an opportunity for authentic relatedness and intersubjectivity. "The process leads one naturally to repeated experiencing of and reflective immersion in the lived phenomena" (Zderad, 1978, p. 8). This immersion into the intersubjective experience and the phenomenological process that one engages in helps guide the nurse in the responsive interchange between the patient and the nurse. During this interchange the nurse calls forth all that she is (education, skills, life experiences, etc.) and integrates it into her response. A common misconception that some students of Humanistic Nursing Theory have is that it asserts that the nurse must provide what it is that the patient is calling for. Remember the response of the nurse is guided by all that she is. This includes her professional role, ethics, and competencies. And so although a response may not actually provide what is being called for, the process of being heard according to this theory is in itself a humanizing experience.

This explanation of Humanistic Nursing Theory calls for elaboration of some of its basic concepts and assumptions. Let's look at the conceptual framework of Humanistic Nursing Theory represented in Figure 12–1.

Humanistic nursing is a moving process that occurs in the living context of human beings, human beings who interface and interact with others and other things in the world. This conceptual framework represents a nonlinear process that, over time, spirals upward. This fluidity may be somewhat dis-

> Nurses respond to calls from a person, family, or community, or from humanity for help with a health-related issue. The nursing is what happens in this dialogue between the nurse and the one being helped. The nursing is the "between."

turbing to the beginning explorer of Humanistic Nursing Theory. It is this fluidity, however, that, once grasped, allows for the generalization to a diversity of practice settings.

In the world of Humanistic Nursing Theory the human beings identified are the patient (i.e., person, family, community, or humanity) and the nurse (Figure 12–2). A patient becomes identified as the patient when he sends a call for help with some health-related problem. The person hearing and recognizing the call is the nurse. The nurse is another human being who by intentionally choosing to become a nurse has made a commitment to help others in relation to their health needs.

It is important to emphasize that the nurse and the patient are both first human beings, or groups of human beings, with their own particular gestalts (Figure 12–3). Gestalt, representing all that those human beings are, includes all their past experiences, all their current being, and all their hopes, dreams, and fears of the future that are experienced in their own space-time dimension. This includes the environmental resources available to them, factors that have increasing import in times of fiscal constraints. In sum, using a humanistic nursing term, they exist "all-at-once." In the context of nursing, when these two human beings encounter and interact with each other, that interaction centers on the call from one person, the patient, for a helpful response from another person, the nurse. Although the call and response is between the nurse and the patient, it is important to understand that all else that makes the individual person who he or she is enters in this interaction too.

This gestalt includes the patient's past and current social relationships, such as the experiences of gender, race, and religion, as well as education, work, and whatever individualized patterns for coping with the experience of living the person has developed. It also includes past experiences with helpers in the health-care system and the patient's image and expectation of what it is that he or she is calling to the nurse for. As incarnate human beings, we exist in this particular space at this particular time, in a physical body that senses, filters, and processes our experiences.

The nurse too brings all that she is. Her expectation is, however, that she be able to respond to the call for help as a nurse. The nurse then interweaves her professional identity and professional education, with all her other life experiences to create her own tapestry, which she projects through her nursing responses. One has only to observe nurses going about their nursing to see how individualized the ex-

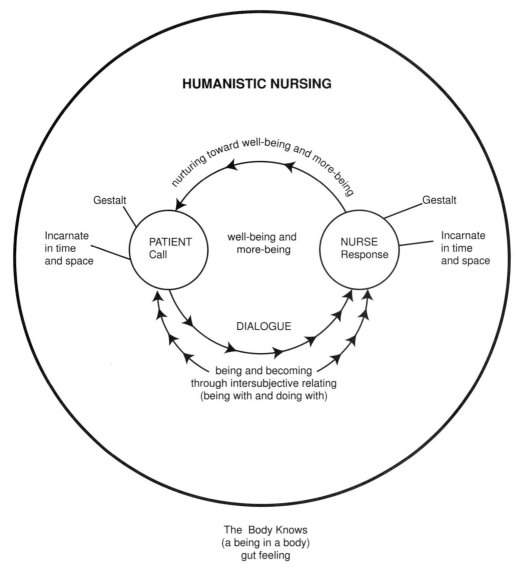

HUMANISTIC NURSING

nurturing toward well-being and more-being

Gestalt

Incarnate
in time
and space

PATIENT
Call

well-being and
more-being

NURSE
Response

Gestalt

Incarnate
in time
and space

DIALOGUE

being and becoming
through intersubjective relating
(being with and doing with)

The Body Knows
(a being in a body)
gut feeling

Figure 12–1 *World of others and things.*

pressed dialogue with a particular patient can be. A very simple example of this may be two nurses performing the same task of suctioning a patient. Depending on the nurse and the patient, I have seen this done with tenderness, with humor, and with masterful technical skills that make the procedure almost unnoticeable. I noticed one nurse who, each time she positioned and suctioned the person she was working with, made sure that she also repositioned the little basket of flowers that the nurse had placed by the patient's bedside. It is this individuality as human beings that makes us alike and provides

one of the threads that unite us throughout this process of living. Being alike in our differences is only one of those core threads, however, and in nursing, humanistic theory attempts to uncover the other unifying threads or essences that make up the human fabric of nursing. The nurse must always be aware that—because in existential theory human beings become through the choices they make and the intersubjective experiences they engage in—the choice to intersubjectively engage and the level of that intersubjective relating are mutually determined by the patient and nurse.

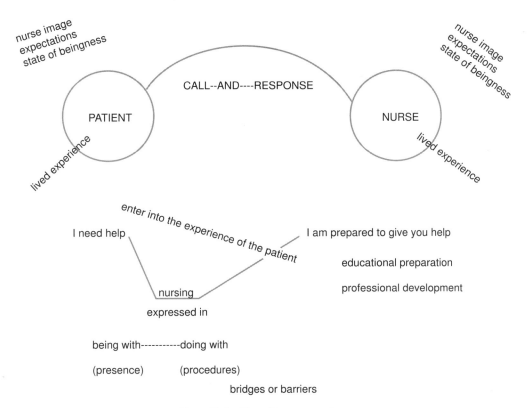

Nursing Is Transactional

nurse image
expectations
state of beingness

CALL--AND----RESPONSE

PATIENT

NURSE

nurse image
expectations
state of beingness

lived experience

lived experience

enter into the experience of the patient

I need help

I am prepared to give you help

educational preparation

professional development

nursing

expressed in

being with-----------doing with

(presence)   (procedures)

bridges or barriers

Figure 12–2 *Shared human experience.*

Philosophical and Methodological Background

The phenomenological movement of the nineteenth century was in response to what its proponents called the dehumanization and objectification of the world by the scientific community. Phenomenologists proposed that human beings, the world, and their experiences of their world are inseparable. You can easily see that a nursing theory that is based in the human context lends itself to phenomenological inquiry rather than reductionism, which attempts to remove subjective humanness and strives to achieve detached objectivity. The early phenomenologists saw their goal as the examination and description of all things, including the human experience of those things, in the particular way that they reveal themselves without preconceived ideas or assumptions. In the early 1960s Josephine Paterson and Loretta Zderad gravitated toward this method to first examine their own nursing. Later they used this method to work with other nurses in examining their nursing

practice to explicate its essences. Today, nursing phenomenologists use variations of phenomenological methods to examine the experiential phenomena of nursing.

There are people, however, who profess that phenomenology is not a philosophy but is at best a method—a method developed by applying phenomenological concepts. In other words, phenomenology is the "experience" of a method that can be integrated into a general approach or way of viewing the world. As I mentioned before, nurses who can relate to this method are inclined to cultivate it and make it a part of their everyday approach to nursing. This method is no less rigorous in its application than the method used in experimental research to build theories. The phenomenological approach is based on description, intuition, analysis, and synthesis. Intuitive openness and accurate description require some aptitude for this conceptual framework. Of importance are training and conscientious self-criticism on the part of the unbiased inquirer as the inquirer investigates the phenomenon as it reveals itself. In phenom-

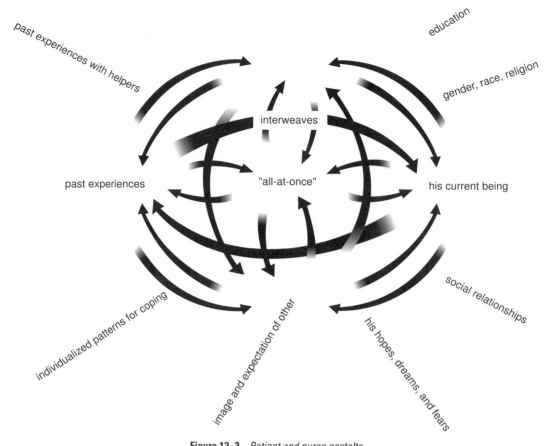

Figure 12–3 *Patient and nurse gestalts.*

enology a statement's validity is based on whether or not it describes the phenomenon accurately. The truth of all the premises resulting from the critical analysis of each phenomenon described can be verified by examining the phenomenon itself.

Dr. Paterson and Dr. Zderad describe five phases to their phenomenological study of nursing. These phases are presented sequentially, but actually in this process they are interwoven, because, as with all of Humanistic Nursing Theory, there is a constant flow between, in all directions, and all-at-once emanating toward a center that is nursing. The phases of humanistic nursing inquiry are:

- preparation of the nurse knower for coming to know
- nurse knowing the other intuitively
- nurse knowing the other scientifically
- nurse complementarily synthesizing known others
- succession within the nurse from the many to the paradoxical one

Enfolded in these five phases are three concepts that are very basic to Humanistic Nursing Theory. They are bracketing, angular view, and noetic loci. These will be taken up as we discuss the phases of inquiry.

Preparation of the Nurse Knower for Coming to Know

In the first phase the inquirer tries to open herself up to the unknown and possibly different. She consciously and conscientiously struggles with understanding and identifying her own "angular view." Angular view involves the gestalt of the human that we spoke about earlier. It includes the conceptual and experiential framework that we bring into any situation with us, a framework that is usually unexamined and casually accepted as we negotiate our everyday world. Angular view is not judged. It is a component of the process and needs to be recognized as such. Later in the process it is called upon to help make sense of and give meaning to the experience of inquiry.

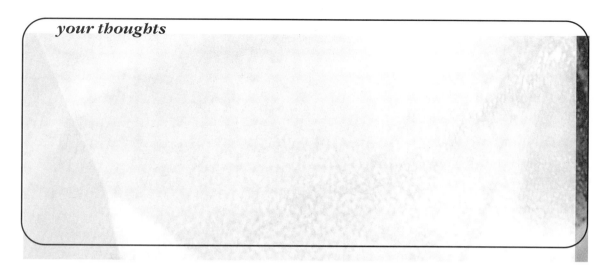
By identifying our angular view we are then able to purposefully bracket it so that we do not superimpose it on the experience we are trying to relate to. When we bracket, we purposefully hold our own thoughts, experiences, and beliefs in abeyance. I reemphasize that this abeyance does not deny our unique selves but suspends them, allowing us to experience the other in its own uniqueness. This is primary to phenomenological inquiry, which calls on us to see that which the phenomenon reveals itself in itself to be.

By becoming aware of and acknowledging what we think is true, we can then attempt to hold these assumptions in abeyance, so that they will not prematurely intrude upon one's attempts to describe the experiences of another. A personal experience that helped me to grasp the concept of bracketing occurred a few years ago when I was traveling in Europe. As I entered each new country, I experienced the excitement of the unknown. I realized at the same time how alert, open, and other directed I was in this uncharted world as compared to my own daily routine at home. Here at times I would kind of fill in the blanks left by my inattentiveness to a routine experience, sometimes anticipating and answering questions even before they were asked. This alertness, openness, and other directedness is the goal of bracketing. According to Husserl (1970), who is considered the father of modern phenomenology, the state desired is that of the perpetual beginner.

Bracketing prepares the inquirer to enter the uncharted world of the other without expectations and preconceived ideas. It helps one to be open to the authentic, in other words to the true experience of the other. Even temporarily letting go of that which shapes our own identity as the self, however, causes anxiety, fear, and uncertainty. Labeling, diagnosing,

and routines add a necessary and very valuable predictability, sense of security, and means of conserving energy to our everyday existence and practice. It may also make us less open, however, to the new and different in a situation. Being open to the new and different is a necessary stance in being able to know of the other intuitively.

Nurse Knowing the Other Intuitively

Knowing the other intuitively is described by Dr. Paterson and Dr. Zderad as "moving back and forth between the impressions the nurse becomes aware of

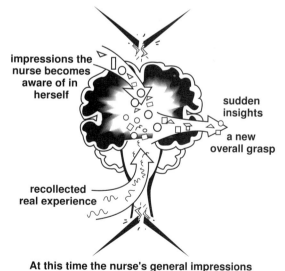

impressions the nurse becomes aware of in herself

sudden insights

a new overall grasp

recollected real experience

At this time the nurse's general impressions are in a dialogue with her unbracketed view

Figure 12–4 *Nurse knowing the other intuitively. Adapted from illustration in Briggs, J., & Peat, D. (1989).* Turbulent Mirror *(p. 176). New York: Harper & Row.*

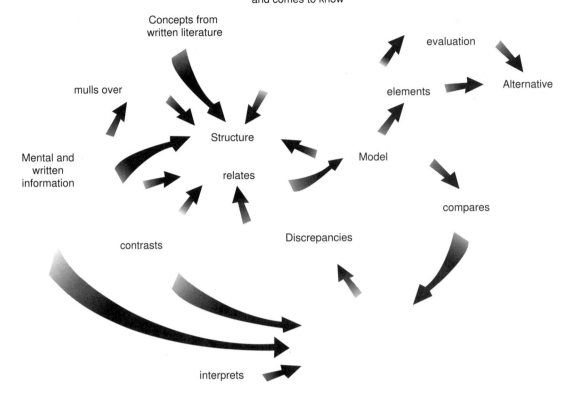

Standing outside the phenomenon, the nurse
examines it through analysis
and comes to know

Concepts from
written literature

mulls over

Mental and
written
information

Structure

relates

contrasts

Discrepancies

interprets

nurse conscious of herself

evaluation

elements

Alternative

Model

compares

Figure 12–5 *Nurse knowing the other scientifically. Adapted from illustration in Briggs, J., & Peat, D. (1989).* Turbulent Mirror *(p. 176). New York: Harper & Row.*

in herself and the recollected real experience of the other" (1976, pp. 88-89), which was obtained through the unbiased being with the other. This process of bracketing versus intuiting is not contradictory. Both are necessary and interwoven parts of the phenomenological process. The rigor and validity of phenomenology are based on the ongoing referring back to the phenomenon itself. It is conceptualized as a dialectic between the impression and the real. This shifting back and forth allows for sudden insights on the part of the nurse, a new overall grasp which manifests itself in a clearer or perhaps a new "understanding of." These understandings generate further development of the process. At this time the nurse's general impressions are in a dialogue with her unbracketed view (Figure 12–4).

Nurse Knowing the Other Scientifically

In the next phase, objectivity is needed as the nurse comes to know the other scientifically. Standing out-

side the phenomenon the nurse examines it through analysis. She comes to know it through its parts of elements that are symbolic and known. This phase incorporates the nurse's ability to be conscious of herself and that which she has taken in, merged with, made part of herself. "This is the time when the nurse mulls over, analyzes, sorts out, compares, contrasts, relates, interprets, gives a name to, and categorizes" (Paterson & Zderad, 1976, p. 79). Patterns and themes are reflective of and rigorously validated by the authentic experience (Figure 12-5).

Nurse Complementarily Synthesizing Known Others

At this point the nurse personifies what has been described by Dr. Paterson and Dr. Zderad as a "noetic locus," a "knowing place" (1976, p. 43). According to this concept, the greatest gift a human being can have is the ability to relate to others, to wonder, search, and imagine about experience, and to create

Section II *Evolution of Nursing Theory: Essential Influences*

out of what has become known. The ability of nurses to see themselves as "knowing places" encourages them to continue to develop their community of world thinkers through their educative processes, which then become a part of their angular view. This self-expansion, through the internalization of what others have come to know, dynamically interrelates with the nurse's human capacity to be conscious of her own lived experiences. Through this interrelationship the subjective and objective world of nursing can be reflected upon by each nurse, who is aware of and values herself as a "knowing place" (Figure 12–6).

Succession within the Nurse from the Many to the Paradoxical One

This is the birth of the new from the existing patterns, themes, and categories. It is in this phase that the nurse "comes up with a conception or abstraction that is inclusive of and beyond the multiplicities and contradictions" (Paterson & Zderad, 1976, p. 81), in a process that corrects and expands her own angular view.

This is the pattern of the dialectic process, which is reflected throughout Humanistic Nursing Theory. In the dialectic process there is a repetitive pattern of organizing the dissimilar into a higher level (Barnum, 1990, p. 44). At this higher level differences are assimilated to create the new. This repetitive dialectic process of humanistic nursing is an approach that feels comfortable and natural for those who think inductively. For me, the pervasive theme of dialectic assimilation speaks to universal interrelatedness from the simplest to the most complex level. Human beings by virtue of their ability to be self-observing have the unique capacity to transcend

themselves and dialectically reflect on their relationship to the universe. This dialectic process has a pattern similar to that of the call and response paradigm of Humanistic Nursing Theory. This paradigm speaks to the interactive dialogue between two different human beings from which a unique yet universal instance of nursing emerges. The nursing interaction is limited in time and space, but the internalization of

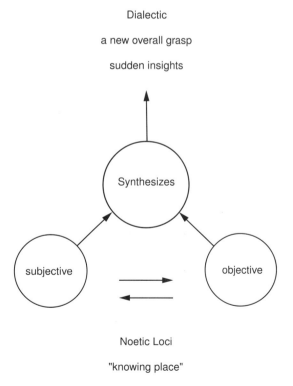

Figure 12–6 *Nurse complementarily synthesizing known others*

> Community is "two or more persons struggling together toward a center." A distinguishing concept of this theory is the obligation of nurses to each other in community.

that experience adds something new to each person's angular view. Neither is the same as before. Each is more because of that coming together. The coming together of the nurse and the patient, the between in the lived world, is nursing. Just as in the double helix of the DNA molecule, this interweaving pattern is what structures the individual. In the fabric of Humanistic Nursing Theory this intentional interweaving between patient and nurse is what also gives nursing its structure, form, and meaning.

Dr. Paterson and Dr. Zderad used this method of phenomenological inquiry and dialectic synthesis in workshops with other nurses. Over 2000 descriptions of nursing were written by more than 120 nurses who shared their lived world of nursing with each other. From the analysis and synthesis of these descriptions, 11 phenomena of nursing were generated. These are awareness, openness, empathy, caring, touching, understanding, responsibility, trust, acceptance, self-recognition, and dialogue. These phenomena were envisioned as the constants in the ever-changing world of patient and nurse interaction.

The Concept of Community

The definition of *community* presented by Drs. Paterson and Zderad is: "Two or more persons struggling together toward a center" (1976, p. 131). They and the other nurses from their workshops were very much a community, a community of nurses struggling toward a center that is nursing. Just as in any community there is the individual and the collective known as the "community." Plato points to the microcosm and the macrocosm and proposes that the one is reflective of the many. In unification theories the emphasis is on recurrent patterns that given enough distance would be found in all the universe. Humanistic Nursing Theory can be considered both a micro- and macrotheory in which the nursing interaction of one is considered to be a reflection of the recurrent pattern of nursing and is therefore worth reflecting upon and valuing. All nurses are members of a community of nurses struggling toward a center that is nursing through dialogue and interaction. A distinguishing concept of Humanistic Nursing Theory is an inherent obligation of nurses to each other in this community. That which enhances one

of us, enhances all of us. Through openness, sharing, and caring, we each will expand our angular views, each becoming more than before. Subsequently we take back into our nursing community these expanded selves, which in turn will touch our patients, other colleagues, and the world of health care.

CLINICAL APPLICATIONS OF HUMANISTIC NURSING THEORY

Nurse's Reflection on Nursing

As an introduction to the clinical applications of Humanistic Nursing Theory, I will share with you two explorations from Dr. Paterson's and Dr. Zderad's nursing experiences. These descriptive explorations are related to the concepts of empathy, comfort, and presence. Dr. Paterson (1977, p. 13) shared her experiences with a terminally ill cancer patient. She describes: "For a while I really beat on myself. I felt nothing, just a kind of indifference and numbness, as Dominic expressed his miseries, fears, and anger. I pride myself on my empathic ability. I felt so inadequate. I could not believe I could not feel with him what he was experiencing. Intellectually I knew his words, his expressions were pain-filled. My feelings of inadequacy, helplessness, and inability to control myself, came through strong. [As] I mulled reflectively about this, suddenly a light dawned amidst my puzzlement. I was experiencing what Dominic was expressing. At this time I was feeling his inadequacy, helplessness, and inability to control his cancer."

This insight brought a greater understanding between Dr. Paterson and this patient, an understanding that brought them closer so that she could endure with him in his fear-filled knowing and unknowing of dying. As his condition deteriorated, she continued to visit at his bedside. "Often after greeting me and saying what he needed he would fall asleep. First, I thought, 'It doesn't matter whether I come or not.' Then I noticed and validated that when I moved his eyes flew open. I reevaluated his sleeping during my visit. I discussed this with him. He felt safe when I sat with him. He was exhausted, staying awake, watching himself to be sure he did not die. When I was there I watched him, and he could sleep. I no longer made any move to leave before my time with him was up. I told him of this intention, so that he could relax more deeply. To alleviate aloneness; this is a most expensive gift. To give this gift of time, and presence in the patient's space, a person has to value, the outcomes of relating."

This gift of presence is poetically described by Dr. Zderad (1978, p. 48):

Section II *Evolution of Nursing Theory: Essential Influences*

Death lifts his scythe
  to swipe down the young man
    misdressed in hospital gown
    displaced in hospital bed.

The cruel cold blade slashes
  the hard mask of his nurse
    silently standing there
    bleeding forth her presence.

The beauty of the articulation of this essence is that it encourages other nurses to reflect, value, and further communicate the essences of their practice. And so Dr. Paterson's and Dr. Zderad's accounts brought back to mind an experience of mine that had stayed with me for years but that I had not truly reflected upon until exposed to the process of humanistic nursing.

Years ago I worked on the night shift in the nursing home portion of a hospital center. One of the patients I worked with was Mrs. W., an 84-year-old woman who had had a major stroke 2 years earlier, as well as several serious infections during that time. Mrs. W. was becoming increasingly compromised in her ability to move and provide any of her own self-care.

Some of the staff had difficulty with Mrs. W. and described her as ornery, nasty, and demanding. She was known to scratch and pull hair if she was displeased with the way she was being positioned during the night. She could speak, but would do so sparingly and seemed to be able to express herself best with four letter words.

One night as I walked through the rooms checking on the patients at the beginning of the shift, I experienced something different immediately upon entering Mrs. W.'s room. It was intuitive. I wasn't sure what it was at first, but upon making eye contact with her I again immediately felt a different sense of connectedness between us. I walked closer and was able to sense a welcoming engagement and a previously not present softness about her. I instinctively touched her hand and she did not respond in her usual combative manner, as somehow I knew she wouldn't. I asked her how she was feeling, and with a barely visible smile, she said softly, "Oh, okay, but do you think I could stay for awhile?" I said, "Of course, you can stay as long as you like." I then told her I'd be back. I went to her chart and there was nothing different noted, but there was something different. I went back and casually did her vital signs, which were all within normal limits for her. There seemed to be no physical indication that she was in any distress. I knew something was happening, though. I felt that she was getting ready to leave.

I made it a point to spend a lot of time with Mrs. W. that night. Fortunately, it was not particularly busy. She let me comb her hair and fuss with her a bit. While I did this she pointed to the picture of her family and for the first time shared some family stories with me. As I was leaving to go home, I stopped in to say good-bye to Mrs. W. She put her hand on mine and weakly smiled good-bye. And I knew we were really saying good-bye for good. Something special had happened between us, so instead of feeling bad, we both seemed to feel quietly good.

Mrs. W. died 2 hours later. It may seem bizarre, but I smiled when I heard. I was glad that we had spent so much time together the night before. I truly believe that I helped Mrs. W. with her inevitable passage with my presence. I know she helped me to experience dying as something that at times is quietly welcome by allowing me to be with her at the beginning of that passage.

Upon reflecting and trying to understand this experience of the patient, I have become better able to share in the final journeys of others. By allowing me to be with her in her experience, she has given me a better understanding of how to offer comfort to those who are dying. I thank her for our experience.

Patient's Reflection on Nursing

It is of great interest to me when I come across reflections by patients of their experiences with nurses. These reflective experiences also help to clarify the essences of nursing. Two years ago I attended a conference on love, intimacy, and connectedness. It was an interdisciplinary conference attended by 300 to 400 people.

One of the opening speakers described the experience that had been related to him by a dear friend. This experience related to his friend, who had just been diagnosed with a serious form of cancer. The speaker described his friend telling him, "In the early evening the family was all around. We talked, but there was the awkwardness of not knowing what to say or what to expect. Later that night, I was in my room all alone. No longer having to be concerned about my family and what they were struggling with, I began to experience some of my own feelings. I felt so alone. Then the evening nurse who had been working with me over the last 2 days of testing came in. We looked at each other—neither of us said a word and she just gently touched my hand. I cried. She stayed there for . . . I don't know how long, until I placed my other hand on top of hers and gently gave it a pat. She left, and I was able to go to sleep. This was one of the most intimate moments in my life. This nurse offered to be with me in the known, and somehow she also conveyed a reassurance that I did not have to go through what was coming, whatever that was, alone."

This ability to be with and endure with the patient in the process of living is frequently taken for granted by us, yet it is what many times differentiates us from other professionals. In my practice as nursing care coordinator I frequently engage in the phenomenological process of humanistic nursing to help me in my everyday interactions. On one occasion the department heads of the day hospital where I work were talking about a program evaluation. This evaluation was partially a result of a study that the nurses of the day hospital had done. I was proposing that it was important to have patients share with us their experience of the groups that they attended. One of the doctors of the day hospital voiced his skepticism that the patients' input was actually necessary. He said that, after all, he was aware of their pathology and diagnosis. Based on this, he believed he could judge the effectiveness of a group by using his clinical skills to assess changes in symptomatology. I took exception to this and must admit I got a little hot under the collar. Upon reflecting on this experience, however, I had an insight related to the angular view. I realized that this doctor was coming from the angular view of medicine rather than the angular view of nursing, which emphasizes that the patients' views and experiences are primary to the treatment process. I felt more tolerant of this doctor at that point. But more important, I had an experience of the difference between doctoring and nursing. Nurses must recognize the difference, respect these differences in the health-care field, and accept the responsibility of meeting the challenges to nursing that those differences entail.

> The ability to be with a patient in his or her process of living is often taken for granted in nursing, yet it may be what differentiates nursing from other professions.

Uses of the Theory in Clinical Supervision

In my clinical supervision with the nurses in the day hospital I use the humanistic nursing approach. In the process of supervision I try to understand the "call" of the nurse when she brings up a clinical issue. This usually is connected to the "call" of the patient to her and some issue that has arisen around the nurse's not being able to hear or respond to that call.

An illustration of this can be seen in one of my nurse supervising experiences. Ms. L. was working with a patient who had recently been told that her HIV test was positive. Although she did not have AIDS, she had been exposed to the AIDS virus, probably through her current boyfriend, who was purportedly an IV drug abuser. The original issue that came up was that the nurse was very concerned that the doctor on the interdisciplinary team, who was also the patient's therapist, was not giving the patient the support that the nurse felt the patient was calling out for. This nurse and I explored her perception that the patient did in fact seem to be reaching out. The nurse and I explored the reaching out in terms of what the patient was reaching for. It had been carefully explained to the patient that she did not have AIDS, but that at some point she might come down with the illness. The patient was told that there were treatments to retard the disease but that there were no cures yet. Given this, the doctor, whose primary function is treatment and cure, was feeling ill prepared to deal with this patient and it was perhaps this sense of inadequacy that fostered avoidant behavior on his part. The nurse and I, however, came to understand that, in fact, the patient was not calling for doctoring; she was calling for nursing care. She was calling for someone to help her get through this experience in her life. When this was clarified, the nurse and I began to explore the nurse's experience of hearing this call. The nurse spoke of the pain of knowing that this young woman who was close to her own age would die prematurely. She spoke of how a friend, who reminded her of this patient, had also died and that when she associated the two she felt sad. This nurse also had had some difficult personal experiences that had elicited a will to survive. By touching on these, she also could relate to this patient.

As we explored what really was the nurse's angular view, we were able to identify areas that were unknown. The nurse had difficulty understanding the need or the role of the patient's relationship with her current boyfriend. We worked on helping the nurse to bracket her own thoughts and judgements, so that she could be open to the patient's experience of this relationship. Subsequently the nurse was able to understand the patient's intense fear of being alone. As the nurse began to understand that choices are humanizing, she began to explore the need for support systems. In the experience of her own angular view, as a part of her being her own "knowing place," the nurse realized that she herself had things to learn in this area. And so to expand her own capability of being a "knowing place" and expanding her angular view, she sought out the help of the nurse practitioner in our gynecology clinic. They worked well together with this patient, who eventually was able to leave our day hospital, get a part-time job, and be all that she could in her current life situation.

The nurse in the day hospital grew from her experience of working with this patient. Although she is usually quite reserved and shies away from public forums, with encouragement she was able to share the experience with this patient in a large public forum. She not only shared with other professionals the role that she as a nurse played in the treatment of this patient, she also acknowledged herself in a group of professionals as a "knowing place." As for me, I was touched by this nurse's experience of struggling through this difficult situation to become more in her nursing realm, and I became more because of her growth.

Another example of the application of Humanistic Nursing Theory in clinical practice involves a nurse working with a patient diagnosed with chronic schizophrenia. The patient had experienced several severe psychotic breaks, with subsequent deterioration in functioning. For certain patients with schizophrenia who experience this downward course, it is heartbreaking to the patient and the family alike. In my supervision with this nurse, it became clear that she was struggling with the threatened decompensation of this patient each time discharge came near. She felt frustrated and at first like the patient was failing. Later she began to see that it was the team that was projecting their own sense of failure at not being able to get the patient to follow through with their discharge plan. By helping this nurse to relate and reflect upon her experience with this patient, she was able to see that he was not noncompliant, one of our favorite labels. When she was with the patient she began to see how hard he really was trying. When asked what she thought he might be calling to her for in their interactions, she suddenly became aware that he was looking for someone to acknowledge how hard he was trying and that he didn't want to disappoint anyone but it was the best he could do.

With this new understanding, the nurse became aware of her need to validate to the patient that she understood. Her further nursing action was to take this information back to the team to help them recognize their own inability to deal with the patient's loss of functioning. For if they were unable to recognize it and deal with it, how could they help the patient to deal with it? Subsequently both the nurse's actions and the team's actions were more attuned to the patient's call rather than their own expectations and needs. This affected not only the attitude of the staff toward the patient but also permitted them to make an appropriate discharge plan that the patient could follow through with. This nurse had the experience of herself as a "knowing place." She exerted her influence with new confidence in her interactions with the team. I, as her supervisor, had a renewed experience in the validity of the process of humanistic nursing.

Although the examples of clinical supervision I have cited were in the psychiatric setting, I do believe using the process enfolded in humanistic nursing theory is beneficial to supervisors and self-reflective practitioners in all areas of nursing. Patients call to us both verbally and nonverbally, with all sorts of health-related needs. It is important to hear the calls and know the process that lets us understand them. In hearing the calls and searching our own experiences of who we are, our personal angular view, we may progress as humanistic nurses.

Use of the Theory in Research

Shifting the application of the theory from the individual nurse to a community of nurses, I would like to share with you a group research project that was conducted in the clinical setting of a psychiatric day hospital. In an effort to better understand why some patients stayed in the day hospital and others left, the nursing staff conducted a phenomenological study that investigated the experiences of patients as they enter and become engaged in treatment in a day hospital system. The initial step in the process, in Dr. Paterson's and Dr. Zderad's terms, is to prepare the nurse knower for coming to know.

Part of the process of preparing the nurses for this study was to expand their angular view by educating them in the phenomenological method and the unstructured interview style. Literature was handed out on this and meetings were held to discuss the articles and any questions about them. We also shared our feelings about this method, our concerns, and other experiences related to this study. As we did this, we began to establish an atmosphere of openness and trust. This open atmosphere was essential to the preparation for gathering descriptions of the patients' experiences. In order to further promote the openness of the interviewers to the experience of the patients, we used our group nursing meetings for the purpose of bracketing our angular views. In these group meetings we raised our consciousness through articulation of our own angular views. In addition, by opening ourselves to each other's experiences and points of view, we were opening ourselves to the world of other possibilities and shaking up the status quo of our own mind sets. Once the descriptions were obtained, we as a group interpreted with the phenomenological method of reflecting, intuiting, analyzing, and synthesizing. We interviewed 15 patients over a period of 8 months, on their day of admission and every 4 weeks thereafter until discharge.

A brief example of the outcome of this study was that we found from our interviews that there were many anxiety-producing experiences on the first day in the day hospital, but very few anxiety-reducing experiences that offered the patient comfort and support. The two patients who left the study at this time found no anxiety-reducing experiences at all. Subsequently recommendations were made that were hypothesized to reduce the anxiety of the patient on the first day. This is an example of how through this method hypotheses are generated that can then be tested in the scientific method.

The concept of research as praxis is also illustrated in this research project. On an individual basis the nurses related that they experienced an increased awareness of the need to be open to the patients' expressions of themselves. The nurses also expressed that they now felt that they had an awareness of a comfortable method that would help them with this openness, as well as a method for analyzing the experience to gain a better understanding of the phenomenon.

After reviewing the interviews of a patient who had had a particularly difficult course of treatment, one of the nurses who was on her treatment team remarked, "We weren't listening to what she was telling us—we just didn't hear the pain." Another nurse had a similar insight into a patient's experiences. She noted with some surprise that her initial impression that a patient she was working with was hostile and withholding had given way to the realization that this patient—as a result of the negative symptoms of schizophrenia—was quite empty and was really giving us all that she had to give. In future interactions with this patient the nurse was empathic and supportive rather than judgmental and angry.

Developing a Community of Nurses

Another group experience in which Humanistic Nursing Theory was utilized was the formation of a community of nurses who were mutually struggling with changes in their nursing roles. You will recall that the inner mandate of Humanistic Nursing Theory is to share with, thereby allowing each to become more. You will also recall that when we spoke of "call," it was indicated that the call, in Humanistic Nursing Theory terms, can be from an individual, a family, a community, or humanity itself. In this instance I became aware of my own experiences as a nursing care coordinator as I struggled with the changes that were happening around me and how these changes were impacting on me.

The nursing shortage, the increased salaries, even government agencies were calling for nurses to be proactive in the current health-care crises. In the report of the Secretary of Health and Human Services' Commission on Nursing (December, 1988) we were told that "the perspective and expertise of nurses are a necessary adjunct to that of other health care professionals in the policy-making, and regulatory, and standard setting process" (p. 31). The challenge being posed to nurses is to help create the changes in the health-care system today. The ability to initiate and cause change is a definition of power (Miller, 1982, p. 2). To be asked to act and to be perceived in a powerful way was a shift for us as nurses, who have historically been reactive rather than proactive. In reflecting and analyzing my own experience of this challenge, I identified some anxiety about this call from the community at large. Recalling my past experience when I was anxious about trying the phenomenological method of inquiry, I identified that going through the process with a group of nurses who were experiencing the same newness was helpful. I called to the community of nurses where I work, and we joined together to struggle with this challenge. For while the importance of organized nursing power cannot be overemphasized, it is the individual nurse in her day-to-day practice who can actualize or undermine the power of the profession.

In settings such as hospitals the time pressure, the unending tasks, the emotional strain, and the conflicts do not allow nurses to relate, reflect, and support each other in their struggle toward a center that is nursing. This isolation and alienation does not allow for the development of either a personal or professional voice. Within our community of nurses it became clear that developing individual voices was clearly our first task. Talking and listening to each other about our nursing worlds allowed us to become more articulate and clear about function and value as nurses. The theme of developing an articulate voice has pervaded and continues to pervade this group. There is an ever-increasing awareness of both manner and language as we interact with each other and those outside the group. The resolve for an articulate voice is even more firm as members of the group experience and share the empowering effect it can have on both one's personal and professional life. It has been said that "[t]hose that express themselves unfold in health, beauty, and human potential.

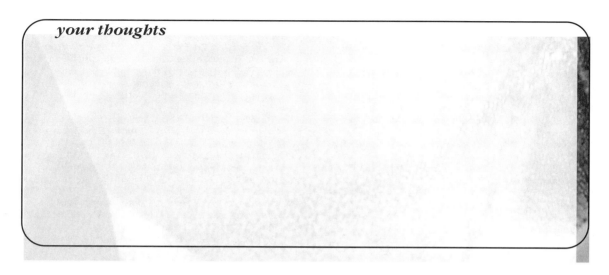
your thoughts

They become unblocked channels through which creativity can flow" (Hills & Stone, 1976, p. 71).

Group members offered alternative approaches to various situations that were utilized and subsequently brought back to the group. In this way each member shared in the experience. That experience therefore became available to all members as they individually formulated their own knowledge base and expanded their angular view. As Dr. Paterson and Dr. Zderad proposed, "[E]ach person might be viewed as a community of the beings with whom she has meaningfully related" (1978, p. 45), and as a potential resource for expanding herself as a "knowing place."

Through openness and sharing we were able to differentiate our strengths. Once the members could truly appreciate the unique competence of each other they were able to reflect that appreciation back. Through this reflection members began to internalize and then project a competent image of themselves. They learned that this positive mirroring did not have to come from outsiders. They can reflect back to each other the image of competence and power. They as a community of nurses can empower each other. This reciprocity is a self-enhancing process, for "the degree to which I can create relationships which facilitate the growth of others as separate persons is a measure of the growth I have achieved in myself" (Rogers, 1976, p. 79). And so by sharing in our community of nurses we can empower each other through mutual confirmation as we help each other move toward a center that is nursing. This is an example of Martin Buber's basic human need (previously described but worth repeating), to be confirmed by others of their kind: "[S]ecretly and bashfully [they] watch for a 'Yes' which allows [them] to be" (1965, p. 71). We as nurses strive to do this with our patients. We as nurses must also strive to do this for each other and the profession of nursing.

The Call of Humanity

Today I perceive another call. This call is resounded in and exemplified by the following description of examining a pregnant woman: "Instead of having to approach the woman, to rest your head near her belly, to smell her skin, to feel her breathing, you could now read the information [on her and her fetus] from across the room, from down the hall" (Rothman, 1987, p. 28).

The call I hear is for nursing. It is the call from humanity to maintain the humanness in the health-care system, which is becoming increasingly sophisticated in technology, increasingly concerned with cost containment, and increasingly less aware of and concerned with the patient as a human being. The context of Humanistic Nursing Theory is humans. The basic question it asks of nursing practice is: Is this particular intersubjective-transactional nursing event humanizing or dehumanizing? Nurses as clinicians, teachers, researchers, and administrators can use the concepts and process of Humanistic Nursing Theory to gain a better understanding of the "calls" we are hearing. Through this understanding we are given direction for expanding ourselves as "knowing places" so that we can fulfill our reason for being which, according to Humanistic Nursing Theory, is nurturing the well-being and more-being of persons in need.

References

Barnum, B. J. S. (1990) .*Nursing theory:Analysis, application, evaluation.* Glenview, IL: Scott, Foresman Co.

Benner, P. (1984). *From novice to expert.* Menlo Park, CA: Addison-Wesley.

Buber, M. (1965). *The knowledge of man.* New York: Harper & Row.

Heidegger, M. (1977). *The question concerning technology.* New York: Harper & Row.

Hills, C., & Stone, R. B. (1976). *Conduct your own awareness sessions: 100 ways to enhance self-concept in the classroom.* Englewood Cliffs, NJ: Prentice-Hall.

Husserl, L. (1970). *The idea of phenomenology.* The Hague, Netherlands: Martinus Nijhoff.

Miller, J. B. (1982). *Toward a new psychology of woman.* Boston: Beacon Press.

May, R. (1995). *The courage to create.* New York: Norton.

Parse, R. (1981). *Man-living-health: A theory of nursing.* New York: Wiley.

Paterson, J. G. (1977). *Living until death, my perspective.* Paper presented at the Syracuse Veteran's Administration Hospital, New York.

Paterson, J. G., & Zderad, L. T. (1976). *Humanistic nursing.* New York: Wiley.

Paterson, J. G., & Zderad, L. T. (1988). *Humanistic nursing.* New York: National League for Nursing.

Rogers, C. R. (1976). *Perceiving, behaving, and becoming: 100 ways to enhance self-concept in the classroom.* Englewood Cliffs, NJ: Prentice-Hall.

Rothman, B. (1987). *The tentative pregnancy: Prenatal diagnosis and the future of motherhood.* New York: Penguin.

U.S. Public Health Services. (1988, December). *Secretary's commission on nursing, final report.* Washington, DC: Department of Health & Human Services.

Watson, J. (1988). *Nursing: Human science and human care.* New York: National League for Nursing.

Zderad, L. T. (1978). "From here-and-now theory: Reflections on 'how'." In *Theory development: What? Why? How?* New York: National League for Nursing.

Section III

Nursing Theory in Nursing
Practice, Education, Research,
and Administration

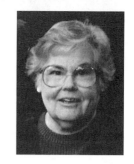

Chapter 13   Part 1

Dorothea E. Orem
The Self-Care Deficit
Nursing Theory

- ❖ Introducing the Theorist
- ❖ Views of Human Beings Specific to Nursing
- ❖ References

Dorothea E. Orem

INTRODUCING THE THEORIST

Dorothea E. Orem is described as a pioneer in the development of distinctive nursing knowledge (Fawcett, 1995, p. 278). Orem contends that the term "care" describes nursing in a most general way, but does not describe nursing in a way that distinguishes it from other forms of care (Orem, 1985). She argues that nursing is distinguished from other human services and other forms of care by the way in which it focuses on human beings. In the 1950s she had the foresight to recognize the need to identify the proper focus of nursing and to clarify the domain and boundaries of nursing as a field of practice in order to enhance nursing's disciplinary evolution. She began her work by seeking an answer to the question of what conditions exist in people when judgements are made about their need for nursing care. She concluded that the human condition associated with the need for nursing is the existence of a health-related limitation in the ability of persons to provide for self the amount and quality of care required (Orem, 1985). This insight provided Orem with an answer to the question, "What is nursing's phenomenon of concern?" She identified nursing's special concern as individuals' needs for self-care and their capabilities for meeting these needs.

> It is nursing's special focus on human beings that distinguishes or differentiates it from other human services.

VIEWS OF HUMAN BEINGS SPECIFIC TO NURSING*

Dorothea E. Orem

Nursing is commonly viewed as a human health service. In this nonspecific generalization the term "human health service" expresses what nursing is. The term implies that there are two categories of human beings, those who need the service nursing and those who produce it; the word "service" implies that nursing is a helpful activity; and the word "health" indicates that the thrust of the service is the structural and functional integrity of persons served. A nursing-specific generalization such as a general concept or theory of nursing gives names and roles to the two categories of human beings, attributes distinct human powers and properties to each, identifies the in-

*Orem, D. E. (1997). Views of human beings specific to nursing. Reprinted with permission from *Nursing Science Quarterly 10*(1) (26–31).

teractions among them, and specifies the broad structural features of the processes of producing nursing. The Nursing Development Conference Group's 1971 general conceptual model of a nursing system demonstrates the foregoing statements (Table 13–1).

In the nursing literature, views of human beings are sometimes represented as distinct from views of nursing. It is true, of course, that one can study and think about the existence, the nature and behaviors of human beings, men, women, children, separate and apart from thoughts about nursing. But it is not true that one can study and think about nursing without incorporating into one's thought processes nursing-specific views of human beings. The integration of views of humankind within views of nursing is the focus of this discussion.

Nursing-Specific Views

The powers and properties of human beings specific to nursing are named in the Nursing Development Conference Group's general concept of nursing systems presented in Table 13–1. They are further developed in Orem's 1995 work and earlier expressions of Self-Care Deficit Nursing Theory with its constituent theories of self-care, self-care deficit, and nursing system. Without question it is individual human beings, through the activation of their powers for result-seeking and result-producing endeavors, who generate the processes and systems of care named "nursing."

Nursing science is knowing and seeking to extend and deepen knowing of both the structure of the processes of nursing and of the internal structure, constitution, and nature of the powers and properties of individuals who require nursing and individuals who produce it. Harré (1970) identifies a theory as a "statement-picture" complex that supplies an account of the constitution and behavior of those entities whose interactions with each other are responsible for the manifested patterns of behaviors. The Nursing Development Conference Group's 1971 Theory of Nursing System and the general theory of nursing named the Self-Care Deficit Nursing Theory express both the nature of the entities and the interactions of the entities responsible for processes, the patterns of behavior, known as nursing. Both theoretical expressions had their beginning in understandings of their formulators about the reasons why individuals need and can be helped through nursing. Such understanding marks the beginning of nursing science.

It is posited that in valid general theories of nursing the named nursing-specific conceptualizations

Concepts of Nursing and Nursing Systems

A *nursing system,* like other systems for the provision of personal services, is the product of a series of relations between persons who belong to different sets (classes), the set A and the set B. From a nursing perspective any member of the set A (legitimate patient) presents evidence descriptive of the complex subsets self-care agency and therapeutic self-care demand and the condition that in A demand exceeds agency due to health or health-related causes. Any member of the set B (legitimate nurse) presents evidence descriptive of the complex subset nursing agency which includes valuation of the legitimate relations between self as *nurse* and instances where, in A, certain values of the component phenomena of self-care agency and therapeutic self-care demand prevail.

B's perceptions of the conditionality of A's subset objective therapeutic self-care demand on the subset self-care agency establishes the conditionality of changes in the states of A's two subsets on the state of and changes in the state of B's subset nursing agency. The activation of the components of the subset nursing agency (change in state) by B to deliberately control or alter the state of one or both of A's subsets—therapeutic self-care demand and self-care agency—is nursing. The perceived relations among the parts of the three subsets (actual system) constitute the organization. The "mapping" of the behaviors in "mathematical or behavioral terms" provides a record of the system.

Source: From *Concept Formalization in Nursing: Process and Product* (1979). (2nd ed., p. 107), by Nursing Development Conference Group (D. E. Orem, Ed.). Boston: Little, Brown. Copyright 1979 by Dorothea E. Orem. Reprinted with permission.

---

are the human points of reference that reveal the human properties and powers, the entities investigated in nursing science. For example, in Self-Care Deficit Nursing Theory individuals throughout their life cycles are viewed as having a continuing demand for engagement in self-care, in care of self; the constituent action components of the demand together are named the therapeutic self-care demand. The Theory of Self-Care (Orem, 1995) offers a theoretical explanation of this continuing action demand. Individuals also are viewed as having the human power (named self-care agency) to develop and exercise capabilities necessary for them to know and meet the components of their therapeutic self-care demands. Nursing is required when individuals' developed and operational powers and capabilities to know and meet their own therapeutic self-care demands, in whole or in part, in time-place frames of reference (that is, their self-care agency), are not adequate because of health state or health-care-related conditions.

The idea central to these nursing-specific views of individuals is that mature human beings have learned and continue to learn to meet some or all components of their own therapeutic self-care demands and the therapeutic self-care demands of their dependents. Engagement of mature and maturing human beings in self-care and dependent-care can be known by others by observing their actions in time-place frames of reference and securing subjective information about what is done and what is not done for self and dependents including the rationales for what is done or what is not done. Both kinds of care are time-specific entities produced by individuals.

It is known that therapeutic self-care demands and self-care agency vary qualitatively and quantitatively in time and over time for individuals. For this reason they are identified in Self-Care Deficit Nursing Theory as *patient variables* dealt with by nurses and persons in need of nursing care within the processes through which nursing is produced. As the values of each vary, the relationship between them varies. When, for health and health-care-associated reasons, self-care agency of individuals is unequal in its development or operability for meeting their existent and changing therapeutic self-care demand, a self-care deficit exists (Orem, 1995). The real or potential existence of such a health-related deficit relationship between the care demand and power of agency is the reason why individuals require nursing care.

Self-Care Deficit Nursing Theory offers the explanation that both internal and external conditions arising from or associated with health states of individuals can bring about action limitation of individuals to engage in care of self, for example, lack of knowledge or developed skills, or lack of energy (Orem, 1995). The presence and nature of such action limitations can set up action deficit relationships between individuals' developed and operational powers of self-care agency and the kinds and frequencies of deliberate actions to be performed to know and meet individuals' therapeutic self-care demands in time and place frames of reference.

The critical power that is operative in nursing is the power of nurses to design and produce nursing care for others. This human power with its constituent capabilities and disposition is named "nursing agency." The centrality of nursing agency as exercised by nurses in the production of nursing care is made clear in the Nursing Development Conference Group's concept of nursing system (see Table 13–1). The identification and development of the power of nurses to design and produce nursing care for others are essential elements in any valid general theory of nursing. The investigation of this power and the capabilities and conditions for its exercise are critical components of nursing science.

Nurses must be knowledgeable about and skilled in investigating and calculating individuals' therapeutic self-care demands, in determining the degrees of development and operability of self-care agency, and in estimating persons' potential for regulation of the exercise or development of their powers of self-care agency. Nurses' capabilities extend to appropriately helping individuals with health-associated self-care deficits to know and meet with appropriate assistance the components of their therapeutic self-care demands and to regulate the exercise and development of their powers of self-care agency. These outcomes of nursing are contributory to the life, health, and well-being of individuals under the care of nurses. Outcomes, of course, are related to the reasons why individuals require nursing care.

Self-Care Deficit Nursing Theory as it has been developed builds from expressed insights about the powers and properties of persons who need nursing care and those who produce it, to the nature and constitution of those properties, to the details of the structure of the processes of providing nursing care for individuals, and to the processes for providing nursing care in multiperson situations, including family and community (Orem, 1995). These are developments of the professional-technological features of nursing. In the initial and later stages of development of this general theory of nursing developers formally recognized that nursing is a triad of interrelated action systems—a *professional-technical system,* the existence of which is dependent on the existence of an *interpersonal system,* and a *societal system* that establishes and legitimates the contractual relationship of nurses and persons who require nursing care.

Nursing students should be helped to understand and recognize in concrete nursing practice situations the tripartite features of nursing systems and the relationships between and among them. Theoretical nursing science differentiates content that is specifically interpersonal from professional-technological content and specifies content that establishes the linkages between interpersonal and professional-technological features of nursing as well as content that establishes the validity or lack of validity of a societal-contractual system.

Societal systems usually begin or are established by specifying the contracting parties and their legitimate relationships. Initial relationships may or may not endure or be legitimate throughout nursing practice situations. There may be or should be changes in both nurses and persons contracting for the care. The societal-contractual system legitimizes the interpersonal relationships of nurses and persons seeking nursing and their next of kin or their legitimate guardians. The interpersonal system is constituted from series and sequences of interaction and communication among legitimate parties necessary for the design and production of nursing in time-place frames of reference. The professional-technological nursing system is the system of action productive of nursing. It is dependent upon the initial and continuing production of an effective interpersonal system.

Comprehensive general theories of nursing address *what* nurses do, *why* they do what they do, *who* does what, and *how* they do what they do. A valid general theory of nursing thus sets forth nursing's professional-technological features specific to the production of nursing. A general theory of nursing that addresses nursing's professional-technological features provides points of articulation with interpersonal features of nursing and sets the standards for safe, effective interpersonal systems. These features also point to the legitimacy of, or need for change in, societal-contractual systems. For the initial expression of the tripartite nature of nursing systems within the frame of Self-Care Deficit Nursing Theory, see the Nursing Development Conference Group's (1979) development of a "Triad of Systems."

Broader Views

Nursing-specific views of individuals fit within one or more broader views of human beings. Consider, for example, the conceptual element self-care agency in Self-Care Deficit Nursing Theory.

Agency within this conceptual element is understood as the human power to deliberate about, make decisions about, and deliberately engage in result-producing actions or refrain from doing so. The *self-care* portion of the conceptual element specifies that agency in this context is specific to deliberating about, making decisions about, and producing the kind of care named self-care. Thus the concept and the term "self-care agency" stand for a specialized form of agency that demands the development of specialized knowledge and action capabilities by humans. However, the power of self-care agency is necessarily attributed to human beings viewed as *persons,* for it is individuals as persons who investigate, reason, decide, and act, exercising their human powers of agency. Thus the view of human beings as self-care agents fits within the view of human beings as persons. The general term attached to persons who act deliberately to produce a foreseen result is the term "agent of action." Within the frame of reference of Self-Care Deficit Nursing Theory, persons who deliberate about and engage in self-care are referred to as "self-care agents" and their power to do so is named "self-care agency." The power of persons who are nurses to produce nursing is named "nursing agency."

The idea is that the specialized powers and characteristic properties of human beings specified in the conceptual elements of general nursing models and theories are necessarily understood within the context of broader views of human beings. Orem (1995) and the Nursing Development Conference Group (1979) suggest five broad views of human beings that are necessary for developing understanding of the conceptual constructs of Self-Care Deficit Nursing Theory and for understanding the interpersonal and societal aspects of nursing systems. The five views are summarized as follows:

1. *The view of person.* Individual human beings are viewed as embodied persons with inherent rights that become sustained public rights who live in coexistence with other persons. A mature human being "is at once a self and a person with a distinctive I and me: . . . with private, publicly viable rights and able to possess changes and pluralities without endangering his [or her] constancy or unity" (Weiss, 1980, p. 128).
2. *The view of agent.* Individual human beings are viewed as persons who can bring about conditions that do not presently exist in humans or in their environmental situations by deliberately acting using valid means or technologies to bring about foreseen and desired results.
3. *The view of user of symbols.* Individual human beings are viewed as persons who use symbols to stand for things and attach meaning to them, to formulate and express ideas, and to communicate ideas and information to others through language and other means of communication.
4. *The view of organism.* Individuals are viewed as unitary living beings who grow and develop exhibiting biological characteristics of homo sapiens during known stages of the human life cycle.
5. *The view of object.* Individual human beings are viewed as having the status of object subject to physical forces whenever they are unable to act to protect themselves against such forces. Inability of individuals to surmount physical forces

such as wind or forces of gravity can arise from both the individual and prevailing environmental conditions.

The person view is central to and an integrating force for understanding and using the other four views. All other views are subsumed by the person view. The person view also is the view essential to understanding nursing as a triad of action systems. It is the view that nurses use (or should use) in all interpersonal contacts with individuals under nursing care and with their family and friends.

The person-as-agent view is the essential operational view in understanding nursing. If there is nursing, nursing agency is developed and operational. If there is self-care on the part of individuals, self-care agency is developed and operational. The agent view incorporates not only discrete deliberate actions to achieve foreseen results and the structure of processes to do so but also the powers and capabilities of persons who are the agents or actors. The internal structure, the constitution, and the nature of the powers of nursing agency and self-care agency are content elements of nursing science. The structure of the processes of designing and producing nursing and self-care is also nursing science content.

The view of person as user of symbols is essential in understanding the nature of interpersonal systems of interaction and communication between nurses and persons who seek and receive nursing. The age and developmental state, culture, and experiences of persons receiving nursing care affect their use of symbols and the meaning they attach to events internal and external to them. The ability of nurses to be with and communicate effectively with persons receiving care and their families incorporates the use of meaningful language and other forms of communication, knowledge of appropriate social-cultural practices, and willingness to search out the meaning of what persons receiving care are endeavoring to communicate.

The user-of-symbol view is relevant to how persons who are nurses communicate with other nurses and other health-care workers. Ideally, persons who are nurses use the language of nursing and at the same time understand and can use the language of disciplines that articulate with nursing. The lack of a nursing language has been a handicap in nurses' communications about nursing to the public as well as to persons with whom they work in the health field. There can be no nursing language until the features of humankind specific to nursing are conceptualized and named and their structure uncovered.

Men, women, and children are unitary beings. They are embodied persons, and nurses must be knowing about their biological and psychobiological features. Viewing human beings as organisms brings into focus the internal structure, the constitution and nature of those human features that are the foci of the life sciences. Knowing human beings as agents or users of symbols has foundations in biology and psychology. Understanding human organic functioning including its aberrations requires knowledge of human physiology and environmental physiology as well as pathology and other developed and developing sciences.

The object view of individual human beings is a view taken by nurses whenever they provide nursing for infants, young children, or adults unable to control their positions and movement in space and contend with physical forces in their environment. This includes the lack of capabilities to ward off physical force exerted against them by other human beings. Taking the object view carries with it a requirement for protective care of persons subject to such forces. The features of protective care are understood in terms of impending or existent environmental forces and known incapacities of individuals to manage and defend themselves in their environments, as well as in the nursing-specific views of individuals that nurses take in concrete nursing practice situations.

These five broad views of human beings not only subsume nursing-specific views, they also aid in understanding them and in revealing their constitution and nature. These broad views point to the sciences and disciplines of knowledge that nurses must be knowing in, and have some mastery of, in order to be effective practitioners of nursing. Establishing the linkages of nursing-specific views of human beings to the named broader views is a task of nursing scholars.

Throughout the processes of giving nursing care to individuals or multiperson units, such as families, nurses use changing combinations of the named views of human beings in accord with presenting conditions and circumstances. Nurses also may need to help individuals under nursing care to take these views about themselves. As previously stated, the person view is the guiding force.

The five described views of individual human beings also come into play when persons who are nurses think about and deal with themselves in nursing situations. They know that they have rights as persons and as persons who are nurses and that they must defend and safeguard these personal and professional rights; their powers of nursing agency must be adequate to fulfill responsibilities to meet nursing requirements of persons under their care; they must know their deficiencies, act to overcome them, or secure help to make up for them; they must be protective of their own biological well-being and act to safeguard themselves from harmful environmental forces. Nurses also have requirements for knowing nursing and articulating fields in a dynamic way. There is also a need for a nursing language that is enabling for thinking nursing within its domain and boundaries and in its articulation with other disciplines and for communicating nursing to others in nursing practice situations.

Model Building and Theory Development

The previously described nursing-specific views of individual human beings are necessary for understanding and identifying (1) when and why individuals need and can be helped through nursing and (2) the structure of the processes through which the help needed is determined and produced. Nurses' continuing development of their knowing about the person, agent, symbolist, organism, and object views of individuals is essential continuing education for themselves as persons who are nurses and nursing scholars.

Such knowing is foundational to model making and theory development in nursing. For example, Louise Hartnett-Rauckhorst (1968) developed models to make explicit what is involved physiologically and psychologically in voluntary, deliberate human action, including motor behaviors. She moved from available authoritative knowledge in the fields of physiology, psychology, and the broad field of human behavior to develop:

1. A basic psychological model of action with three submodels:
   a. The personal frame of reference of the basic psychologic model of action.
   b. The veridical (coinciding with reality) frame of reference of the basic psychologic model of action.
   c. The sociocultural frame of reference of the basic psychologic model of action.
2. A physiologic model of action.

The Hartnett-Rauckhorst theoretical models set forth structural features of the process of voluntary human action (that is, deliberate action). These models develop the agent view; however, their structure reflects the person, the user of symbols, and the organism views of individual human beings (Nursing Development Conference Group, 1979).

The study of these and other general theoretical models of deliberate action stimulated some members of the Nursing Development Conference Group to investigate and formalize the conceptual structure of self-care agency, conceptualizing it as the developed power to engage in a specific kind of deliberate action. The goal of these efforts was the construction of models to identify types of relevant information and to aid in the development of techniques for collection and analysis of data about self-care agency. By 1979, the following theoretical models were developed:

1. A model of self-care operations, estimative, decision making, and productive operations and their results.
2. A model of power components operationally involved with and enabling for performance of self-care operations.
3. A model of human capabilities and dispositions foundational for:
   a. the development and operability of the power components.
   b. the performance of the self-care operations in time and place frames of reference.

(Refer to Orem, 1995, for descriptions of these models and highlights of their development.) The three theoretical models descriptive and explanatory of self-care agency when considered together in their articulations constitute the elements for process models of the operation of self-care agency, a process with a specified structure. The first model, the self-care operations model, is modeled on deliberate action. The power component model names specific enabling capabilities necessary for performing each of the named operations. *Capabilities* are powers that can be developed or lost without a substantial change in the possessor of the power. The foundational capabilities and dispositions model expresses physiologically or psychologically described capabilities and dispositions that permit for or facilitate or hinder persons' performance of self-care operations or the development or adequacy of the power components.

The nursing-specific view that each and every individual human being has a therapeutic self-care demand to be met continuously over time was conceptually developed through the construction of theoretical models using the broad views of human beings. Models of categories of constituent care requisites within the demand (universal, developmental, and health deviation types) were developed as well as a model to show the constituent content elements of a therapeutic self-care demand and their derivation (Orem, 1995). A process model of the structural elements of an action system to meet a specific self-care requisite particularized for an individual was developed as an example of what actions must be performed to meet each of the self-care requisites of individuals.

These models express the content elements of the conceptual entity therapeutic self-care demand. The models also express the derivation of the content elements, the relationships among them, and the regulatory results sought. The therapeutic self-care demand models represent what is to be known and met by individuals through their exercise of self-care agency or met for them when required by reason of self-care agency limitations.

These examples of models demonstrate that nursing theorists and scholars involved in development of Self-Care Deficit Nursing Theory used both nursing-specific and more general views of individual human beings in the processes of model building. The examples also demonstrate that in model development theorists used knowledge from more than one science or discipline of knowledge. The subjects of the models, namely, nursing systems, deliberate action, self-care agency, and therapeutic self-care demand, also differed from the sources and content elements of the respective models.

The models are offered as a means toward understanding the reality of the named entities in concrete nursing practice situations. Despite the diversity of these models, they are all directed toward knowing the structure of the processes that are operational or become operational in the production of nursing systems, systems of care for individuals or for dependent-care units or multiperson units served by nurses.

For information about models and scientific growth involving growth of knowledge in individual scientists the reader is referred to Wallace (1983) and Harré (1970). Black's *Models and Metaphors* (1962) was the source first used by the writer.

Conclusions

The use of specific views of human beings by nurses or persons in other disciplines does not negate their acceptance of the unity, the oneness of each individual man, woman, or child. In human sciences, specific views of human beings identify the domain and boundaries of the science within the broad frames of humanity and society. In nursing, for example, the views of human beings expressed in Self-Care Deficit Nursing Theory identified the proper object of nursing and were enabling for the development and structuring of nursing knowledge.

Science, including models and theories, is about existent entities. A valid comprehensive theory of nursing has as its reality base individuals who need and receive nursing care and those who produce it, as well as the events of its production. Nursing does exist in human societies. Nursing is something produced by human beings for other human beings when known conditions and relationships prevail. It is posited that the life experiences of nursing theorists, their observations and judgments about the world of nurses, can and do result in insights about nursing that can lead to descriptions and explanations of the human health-care service, nursing.

Nurses and nursing students who are confronted with tasks of reviewing, studying, mastering, or taking positions about extant general models or theories of nursing should look for and identify the view(s) of human beings being expressed or implicit in them. The adequacy of the theories should be explored. Models and theories that purport to be general models of nursing can be adequate or deficient in their scope as related to expressing why people need and can be helped through nursing or in describing and explaining the structure of nursing processes.

In any practice field a general model or theory incorporates not only the what and the why, but also the who and the how. The adequacy of a general theory comes into question when there is omission of any one of the named elements. The validity and specificity of theories referred to as nursing theories are in question when there is no reference to the human condition that gives rise to needs for nursing on the part of individuals, to the presence and the powers of persons qualified as nurses, to the structure of processes of production of nursing, and to the results sought.

What comes first, the view of humankind or the view of nursing in the cognitional processes of theorists, is a moot question. The writer's position is that a theorist's life experiences in and accumulated knowledge of nursing practice situations support the recognition and naming of nursing-specific views of human beings. Nursing-specific views of individual human beings are differentiated from those general views that are relevant to all the health services or even to human existence. Such general views include the view of human beings as energy fields, or as living health, as culture-oriented, or as caring beings. Such general views, however helpful in understanding humankind or in identifying approaches to data collection, do not and cannot support viable nursing science, theoretical and practical.

References

Black, M. (1962). *Models and metaphors.* Ithaca, NY: Cornell University Press.

Harré, R. (1970). *The principles of scientific thinking.* Chicago: University of Chicago Press.

Hartnett-Rauckhorst, L. (1968). *Development of a theoretical model for the identification of nursing requirements in a selected aspect of self-care.* Unpublished master's thesis, Catholic University of America, Washington, DC.

Nursing Development Conference Group. (1979). *Concept formalization in nursing: Process and product* (2nd ed., D. E. Orem, Ed.). Boston: Little, Brown.

Orem, D. E. (1995). *Nursing: Concepts of practice.* St. Louis: Mosby-Year Book.

Wallace, W. A. (1983). *From a realist point of view: Essays on the philosophy of science.* Washington, DC: University Press of America.

Weiss, P. (1980). *You, I, and the others.* Carbondale, IL: Southern Illinois University Press.

Chapter 13 Part 2

Self-Care Deficit Nursing Theory: Directions for Advancing Nursing Science and Professional Practice

Marjorie A. Isenberg

Orem's General Theory of Nursing

According to Orem (1985), it is the special focus on human beings that distinguishes or differentiates nursing from other human services. From this point of view, the role of nursing in society is to enable individuals to develop and exercise their self-care abilities to the extent that they can provide for themselves the amount and quality of care required. According to the theory, individuals whose requirements for self-care exceed their capabilities for engaging in self-care are said to be experiencing a self-care deficit. Moreover, it is the presence of an existing or potential self-care deficit that identifies those persons in need of nursing. Thus, Orem's Self-Care Deficit Nursing Theory explains when and why nursing is required. Clearly, the work of this theorist differentiates nursing as a discipline and provides a basis for structuring nursing knowledge and nursing practice.

Orem (1995) describes the Self-Care Deficit Nursing Theory as a general theory of nursing. General theories of nursing are those that are applicable across all practice situations in which persons are in need of nursing care. As such, the Self-Care Deficit Nursing Theory describes and explains the key concepts common to all nursing practice situations (Orem, 1995, p. 167). The theory consists of four concepts about persons under the care of nurses, two nurse-related concepts, and three interrelated theories: the Theory of Nursing Systems, the Theory of Self-Care Deficit, and the Theory of Self-Care. Concepts in the general theory include: self-care, self-care agency, therapeutic self-care demand, self-care deficit, nursing agency, and nursing systems. The theory describes and explains the relationship between the *capabilities of individuals to engage in self-care* (self-care agency) and *their requirements for self-care* (therapeutic self-care demand). The term "deficit" refers to a particular *relationship* between *self-care agency* and *self-care demand* that is said to exist when capabilities for engaging in self-care are *less than* the demand for self-care.

Self-care is defined by Orem (1995, p. 104) as the practice of activities that individuals initiate and perform on their own behalf in maintaining life, health, and well-being. Meeting the self-care requisites (requirements) is identified as the purpose of self-care. Self-care requisites are expressed by Orem (1995, p. 191) as actions to be performed by individuals that are regulatory of human functioning and development. As one would expect in a general theory of nursing, the concepts of the Self-Care Deficit Nursing Theory are developed comprehensively. The sub-

stantive structure of the self-care requisites provides a good example of the scope of the theory. In the initial description of the requisites, only two categories were identified: universal and health deviation (Orem, 1971). Since the initial description of the self-care requisites, Orem has expanded the categories to include developmental as well as universal and health-deviation self-care requisites (1995, p. 192).

Meeting of the universal self-care requisites contributes to maintenance of human structure and function, which, in turn, fosters positive health and well-being (Orem, 1995, p. 192). Meeting of the developmental self-care requisites promotes human development and prevents or overcomes conditions and situations encountered throughout the life cycle that can adversely affect human development (Orem, 1995, p. 197). Health-deviation self-care requisites relate to the health states of individuals. According to the theory, health deviation self-care requisites exist for persons who are ill or injured, have specific forms of pathology, have a predisposition to specific diseases, or are under medical diagnosis and treatment (Orem, 1995, p. 201). Meeting of the health-deviation self-care requisites contributes to the goals of health maintenance, health restoration, and the prevention of disease. As can be seen from this description, the comprehensive development of the three types of self-care requisites enhances the usefulness of the Self-Care Deficit Nursing Theory as a guide to nursing practice situations involving individuals across the life span who are experiencing health or illness, and nurse-client situations aimed at health promotion, health restoration, or health maintenance.

> Self-care is the practice of activities that individuals initiate and perform on their own behalf in maintaining life, health, and well-being.

According to this theory, nurses use their specialized capabilities to create a helping system in situations where persons are deemed to have an existent or potential self-care deficit. Three variations in nursing systems are described: wholly compensatory, partly compensatory, and supportive-educative nursing systems (Orem, 1995, p. 309). Decisions about what type of nursing system is appropriate in a given nursing practice situation rests with the answer to the question "Who can and should perform the self-care operations that require movement in space and controlled manipulations?" (Orem, 1995, p. 306). When the answer to the question is the nurse, a

Section III *Nursing Theory in Nursing Practice, Education, Research, and Administration*

wholly compensatory system of helping is appropriate. When it is concluded that the patient can and should perform all self-care actions, the nurse assumes a supportive-educative role and designs a nursing system accordingly. In each of the three nursing practice situations the goal of nursing is to empower the person to meet their self-care requirements by doing for (wholly compensatory system), doing with (partly compensatory system), or developing agency (supportive-educative system). Clearly, these three variations in the types of nursing systems to be employed in practice situations enhances the breadth or scope of the Self-Care Deficit Nursing Theory.

The Development of Nursing Science

This chapter focuses on the extent to which Orem's theory is offering direction to nurse scholars and scientists in advancing nursing science and professional practice. Dorothy Johnson (1959), in her treatise on the development of nursing theory, viewed this attribute of a theory as its value for the profession, its *social utility*. The social utility of a theory is assessed by the extent to which it provides clear direction for nursing practice and research.

It is important to note that Dorothea Orem's theory is offering clear direction to nurses in the advancement of nursing science in the new millennium. Recall that when she began her theoretical work in the 1950s, Orem's goal was to identify the domain and boundaries of nursing as a field of knowledge. She recognized the need to clarify the issue of what is it that nurses study in order for the discipline to evolve. Orem set forth the Self-Care Deficit Nursing Theory as the foundation for the development of nursing science. Moreover, men, women, and children who have existent or potential self-care deficits are identified as the focus of inquiry of nurse scientists (Orem, 1995, p. 167).

Orem describes nursing as a practical science that is comprised of both theoretical and practical knowledge, a point of view that is grounded in modern realism (1995, p. 167). Parallels can be seen between Orem's description of nursing as a practical science and Donaldson and Crowley's discussion of nursing as a professional discipline. Recall that Donaldson and Crowley (1978) stated that the aim of professional disciplines is to know and to *use* knowledge to achieve the practical goal of the discipline. Both per-

spectives address the need for nurses to develop both theoretical and practical knowledge.

A model comprised of five stages for development of nursing science has been identified by Orem (1995, p. 178). Each stage is intended to yield different kinds of knowledge about persons with existent or potential health-related self-care deficits. Stage 1 and Stage 2 of this developmental schema for science focus on the advancement of the theoretical component of nursing science. The theory is the result of Stage 1. Stage 2 is described as the study of concurrent variations between the concepts proposed within the Self-Care Deficit Nursing Theory (Orem 1995, p. 179) for the purpose of verifying and further explicating the propositions. Clearly, the propositions of the Self-Care Deficit Nursing Theory provide direction to nursing researchers who aim to focus their inquiry in theory-based research.

Numerous examples of research illustrating scientific inquiry at the Stage 2 level of development can be found in the nursing literature. The aspect of the Self-Care Deficit Nursing Theory that has generated the most research of this type is the relationship posited between basic conditioning factors and self-care agency. The basic conditioning factors were identified initially by the Nursing Development Conference Group (1979) and were formalized later in a proposition linking them to self-care agency. The second proposition listed in the Self-Care Deficit Theory states that individuals' abilities to engage in self-care (self-care agency) are conditioned by age, developmental state, life experiences, sociocultural orientation, health, and available resources (Orem, 1995, p. 175). This proposition offers direction to nurses with an interest in engaging in theory-based research.

Basic conditioning factors are defined as "[c]onditions or events in a time-place matrix that affect the value of person's abilities to care for themselves" (Orem, 1995). It is important to note that the influence of the basic conditioning factors on self-care agency is not assumed to be operative at all times. Nor are all the basic conditioning factors assumed to be operative at all times. Because the influence of these factors occurs within a time-place matrix, research is necessary to identify those nursing practice situations in which the factors are operative and to explain the nature of their influence on self-care agency. Based upon research findings, relationships between the basic conditioning factors and the substantive structure of self-care agency can then be made explicit. Programs of research designed in this way can verify the existence of linkages between these concepts and can explain the nature of the linkages. Scholarly work of this type is vital to the advancement of the theoretical knowledge of nursing science.

Over the past decade, nurse researchers have studied the influence of basic conditioning factors, singularly and in combination, on individuals' self-care abilities. Foremost among the basic conditioning factors studied is health state. Several studies designed to determine the nature of the influence of variations in health state on self-care abilities are reported in the research literature. Research suggests that this relationship is particularly salient in practice situations with persons experiencing chronic health problems. The work of selected investigators is presented here to exemplify this line of inquiry. The influence of change in health state on the self-care abilities of persons with coronary artery disease has been studied with both American and Dutch adult patient populations (Isenberg et al., 1987, 1991). Across these studies, changes in health state were found to be critical determinants of the quality of the self-care abilities of this patient population. As the health state of patients improved as manifested by absence of chest pain, so did their capabilities for self-care. Conversely, self-care capabilities tended to decline as patients experienced recurrence of chest pain and declining health. The findings revealed a positive relationship between health state and self-care agency in patients with cardiac disease.

In addition to the study of variation in health state due to pathophysiology, the conditioning influence of health state on self-care agency has also been explored in situations in which the variation in health state is due to psychopathology. West (1993) investigated the influence of clinical variations in the level of depression, conceptualized as a health-state factor, on the self-care abilities of young American women.

West (1993) reported that of the basic conditioning factors studied, the level of depression (health state) was the dominant predictor of the quality of the self-care abilities of her sample. In a study with Dutch psychiatric patients, Brouns (1991) also reported that variations in mental health state significantly influenced patients' self-care capabilities. In both studies a positive relationship between health state and self-care agency was revealed. Higher levels of mental health were correlated with higher self-care agency scores. These findings verified the conditioning influence of health state on the self-care agency of patients' experience variations in physical and mental health. Moreover, the research findings clarified the nature of the influence of health state on self-care agency.

The conditioning influence of other basic factors on the self-care abilities of clinical and nonclinical populations has been the focus of inquiry of several nurse scholars. For example, Brugge (1981) studied the influence of family as a social support system on the self-care agency of adults with diabetes mellitus. Vannoy (1989) explored the influence of basic conditioning factors on the self-care agency of persons enrolled in a weight-loss program. Schott-Baer (1989) studied the influence of family variables and caregiver variables on the self-care abilities of the spouses of patients with a diagnosis of cancer. Baker (1991) explored the predictive effect of basic conditioning factors on the self-care agency and self-care in adolescents with cystic fibrosis. McQuiston (1993) investigated the influence of basic conditioning factors on the self-care capabilities of unmarried women at risk for sexually transmitted disease. Horsburgh (1994) conceptualized personality as a basic conditioning factor and tested the model with a healthy popula-

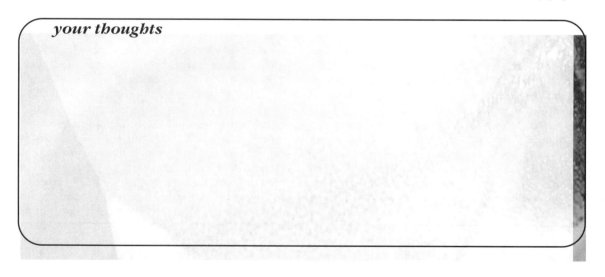

your thoughts

tion and a comparative clinical population with chronic renal disease. Two personality factors—neuroticism and extroversion—were reported to have a conditioning effect on self-care agency (Horsburgh, 1994). O'Connor (1995) studied the influence of basic conditioning factors on the self-care abilities of a healthy and clinical adult population enrolled in a nurse-managed primary care clinic. In this study health state, adult developmental status, and age were found to be the strongest predictors of self-care agency (O'Connor, 1995). Baiardi (1997) explored the influence of health state and caregiving factors on the self-care agency of the caregivers of cognitively impaired elders. Health status of the caregiver and the degree of burden associated with caregiving were shown to influence the self-care abilities of the caregivers (Baiardi, 1997).

Opportunities to test elements of the Self-Care Deficit Nursing Theory have been greatly enhanced by the measurement work with self-care concepts that has transpired over the past 20 years. It is important to note that the theory-testing studies cited above were made possible by the development and psychometric testing of instruments to measure the theoretical concepts. Instruments are currently available to measure the self-care agency of adolescent populations (Denyes, 1982), adult populations (Evers et al., 1993; Geden & Taylor, 1991; Hanson & Bickel, 1985), and elderly populations (Biggs, 1990). The availability of valid and reliable measures of self-care agency has been vital to the advancement of the theoretical component self-care nursing science.

In addition to the theory verification line of research, the Self-Care Deficit Nursing Theory is being used to guide programs of research to identify the self-care requisites and self-care behaviors of specific clinical populations. Intervention studies designed to enhance self-care performance are also under way. The work of Marylin J. Dodd exemplifies this line of inquiry. Since completing her dissertation in 1980, Dodd has launched a program of research focused on the self-care of cancer patients who were receiving chemotherapy or radiation therapy. Her early descriptive studies clarified the health-deviation self-care requisites of this population and documented the therapeutic self-care demand (Dodd 1982, 1984). More recent work described specific self-care behaviors initiated by patients receiving these therapies and led to the identification of a patient profile of self-care that can be used in practice to target specific patient groups who are in most need of nursing interventions (Dodd, 1997). Dodd's intervention studies demonstrated that with targeted information, patients can learn more about their treatment and

can perform more effective self-care behaviors (Dodd, 1997). Her work has advanced to the point of conducting randomized control trials to test a self-care intervention called PRO-SELF© to decrease chemotherapy-related morbidity (Dodd, 1997). Through her 20-year program of descriptive, predictive, and intervention studies based on self-care theory, Dodd's research has demonstrated how to enhance patients' knowledge of their treatment and how to increase effective self-care activities. Dodd clearly qualifies as a pioneer in self-care theory-based research.

Investigators have used Orem's theory to identify the self-care requisites and self-care capabilities of patients across a broad range of health deviations. Based on the theory, Utz and Ramos (1993) have conducted a sequence of studies to explore and describe the self-care needs of people with symptomatic mitral valve prolapse. The self-care capabilities and the self-care needs (requisites) of persons with rheumatoid arthritis have also been described. The most frequently reported universal self-care requisites for these clients were the maintenance of a balance between activity and rest, the promotion of normalcy, and the prevention of hazards (Ailinger & Dear, 1997). Duration of illness (health state) and educational level were found to be related to self-care agency (Ailinger & Dear, 1993). Aish (1993) tested the effect of an Orem-based nursing intervention on the nutritional self-care of myocardial infarction patients. A supportive-educative nursing system was reported to be effective in promoting healthy low-fat eating behavior (Aish, 1993). Metcalfe (1996) studied the therapeutic self-care demand, self-care agency, and the self-care actions of individuals with chronic obstructive lung disease. Health state was found to offer significant explanation of variations in the self-care actions of this population. Based on the universal, developmental, and health deviation self-care requisites, Riley (1996) developed a tool to measure the performance and frequency of the self-care actions of patients with chronic obstructive lung disease. This tool has the potential to be useful as an outcome measure in future intervention studies designed to enhance the self-care abilities of this population.

Moore (1995) has used Self-Care Deficit Nursing Theory as the basis for her program of research with children. She has developed the Child and Adolescent Self-Care Practice Questionnaire, which can be used to assess the self-care performance of children and adolescents. In a study of children with cancer, Mosher and Moore (1998) reported a significant relationship between self-concept and self-care. Children with higher self-concept scores were found to perform more self-care activities than children with low self-concept scores (Mosher & Moore, 1998).

The Cross-Cultural and International Scope of Nursing Research

In contrast to these studies focused on clinical populations experiencing health-deviation self-care requisites, Hartweg's research centers on *health promotion*. Hartweg (1990) conceptualized health promotion self-care within Orem's Self-Care Deficit Nursing Theory and went on to explore through a descriptive study the self-care actions performed by healthy middle-aged women to promote well-being. The women studied were able to identify over 8000 diverse self-care actions, the majority of which were related to the universal self-care requisites (Hartweg, 1993). The interview guide used with this American population has recently been validated with healthy, middle-aged Mexican-American women in a comparative study (Hartweg & Berbiglia, 1996). Whetstone (1987) and Whetstone and Hansson (1989) also conducted cross-cultural comparative studies using self-care concepts. They compared the meanings of self-care among Americans, German, and Swedish populations.

In addition to the cross-cultural comparative research, the Self-Care Deficit Nursing Theory is being applied in studies with specific cultural groups. In an ethnographic study based on concepts within Orem's theory, Villarruel (1995) explored the cultural meanings, expressions, self-care, and dependent care actions related to pain with a Mexican-American population and commented on the use of the theory with this population. Dashiff (1992) applied Orem's theory in her description of the self-care capabilities of young African-American women prior to menarche.

Nurse scientists beyond our national borders are currently using Self-Care Deficit Nursing Theory as a basis for their research. Professor Georges Evers at the Catholic University of Leuven in Belgium has developed an extensive program of research based on the theory. His program includes descriptive and explanatory studies of the self-care requisites and self-care capabilities of diverse clinical populations, the development and psychometric testing of instruments to measure self-care concepts, and the testing of interventions to enhance self-care performance (Evers, 1998).

Orem's theory is also being applied by Jaarsma and colleagues as a basis for an ongoing program of research with cardiac patients in the Netherlands. Using a questionnaire derived from the self-care req-

uisites described in the Self-Care Deficit Nursing Theory, Jaarsma et al. (1995) identified problems frequently encountered by cardiac patients in the early recovery phase from coronary artery bypass surgery or myocardial infarction. Factors influencing the self-care agency of Dutch patients with coronary artery disease are also being studied (Lukkarinen, 1997).

Hanucharurnkul (1989) used Orem's theory as a basis for her work with Thai patients who were receiving chemotherapy for the treatment of cancer. She developed and tested a model to predict the self-care behaviors of cancer patients. Similar to the early work of Ream (1984), she conducted a descriptive study of the self-care behaviors used by a population of British patients to cope with chemotherapy-induced fatigue.

The utility of Self-Care Deficit Nursing Theory beyond our national borders can be explained in part by the fact that Orem's intention was to develop a general theory of nursing that would be useful in describing and explaining universal nursing knowledge. The applicability of the theory beyond Western civilizations may be further explained by the inclusion of culture as a primary influence on people's care beliefs and practices. According to the theory, "self-care" is described as learned behavior, and the activities of self-care are learned according to the beliefs and practices that characterize the cultural way of life of the group to which the individual belongs (Orem, 1985). The individual first learns about cultural standards within the family. Thus, the self-care practices that individuals employ should be understood and examined by nurses within the cultural context of social groups and within the health-care systems of societal groups. Clearly, the theory provides a means to study the types of self-care needs identified by specific cultural groups and the acceptable cultural self-care practices to meet the needs (Meleis, Isenberg, Koerner, Lacey, & Stern, 1995).

The Self-Care Deficit Nursing Theory is grounded in the premise that individuals have the potential to develop their intellectual and practical skills and the motivation essential for self-care (Orem, 1995). The goal of nursing within this perspective is to empower persons to meet their self-care needs by helping them to develop and exercise their self-care capabilities (agency). The theory offers direction in the study of factors that condition the development, operability, and adequacy of individuals' self-care capabilities and the quality of self-care performed. The inclusion of sociocultural orientation as one of the conditioning factors enhances the generality of the theory and in turn its global utility.

The book *Nursing: Concepts of Practice* has been translated into Dutch, French, German, Italian, and Spanish. Records cited in a CINAHL index search of the nursing literature included publications describing the application of Self-Care Deficit Nursing Theory in nursing situations in Australia, Belgium, Denmark, Finland, Germany, the Netherlands, Norway, Portugal, Sweden, Switzerland, the United Kingdom, Hong Kong, Taiwan, Thailand, Turkey, Canada, Mexico, the United States, and Puerto Rico. Cultural groups are being studied independently, such as the work of Villarruel (1995) and Hartweg and Berbiglia (1996) with Mexican-American populations or in comparison with other groups (Van Achterberg et al., 1991) to discover culturally specific self-care abilities needs and practices. Both types of research are currently under way on national and global levels.

> The use of Orem's theory beyond national borders can be explained by the fact that her intention was to develop a general theory that would be useful in describing universal nursing knowledge.

Over the past 15 years, the author has been privileged to be a part of an international network of nurse scholars and scientists focused on the development of disciplinary knowledge derived from Self-Care Deficit Nursing Theory. Our collaborative work began in 1983 when the author was invited as a consultant to the faculty of health sciences at the University of Maastricht in the Netherlands to assist faculty and students in developing programs of nursing theory-based research. Initially, our work focused primarily on the teaching of nursing science seminars for nurses throughout the Netherlands. In 1986, we extended the seminars to include nurses from all parts of Europe. Over the subsequent 5 years, approximately 200 nurses from 12 European countries participated in the seminars. The participants studied the Self-Care Deficit Nursing Theory, research methodology, and the interrelatedness of theory and research. Each participant developed a self-care theory-based research project that could be implemented in his or her home settings.

Our first collaborative research project involved the development of an instrument to measure Orem's theoretical concept of self-care agency. The English and Dutch versions of the Appraisal of Self-Care Agency (ASA) Scale were the products of this endeavor. The team that participated in the development and psychometric testing of the ASA Scale included Professor Hans Philipsen, Professor Georges Evers, Ger Brouns, Harrie Smeets, and the author. Soon, nurse scientists from other countries (Canada, Denmark, Finland, Norway, Sweden, Switzerland, Thailand, and Mexico) joined the team with a desire to translate the ASA Scale into their native language and to validate the instrument within their culture. To date the ASA Scale has been translated and validated for research use with populations in the following countries: Belgium, Denmark, Finland, Canada (French-speaking), Germany, Norway, Sweden, Switzerland (German-speaking), Japan, Korea, Thailand, Turkey, and Mexico.

This collaborative project provided the team with the opportunity to identify universal nursing knowledge and, by means of transnational comparisons, identify culture-specific knowledge. The current shared programs of research focus on: (1) influences of aging on the self-care abilities of Americans (Jirovec & Kasno, 1990), Canadians (Ward-Griffin & Bramwell, 1990), Danes (Lorensen, Holter, Evers, Isenberg, & Van Achterberg, 1993), Dutch (Evers, Isenberg, Philipsen, Senten, & Brouns, 1993), Finns (Katainen, Merlainen, & Isenberg, 1993), Norwegians (Van Achterberg et al., 1991), and Swedes (Soderhamn, Evers, & Hamrin, 1996); and (2) influence of chronic health problems such as coronary artery disease on the self-care abilities of Americans (Isenberg, 1987, 1993), Canadians (Aish & Isenberg, 1996), and Dutch clients (Isenberg, 1993; Isenberg, Evers, & Brouns, 1987; Senten, Evers, Isenberg, & Philipsen, 1991). Using the Mexican version of the ASA Scale to measure self-care agency, Professor Esther Gallegos at the University of Nuevo Leon in Monterrey, Mexico, recently completed a study of the influence of social, family, and individual conditioning factors on the self-care abilities and practices of Mexican women. The results of her study indicated that health state was the predominant predictor of women's self-care agency and self-care performance (Gallegos, 1997). The level of poverty experienced by the Mexican women also had a significant influence on their self-care performance.

One of the challenges of international collaborative research deals with establishing sources for funding to carry out the scientific work. The research work cited above was funded in part by a variety of agencies: the Netherlands Heart Foundation, the Swiss National Fund, Fulbright Scholarship, Finnish Academy of Science, and the Kellogg Foundation. Our collaborative work was further enhanced by the generous support that each of us received from our respective institutions: Wayne State University, United States; University of Maastricht, the Netherlands;

Catholic University of Leuven, Belgium; University of Oslo, Norway; University of Nuevo Leon, Mexico; St. Gallen Hospital, Switzerland; and University of Kuopio, Finland.

To this network of nurse scientists, international collaboration has provided an opportunity and a means to pursue a shared vision and address a shared challenge. By means of shared ideas, resources, research designs, and instruments, we are advancing nursing science derived from Self-Care Deficit Nursing Theory. To date, specific propositions of the theory have been tested in nine countries. Through this theory testing program of research, data are being accrued that will provide answers to the question "To what extent is Self-Care Deficit Nursing Theory relevant to the global community?" The findings of the transnational comparative studies are identifying universal elements of the theory and suggest that the translated versions of the ASA Scale are cross-nationally valid.

Our experience supports the idea that the testing of nursing theories in diverse countries by means of collaborative international research programs is an effective strategy for nurse scientists to face the challenge of developing globally relevant nursing science. The idea to organize a forum for self-care scientists and scholars originated with this group. In 1991, the International Orem Society for Nursing Science and Scholarship was founded. The mission of the society is to advance nursing science and scholarship through the use of Dorothea E. Orem's nursing conceptualizations in nursing education, practice, and research. The society publishes a quarterly newsletter and cosponsors a Biennial International Self-Care Conference with the University of Columbia, Missouri.

The Uses of Orem's Theory in Nursing Practice: An Overview

I chose to focus this chapter on the ways in which the Self-Care Deficit Nursing Theory is guiding nursing research. This choice was made in full awareness that the utility of the theory to nursing practice is well-documented in the literature. However, it would be remiss not to comment on the extensive applications of the theory to nursing practice. Since the pioneering efforts of Crews (1972) and Backscheider (1974) in the use of the theory in the structuring and organization of nursing care to patients in nurse-managed clinics, nurse scholars have been proclaiming the usefulness of the theory as a guide to practice. The theory has been used to guide practice across a wide range of nursing situations in all types of care settings, ranging from neonatal intensive care units (Tolentino, 1990) to nursing home facilities (Anna et al., 1978). The relevance of the theory to the care of patients in intensive care units has also been examined. Jacobs (1990) concluded that although most patients require wholly compensatory systems of care, patient situations do exist in which partly compensatory or supportive-educative systems of care are more appropriate. Orem-based nursing practice has been extensively described in the care of patients of various ages with all kinds of health-deviation self-care requisites and developmental requisites. For example, the theory has been applied to the long-term care of ambulatory adolescent transplant recipients. Nursing services based on Orem's theory were found to enhance the quality of life of this adolescent population significantly (Norris, 1991). Haas (1990) also reported on the usefulness of Self-Care Deficit Nursing Theory as a basis for

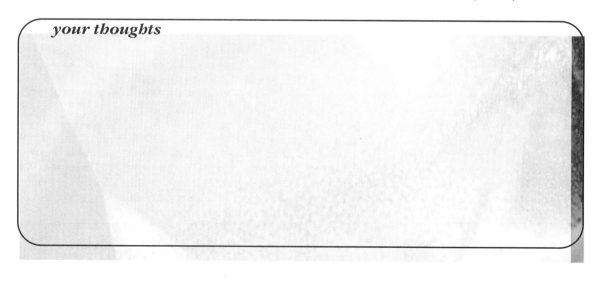

your thoughts

nursing practice aimed at meeting the care demands of children with long-term chronic health problems. Clearly, the extent of the documentation of this work far exceeds the scope of this chapter. Selected citations appear in the bibliography.

Summary

I began this chapter by describing Dorothea E. Orem's quest for understanding of the proper focus of nursing. She contended that identification of nursing's focus would enhance the productivity of nurse scholars and scientists. She set forth the premise that the Self-Care Deficit Nursing Theory was the foundation for developing nursing science, and then described her views of nursing science. The abundance of Orem-based research documented in the literature today speaks of the validity of her convictions and the utility of the theory in guiding the research and scholarship of nurses worldwide. Clearly, the Self-Care Deficit Nursing Theory is playing, and is expected to continue to play, a pivotal role in the advancement of nursing science and professional practice.

References

Ailinger, R. L., & Dear, M. R. (1993). Self-care agency in persons with rheumatoid arthritis. *Arthritis Care and Research, 6*(3), 134–140.

Ailinger, R. L., & Dear, M. R. (1997). An examination of the self-care needs of clients with rheumatoid arthritis . . . including commentary by Popovich, J. *Rehabilitation Nursing, 22*(3), 135–140.

Aish, A. E. (1993). *An investigation of a nursing system to support nutritional self-care in post myocardial infarction patients.* Unpublished doctoral dissertation, Wayne State University, Detroit.

Aish, A. E., & Isenberg, M. A. (1996). Effects of Orem-based nursing intervention on nutritional self-care of myocardial infarction patients. *International Journal of Nursing Studies, 33*(3), 259–270.

Anna, D. J., Christensen, D. G., Hohon, S. A., Ord, L., & Wells, S. R. (1978). Implementing Orem's conceptual framework. *Journal of Nursing Administration, 8*(11), 8–11.

Backscheider, J. E. (1974). Self-care requirements, self-care capabilities and nursing systems in the diabetic nurse management clinic. *American Journal of Public Health, 64,* 1138–1146.

Baiardi, J. (1997). *The influence of health status, burden, and degree of cognitive impairment on the self-care agency and dependent-care agency of caregivers of elders.* Unpublished doctoral dissertation, Wayne State University, Detroit.

Baker, L. K. (1991). *Predictors of self-care in adolescents with cystic fibrosis: A test and explication of Orem's theories of self-care and self-care deficit.* Un-

published doctoral dissertation, Wayne State University, Detroit.

Biggs, A. J. (1990). Family caregiver versus nursing assessments of elderly self-care abilities. *Journal of Gerontological Nursing, 16*(8), 11–16.

Brouns, G. (1991). *Self-care agency of psychiatric patients: A validity and reliability study of the ASA-Scale.* Unpublished master's thesis, University of Limburg, Maastricht, the Netherlands.

Brugge, P. (1981). *The relationship between family as a social support system, health status, and exercise of self-care agency in the adult with a chronic illness.* Unpublished doctoral dissertation, Wayne State University, Detroit.

Crews, J. (1972). Nurse-managed cardiac clinics. *Cardio-Vascular Nursing, 8,* 15–18.

Dashiff, C. J. (1992). Self-care capabilities in black girls in anticipation of menarche. *Health Care for Women International, 13*(1), 67–76.

Denyes, M. J. (1982). Measurement of self-care agency in adolescents. *Nursing Research, 31,* 63.

Dodd, M. J. (1982). Assessing patient self-care for side effects of cancer chemotherapy—part 1. *Cancer Nursing, 5,* 447–451.

Dodd, M. J. (1984). Patterns of self-care in cancer patients receiving radiation therapy. *Oncology Nursing Forum, 11,* 23–27.

Dodd, M. J. (1997). Self-care: Ready or not! *Oncology Nursing Forum, 24*(6), 983–990.

Donaldson, S. K., & Crowley, D. M. (1978). The discipline of nursing. *Nursing Outlook, 26*(2), 113–120.

Evers, G. (1998). *Meten van zelfzorg: Verpleegkundige instrumenten voor onderzoek en klinische praktijk.* [Measurement of Self-Care: Nursing instruments for research in clinical practice]. Belgium: Universitaire Pers Leuven.

Evers, G. C. M., Isenberg, M. A., Philipsen, H., Senten, M., & Brouns, G. (1993). Validity testing of the Dutch translation of the appraisal of the self-care agency ASA-scale. *International Journal of Nursing Studies, 30*(4), 331–342.

Fawcett, J. (1995). *Analysis and evaluation of conceptual models of nursing.* Philadelphia: F. A. Davis.

Gallegos, E. (1997). *The effect of social, family and individual conditioning factors on self-care agency and universal self-care of adult Mexican women.* Unpublished doctoral dissertation, Wayne State University, Detroit.

Geden, E., & Taylor, S. (1991). Construct and empirical validity of the self-as-carer inventory. *Nursing Research, 40*(1), 47–50.

Haas, D. L. (1990). Application of Orem's Self-Care Deficit Theory to the pediatric chronically ill population. *Issues in Comprehensive Pediatric Nursing, 13,* 253–264.

Hanson, B. R., & Bickel, L. (1985). Development and testing of the questionnaire on perception of self-care agency. In Riehl-Sisca, J. (Ed.), *The science and art of self-care* (pp. 271–278). Norwalk, CT: Appleton-Century-Crofts.

Hanucharurnkul, S. (1989). Predictors of self-care in cancer patients receiving radiotherapy. *Cancer Nursing, 12*(1), 21–27.

Hartweg, D. L. (1993). Self-care actions of healthy, middle-aged women to promote well-being. *Nursing Research, 42*(4), 221–227.

Hartweg, D. L. (1990). Health promotion self-care within Orem's general theory of nursing. *Journal of Advanced Nursing, 15*(1), 35–41.

Hartweg, D. L., & Berbiglia, V. A. (1996). Determining the adequacy of a health promotion self-care interview guide with healthy, middle-aged, Mexican-American women: A pilot study. *Health Care for Women, 17*(1), 57–68.

Horsburgh, M. E. (1994). *The contribution of personality to adult well-being: Test and explication of Orem's theory of self-care.* Unpublished doctoral dissertation, Wayne State University, Detroit.

Isenberg, M. (1987). International research project to test Orem's Self-Care Deficit Theory of Nursing. *Proceedings of scientific session of the 29th Biennial Convention of Sigma Theta Tau International.* Sigma Theta Tau, San Francisco, California.

Isenberg, M. (1993). The influence of health state on the self-care agency of persons with coronary artery disease. *Proceedings of Sigma Theta Tau International Research Congress* (Madrid, Spain). Indianapolis: Sigma Theta Tau.

Isenberg, M., Evers, G. C. M., & Brouns, G. (1987). An international research project to test Orem's Self-Care Deficit Theory. *Proceedings of the International Research Congress.* Edinburgh, United Kingdom: University of Edinburgh.

Isenberg, M. A. (1991). Insights from Orem's nursing theory on differentiating nursing practice. In Goertzen, E. E. (Ed.), *Differentiating nursing practice: Into the twenty-first century* (pp. 45–49). Kansas City, MO: American Academy of Nursing.

Jaarsma, T., Kastermans, M., Dassen, T., & Philipsen, H. (1995). Problems of cardiac patients in early recovery. *Journal of Advanced Nursing, 21*(1), 21–27.

Jacobs, C. J. (1990). Orem's self-care model: Is it relevant to patients in intensive care? *Intensive Care Nursing, 6*(2), 100–103.

Jirovec, M. M., & Kasno, J. (1990). Self-care agency as a function of patient-environmental factors among nursing home residents. *Research in Nursing and Health, 13,* 303–309.

Johnson, D. E. (1959). The nature of a science of nursing. *Nursing Outlook, 7*(5), 291–294.

Katainen, A. L., Merlainen, P., & Isenberg, M. (1993). Reliability and validity testing of Finnish version of the appraisal of self-care agency (ASA) scale. *Proceedings of the Sigma Theta Tau International Research Congress* (Madrid, Spain). Indianapolis: Sigma Theta Tau.

Lorensen, M., Holter, I. M., Evers, G. C. M., Isenberg, M. A., & Van Achterberg, T. (1993). Cross-cultural testing of the "Appraisal of Self-Care Agency: ASA Scale" in Norway. *International Journal of Nursing Studies, 30*(1), 15–23.

Lukkarinen, H. (1997). Self-care agency and factors related to this agency among patients with coronary heart disease. *International Journal of Nursing Studies, 34*(4), 295–304.

McQuiston, C. M. (1993). *Basic conditioning factors and self-care agency of unmarried women at risk for sexually transmitted disease.* Unpublished doctoral dissertation, Wayne State University, Detroit.

Meleis, A. I., Isenberg, M. A., Koerner, J. E., Lacey, B., & Stern, P. (1995). *Diversity, marginalization, and culturally competent health care issues in knowledge development.* Washington, DC: American Academy of Nursing.

Metcalfe, S. A. (1996). *Self-care actions as a function of therapeutic self-care demand and self-care agency in individuals with chronic obstructive pulmonary disease.* Unpublished doctoral dissertation, Wayne State University, Detroit.

Moore, J. B. (1995). Measuring the self-care practice of children and adolescents: Instrument development. *Maternal Child Nursing Journal, 23*(3), 101–108.

Mosher, R. B., & Moore, J. B. (1998). The relationship of self-concept and self-care in children with cancer. *Nursing Science Quarterly, 11*(3), 116–122.

Norris, M. K. G. (1991). Applying Orem's theory to the long-term care of adolescent transplant recipients. *American Nephrology Nurses Association Journal, 18,* 45–47, 53.

Nursing Development Conference Group. (1979). *Concept formalization in nursing: Process and product* (2nd ed.). Boston: Little, Brown.

O'Connor, N. A. (1995). *Maieutic dimensions of self-care agency: Instrument development.* Unpublished doctoral dissertation, Wayne State University, Detroit.

Orem, D. E. (1971). *Nursing: Concepts of practice.* New York: McGraw-Hill.

Orem, D. E. (1985). *Nursing: Concepts of practice* (3rd ed.). New York: McGraw-Hill.

Orem, D. E. (1995). *Nursing: Concepts of practice* (5th ed.). New York: McGraw-Hill.

Richardson, A., & Ream, E. K. (1997). Self-care behaviours initiated by chemotherapy patients in response to fatigue. *International Journal of Nursing Studies, 34*(1), 35–43.

Riley, P. (1996). Development of a COPD self-care action scale. *Rehabilitation Nursing Research, 5*(1), 3–8.

Schott-Baer, D. (1989). *Family culture, family resources, dependent care, caregiver burden and self-care agency of spouses of cancer patients.* Unpublished doctoral dissertation, Wayne State University, Detroit.

Senten, M. C., Evers, G. C. M., Isenberg, M., & Philipsen, H. (1991). Veranderingen in selfsorg na coronair bypass operatie, een prospectieve stude [Changes in self-care following coronary artery bypass surgery, a prospective study]. *Verplegkuude, 5*(1), 34–43.

Soderhamn, O., Evers, G., & Hamrin, E. (1996). A Swedish version of the Appraisal of Self-Care Agency (ASA) scale. *Scandinavian Journal of Caring, 10*(1), 3–9.

Tolentino, M. B. (1990). The use of Orem's self-care model in the neonatal intensive care unit. *Journal of Obstetric, Gynecologic, and Neonatal Nursing, 19,* 496–500.

Utz, S. W., & Ramos, M. C. (1993). Mitral valve prolapse and its effects: A programme of inquiry within Orem's Self-Care Deficit Theory of Nursing. *Journal of Advanced Nursing, 18,* 742–751.

Van Achterberg, T., Lorensen, M., Isenberg, M., Evers, G. C. M., Levin, E., & Philipsen, H. (1991). The Norwegian, Danish and Dutch version of the appraisal of self-care agency scale: Comparing reliability aspects. *Scandinavian Journal of Caring Science, 5*(1), 1–8.

Vannoy, B. (1989). *The relationship among motivational dispositions, basic conditioning factors, and the power element of self-care agency in people beginning a weight loss program.* Unpublished doctoral dissertation, Wayne State University, Detroit.

Villarruel, A. M. (1995). Mexican-American cultural meanings, expressions, self-care and dependent care actions associated with experiences of pain. *Research in Nursing & Health, 18*(5), 427–436.

Ward-Griffin, C., & Bramwell, L. (1990). The congruence of elderly client and nurse perceptions of the clients' self-care agency. *Journal of Advanced Nursing, 15*(9), 1070–1077.

West, P. (1993). *The relationship between depression and self-care agency in young adult women.* Unpublished doctoral dissertation, Wayne State University, Detroit.

Whetstone, W. R. (1987). Perceptions of self-care in East Germany: A cross-cultural empirical investigation. *Journal of Advanced Nursing, 12,* 167–176.

Whetstone, W. R., & Hansson, A. M. O. (1989). Perceptions of self-care in Sweden: A cross-cultural replication. *Journal of Advanced Nursing, 14*(11), 962–969.

Bibliography

Ailinger, R. L. (1993). Patient's explanations of rheumatoid arthritis. *Western Journal of Nursing Research, 15*(3), 340–351.

Allison, S. E. (1985). *Structuring nursing practice based on Orem's theory of nursing: A nurse administrator's perspective.* Norwalk, CT: Appleton-Century-Crofts.

Allison, S. E., McLaughlin, K., & Walker, D. (1991). Nursing theory: A tool to put nursing back into nursing administration. *Nursing Administration Quarterly, 15*(3), 72–78.

Angeles, D. M. (1991). An Orem-based NICU orientation checklist, *Neonatal-Nater, 9*(7) 43–48.

Berbiglia, V. A. (1991). A case study: Perspectives on a self-care deficit nursing theory-based curriculum. *Journal of Advanced Nursing, 16,* 1158–1163.

Bidigare, S. A., & Oermann, M. H. (1991). Attitudes and knowledge of nurses regarding organ procurement. *Heart and Lung, 20,* 20–24.

Biley, F., & Dennerley, M. (1990). Orem's model: A critical analysis . . . part 2. *Nursing (London): The Journal of Clinical Practice, Education and Management, 4*(13), 21–22.

Bliss-Holtz, V. J. (1988). Primiparas' prenatal concern for learning infant care. *Nursing Research, 37,* 20–24.

Bliss-Holtz, V. J. (1991). Developmental tasks of pregnancy and prenatal education. *International Journal of Childbirth Education, 6*(1), 29–31.

Bottorff, J. L. (1988). Assessing an instrument in a pilot project: The self-care agency questionnaire. *Canadian Journal of Nursing Research, 20,* 7–16.

Campbell, J. C. (1986). Nursing assessment for risk of homicide with battered women. *Advances in Nursing Science, 8*(4), 36–51.

Campbell, J. C. (1989). A test of two explanatory models of women's responses to battering. *Nursing Research, 38,* 18–24.

Comley, A. L. (1994). A comparative analysis of Orem's self-care model and Peplau's interpersonal theory. *Journal of Advanced Nursing, 20*(4), 755–760.

Conn, V. (1991). Self-care actions taken by older adults for influenza and colds. *Nursing Research, 40,* 176–181.

Conn, V. S., Taylor, S. G., & Kelley, S. (1991). Medication regimen complexity and adherence among older adults. *Image: Journal of Nursing Scholarship, 23,* 231–235.

Dellasega, C. (1995). SCOPE: A practical method for assessing the self-care status of elderly persons. *Rehabilitation Nursing Research, 4*(4), 128–135.

Denyes, M. J. (1988). Orem's model used for health promotion: Directions from research. *Advances in Nursing Science Research, 11*(1), 13–21.

Denyes, M. J. (1993). Response to "Predictors of children's self-care performance: Testing the theory of self-care deficit." *Scholarly Inquiry for Nursing Practice, 7,* 213–217.

Denyes, M. J., Neuman, B. M., & Villarruel, A. M. (1991). Nursing actions to prevent and alleviate pain in hospitalized children. *Issues in Comprehensive Pediatric Nursing, 14,* 31–48.

Denyes, M. J., O'Connor, N. A., Oakley, D., & Ferguson, S. (1989). Integrating nursing theory, practice and research through collaborative practice. *Journal of Advanced Nursing, 14,* 141–145.

Dodd, M. J. (1983). Self-care for side effects in cancer chemotherapy: An assessment of nursing interventions—part 2. *Cancer Nursing, 6,* 63–67.

Dodd, M. J. (1984). Measuring informational intervention for chemotherapy knowledge and self-care behavior. *Research in Nursing and Health, 7,* 43–50.

Dodd, M. J. (1987). Efficacy of proactive information on self-care in radiation therapy patients. *Heart and Lung, 16,* 538–544.

Dodd, M. J. (1988a). Efficacy of proactive information on self-care in chemotherapy patients. *Patient Education and Counseling, 11,* 215–225.

Dodd, M. J. (1988b). Patterns of self-care in patients with breast cancer. *Western Journal of Nursing Research, 10,* 7–24.

Dodd, M. J. (1997). Self-Care: Ready or not! *Oncology Nursing Forum, 24*(6), 983–990.

Dowd, T. (1993). *Relationships among health state factors, foundational capabilities, and urinary incontinence self-care in women.* Unpublished doctoral dissertation, Wayne State University, Detroit.

Dowd, T. T. (1991). Discovering older women's experience of urinary incontinence. *Research in Nursing and Health, 14,* 179–186.

Evers, G. (1989). *Appraisal of self-care agency scale: Validity and reliability testing with Dutch populations.* Van Gorcum: Assen/Maastricht.

Ewing, G. (1989). The nursing preparation of stoma patients for self-care. *Journal of Advanced Nursing, 14,* 411–420.

Fawcett, J., Ellis, V., Underwood, P., Naqvi, A., & Wilson, D. (1990). The effect of Orem's self-care model on nursing care in a nursing home setting. *Journal of Advanced Nursing, 15,* 659–666.

Frey, M. A., & Denyes, M. J. (1989). Health and illness self-care in adolescents with IDDM: A test of Orem's theory. *Advances in Nursing Sciences, 12*(1), 67–75.

Frey, M. A., & Fox, M. A. (1990). Assessing and teaching self-care to youths with diabetes mellitus. *Pediatric Nursing, 16,* 597-800.

Furlong, S. (1996). Self-care: The application of a ward philosophy. *Journal of Clinical Nursing, 5*(2), 85-90.

Gammon, J. (1991). Coping with cancer: The role of self-care. *Nursing Practice, 4*(3), 11-15.

Gast, H. L., Denyes, M. J., Campbell, J. C., Hartweg, D. L., Schott-Baer, D., & Isenberg, M. (1989). Self-care agency: Conceptualizations and operationalizations. *Advances in Nursing Science, 12*(1), 26-38.

Gaut, D. A., & Kieckhefer, G. M. (1988). Assessment of self-care agency in chronically ill adolescents. *Journal of Adolescent Health Care, 9,* 55-60.

Gulick, E. E. (1987). Parsimony and model confirmation of the ADL Self-Care Scale for multiple sclerosis persons. *Nursing Research, 36,* 278-283.

Gulick, E. E. (1988). *The self-administered ADL scale for persons with multiple sclerosis.* New York: Springer.

Gulick, E. E. (1989). Model confirmation of the MS-related symptom checklist. *Nursing Research, 38,* 147-153.

Gullifer, J. (1997). The acceptance of a philosophically based research culture? *International Journal of Nursing Practice, 3*(3), 154-158.

Hanucharurnkul, S. (1989). Comparative analysis of Orem's and King's theories. *Journal of Advanced Nursing, 15,* 35-41.

Hanucharurnkul, S., & Vinya-nguag, P. (1991). Effects of promoting patients' participation in self-care on postoperative recovery and satisfaction with care. *Nursing Science Quarterly, 4*(1), 14-20.

Harper, D. (1984). Application of Orem's theoretical constructs to self-care medication behaviors in the elderly. *Advances in Nursing Science, 6*(3), 29-46.

Harris, J. L., & Williams, L. K. (1991). Universal self-care requisites as identified by homeless elderly men. *Journal of Gerontological Nursing, 17*(6), 39-43.

Hartweg, D. L. (1991). *Dorothea Orem: Self-care Deficit Theory.* Newbury Park, CA: Sage.

Hartweg, D. L., & Metcalfe, S. (1986). Self-care attitude changes of nursing students enrolled in a self-care curriculum—a longitudinal study. *Research in Nursing and Health, 9,* 347-353.

Hautman, M. A. (1987). Self-care responses to respiratory illnesses among Vietnamese. *Western Journal of Nursing Research, 9,* 223-243.

Hiromoto, B. M., & Dungan, J. (1991). Contract learning for self-care activities: A protocol study among chemotherapy outpatients. *Cancer Nursing, 14,* 148-154.

Holzemer, W. L. (1992). Linking primary health care and self-care through case management. *International Nursing Review, 39*(3), 83-89.

Horsburgh, M. E. (1994). *The contribution of personality to adult well-being: Test and explication of Orem's theory of self-care.* Unpublished doctoral dissertation, Wayne State University, Detroit.

Humphreys, J. (1991). Children of battered women: Worries about their mothers. *Pediatric Nursing, 17,* 342-345, 354.

Ip, W., Chau, J., Leung, M., Leung, Y., Foo, Y., & Chang, A. M. (1996). Research forum: Relationship between self-concept and perception of self-care ability of elderly in a Hong Kong hostel. *Hong Kong Nursing Journal, 72,* 6-12.

Jenny, J. (1991). Self-care deficit theory and nursing diagnosis: A test of conceptual fit. *Journal of Nursing Education, 30*(5), 227-232.

Jirovec, M. M., & Kasno, J. (1993). Predictors of self-care abilities among the institutionalized elderly. *Western Journal of Nursing Research, 15,* 314-326.

Jopp, M., Carroll, M. C., & Waters, L. (1993). Using self-care theory to guide nursing management of the older adult after hospitalization. *Rehabilitation Nursing, 18,* 91-94.

Kearney, B. Y., & Fleischer, B. J. (1979). Development of an instrument to measure exercise of self-care agency. *Research in Nursing and Health, 2,* 25-34.

Kerkstra, A., Castelein, E., & Philipsen, H. (1991). Preventive home visits to elderly people by community nurses in the Netherlands. *Journal of Advanced Nursing, 16,* 631-637.

Kirkpatrick, M. K., Brewer, J. A., & Stocks, B. (1990). Efficacy of self-care measures for perimenstrual syndrome (PMS). *Journal of Advanced Nursing, 15,* 281-285.

Leininger, M. (1992). Self-care ideology and cultural incongruities: Some critical issues. *Journal of Transcultural Nursing, 4*(1), 2-4.

Lev, E. L. (1995). Triangulation reveals theoretical linkages and outcomes in a nursing intervention study. *Clinical Nurse Specialist, 9*(6), 300-305.

Malik, U. (1992). Women's knowledge, beliefs, and health practices about breast cancer, and breast self-examination. *Nursing Journal of India, 83,* 186-190.

McBride, S. (1987). Validation of an instrument to measure exercise of self-care agency. *Research in Nursing and Health, 10,* 311-316.

McDermott, M. A. N. (1993). Learned helplessness as an interacting variable with self-care agency: Testing a theoretical model. *Nursing Science Quarterly, 6,* 28-38.

McQuiston, C. M., & Campbell, J. C. (1997). Theoretical substruction: A guide for theory testing research. *Nursing Science Quarterly, 10*(3), 117-123.

Moore, J. B. (1993). Predictors of children's self-care performance: Testing the theory of self-care deficit. *Scholarly Inquiry for Nursing Practice, 7,* 199-212.

Moore, J. B., & Gaffney, K. F. (1989). Development of an instrument to measure mothers' performance of self-care activities for children. *Advances in Nursing Science, 12*(1), 76-83.

Morales-Mann, E. T., & Jiang, S. L. (1993). Applicability of Orem's conceptual framework: A cross-cultural point of view. *Journal of Advanced Nursing, 18,* 737-741.

Nursing Development Conference Group. (1973). *Concept formalization in nursing: Process and product.* Boston: Little, Brown.

Orem, D. E. (1980). *Nursing: Concepts of practice* (2nd ed.). New York: McGraw-Hill.

Orem, D. E. (1983a). *The family coping with a medical illness: Analysis and application of Orem's theory.* New York: Wiley.

Orem, D. E. (1983b). *The family experiencing emotional crisis: Analysis and application of Orem's Self-Care Deficit Theory.* New York: Wiley.

Orem, D. E. (1983c). *The Self-Care Deficit Theory of Nursing: A general theory.* New York: Wiley.

Orem, D. E. (1987). *Orem's general theory of nursing.* Philadelphia: W. B. Saunders.

Orem, D. E. (1990). A nursing practice theory in three parts, 1956-1989. In Parker, M. (Ed.), *Nursing theories in practice.* New York: National League for Nursing.

Orem, D. E. (1991). *Nursing: Concepts of practice* (4th ed.). New York: McGraw-Hill.

Orem, D. E., & Taylor, S. G. (1986). *Orem's general theory of nursing.* New York: National League for Nursing.

Rhodes, V. A., Watson, P. M., & Hanson, B. M. (1988). Patients' descriptions of the influence of tiredness and weakness on self-care abilities. *Cancer Nursing, 11,* 186-194.

Richardson, A. (1992). Studies exploring self-care for the person coping with cancer treatment: A review. *International Journal of Nursing Studies, 29,* 191-204.

Richardson, A., & Ream, E. K. (1997). Self-care behaviours initiated by chemotherapy patients in response to fatigue. *International Journal of Nursing Studies, 34*(1), 35-43.

Riesch, S. K. (1988). Changes in the exercise of self-care agency. *Western Journal of Nursing Research, 10,* 257-273.

Riesch, S. K., & Hauck, M. R. (1988). The exercise of self-care agency: An analysis of construct and discriminant validity. *Research in Nursing and Health, 11,* 245-255.

Roberson, M. R., & Kelley, J. H. (1996). Using Orem's theory in transcultural settings: A critique. *Nursing Forum, 31*(3), 22-28.

Rosenbaum, J. (1986). Comparison of two theorists on care: Orem and Leninger. *Journal of Advanced Nursing, 11,* 409-411.

Schott-Baer, D. (1993). Dependent care, caregiver burden, and self-care agency of spouse caregivers. *Cancer Nursing, 16,* 230-236.

Simmons, S. J. (1990a). The health-promoting self-care system model: Directions for nursing research and practice. *Journal of Advanced Nursing, 15*(10), 1162-1166.

Simmons, S. J. (1990b). The health-promoting self-care system model: Directions for nursing research and practice. *Journal of Advanced Nursing, 15*(10), 1162-1166.

Smith, M. C. (1979). Proposed metaparadigm for nursing research and theory development: An analysis of Orem's self-care theory. *Image, 11,* 75-79.

Smits, J., & Kee, C. C. (1992). Correlates of self-care among the independent elderly: Self-concept affects well-being. *Journal of Gerontological Nursing, 18*(9), 13-18.

Spearman, S. A., Duldt, B. W., & Brown, S. (1993). Research testing theory: Selective review of Orem's Self-Care Theory. *Journal of Advanced Nursing, 18*(10), 1626-1631.

Spitzer, A., Bar-Tal, Y., & Ziv, L. (1996). The moderating effect of age on self-care. *Western Journal of Nursing Research, 18*(2), 136-148.

Underwood, P. R. (1980). Facilitating self-care. In Pothier, P. (Ed.). *Psychiatric Nursing* (pp. 115-144). Boston: Little, Brown.

Urbancic, J. C. (1992a). Empowerment support with adult female survivors of childhood incest: Part I—Theories and research. *Archives of Psychiatric Nursing, 6,* 275-281.

Urbancic, J. C. (1992b). Empowerment support with adult female survivors of childhood incest: Part II—Application of Orem's method helping. *Archives of Psychiatric Nursing, 6,* 282-286.

Utz, S. W. (1990). Motivating self-care: A nursing approach. *Holistic Nursing Practice, 4*(2), 13-21.

Utz, S. W., Hammer, J., Whitmire, V. M., & Grass, S. (1990). Perceptions of body image and health status in persons with mitral valve prolapse. *Image: Journal of Nursing Scholarship, 22,* 18-22.

Villarruel, A. M., & Denyes, M. J. (1991). Pain assessment in children: Theoretical and empirical validity. *Advances in Nursing Science, 14*(2), 32-41.

Villarruel, A. M., & Denyes, M. J. (1997). International scholarship: Testing Orem's theory with Mexican Americans. *Image: Journal of Nursing, 29*(3), 283-288.

Wagnild, G., Rodriguez, W., & Pritchett, P. (1987). Orem's self-care theory: A tool for education and practice. *Journal of Nursing Education, 26,* 343.

Wang, C. (1997). The cross-cultural applicability of Orem's conceptual framework. *Journal of Cultural Diversity, 4*(2), 44-48.

Weaver M. T. (1987). Perceived self-care agency: A LISREL factor analysis of Bickel and Hanson's questionnaire. *Nursing Research, 36,* 381-387.

Woodtli, A. O. (1988). Changes in the exercise of self-care agency. *Western Journal of Nursing, 10*(3), 269-271.

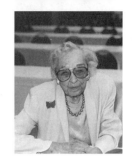

Chapter 14 Part 1

Martha E. Rogers
Science of Unitary Human Beings

Violet M. Malinski

INTRODUCING THE THEORIST

Martha E. Rogers, one of nursing's foremost scientists, was a staunch advocate for nursing as a basic science. She believed that the art of practice could be developed only as the science of nursing evolved. A common refrain throughout her career was the need to differentiate skills, techniques, and ways of using knowledge from the body of knowledge that guides practice to promote health and well-being for humankind. "The practice of nursing is not nursing. Rather, it is the use of nursing knowledge for human betterment" (Rogers, 1994a, p. 34). Rogers identified the unitary human being and the environment as the central concern of nursing, rather than health and illness. She repeatedly emphasized the need for nursing science to encompass beings in space as well as on Earth. Who was this visionary who introduced a new worldview to nursing?

Martha Elizabeth Rogers was born in Dallas, Texas, on May 12, 1914, a birthday she shared with Florence Nightingale. Her parents soon returned home to Knoxville, Tennessee, where Martha and her three siblings grew up, surrounded by a close-knit extended family of grandparents, aunts, uncles, and cousins. She loved to read, and became a frequent visitor to the public library before age 6 (Hektor, 1989/1994). Rogers found ways to share what she learned with others at an early age. Jane Rogers Coleman, her youngest sister, recalled plays Martha composed for her sisters and brother to act out for different audiences, particularly one called "Nutrition and Health" (Malinski, 1994).

Rogers spent two years at the University of Tennessee in Knoxville before entering the nursing program at Knoxville General Hospital. Next, she attended George Peabody College in Nashville, Tennessee, where she earned her bachelor of science degree in public health nursing, choosing that field as her professional focus.

Rogers spent the next 13 years in rural public health nursing in Michigan, Connecticut, and Arizona, where she established the first Visiting Nurse Service in Phoenix, serving as its executive director (Hektor, 1989/1994). Recognizing the need for advanced education, she took a break during this period and returned to academia, earning her master's degree in nursing from Teachers College, Columbia University, in the program developed by another nurse theorist, Hildegard Peplau. In 1951 she returned to academia, this time earning a master's of public health and doctor of science degree from Johns Hopkins University in Baltimore, Maryland.

In 1954 Rogers was appointed head of the Division of Nursing at New York University (NYU), beginning the second phase of her career overseeing baccalaureate, master's, and doctoral programs in nursing and developing the nursing science she knew was integral to the knowledge base nurses needed. She articulated the need for a "valid baccalaureate education" that would serve as the base for graduate and doctoral studies in nursing. Such a program, she believed, required 5 years of study in theoretical content in nursing as well as liberal arts and the biological, physical, and social sciences. Under her leadership, NYU established such a program. At the doctoral level, Rogers opposed the federally funded nurse-scientist doctoral programs that prepared nurses in other disciplines rather than in the science of nursing. During the 1960s she successfully shifted the focus of doctoral research from nurses and their functions to human beings in mutual process with the environment. She wrote three books that explicated her ideas: *Educational Revolution in Nursing* (1961), *Reveille in Nursing* (1964), and the landmark *An Introduction to the Theoretical Basis of Nursing* (1970). From 1963 to 1965 she edited a journal that was far ahead of its time, *Nursing Science,* which offered content on theory development and the emerging science of nursing plus research and issues in education and practice.

Rogers recognized the need to combine both professional and political activism. Throughout her career she participated in regional, state, national, and international organizations, both nursing and non-nursing. She helped draft the revised Nurse Practice Act in New York State, lobbied for its passage, and participated in the nurses' march on the state capitol in 1970 to urge its passage, which occurred in 1972.

Along with a number of nursing colleagues, Rogers established the Society for Advancement in Nursing in 1974. Among other issues, this group supported differentiation in education and practice for professional and technical careers in nursing. They drafted legislation to amend the Education Law in New York State proposing licensure as an Independent Nurse (IN) for those who had a minimum of a baccalaureate degree and introduced a new exam and licensure as a Registered Nurse (RN) for those with either a diploma or an associate degree in nursing who passed the traditional boards (Governing Council of the Society for Advancement in Nursing, 1977/1994). Differentiation of practice according to educational preparation remains a contentious issue today.

Rogers is best remembered for the paradigm she introduced to nursing, the Science of Unitary Human Beings, which displays her visionary, future-oriented perspective. Her theoretical ideas appeared in embryonic form in her two earlier books and were fleshed out in the 1970 book, then revised and refined in a number of articles and book chapters written between 1980 and 1994. She helped create the Society of Rogerian Scholars, Inc., chartered in New York in 1988, as one avenue for furthering the development of this nursing science.

In her personal life Rogers was devoted to her extended family, who remember her as a treasured sister, aunt, and cousin who gave unstintingly of her time and affection. Every summer Rogers returned by car to her home in Phoenix, each time with assorted family members. They traveled the scenic routes so Martha could introduce different nieces, nephews, and cousins to sites like the Grand Canyon, Yellowstone, and Lake Louise. She gifted her nieces and nephews with books of all genres and with trips to Europe following high school graduation. In the words of one niece, the Reverend Nancy J. Wilhite, "Aunt Martha was the Auntie Mame of all her nieces and nephews!" (Malinski, 1994, p. 7).

> The unique focus of nursing is the irreducible human being and its environment, both identified as energy fields.

Rogers died in 1994, leaving a rich legacy in her writings on nursing science, the space age, research, education, and professional/political issues in nursing. Readers interested in further information on her life and reprints of her seminal works will find them in *Martha E. Rogers: Her Life and Her Work,* edited by Malinski and Barrett (1994).

THE SCIENCE OF UNITARY HUMAN BEINGS: OVERVIEW

The historical evolution of the Science of Unitary Human Beings has been described by Malinski and Barrett (1994). This chapter presents the science in its current form and identifies work in progress to expand it further.

Rogers (1994a) identified the unique focus of nursing as "the irreducible human being and its environment, both identified as energy fields" (p. 33). "Human" encompasses both *Homo sapiens* and *Homo spatialis,* the evolutionary transcendence of humankind as we voyage into space, and environment encompasses outer space. This perspective ne-

cessitates a new worldview, out of which emerges the Science of Unitary Human Beings, "a pandimensional view of people and their world" (Rogers, 1992/1994, p. 257).

Rogers' Worldview

Rogers described the new worldview underpinning her conceptual system to students and colleagues beginning in 1968. It has been available in print with some revisions in language since 1986 (Madrid & Winstead-Fry, 1986; Malinski, 1986; Rogers, 1990a, 1990b, 1992, 1994a, 1994b). Rogers (1992) described the evolution from older to newer worldviews in such shifting perspectives as cell theory to field theory, entropic to negentropic universe, three dimensional to pandimensional, person-environment as dichotomous to person-environment as integral, causation and adaptation to mutual process, dynamic equilibrium to innovative growing diversity, homeostasis to homeodynamics, waking as a basic state to waking as an evolutionary emergent, and closed to open systems. She pointed out that in a universe of open systems, energy fields are continuously open, infinite, and integral with each other. Change that is predictable, brought about by a linear, causal chain of events, gives way to change that is diverse, creative, innovative, and unpredictable. In addition to her own worldview as an example of this paradigm change, Rogers (1992) identified other examples, such as synthesis and holism, represented in the works of people like Buckminster Fuller, James Lovelock, David Bohm, Fritjof Capra, and Rupert Sheldrake.

> In a universe of open systems, energy fields are continuously open, infinite, and integral with each other.

Rogers was aware that the world looks very different from the vantage point of the newer view as contrasted with the older, traditional worldview. She pointed out that we are already living in a new reality, one that is "a synthesis of rapidly evolving, accelerating ways of using knowledge" (Rogers, 1994a, p. 33), even if people are not always fully aware that these shifts have occurred or are in process. She urged that nurses be visionary, looking forward and not backward, not allowing themselves to become stuck in the present, in the details

> The four fundamental postulates of Rogerian nursing science are energy fields, openness, pattern, and pandimensionality.

of how things are now, but envision how they might be in a universe where continuous change is the only given. Rogers (1994b) cautioned that, although traditional modalities of practice and methods of research serve a purpose, they are inadequate for the newer worldview, which urges nurses to use the knowledge base of Rogerian nursing science creatively in order to develop innovative new modalities and research approaches that would promote the betterment of humankind.

Postulates of Rogerian Nursing Science

Rogers (1992) identified four fundamental postulates: energy fields, openness, pattern, and pandimensionality, formerly called both four-dimensionality and multidimensionality. In their irreducible unity they form reality as experienced in this worldview. Rogers (1990a, 1994a, 1994b) defined the energy field as "the fundamental unit of the living and the non-living," noting that the energy field is infinite and dynamic, meaning that it is continuously moving and flowing (1990a, p. 7). She identified two energy fields of concern to nurses, which are distinct but not separate: the human field, or unitary human being; and the environmental field. The human field can be conceptualized as one person or a group, family, or community. The human and environmental fields are irreducible; they cannot be broken down into component parts or subsystems. Parts have no meaning in unitary science. For example, the unitary human is not described as a bio-psycho-sociocultural or body-mind-spirit entity. Rogers interpreted such designations as representative of current uses of "holistic," meaning a summation of parts to arrive at the whole, where a nurse would assess the domains, subsystems, or components identified, then synthesize the accumulated data to arrive at a picture of the total person. Instead, Rogers maintained that each field, human and environmetal, is identified by pattern, defined as "the distinguishing characteristic of an energy field perceived as a single wave" (Rogers, 1990a, p. 7). Pattern manifestations and characteristics are specific to the whole.

Because human and environmental fields are integral with each other, they cannot be separated. They are always in mutual process. A concept like adaptation, a change in one preceding change in another, loses meaning in this nursing science. Change occurs simultaneously for human and environment.

The fields are pandimensional, defined as "a non-linear domain without spatial or temporal attributes" (Rogers, 1992, p. 28). Pandimensional reality transcends traditional notions of space and time, which can be understood as perceived boundaries only. Examples of pandimensionality include phenomena commonly labeled "paranormal" that are, in Rogerian nursing science, manifestations of the changing diversity of field patterning and examples of pandimensional awareness.

It is possible for people who are not in the same room or in contact via phone with family members to know suddenly that the latter are in trouble and need help. It is not unusual to think of a friend, who may live in another town, state, or country, decide to call that person, and go to the phone only to have it ring and hear that very friend on the other end.

The postulate of openness resonates throughout the above discussion. In an open universe, there are no boundaries other than perceptual ones. Therefore, human and environment are not separated by boundaries. The energy of each flows continuously through the other in an unbroken wave. Rogers repeatedly emphasized that person and environment are energy fields—but they do not have energy fields, such as auras, surrounding them. In an open universe, there are multiple potentials and possibilities. Nothing is predetermined or foreordained. Causality breaks down, paving the way for a creative, unpredictable future. People experience their world in multiple ways, evidenced by the diverse manifestations of field patterning that continuously emerge.

Rogers (1992, 1994a) described pattern as changing continuously while giving identity to each unique human-environmental field process. Although pattern is an abstraction, not something that can be observed directly, "it reveals itself through its manifestations" (Rogers, 1992, p. 29). Individual characteristics of a particular person are not characteristics of field patterning. Pattern manifestations reflect the human-environmental field mutual process as a unitary, irreducible whole. Person and environment cannot be examined or understood as separate entities. Pattern manifestations reveal the relative diversity, lower frequency, and higher frequency patterning of this human-environmental mutual field process. Rogers identified some of these manifestations as lesser and greater diversity; longer, shorter, and seemingly continuous rhythms; slower, faster, and seemingly continuous motion; time experienced as slower, faster, and timelessness; pragmatic, imaginative, and visionary; and longer sleeping, longer waking, and beyond waking. She explained "seems continuous" as "a wave frequency so rapid that the observer perceives it as a single, unbroken event" (Rogers, 1990a, p. 10). This view of the ongoing process of change is captured in Rogers' Principles of Homeodynamics.

your thoughts

Principles of Homeodynamics

Like adaptation, homeostasis—maintaining balance or equilibrium—is an outdated concept in the worldview represented in Rogerian nursing science. Rogers chose "homeodynamics" to convey the dynamic, ever-changing nature of life and the world. Her three principles of homeodynamics—resonancy, helicy, and integrality—describe the nature of change in the human-environmental field process. *Resonancy* specifies the "continuous change from lower to higher frequency wave patterns in human and environmental fields" (Rogers, 1990a, p. 9). Resonancy presents the way change occurs. Although Rogers stated that this process is nonlinear, she was unable to move away from the language of "from lower to higher" in the principle itself that seems to indicate a linear progression. Rogers (1990b, p. 10) elaborated: "[I]ndividuals experience lesser diversity and greater diversity . . . time as slower, faster, or unmoving. Individuals are sometimes pragmatic, sometimes imaginative, and sometimes visionary. Individuals experience periods of longer sleeping, longer waking, and periods of beyond waking."

Resonancy, then, specifies change flowing in lower and higher frequencies that continually fluctuate, rather than flowing from lower to higher frequencies. Both lower and higher frequency awareness and experiencing are essential to the wholeness of rhythmical patterning. As Phillips (1994, p. 15) described it, "[W]e may find that growing diversity of pattern is related to a dialectic of low frequency–high frequency, similar to that of order-disorder in chaos theory. When the rhythmicities of lower-higher frequencies work together, they yield innovative, diverse patterns."

Helicy is the "continuous innovative, unpredictable, increasing diversity of human and environmental field patterns" (Rogers, 1990a, p. 8). This principle describes the nature of change. *Integrality* is "continuous mutual human field and environmental field process" (Rogers, 1990a, p. 8). It specifies the context of change as the integral human-environmental field process where person and environment are inseparable.

Together the principles suggest that the mutual patterning process of human and environmental fields changes continuously, innovatively, and unpredictably, flowing in lower and higher frequencies. Rogers (1990a, p. 9) believed that they serve as guides both to the practice of nursing and to research in the science of nursing.

THEORIES IDENTIFIED BY ROGERS

Rogers clearly stated her belief that multiple theories can be derived from the Science of Unitary Human Beings. They are specific to nursing and reflect not what nurses do, but an understanding of people and our world (Rogers, 1992). Nursing education is identified by transmission of this theoretical knowledge, and nursing practice is the creative use of this knowledge. Nursing research uses it to illuminate the nature of the human-environmental field change process and its many unpredictable potentials.

The theory of accelerating evolution suggests that the only "norm" is accelerating change. Higher frequency field patterns that manifest growing diversity open the door to wider ranges of experiences and behaviors, calling into question the very idea of "norms" as guidelines. Human and environmental field rhythms are speeding up. We experience faster environmental motion now than ever before, in cars

and high-speed trains and planes, for example. It is common for people to experience time as rapidly speeding by. People are living longer. Rather than viewing aging as a process of decline or a "running down," as in an entropic worldview, this theory views aging as a creative process whereby field patterns show increasing diversity in such manifestations as sleeping, waking, and dreaming. Rogers hypothesized that hyperactive children provide a good example of speeded-up rhythms relative to other children. They would be expected to show indications of faster rhythms, increased motion, and other behaviors indicative of this shift. She expected that relative diversity would manifest in different patterns for individuals within any age cohort, concluding that chronological age is not a valid indicator of change in this system: "[I]n fact, as evolutionary diversity continues to accelerate, the range and variety of differences between individuals also increase; the more diverse field patterns evolve more rapidly than the less diverse ones" (Rogers, 1992, p. 30).

The theory of the emergence of paranormal phenomena suggests that experiences commonly labeled "paranormal" are actually manifestations of the changing diversity and innovation of field patterning. They are pandimensional forms of awareness, examples of pandimensional reality that manifest visionary, beyond waking potentials. Meditation, for example, transcends traditionally perceived limitations of time and space, opening the door to new and creative potentials. Therapeutic touch provides another example of such pandimensional awareness. Both participants often share similar experiences during therapeutic touch, such as a visualization sharing common features that evolves spontaneously for both, a shared experience arising within the mutual process both are experiencing, with neither able to lay claim to it as a personal, private experience. Precognition, déjà vu, and clairvoyance become normal rather than paranormal experiences.

McEvoy (1990) hypothesized that the process of dying exemplifies four-dimensional awareness and thus encompasses paranormal events such as out-of-body and apparitional experiences. She cited Margeneau's discussion in "Science, Creativity, and Psi," identifying paranormal experiences as ability to perceive within a four-dimensional world: "It is our human lot to look at the four-dimensional world through a slit-like opening. . . . Whenever the slit opens, and for some people the slit only opens at the time of death, you see more than a segmented three-dimensional slice of the four-dimensional universe" (cited in McEvoy, 1990, p. 211). Death itself is a transition, not an end, a manifestation of increasing diversity as energy fields transform.

Rogers' third theory, rhythmical correlates of change, was changed to manifestations of field patterning in unitary human beings, discussed earlier. Here Rogers suggested that evolution is an irreducible, nonlinear process characterized by increasing diversity of field patterning. She offered some manifestations of this relative diversity, including the rhythms of motion, time experience, and sleeping-waking, encouraging others to suggest further examples.

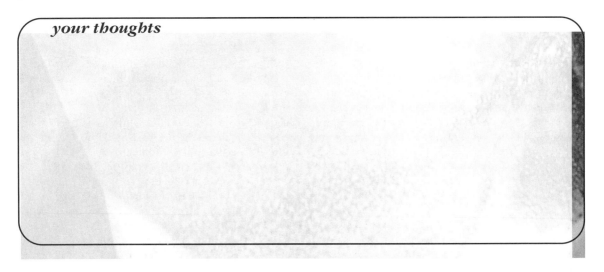

your thoughts

Barrett's Theory of Power as Knowing Participation in Change

Change is ongoing in Rogerian nursing science. Rogers maintained that one cannot stop or start the change process; it simply is. However, one is capable of knowing participation in that change. Barrett (1986, 1990) took that assumption and looked at how people can change the nature of their participation in change. She developed both a theory of and a tool to measure power as knowing participation in change. Barrett (1990, p. 108) defined power as "the capacity to participate knowingly in the nature of change characterizing the continuous patterning of the human and environmental fields as manifested by awareness, choices, freedom to act intentionally, and involvement in creating change." She continued, "Power is being aware of what one is choosing to do, feeling free to do it, and doing it intentionally. Depending on the nature of the awareness, the choices one makes, and the freedom to act intentionally, the range of situations in which one is involved in creating change varies" (Barrett, 1986, p. 174). Rather than good or bad power, more power or less power, power is a lower and higher frequency phenomenon. Higher frequency power or knowing participation in change may be descriptive of the accelerating change theorized by Rogers.

The power tool is one of the most widely used in Rogerian science–based research to explore power and variables such as leadership, human field motion, creativity, purpose in life, well-being, chronic pain, reminiscence, empathy, feminism, and spirituality. Caroselli and Barrett (1998) and Barrett and Caroselli (1998) have critically reviewed the research literature and discussed methodological issues raised and insights gained from this body of work.

EXAMPLES OF PROPOSED THEORIES BEING DEVELOPED BY OTHER ROGERIAN SCHOLARS

Theory of Perceived Dissonance

Bultemeier (1997) explored health concerns labeled as abnormal or illness processes, offering a theoretical perspective for pattern appraisal of these field manifestations. "The inherent rhythmicity of fields can evolve into rhythms that vary and may manifest as discordant . . . perceived as nonharmonic and as uncomfortable or unsettling to the person; thus the person views himself/herself as out of harmony or 'ill'" (Bultemeier, 1997, p. 158). She linked her theory with Barrett's and the steps of the health patterning process to show how nurses can use clients' perceptions and feelings to highlight areas of harmony and dissonance in pattern appraisal, then identify possible patterning activities such as meditation, therapeutic touch, light and color, affirmations, and humor.

The Theory of Sentience Evolution

Parker (1989) proposed this theory of sleeping, waking, and beyond waking, building on the concept of *sentience* (the capability to think, feel, and perceive) introduced by Rogers in her 1970 book. Although Rogers dropped this concept in later writings, the sleeping-waking-beyond waking manifestations of change are well established. Parker proposed that beyond waking is "sentience experienced as a higher frequency phenomenon" and that "sentience evolution is thinking, feeling, and perceiving in the sleeping, waking, and beyond waking states" (p. 5). Reiterating that this is a nonlinear process, Parker suggested that changes in sleeping-waking-beyond waking patterning occur continuously and change in association with different life events and circumstances. Drawing on Barrett's Power Theory, she proposed that this process involves and can be enhanced by knowing participation in change. She used the example of sleep management to illustrate the implications of this theory for practice. Nurses would work with clients to describe sleep pattern changes, dreams, out-of-body experiences, and other manifestions of beyond waking experiences. Journaling, imagery, sleep hygiene, dietary changes, and the alleviation of anxiety, stress, and depression become alternatives to sedatives and hypnotics.

Theory of Healthiness

Leddy (Leddy & Fawcett, 1997) proposed that "greater perceived ease and expansiveness of human-environmental mutual process (participation) is associated with less perceived change," which, in turn, is associated with greater perceived energy contributing to healthiness (p. 76). She defined *healthiness* as characterized by purpose, "the perception of being energized by meaningful and significant goals," connections, "perception of having rewarding mutual process with others," and power to achieve goals (p. 77). She developed power along the dimensions of challenge-curiosity, confidence-assurance, capacity, choice-creativity, and capability. Leddy and Fawcett present the conceptual and methodological problems associated with the proposed derivation of this theory from Rogerian nursing science.

Enfolding Health-as-Wholeness-and-Harmony

Carboni (1995a) synthesized concepts and principles from Rogerian nursing science and the holonomic (meaning whole) theory of physicist David Bohm to derive a Rogerian practice theory whereby nurse and client have the potential to participate knowingly in evolutionary change for the betterment of humankind. Carboni encapsulates this process as "the evolutionary movement of fragmentation and disharmony to wholeness and harmony" (p. 77), which becomes the focus of knowing participation in patterning for Rogerian nursing practice. Identifying the mutual human/environmental field pattern involves changing configurations of lower frequency and lesser complexification, such as a "fragmenting human field–environmental field relationship," and higher frequency and greater complexification such as a "healing human field–environmental field relationship" (p. 76). Awareness can manifest as unitary knowing or fragmented knowing, action as unitary or fragmented action. The field pattern of place can reflect a healing place or a fragmented place. The nature of health and illness can reflect a pattern of health-within-illness or disease. The purpose of nursing practice is coparticipation "in the evolutionary change of patterns of disease and fragmenting place to new syntheses of patterns of health-within-illness and healing place," perhaps involving such experiences as peace, sacredness, and belonging (p. 78).

ROGERIAN SCIENCE-BASED PRACTICE AND RESEARCH

Practice

Rogers identified noninvasive modalities as the basis for nursing practice now and in the future. She said that nurses must use "nursing knowledge in noninvasive ways in a direct effort to promote well-being" (Rogers, 1994a, p. 34). This focus gives nurses a central role in health care rather than medical care. She also noted that health services should be community-based, not hospital-based. Hospitals are properly used to provide satellite services in specific instances of illness and trauma; they do not provide health services. In a 1990 panel discussion among Rogers and five other theorists, she

> Rogers stated that nurses must use knowledge in noninvasive ways in a direct effort to promote well-being.

maintained that "[o]ur primary concern . . . is to focus on people wherever they are and to help them get better, whatever that means. . . . Our job is better health, and people do better making their own choices. The best prognosis is for the individual who is non-compliant" (Randell, 1992, p. 181). In yet another panel discussion in 1991, she explained that greater diversity necessitates "services that are far more individualized than we have ever provided" (Takahashi, 1992, p. 89), and went on to reiterate her lack of support for nursing diagnosis.

Rogers consistently identified the need for individualized, community-based health services incorporating noninvasive modalities. She offered examples from those currently in use, such as therapeutic touch, meditation, imagery, humor, and laughter, while stating her belief that new ones will emerge out of the evolution toward spacekind (Rogers, 1994b). The principles of homeodynamics provide a way to understand the process of human-environmental change and, therefore, can serve as guidelines for developing nursing practice.

Multiple examples of practice based on Rogerian nursing science exist in the literature. For example, Morwessel (1994) and Tudor, Keegan-Jones, & Bens (1994) presented the way they and their colleagues implement Rogerian science–based nursing at the Children's Hospital Medical Center in Cincinnati, Ohio. Heggie, Garon, Kodiath, and Kelly (1994) and Woodward and Heggie (1997) discussed its use to guide nursing practice at the San Diego Veterans Affairs Medical Center. Andersen and Smereck (1989, 1992) developed the Personalized Nursing LIGHT Model for use with hard-to-reach clients, including those actively involved in substance abuse and at risk for AIDS/HIV.

Barrett (1988, 1990) developed a blueprint for Rogerian-based practice designed to assist clients with knowing participation in change, calling it "health patterning." The first phase, pattern manifestation knowing, involves "the continuous process of identifying manifestations of the human and environmental fields that relate to current health events" (Barrett, 1988, p. 50; Barrett, 1998). The second, voluntary mutual patterning, is "the process whereby the nurse with the client patterns the environmental field to promote harmony related to health events" (Barrett, 1988, p. 50; Barrett, 1998). The nurse assists clients to knowingly participate in their own well-being. One health-patterning modality Barrett (1992) specifically developed to assist in this process is a particular form of imagery—innovative imagery—where the content reflects this power theory and thus the Science of Unitary Human Beings.

Cowling (1990, 1997) has offered a template of unitary pattern appreciation to guide both practice and research. Pattern information derived from a person's experiences, perceptions, and expressions is used to compose a pattern appreciation profile. This is a coparticipatory process involving nurse and client. The client provides information in various forms that may involve speaking, journaling, music, art, poetry, photographs, and audio and/or visual recordings. The nurse records the process in journal forms such as reflective notes, theoretical and/or methodological notes, and peer review notes. The synthesized pattern profile is verified by the client and used by the nurse to suggest and reflect on possibilities for facilitating change, with the client appraising and reflecting on how these potential strategies fit or do not fit with personal experiences. Cowling describes pattern appreciation as a transformative process, both in offering clients a context for new awareness and in helping them access the infinite potentials for change inherent in pandimensionality. He also describes how his pattern appreciation fits with Barrett's pattern appraisal and deliberative mutual patterning (Cowling, 1990).

Research

Rogers maintained that both qualitative and quantitative methods were appropriate for Rogerian science–based research, with the nature of the question and the phenomena under investigation guiding the selection. However, she cautioned that neither is totally adequate for the new worldview and encouraged the development of new methods.

Pattern manifestations have provided a common research focus, highlighting the need for tools by which they can be measured. The earliest such tool, developed by Ference (1986) in her 1979 dissertation, is the Human Field Motion Tool, a semantic differential scale rating two concepts, "my motor is running" and "my field expansion."

Barrett (1986, 1990) developed the next tool in her 1983 dissertation. The Power as Knowing Participation in Change Tool (PKPCT) uses the semantic differential technique to rate the four concepts of her power theory—awareness, choices, freedom to act intentionally, and involvement in creating changes.

Paletta (1990) developed the Temporal Experience Scales using metaphors to capture the experiences of time dragging, time racing, and timelessness. Johnston (1994; Watson et al., 1997) developed the Human Field Image Metaphor Scale to measure awareness of the infinite wholeness of the human field. Gueldner (cited in Watson et al., 1997) developed the Index of Field Energy, composed of 18 pairs of line drawings judged to represent low and high frequency descriptions of a concept. Respondents indicate how they feel now along a 7-point scale. Hastings-Tolsma's (Watson et al., 1997) Diversity of Human Field Pattern Scale explores diverse pattern changes and personal preferences for participation in change. Watson's (Watson et al., 1997) Assessment of Dream Experience Scale explores dreaming as a beyond-waking experience. Leddy (1995) developed the Person-Environment Parti-

> Rogers noted that qualitative and quantitative research methods were appropriate for Rogerian nursing science, depending on the nature of the question and the phenomena under investigation.

cipation Scale and the Leddy Healthiness Scale (1996).

Carboni (1992) developed an interview guide designed to reflect the mutuality of the nurse-client relationship as well as the unitary nature of the human-environment patterning process. The Mutual Exploration of the Healing Human Field–Environmental Field Relationship asks for narrative descriptions of this relationship, including thoughts and feelings as well as any spiritual qualities that surfaced for the participants. Each is asked to express the relationship metaphorically, artistically, and through evocative words such as flowing, peace, partnership, harmonize, or healing. Together, nurse and client explore their perceptions of the relationship.

Two examples of new research methods developed in Rogerian nursing science come from Butcher and Carboni. Butcher (1994, 1998) created the Unitary Field Pattern Portrait research method, a new qualitative research method that assists in illuminating well-being from a unitary perspective. Carboni (1995b) developed a qualitative Rogerian process of inquiry to explore the enfolding-unfolding change of human-environmental field patterning.

Currently researchers are using Rogerian tools such as those described in multiple investigations, while other tools are in various stages of development. Innovative potentials for promoting the well-being of people and their environment emerge daily as nurses apply the knowledge gained through Rogerian nursing science. Rogers' challenge has been eagerly taken up by a community of committed scholars.

The Science of Unitary Human Beings reflects Rogers' optimism and hope for the future. She envisioned humankind poised "on the threshold of a fantastic and unimagined future" (Rogers, 1992, p. 33), looking toward space while simultaneously engaging in a transformative Rogerian revolution in health care on Earth. One manifestation will surely be the establishment of autonomous Rogerian nursing centers here on Earth and ultimately in space.

References

Andersen, M. D., & Smereck, G. A. D. (1989). Personalized nursing LIGHT model. *Nursing Science Quarterly, 2,* 120-130.

Andersen, M. D., & Smereck, G. A. D. (1992). The consciousness rainbow: An explication of Rogerian field pattern manifestation. *Nursing Science Quarterly, 5,* 72-79.

Barrett, E. A. M. (1986). Investigation of the principle of helicy: The relationship of human field motion and power. In Malinski, V. M. (Ed.), *Explorations on Martha Rogers' science of unitary human beings* (pp. 173-184). Norwalk, CT: Appleton-Century-Crofts.

Barrett, E. A. M. (1988). Using Rogers' science of unitary human beings in nursing practice. *Nursing Science Quarterly, 1,* 50-51.

Barrett, E. A. M. (1990). Health patterning with clients in a private practice environment. In Barrett, E. A. M. (Ed.), *Visions of Rogers' science-based practice* (pp. 105-115). New York: National League for Nursing.

Barrett, E. A. M. (1992). Innovative imagery: A health patterning modality for nursing practice. *Journal of Holistic Nursing, 10,* 154-166.

Barrett, E. A. M. (1998). A Rogerian practice methodology for health patterning. *Nursing Science Quarterly, 11,* 136-138.

Barrett, E. A. M., & Caroselli, C. (1998). Methodological ponderings related to the power as knowing participation in change tool. *Nursing Science Quarterly, 11,* 17-22.

Bultemeier, K. (1997). Rogers' science of unitary human beings in nursing practice. In Alligood, M. R. & Marriner-Tomey, A. (Eds.), *Nursing theory utilization and practice* (pp. 153-174). St. Louis: Mosby.

Butcher, H. K. (1994). The unitary field portrait method: Development of a research method for Rogers' science of unitary human beings. In Madrid, M., & Barrett, E. A. M. (Eds.), *Rogers' scientific art of nursing practice* (pp. 397-429). New York: National League for Nursing.

Butcher, H. K. (1998). Crystallizing the process of the unitary field portrait research method. *Visions: The Journal of Rogerian Nursing Science, 6,* 13-26.

Carboni, J. (1992). Instrument development and the measurement of unitary constructs. *Nursing Science Quarterly, 5,* 134-142.

Carboni, J. (1995a). Enfolding health-as-wholeness-and-harmony: A theory of Rogerian nursing practice. *Nursing Science Quarterly, 8,* 71-78.

Carboni, J. (1995b). A Rogerian process of inquiry. *Nursing Science Quarterly, 8,* 22-37.

Caroselli, C., & Barrett, E. A. M. (1998). A review of the power as knowing participation in change literature. *Nursing Science Quarterly, 11,* 9-16.

Cowling, W. R. (1990). A template for unitary pattern-based nursing practice. In Barrett, E. A. M. (Ed.), *Visions of Rogers' science-based practice* (pp. 45-65). New York: National League for Nursing.

Cowling, W. R. (1997). Pattern appreciation: The unitary science/practice of reaching for essence. In Madrid, M. (Ed.), *Patterns of Rogerian knowing* (pp. 129-142). New York: National League for Nursing.

Ference, H. M. (1986). The relationship of time experience, creativity traits, differentiation, and human field motion. In Malinski, V. M. (Ed.), *Explorations on Rogers' science of unitary human beings* (pp. 95-105). Norwalk, CT: Appleton-Century-Crofts.

Governing Council of the Society for the Advancement of Nursing (SAIN) (1977/1994). SAIN Perspective. In Malinski, V. M. & Barrett, E. A. M. (Eds.), *Martha E. Rogers: Her life and her work* (pp. 182-191). Philadelphia: F. A. Davis. (Reprinted from *SAIN Newsletter,* pp. 4-6, 1977, January.)

Heggie, J., Garon, M., Kodiath, M., & Kelly, A. (1994). Implementing the science of unitary human beings at the San Diego Veterans Affairs Medical Center. In Madrid, M. & Barrett, E. A. M. (Eds.), *Rogers' scientific art of nursing practice* (pp. 285-304). New York: National League for Nursing.

Hektor, L. M. (1989/1994). Martha E. Rogers: A life history. In Malinski, V. M. & Barrett, E. A. M. (Eds.), *Martha E. Rogers: Her life and her work* (pp. 10-27). Philadelphia: F. A. Davis. (Reprinted from *Nursing Science Quarterly, 2,* 63-73).

Johnston, L. W. (1994). Psychometric analysis of Johnston's human field image metaphor scale. *Visions: The Journal of Rogerian Nursing Science, 2,* 7-11.

Leddy, S. K. (1995). Measuring mutual process: Development and psychometric testing of the person-environment participation scale. *Visions: The Journal of Rogerian Nursing Science, 3,* 20-31.

Leddy, S. K. (1996). Development and psychometric testing of the Leddy Healthiness Scale. *Research in Nursing and Health, 19,* 431-440.

Leddy, S. K., & Fawcett, J. (1997). Testing the theory of healthiness: Conceptual and methodological issues. In M. Madrid (Ed.), *Patterns of Rogerian knowing* (pp. 75-86). New York: National League for Nursing.

Madrid, M., & Winstead-Fry, P. (1986). Rogers' conceptual model. In Winstead-Fry, P. (Ed.), *Case studies in nursing theory* (pp. 73-102). New York: National League for Nursing.

Malinski, V. M. (1986). Further ideas from Martha Rogers. In Malinski, V. M. (Ed.), *Explorations on Martha Rogers' science of unitary human beings* (pp. 9-14). Norwalk, CT: Appleton-Century-Crofts.

Malinski, V. M. (1994). A family of strong-willed women. In Malinski, V. M. & Barrett, E. A. M. (Eds.), *Martha E. Rogers: Her life and her work* (pp. 3-9). Philadelphia: F. A. Davis.

Malinski, V. M., & Barrett, E. A. M., (Eds.) (1994). *Martha E. Rogers: Her life and her work*. Philadelphia: F. A. Davis.

McEvoy, M. D. (1990). The relationships among the experience of dying, the experience of paranormal events, and creativity in adults. In Barrett, E. A. M. (Ed.), *Visions of Rogers' science-based nursing* (pp. 209-228). New York: National League for Nursing.

Morwessel, N. J. (1994). Developing an effective pattern appraisal to guide nursing care of children with heart variations and their families. In Madrid, M. & Barrett, E. A. M. (Eds.), *Rogers' scientific art of nursing practice* (pp. 147-161). New York: National League for Nursing.

Paletta, J. L. (1990). The relationship of temporal experience to human time. In Barrett, E. A. M. (Ed.), *Visions of Rogers' science-based nursing* (pp. 239-253). New York: National League for Nursing.

Parker, K. P. (1989). The theory of sentience evolution: A practice-level theory of sleeping, waking, and beyond waking patterns based on the science of unitary human beings. *Rogerian Nursing Science News, 2*(1), 4-6.

Phillips, J. R. (1994). The open-ended nature of the science of unitary human beings. In Madrid, M. & Barret, E. A. M. (Eds.), *Rogers' scientific art of nursing practice* (pp. 11-25). New York: National League for Nursing.

Randell, B. P. (1992). Nursing theory: The 21st century. *Nursing Science Quarterly, 5,* 176-184.

Rogers, M. E. (1990a). Nursing: Science of unitary, irreducible human beings: Update 1990. In Barrett, E. A. M. (Ed.), *Visions of Rogers' science-based nursing* (pp. 5-11). New York: National League for Nursing.

Rogers, M. E. (1990b). Space-age paradigm for new frontiers in nursing. In Parker, M. E. (Ed.), *Nursing theories in practice* (pp. 105-113). New York: National League for Nursing.

Rogers, M. E. (1992). Nursing science and the space age. *Nursing Science Quarterly, 5,* 27-34.

Rogers, M. E. (1994a). The science of unitary human beings: Current perspectives. *Nursing Science Quarterly, 7,* 33-35.

Rogers, M. E. (1994b). Nursing science evolves. In Madrid, M. & Barrett, E. A. M. (Eds.), *Rogers' scientific art of nursing practice* (pp. 3-9). New York: National League for Nursing.

Takahashi, T. (1992). Perspectives on nursing knowledge. *Nursing Science Quarterly, 5,* 86-91.

Tudor, C. A., Keegan-Jones, L., & Bens, E. M. (1994). Implementing Rogers' science-based nursing practice in a pediatric nursing service setting. In M. Madrid & E. A. M. Barrett (Eds.), *Rogers' scientific art of nursing practice* (pp. 305-322). New York: National League for Nursing.

Watson, J., Barrett, E. A. M., Hastings-Tolsma, M., Johnston, L., & Gueldner, S. (1997). Measurement in Rogerian science: A review of selected instruments. In M. Madrid (Ed.), *Patterns of Rogerian knowing* (pp. 87-99). New York: National League for Nursing.

Woodward, T. A., & Heggie, J. (1997). Rogers in reality: Staff nurse application of the science of unitary human beings in the clinical setting following changes in an orientation program. In M. Madrid (Ed.), *Patterns of Rogerian knowing* (pp. 239-248). New York: National League for Nursing.

Bibliography

Rogers, M. F. (1961). *Educational revolution in nursing*. New York: Macmillan.

(1963). Building a strong educational foundation. *American Journal of Nursing, 63*(6), 94-95.

(1963). Courage of their convictions. *Nursing Science, 1,* 44-47.

(1963, April-May). Some comments on the theoretical basis of nursing practice. *Nursing Science, 1.*

(1964). *Reveille in nursing*. Philadelphia: F. A. Davis.

(1965, January). What the public demands of nursing today. *RN. 28*:80.

(1966, January). Research in nursing. *Nursing Forum.*

(1967, December). Professional commitment. *Image.*

(1968). Nursing science: Research and researchers. *Teachers College Record, 69,* 469-476.

(1968). For public safety: Higher education's responsibility for professional education in nursing. *Hartwick Review, 5*(1), 21-25.

(1969). Nursing research: Relevant to practice. *Proceedings of the fifth nursing research conference.* New York: American Nurses' Association.

(1969). Regional planning for graduate education in nursing. *Proceedings of the National Committee of Deans of Schools of Nursing having accredited graduate programs in nursing.* New York: National League for Nursing.

(1970). *An introduction to the theoretical basis of nursing.* Philadelphia: F. A. Davis.

(1970). Yesterday a nurse—today a manager—what now? *Journal of the New York State Nurses' Association 1*(1), 15-21.

(1972). Nurses' expanding role and other euphemisms. *Journal of the New York State Nurses' Association, 3*(4), 5-10.

(1972). Nursing: To be or not to be? *Nursing Outlook, 20,* 42-46.

(1975). Euphemisms and nursing's future. *Image, 7*(2), 3-9.

(1975). Nursing is coming of age. *American Journal of Nursing, 75*(10), 1834-1843, 1859.

(1977). Nursing: To be or not to be. In Bullough, B. & Bullough, V. (Eds.), *Expanding horizons for nursing.* New York: Springer.

(1978). Emerging patterns in nursing education. In *Current perspectives in nursing education* (Vol. II, pp. 1-8). St. Louis: Mosby.

(1978). Legislative and licensing problems in health care. *Nursing Administration Quarterly, 2*(3).

(1978, January–February). A 1985 dissent. *Health/PAC Bulletin, 80,* 32-34.

(1980). Nursing: A science of unitary man. In Riehl, J. P. & Roy, C. (Eds.), *Conceptual models for nursing practice* (2nd ed., pp. 329-337). New York: Appleton-Century-Crofts.

(1981). Science of unitary man: A paradigm for nursing. In Laskar, G. E. (Ed.), *Applied systems and cybernetics, Vol. 4. Systems research in health care, biocybernetics and ecology* (pp. 1719-1722). New York: Pergamon.

(1983). The family coping with a surgical crisis: Analysis and application of Rogers' theory of nursing. In Clements, I. W. & Roberts, F. B. (Eds.), *Family health: A theoretical approach to nursing care* (pp. 390-391). New York: Wiley.

(1983). Science of unitary human beings: A paradigm for nursing. In Clements, I. W. & Roberts, F. B. (Eds.), *Family health: A theoretical approach to nursing care* (pp. 219-227). New York: Wiley.

(1985). The nature and characteristics of professional education for nursing. *Journal of Professional Nursing, 1,* 381-383.

(1985). The need for legislation for licensure to practice professional nursing. *Journal of Professional Nursing, 1,* 384.

(1985). Nursing education: Preparation for the future. In *Patterns in education: The unfolding of nursing* (pp. 11-14). New York: National League for Nursing.

(1985). Science of unitary human beings: A paradigm for nursing. In Wood, R. & Kekahbah, J. (Eds.), *Examining the cultural implications of Martha E. Rogers' science of unitary human beings* (pp. 13-23). Pawhuska, OK: Wood-Kekahbah Associates.

(1986). Science of unitary human beings. In Malinski, V. M. (Ed.), *Explorations on Martha Rogers' science of unitary human beings* (pp. 3-8). Norwalk, CT: Appleton-Century-Crofts.

(1987). Nursing research in the future. In Roode, J. (Ed.), *Changing patterns in nursing education* (pp. 121-123). New York: National League for Nursing.

(1987). Rogers' science of unitary human beings. In Parse, R. R. (Ed.), *Nursing science: Major paradigms, theories, and critiques* (pp. 139-146). Philadelphia: Saunders.

(1988). Nursing science and art: A prospective. *Nursing Science Quarterly, 1,* 99-102.

(1989). Nursing: A science of unitary human beings. In Riehl-Sisca, J. P. (Ed.), *Conceptual models for nursing practice* (3rd ed., pp. 181-188). Norwalk, CT: Appleton & Lange.

(1992). Nightingale's *Notes on Nursing:* Prelude to the 21st century. In Nightingale, F. N. *Notes on nursing: What it is, and what it is not* (Commemorative edition, pp. 58-62). Philadelphia: Lippincott. (Originally published in 1854)

(1994). The science of unitary human beings: Current perspectives. *Nursing Science Quarterly, 7,* 33-35.

Chapter *14*

Nursing Science in the New Millennium: Practice and Research within Rogers' Science of Unitary Human Beings

Howard K. Butcher

Nursing practice and research guided by nursing theory *distinguishes* nursing care from other healthcare disciplines. Because nursing theory is the scientific core of the nursing discipline, nursing theory needs to: (1) be integrated into all aspects of nursing education; (2) serve as the conceptual guide for nursing practice; and 3) function as the conceptual orientation of nursing research. Rogers' (1970, 1980, 1988, 1992) Science of Unitary Human Beings is a major conceptual system unique to nursing that offers nurses a radically new way of viewing persons and their universe concordant with the most contemporary emerging scientific theories describing a worldview of wholeness (Bohm, 1980; Briggs & Peat, 1984; Capra, 1982; Lovelock, 1979; Sheldrake, 1988; Woodhouse, 1996). New worldviews require new ways of thinking, sciencing, languaging, and practicing. Rogers' nursing science postulates a pandimensional universe of mutually processing human and environmental energy fields manifesting as continuously innovative, increasingly diverse, creative, and unpredictable unitary field patterns.

A hallmark of a maturing scientific practice discipline is the development of specific practice and research methods evolving from the discipline's extant conceptual systems. Over the past decade, practice and research methods have been derived from specific nursing conceptual systems. Rogers (1992) asserted that practice and research methods must be consistent with the Science of Unitary Human Beings in order to study irreducible human beings in mutual process with a pandimensional universe. Therefore, Rogerian practice and research methods must be congruent with Rogers' postulates and principles if they are to be consistent with Rogerian science. The purpose of this chapter is to present recent innovations in the development of practice and research methods derived from Rogers' postulates and principles.

> New worldviews require new ways of thinking, sciencing, languaging, and practicing.

ROGERIAN PRACTICE MODELS

Nursing exists as a human service. The goal of nursing practice is the promotion of well-being and human betterment. Nursing is a service to people wherever they may reside. Nursing practice—the art of nursing—is the application of substantive scientific knowledge developed through research. Since the 1960s, the nursing process has been the dominant nursing practice method. The nursing process is

an appropriate practice methodology for many nursing theories, including Roy's Adaptation Model, King's Theory of Goal Attainment, and Orem's Theory of Self-Care Deficit. However, there has been some confusion in the nursing literature concerning the use of the nursing process within Rogers' Nursing Science.

In early writings, Rogers (1970) did make reference to nursing process and nursing diagnosis. But in later years she asserted that nursing diagnoses were not consistent with her scientific system. Rogers (quoted in Smith, 1988, p. 83) stated:

> Nursing exists as a human service; practice methods have been derived from Rogers' postulates and principles.

> [N]ursing diagnosis is a static term that is quite inappropriate for a dynamic system ... it [nursing diagnosis] is an outdated part of an old worldview, and I think by the turn of the century, there is going to be new ways of organizing knowledge.

Furthermore, nursing diagnoses are particularistic and reductionistic labels describing cause and effect (i.e., "related to") relationships inconsistent with a "nonlinear domain without spatial or temporal attributes" (Rogers, 1992, p. 29). The nursing process is a stepwise sequential process inconsistent with a nonlinear or pandimensional view of reality. In addition, the term "intervention" is not consistent with Rogerian science. *Intervention* means to "come, appear, or lie between two things" (American Heritage Dictionary, 1992, p. 944). The principle of integrality describes the human and environmental field as integral and in mutual process. Energy fields are open, infinite, dynamic, and constantly changing. The human and environmental fields are inseparable, so one cannot "come between." The nurse and the client are already inseparable and interconnected. Outcomes are also inconsistent with Rogers' principle of helicy: that expected outcomes infer predictability. The principle of helicy describes the nature of change as being unpredictable. Within an energy field perspective, nurses in mutual process assist clients in actualizing their field potentials by enhancing their ability to participate knowingly in change (Butcher, 1997).

Given the inconsistency of the traditional nursing process with Rogers' postulates and principles, the Science of Unitary Human Beings requires the development of new and innovative practice methods derived from and consistent with the conceptual system. Over the last decade, a number of practice methods have been derived from Rogers' postulates and principles.

Barrett's Rogerian Practice Methodology for Health Patterning

Barrett's two-phase Rogerian practice methodology for health patterning is the accepted alternative to the nursing process for Rogerian practice and is currently the most widely used Rogerian practice model. Barrett's (1988) practice model was derived from the Science of Unitary Human Beings and consisted of two phases: pattern manifestation appraisal and deliberative mutual patterning. Barrett (1998) expanded and updated the methodology by refining each of the phases, now more appropriately referred to as "processes." Each of the processes have also been renamed for greater clarity and precision. *Pattern manifestation knowing* is the continuous process of apprehending the human and environmental field (Barrett, 1998). "Appraisal" means to estimate an amount or to judge the value of something, negating the egalitarian position of the nurse, whereas "knowing" means to recognize the nature, achieve an understanding, or become familiar or acquainted with something. *Voluntary mutual patterning* is the continuous process whereby the nurse assists clients in freely choosing—with awareness—ways to participate in their well-being (Barrett, 1998). The change to the term "voluntary" emphasizes freedom, spontaneity, and choice of action. The nurse does not invest in changing the client in a particular direction, but rather facilitates and mutually explores with the client options and choices, and provides information and resources so the client can make informed decisions regarding his or her health and well-being. Thus, clients feel free to choose with awareness how they want to participate in their own change process.

The two processes are continuous and nonlinear, and therefore not necessarily sequential. Patterning is continuous and occurs simultaneously with knowing. Control and predictability are not consistent with Rogers' postulate of pandimensionality and principles of integrality and helicy. Rather, acausality allows for freedom of choice, and means outcomes are unpredictable. The goal of voluntary mutual patterning is the actualization of *potentialities* for well-being through knowing participation in change.

Cowling's Pattern Appreciation Practice Method

Cowling (1990) expanded Barrett's original practice methodology by proposing a template comprising ten constituents for the development of Rogerian practice models consistent with the postulates and principles of Rogerian science. Cowling (1993b, 1997) refined the template and proposed that "pattern appreciation" was a method for unitary knowing in both Rogerian nursing research and practice. Cowling preferred the term "appreciation" rather than "assessment" or "appraisal" because *appraisal* is associated with evaluation. *Appreciation* has broader meaning, which includes "being full aware or sensitive to or realizing; being thankful or grateful for; and enjoying or understanding critically or emotionally" (Cowling, 1997, p. 130). Pattern appreciation is approached with gratefulness, enjoyment, and understanding and reaches for the essence of pattern. Pattern appreciation has a potential for deeper understanding.

The first constituent for unitary pattern appreciation identifies the human energy field emerging from the human/environment mutual process as the basic referent. Pattern manifestations emerging from the human/environment mutual process are the focus of nursing care. Next, the person's experiences, perceptions, and expressions are unitary manifestations of pattern and provide a focus for pattern appreciation. Third, "pattern appreciation requires an inclusive perspective of what counts as pattern information (energetic manifestations)" (Cowling, 1993b, p. 202). Thus, any information gathered from and about the client, family, or community, including sensory information, feelings, thoughts, values, introspective insights, intuitive apprehensions, lab values, and physiological measures, are viewed as "energetic manifestations" emerging from the human/environmental mutual field process.

The fourth constituent is that the nurse uses pandimensional modes of awareness when appreciating pattern information. In other words, intuition, tacit knowing, and other forms of awareness beyond the five senses are ways of apprehending manifestations of pattern. Fifth, all pattern information has meaning only when conceptualized and interpreted within a unitary context. Synopsis and synthesis are requisites to unitary knowing. *Synopsis* is a process of deliberately viewing together all aspects of a human experience (Cowling, 1997). Interpreting pattern information within a unitary perspective means that all phenomena and events are related nonlinearly. Also, phenomena and events are not discrete or separate but rather coevolve together in mutual process. Furthermore, all pattern information is a reflection of the human/environment mutual field process. The human and environmental fields are inseparable. Thus, any information from the client is also a reflection of his or her environment. Physiological and

other reductionistic measures have new meaning when interpreted within a unitary context. For example, a blood pressure interpreted within a unitary context means the blood pressure is a manifestation of pattern emerging from the entire human/environmental field mutual process rather than simply a physiological measure. Thus, any expression from the client is unitary and not particular by reflecting the unitary field from which it emanates (Cowling, 1993b).

The sixth constituent in Cowling's practice method describes the format for documenting and presenting pattern information. Rather than stating nursing diagnoses and reporting "assessment data" in a format that is particularistic and reductionistic by dividing the data into categories or parts, the nurse constructs a "pattern profile." Usually the pattern profile is in the form of a narrative summarizing the client's experiences, perceptions, and expression inferred from the pattern appreciation process. The pattern profile tells the story of the client's situation and should be expressed in as many of the client's own words as possible. Relevant particularistic data such as physiological data interpreted within a unitary context may be included in the pattern profile. Cowling (1990, 1993b) also identified additional forms of pattern profiles, including single words or phrases; and listing pattern information, diagrams, pictures, photographs, or metaphors that are meaningful in conveying the themes and essence of the pattern information.

Seventh, the primary source for verifying pattern appreciation and profile is the client. Verifying can occur by sharing the pattern profile with the client for revision and confirmation. During verification, the nurse also discusses options, mutually identifies

goals, and plans mutual patterning strategies. Sharing the pattern profile with the client enhances participation in the planning of care and facilitates the client's knowing participation in the change process (Cowling, 1997).

The eighth constituent identifies knowing participation in change as the foundation for health patterning. Knowing participation in change is being aware of what one is choosing to do, feeling free to do it, doing it intentionally, and being actively involved in the change process. The purpose of health patterning is to assist clients in knowing participation in change (Barrett, 1988). Ninth, pattern appreciation incorporates the concepts and principles of unitary science, and approaches for health patterning are determined by the client. Last, knowledge derived from pattern appreciation reflects the unique patterning of the client (Cowling, 1997).

Toward a Synthesis of Rogerian Practice Models

Butcher (1993, 1997), and Martin, Forchuk, Santopinto, and Butcher (1992) synthesized Cowling's Rogerian practice model with Barrett's practice methodology to develop an inclusive and comprehensive Rogerian practice model. The more detailed model presented below incorporates both Barrett's and Cowling's recent refinements and clarifications. In addition, in an ethical analysis of Rogers' life and science, Butcher (1999) identified a constellation of values intrinsic to the Science of Unitary Human Beings and asserted that Rogerian practice also includes making the following cherished values of Rogerian ethics intentional in the mutual patterning process: reverence, human betterment, generosity, commitment, diversity, responsibility, compassion, wisdom, justice-creating, openness, courage, optimism, humor, unity, transformation, and celebration.

The focus of nursing care guided by Rogers' nursing science is on recognizing manifestations of patterning through *pattern manifestation knowing and appreciation,* and facilitating the client's ability to participate knowingly in change, harmonizing person/environment integrality, and promoting healing potentialities and well-being using noninvasive modalities through *voluntary mutual patterning.*

Pattern Manifestation Knowing and Appreciation

Pattern manifestation knowing and appreciation is the process of identifying manifestations of patterning emerging from the human/environmental field mutual process and involves focusing on the client's experiences, perceptions, and expressions. "Knowing" refers to apprehending pattern manifestations (Barrett, 1988), whereas "appreciation" seeks for a perception of the "full force of pattern" (Cowling, 1997). Appreciation requires sensitivity, recognition of the excellence of the meaning of energy field patterning, and is approached with gratefulness, enjoyment, and understanding. Appreciation is reaching for the essence of pattern and has the potential to deepen understanding in the service to the client's process of knowing participation in change and transformation (Cowling, 1997).

Pattern is the distinguishing feature of the human/environmental field. Everything experienced, perceived, and expressed is a manifestation of patterning. During the process of pattern manifestation knowing and appreciation, the nurse and client are co-equal participants. Clients may be persons, families, and/or communities. Intentionality is expressed by approaching nursing situations with the intent to facilitate human betterment guided by a scientific base for practice and a commitment to enhance the client's potentialities for well-being. It is also important to create an atmosphere of openness and freedom so clients can freely participate in the process of knowing participation in change. Approaching the nursing situation with an appreciation of the uniqueness of each person, unconditional love, compassion, and empathy can help create an atmosphere of openness and healing patterning.

> Pattern is the distinguishing feature of the human/environmental field. The focus of nursing is on recognizing manifestations of patterning through knowing and appreciation.

Pattern manifestation knowing and appreciation involves focusing on the experiences, perceptions, and expressions of a health situation, revealed through a rhythmic flow of communion and dialogue. In most situations, the nurse can initially ask the client to describe his or her health situation and concern. The dialogue is guided toward focusing on uncovering the client's experiences, perceptions, and expressions related to the health situation as a means to reaching a deeper understanding of unitary field pattern. Humans are constantly all-at-once experiencing, perceiving, and expressing (Cowling, 1993a). Experience involves the rawness of living through sensing and being aware as a source of knowledge and includes any item or ingredient the client senses (Cowling, 1997). The client's own observations and description of his or her health situation includes his or her experiences. "Perceiving is the apprehending of experience or the ability to reflect while experiencing" (Cowling, 1993a, p. 202). Perception is making sense of the experience through awareness, apprehension, observation, and interpreting. Asking clients about their concerns, fears, observations is a way of apprehending their perceptions. Expressions are manifestations of experiences and perceptions that reflect human field patterning. In addition, expressions are any form of information that comes forward in the encounter with the client. All expressions are energetic manifestations of field pattern. Body language, communication patterns, gait, behaviors, lab values, and vital signs are examples of energetic manifestations of human/environmental field patterning.

Throughout pattern manifestation knowing and appreciating, the nurse is open to and uses multiple forms of knowing, including pandimensional modes of awareness (intuition, meditative insights, tacit knowing). Since all information about the client/environment/health situation is relevant, various health assessment tools such as the comprehensive holistic assessment tool developed by Dossey, Keegan, Guzzetta, and Kolkmeirer (1995) may also be useful in pattern knowing and appreciation. However, all information must be interpreted within a unitary context. A unitary context refers to conceptualizing all information as energetic/dynamic manifestations of pattern emerging from a pandimensional human/environment mutual process. All information is interconnected, inseparable from environmental context, unfolds rhythmically and acausally, and reflects the whole. Data are not divided or understood by dividing information into physical, psychological, social, spiritual, or cultural categories. Rather, a focus on experiences, perceptions, and expressions is a synthesis more than and different from the sum of parts.

More importantly, a unitary perspective in nursing practice leads to an appreciation of new kinds of information that may not be considered within other conceptual approaches to nursing practice. For example, pattern information concerning time perception, sense of rhythm or movement, sense of connectedness with the environment, ideas of one's own personal myth, and sense of integrity are relevant indicators of human/environment/health potentialities (Madrid & Winstead-Fry, 1986). A person's hopes and dreams, communication patterns, sleep-rest rhythms, comfort-discomfort, waking-beyond waking experiences, and degree of knowing participation in change provide important information regarding each client's thoughts and feelings concerning a health situation.

The nurse can also use a number of tools derived from Rogers' postulates and principles to enhance the collecting and understanding of relevant information specific to Rogerian science. Barrett (1989) developed the Power as Knowing Participation in Change Tool (PKPCT) as a way of knowing the client's energy field pattern in relation to his or her capacity to knowingly participate in the continuous patterning of human and environmental fields as manifested in frequencies of awareness, choice-making ability, sense of freedom to act intentionally, and degree of involvement in creating change. A score on each of the four scales is an indicator of human/environmental field patterning in relation to the client's sense of how he or she is participating in his or her own change process. The Hastings-Tolsma Diversity of Human Field Pattern Scale (Hastings-Tolsma, 1992) may be used as a means of knowing and appreciating clients' perceptions of the diversity of their energy field patterns, and Johnson's Human Image Metaphor Scale (Johnson, 1994) can be used as a way of knowing and appreciating the clients' perceptions of the wholeness of their energy fields. Watson's Assessment of Dream Experience Scale (Watson, 1993) can be used to know and appreciate each client's dream experiences and Ference's Human Field Motion Tool (Ference, 1979) is an indicator of the wave frequency pattern of the energy field. Paletta (1990) developed a tool consistent with Rogerian science that measures the subjective awareness of temporal experience. Leddy's (1995) Person-Environment Participation Scale may be used to know and appreciate expansiveness and ease of a person's participation in the human/environment/ health process. Disturbances are energy field patterning and may manifest as a low score in either power, human field motion, diversity of pattern, or human field image.

When initial pattern manifestation knowing and appreciation is complete, the nurse synthesizes all the pattern information into a meaningful pattern profile. Usually the pattern profile will be in the form of a narrative that describes the essence of the properties, features, and qualities of the human/environment/health situation. The pattern profile reflects the essence of the client's experiences, perceptions, and expressions, and, in addition to a narrative form, the pattern profile may also include diagrams, poems, listings, phrases, and/or metaphors. Interpretations of any measurement tools may also be incorporated into the pattern profile.

> Middle-range Rogerian practice theories are useful for pattern manifestation knowing and appreciation, and voluntary mutual patterning processes.

Voluntary Mutual Patterning

Voluntary mutual patterning is a process of transforming human/environmental field patterning. The goal of voluntary mutual patterning is to facilitate each client's ability to participate knowingly in change, harmonize person/environment integrality, and promote healing potentialities, lifestyle changes, and well-being in the client's desired direction of change or attachment to predetermined outcomes. The process is mutual in that both the nurse and the client are changed with each encounter, each patterning one another and coevolving together. The process is voluntary and intentional in that the nurse approaches each nursing situation with the *intention* of promoting well-being and human betterment. Intentionality is an active process of desiring action and is the volitional propagation of energy. Action is a process of movement or transformation of energy (Butcher, 1998a). "Voluntary" signifies freedom of choice or action without external compulsion (Barrett, 1998). The nurse has no investment in changing the client in a particular way.

Whereas patterning is continuous, voluntary mutual patterning may begin by sharing the pattern profile with the client. Sharing the pattern profile with the client is a means of validating the interpretation of pattern information and may spark further dialogue, revealing new and more in-depth information. Sharing the pattern profile with the client facilitates

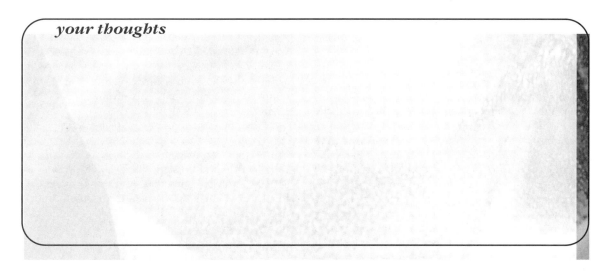

your thoughts

pattern recognition and also may enhance the client's knowing participation in his or her own change process. An increased awareness of one's own pattern may offer new insight and increase one's desire to participate in the change process. In addition, the nurse and client can continue to mutually explore goals, options, choices, and voluntary mutual patterning strategies as a means to facilitate the client's actualization of his or her human/environmental field potentials.

A wide variety of mutual patterning strategies may be used in Rogerian practice, including many "interventions" identified in the Nursing Intervention Classification (McCloskey & Bulechek, 1996). However, interventions are reconceptualized within a unitary perspective as voluntary mutual patterning strategies. Furthermore, Rogers (1988, 1992, 1994) placed great emphasis on modalities that are traditionally viewed as holistic and noninvasive. In particular, therapeutic touch, guided imagery, and the use of humor, sound, dialogue, affirmations, music, massage, journaling, exercise, nutrition, reminiscence, aroma, light, color, artwork, meditation, storytelling, literature, poetry, movement, and dance are just a few of the voluntary mutually patterning strategies consistent with a unitary perspective. Sharing of knowledge through health education, and providing health education literature and teaching also have the potential to enhance knowing participation in change. These and other noninvasive modalities are well described and documented in both the Rogerian literature (Barrett, 1990; Madrid, 1997; Madrid & Barrett, 1994) and in the holistic nursing practice literature (Dossey, 1997; Dossey, Keegan, Guzzetta, & Kolkmeirer, 1995; Guzzetta, 1998). Evaluation is continuous and is integral both to pattern manifesta-

tion knowing and appreciation and to voluntary mutual patterning. The nurse is continuously evaluating changes in patterning emerging from the human/environmental field mutual process. Regardless of which combination of voluntary patterning strategies is used, the intention is for clients to actualize their potentials related to human well-being and betterment.

Selected Mid-range Rogerian Practice Theories

In addition to the processes of the practice model, a number of mid-range Rogerian practice theories have been developed that are useful in informing the pattern manifestation knowing and appreciation and voluntary mutual patterning processes. Nursing science is advanced when mid-range theory development evolves from nursing's conceptual models. Each of the selected mid-range Rogerian practice theories is briefly described below.

Theory of Power as Knowing Participation in Change

Barrett's (1989) Theory of Power as Knowing Participation in Change was derived directly from Rogers' postulates and principles and interweaves awareness, choices, freedom to act intentionally, and involvement in creating changes. Power is a natural continuous theme in the flow of life experiences and dynamically describes how human beings participate with the environment to actualize their potential. Barrett (1983) pointed out that most theories of power are causal and define power as the ability to influence, prevent, or cause change with dominance, force, and hierarchy. Power, within a Rogerian perspective, is being aware of what one is choosing to do, feeling free to do it, doing it intentionally, and being actively involved in the change process. A person's ability to participate knowingly in change varies in given situations. Thus, the intensity, frequency, and form that power manifests vary. Power is neither inherently good nor evil; however, the form in which power manifests may be viewed as either constructive or destructive depending on one's value perspective (Barrett, 1989). Barrett (1989) stated that her theory does not value different forms of power, but instead recognizes differences in power manifestations. The Power as Knowing Participation in Change Tool (PKPCT), mentioned earlier, is a measure of one's relative frequency of power. Barrett (1989) suggests that the Power Theory and PKPCT may be useful in a wide variety of nursing situations. Barrett's Power Theory is useful with clients who are experiencing hopelessness, suicidal ideation, hypertension and obesity, drug and alcohol dependence, grief and loss, self-esteem issues, adolescent turmoil, career conflicts, marital discord, cultural relocation trauma, or the desire to make a lifestyle change. In fact, all health/illness experiences involve issues concerning knowing participation in change.

During pattern manifestation knowing and appreciation, the nurse invites the client to complete the PKPCT as a means to identify the client's power pattern. To prevent biased responses, the nurse should refrain from using the word "power." The power score is determined on each of the four subscales (manifestations of power): awareness, choices, freedom to act intentionally, and involvement in creating changes. The scores are documented as part of the client's pattern profile and shared with the client during voluntary mutual patterning. Scores are considered as a tentative and relative measure of the ever-changing nature of one's field pattern in relation to power. At this time the nurse can explain the meaning of the scores and the power theory and continues until the client understands each of the four manifestations of power. Misinterpretations are clarified, judgements are suspended, and understanding is validated. Power is viewed acausally. Instead of focusing on issues of control, the nurse helps the client identify the changes and the direction of change the client desires to make. Exploring aspects of the situation potentially increases the client's awareness. Using open-ended questions, the nurse and the client mutually explore choices and options and identify barriers preventing change, strategies, and resources to overcome barriers; the nurse facilitates the client's active involvement in creating the changes. For example, asking the ques-

tions "What do you want?" "What choices are open to you now?" "How free do you feel to do what you want to do?" and "How will you involve yourself in creating the changes you want?" can enhance the client's awareness, choice-making, freedom to act intentionally, and his or her involvement in creating change (Barrett, 1998).

A wide range of voluntary mutual patterning strategies may be used to enhance knowing participation in change, including meaningful dialogue, dance/movement/motion, sound, light, color, music, rest/activity, imagery, humor, nutrition, therapeutic touch, bibliotherapy, journaling, drawing, and nutrition (Barrett, 1998). The PKPCT can be used at intervals to evaluate the client's relative changes in power.

Theory of Perceived Dissonance

Bultemeier (1997) derived a mid-range theory from Rogers' postulates and principles that is also useful in a wide variety of nursing practice situations. The Theory of Perceived Dissonance proposes that experiences labeled as "illness" or as "abnormal processes" are manifestations of human/environmental field patterning characterized by nonharmonic, uncomfortable, unsettling, discordant rhythmicities perceived as dissonance (Bultemeier, 1997). Pain, anxiety, fear, anger, and depression are just a few human experiences relevant to nursing practice that may be conceptualized as dissonance. During pattern manifestation knowing and appreciation, the nurse identifies human and environmental field patterns of dissonance and harmony. Barrett's Theory of Power and Bultemeier's Theory of Perceived Dissonance can be used together in a client situation. During voluntary mutual patterning, the nurse and client mutually design and participate together in patterning activities to strengthen the coherence, harmony, and integrity of the human/environmental field.

Theory of Kaleidoscoping in Life's Turbulence

Butcher's (1993) mid-range practice theory of Kaleidoscoping in Life's Turbulence was derived from Rogers' Science of Unitary Human Beings, chaos theory (Briggs & Peat, 1989; Peat, 1991), and Csikszentmihalyi's (1990) Theory of Flow. It focuses on facilitating well-being and harmony amid turbulent life events. Turbulence is a dissonant commotion in the human/environmental field characterized by chaotic and unpredictable change. Any crisis may be viewed as a turbulent event in the life process. Nurses often work closely with clients who are in a "crisis." The turbulent life event may be an illness, the uncertainty of a medical diagnosis, marital discord, or loss of a loved one. Turbulent life events are often chaotic in nature, unpredictable, and always transformative.

Kaleidoscoping is a way of engaging in mutual process with clients who are in the midst of experiencing a turbulent life event by mutually *flowing with turbulent manifestations of patterning* (Butcher, 1993). *Flow* is an intense harmonious involvement in the human/environment mutual field process. The term "kaleidoscoping" was used because it evolves directly from Rogers' writings and conveys the unpredictable continuous flow of patterns, sometimes turbulent, that one experiences when looking through a kaleidoscope. Rogers (1970, p. 62) explained that the "organization of the living system is maintained amidst kaleidoscopic alterations in the patterning of system."

The Theory of Kaleidoscoping with Turbulent Life Events is used in conjunction with the pattern manifestation knowing and appreciation and voluntary mutual patterning processes. In addition to engaging in the processes already described in pattern manifestation knowing and appreciation, the nurse identifies manifestations of patterning and mutually explores the meaning of the turbulent situation with the client. A pattern profile describing the essence of the client's experiences, perceptions, and expressions related to the turbulent life event is constructed and shared with the client.

In the theory of kaleidoscoping, voluntary mutual patterning also incorporates the processes of transforming turbulent events by *cultivating purpose, forging resolve, and recovering harmony* (Butcher, 1993). *Cultivating purpose* involves assisting clients in identifying goals and developing an action system.

The action system is comprised of patterning strategies designed to promote harmony amid adversity and facilitate the actualization of the potential for well-being.

In moments of turbulence, clients may want to increase their awareness of the complexity of the situation. Creative suspension is a technique that may be used to facilitate comprehension of the situation's complexity (Peat, 1991). Guided imagery is a useful strategy for facilitating creative suspension because it potentially enhances the client's ability to enter a timeless suspension directed toward visualizing the whole situation and facilitating the creation of new strategies and solutions. *Forging resolve* is assisting the clients in becoming involved and immersed in their action system. Since chaotic and turbulent systems are infinitely sensitive, actions are "gentle" or subtle in nature and distributed over the entire system involved in the change process. Entering chaotic systems with a "big splash" or trying to force a change in a particular direction will likely lead to increased turbulence (Butcher, 1993).

Forging resolve involves incorporating flow experiences into the change process. Flow experiences promote harmonious human/environmental field patterns. There are a wide range of flow experiences that can be incorporated into the daily activities: art, music, exercise, reading, gardening, meditation, dancing, sports, sailing, swimming, carpentry, sewing, yoga, or any activity that is a source of enjoyment, concentration, and deep involvement. The incorporating of flow experiences into daily patterns potentiates the recovering of harmony. *Recovering harmony* is achieving a sense of courage, balance, calm, and resilience amid turbulent and threatening live events.

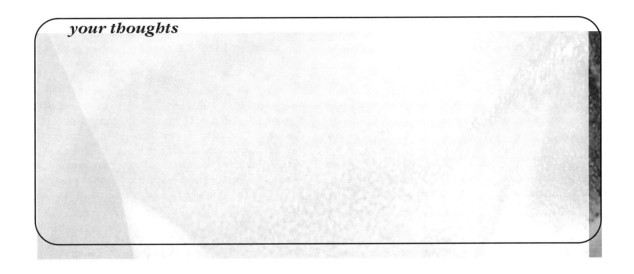

your thoughts

The art of kaleidoscoping with turbulence is a mutual creative expression of beauty and grace and is a way of enhancing perseverance through difficult times.

Enfolding Health-as-Wholeness-and-Harmony

Carboni (1995a) defined *Rogerian nursing practice* as the nurse and the client knowingly participating in evolutionary patterning of the human and environmental fields for the purpose of enfolding health-as-wholeness-and-harmony. Carboni derived the Enfolding Health-as-Wholeness-and-Harmony practice theory from a synthesis of Bohm's (1980) theory of the implicate-explicate order with Rogers' postulates and principles. According to Carboni, the three guiding principles of Rogerian nursing practice are: (1) knowingly participating, (2) evolutionary patterning of human and environmental fields, and (3) enfolding health-as-wholeness-and-harmony (Carboni, 1995a). Carboni defined each of the major concepts.

Knowingly participating is "enfolding the subtle configurations of patterning of healing human-environmental field relationship and unitary knowing within a pandimensional field of nonlinearity and acausality" (Carboni, 1995a, p. 76). *Evolutionary patterning of the human and environmental fields* is "enfolding the subtle configurations of patterning of unitary action while co-participating in the nonlinear and acausal transforming of the gross configurations of patterning of dis-ease and fragmenting place to a new synthesis of subtle configurations of patterning of health-within-illness healing place" (Carboni, 1995a, pp. 76–77). *Enfolding health-as-wholeness-and-harmony* is "enfolding the dynamic matrix of subtle configurations of patterning of the healing human field–environmental field relationship, unitary knowing, unitary action, health-within-illness and healing place within increasingly complex and diverse pandimensional human field–environmental field mutual process of higher wave frequency patterns of wholeness-and-harmony-in-process" (Carboni, 1995a, p. 77).

Carboni goes on to define each of the subconcepts, including unitary knowing and unitary action. Carboni's model has wide application in nursing practice. Any illness or "dis-ease" is understood as experiences, perceptions, and expressions reflecting an unfolding of disharmony or "fragmenting" of the integrity of human and environmental fields. Within this enfolding of subtle configurations of patterning, the nurse and the client participate together in patterning fragmented field patterns to a new synthesis and harmony in human–environmental field patterns. A wide variety of noninvasive voluntary mutual patterning strategies may be used to create a sense of unity, harmony, peace, sacredness, belonging, and home.

Personalized Nursing LIGHT Practice Model

The final mid-range Rogerian practice theory discussed in this overview is the successful Personalized Nursing LIGHT Practice Model (Anderson & Smereck, 1989, 1992, 1994). For more than 10 years the model has been used by the Personalized Nursing Corporation, an independent, nurse-owned, nurse-managed company providing outreach nursing care to high-risk and active drug users in Detroit, Michigan. The goal of the LIGHT model is to assist clients in improving their sense of well-being. With a higher sense of well-being, clients are less likely to continue to engage in high-risk drug-related behaviors. Drug-addicted behaviors are postulated to be a painful means to experience an awareness of integrality. During the pattern manifestation knowing and appreciation process, clients are asked to name a painful experience, encouraged to "be in the moment" in a safe place with the experience/feeling, asked to identify the choices they usually make during the painful experience, and then asked to identify pattern manifestations associated with their usual choices. Well-being (global and current), life pattern manifestations, and talents are also assessed using a heuristic teaching tool.

The acronym LIGHT guides the voluntary mutual patterning process. Nurses **L**—love the client, **I**—intend to help, **G**—give care gently, **H**—help the client improve well-being, and **T**—teach the healing process of the LIGHT model. Clients make progress toward well-being as they learn to **L**—love themselves, **I**—identify concerns, **G**—give themselves goals, **H**—have confidence and help themselves, and **T**—take positive action. In a three-year pre- and postcontrol treatment group study involving 744 participants, clients who received nursing care with the LIGHT model improved their sense of well-being associated with a decrease in high-drug behaviors (Anderson & Hockman, 1997).

Nursing practice *is* the application of nursing theory. Together, the mid-range practice theories briefly described offer a rich tapestry of theoretical guides for unitary practice in any nursing situation. Practicing nursing from a unitary perspective is a creative leap into a new worldview in concert with contemporary and progressive scientific theories of wholeness. Shifting one's perspective from an old worldview to a new one requires immersion and serious study. Readers are encouraged to study the original works cited for each of the mid-range theories. For students and nurses wishing to advance Rogerian science, each of the practice theories is an abounding source for theory-testing research.

RESEARCH WITHIN THE SCIENCE OF UNITARY HUMAN BEINGS

Research is the bedrock of nursing practice. The Science of Unitary Human Beings has a long history of theory-testing research. As new practice theories and health patterning modalities evolve from the Science of Unitary Human Beings, there remains a need to test the viability and usefulness of mid-level theories and voluntary health patterning strategies. The mass of Rogerian research has been reviewed in a number of publications (Caroselli & Barrett, 1998; Dykeman & Loukissa, 1993; Fawcett, 1995; Malinski, 1986, 1994; Phillips, 1989b; Watson, Barrett, Hastings-Tolsma, Johnson, & Gueldner, 1997). Rather than repeat the reviews of Rogerian research, the following section describes current methodological trends within the Science of Unitary Human Beings to assist researchers interested in Rogerian science in making methodological decisions.

> Research is the bedrock of nursing practice. Criteria for research methods guide, the design of investigations.

Methodological Issues

Although there is some debate among Rogerian scholars and researchers concerning the choice of an appropriate methodology in Rogerian research, Rogers (1994) maintained that both quantitative and qualitative methods may be useful for advancing Rogerian science. Similarly, Barrett (1996), Barrett and Caroselli (1998), Barrett, Cowling, Carboni, and Butcher (1997), Cowling (1986), and Rawnsley (1994) have all advocated for the appropriateness of multiple methods in Rogerian research. Conversely, Butcher (cited in Barrett et al., 1997); Butcher (1994), and Carboni (1995b) have argued that the ontological and epistemological assumptions of causality, reductionism, particularism, control, prediction, and linearity of quantitative methodologies are inconsistent with Rogers' unitary ontology and participatory epistemology. For the purpose of this chapter, an inclusive view of methodologies is advocated. However, the researcher needs to present an argument as to how the design of the study and interpretations of results are congruent with Rogers' postulates and principles. Furthermore, nurses interested in engaging in Rogerian research are encouraged to use, test, and refine the research methods and tools that have been developed consistent with the ontology and epistemology of the Science of Unitary Human Beings. Most importantly, since the development of unique research methods is a route toward disciplinary definition, there continues to be a great need to develop new research methods and tools consistent with Rogerian science (Barrett et al., 1997; Butcher, 1994; Carboni, 1992; Phillips, 1988; Rogers, 1994).

Criteria for Rogerian Inquiry

The criteria for developing Rogerian research methods presented in this chapter are a synthesis and modification of the Criteria of Rogerian Inquiry developed by Butcher (1994) and the Characteristics of Operational Rogerian Inquiry developed by Carboni (1995b). The criteria may be a useful guide in design-

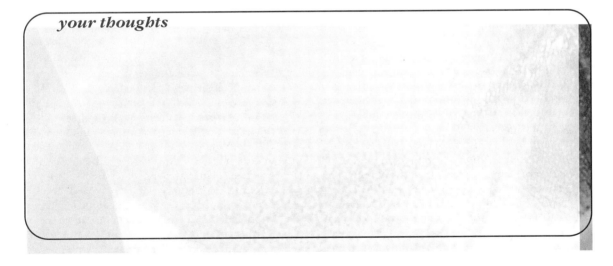

your thoughts

ing research investigations guided by the Science of Unitary Human Beings.

1. *A Priori Nursing Science:* All research flows from a theoretical perspective. Every step of the inquiry, including the type of questions asked, the conceptualization of phenomena of concern, choice of research design, selection of participants, selection of instruments, and interpretation of findings is guided by the Science of Unitary Human Beings. The researcher explicitly identifies the Science of Unitary Human Beings as the conceptual orientation of the study. Nursing research must be grounded in a theoretical perspective unique to nursing in order for the research to contribute to the advance of nursing science.

2. *Creation:* The Rogerian research endeavor is a creative and imaginative process for discovering new insights and knowledge concerning unitary human beings in mutual process with their environment.

3. *Irreducible Human-Environmental Energy Fields Are the Focus of Rogerian Inquiry:* Energy fields are postulated to constitute the fundamental unit of the living and nonliving. Both human beings and the environment are understood as dynamic energy fields that cannot be reduced to parts.

4. *Pattern Manifestations Are Indicators of Change:* Pattern is the distinguishing characteristic of an energy field and gives identity to the field. Pattern manifestations are the source of information emerging from the human/environmental mutual field process and are the only valid reflections of the energy field. The phenomenon of concern in Rogerian inquiry is conceptualized and understood as manifestations of human/environmental energy mutual process.

5. *Pandimensional Awareness:* Rogerian inquiry recognizes the pandimensional nature of reality. All forms of awareness are relevant in a pandimensional universe. Thus, intuition, both tacit and mystical, and all forms of sensory knowing are relevant ways of apprehending manifestations of patterning.

6. *Human Instrument Is Used for Pattern Knowing and Appreciation:* The researchers use themselves as the primary pattern-apprehending instrument. The human instrument is the only instrument sensitive to, and which has the ability to interpret and understand, pandimensional potentialities in human/environmental field patterning. Pattern manifestation knowing and ap-

preciation is the process of apprehending information or manifestations of patterning emerging from the human/environmental field mutual process. The process of pattern knowing and appreciation is the same in the research endeavor as described earlier in the Rogerian practice methodology.

7. *Both Quantitative and Qualitative Methods Are Appropriate:* Quantitative methods may be used when the design, concepts, measurement tools, and results are conceptualized and interpreted in a way consistent with Rogers' nursing science. It is important to note, that because of the incongruency between ontology and epistemology of Rogerian science with assumptions in quantitative designs, Carboni (1995b) argues that the researcher must select qualitative methods exclusively over quantitative methods. Barrett and Caroselli (1998), however, recognize the inconsistencies of quantitative methods with Rogerian science, and argue that the "research question drives the choice of method; hence, both qualitative and quantitative methods are not only useful but necessary" (p. 21). The ontological and epistemological congruence is reflected in the nature of questions asked and their theoretical conceptualization (Barrett, 1996). However, qualitative designs, particularity those that have been derived from the postulates and principles of the Science of Unitary Human Beings, are *preferred* because the ontology and epistemology of qualitative designs are more congruent with Rogers' notions of unpredictability, irreducibility, acausality, integrality, continuous process, and pattern (Barrett et al., 1997; Butcher, 1994).

8. *Natural Setting:* Rogerian inquiry is pursued in the natural settings where the phenomenon of inquiry occurs naturally, because the human field is inseparable and in mutual process with the environmental field. Any "manipulation" of "variables" is inconsistent with mutual process, unpredictability, and irreducibility.

9. *The Researcher and the Researcher-Into Are Integral:* The principle of integrality implies that the researcher is inseparable and in mutual process with the environment and the participants in the study. Each evolves during the research process. The researcher's values are also inseparable from the inquiry. "Objectivity" and "bracketing" are not possible when the human and environmental field are integral to one another.

10. *Purposive Sampling:* The researcher uses purposive sampling to select participants who mani-

fest the phenomenon of interest. Recognition of the integrality of all that is tells us that information about the whole is available in individuals, groups, and settings; therefore, representative samples are not required to capture manifestations of patterning reflective of the whole.

11. *Emergent Design:* The Rogerian researcher is aware of dynamic unpredictability and continuous change, and is open to the idea that patterns in the inquiry process may change in the course of the study that may not have been envisioned in advance. Rather than adhere to preordained rigid patterns of inquiry, the research design may change and evolve during the inquiry. It is essential that the researcher document and report any design changes.

12. *Pattern Synthesis:* Rogerian science emphasizes synthesis rather than analysis. Analysis is the separation of the whole into its constituent parts. The separation of parts is not consistent with Rogers' notion of integrality and irreducible wholes. Patterns are manifestations of the whole emerging from the human/environmental mutual field process. Synthesis allows for creating and viewing a coherent whole. Therefore, data are not "analyzed" within Rogerian inquiry, but "synthesized." Data processing techniques that put emphasis on information or pattern synthesis are preferred over techniques that place emphasis on data "analysis."

13. *Shared Description and Shared Understanding:* Mutual process is enhanced by including participants in the process of inquiry where possible. For example, sharing of results with participants in the study enhances shared awareness, understanding, and knowing participation in change. Furthermore, participants are the best judges of the authenticity and validity of their own experiences, perceptions, and expressions. Participatory action designs and focus groups conceptualized within Rogerian science may be ways to enhance mutual exploration, discovery, and knowing participation in change.

14. *Evolutionary Interpretation:* The researcher interprets all the findings within the perspective of the Science of Unitary Human Beings. Thus, the findings are understood and presented within the context of Rogers' postulates of energy fields, pandimensionality, openness, pattern, and the principles of integrality, resonancy, and helicy. Evolutionary interpretation provides *meaning* to the findings within a Rogerian science perspective. Interpreting the findings within a Rogerian perspective advances Rogerian science, practice, and research.

Potential Rogerian Research Designs

Cowling (1986) was among the first to suggest a number of research designs that may be appropriate for Rogerian research, including philosophical, historical, and phenomenological ones. There is strong support for the appropriateness of phenomenological methods in Rogerian science. For example, Rogers, quoted in Malinski (1986), stated: "[A]nother resource in terms of research we haven't used much yet [is] phenomenology. . . . Description and phenomenology both provide further ways of trying to look at things" (p. 14). According to Reeder (1986), phenomenological methods better reflect the Rogerian paradigm because they are not limited to sensory experience, but include multiple modes of awareness inherent in a pandimensional universe. Reeder (1986) provided a convincing argument demonstrating the congruence between Husserlian phenomenology and the Rogerian Science of Unitary Human Beings, stating:

> [G]iven the congruency between Husserlian phenomenology and the Rogerian conceptual system, a sound, convincing rationale is established for the use of this philosophy of science as an alternative for basic theoretical studies in Rogerian nursing science . . . Nursing research in general requires a broader range of human experience than sensory experience (whether intuitive or perceptive) in the development and testing of conceptual systems for gaining better access to multifaceted phenomena. . . . Husserlian phenomenology as a rigorous science provides just such an experience. (p. 62)

Phillips (1989b, p. 52) asserted that phenomenological research leads to knowledge about the whole by uncovering meaning of the human/environmental mutual field process. In phenomenological research, there is "no need to deal with such polarities as subjective-objective, since the living experience emerges from the interconnectedness of the two, where reality is experienced as a whole."

Experimental and quasi-experimental designs are problematic because of assumptions concerning causality; however, these designs may be appropriate for testing propositions concerning differences in the change process in relation to "introduced environmental change" (Cowling, 1986, p. 73). The researcher must be careful to interpret the findings in a way that is consistent with Rogers' notions of unpredictability, integrality, and nonlinearity. Emerging

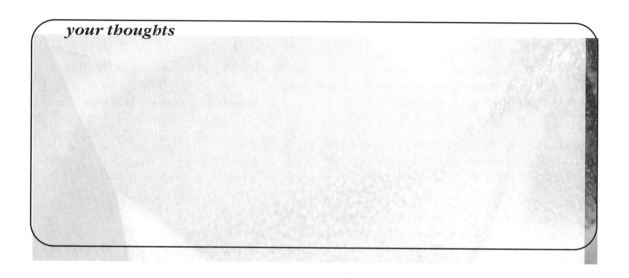

interpretive evaluation methods, such as Guba and Lincoln's (1989) Fourth Generation Evaluation, offer an alternative means for testing for differences in the change process within and/or between groups more consistent with the Science of Unitary Human Beings.

Cowling (1986) contended that in the early stages of theory development designs that generate descriptive and explanatory knowledge are relevant to the Science of Unitary Human Beings. For example, correlational designs may provide evidence of patterned changes among indices of the human field. Advanced and complex designs with multiple indicators of change that may be tested using "linear structural relations" (LISREL) statistical analysis may also be a means to uncover knowledge about the pattern of change rather than just knowledge of parts of a change process (Phillips, 1990). Barrett (1996) suggests that canonical correlation may be useful in examining relationships and patterns across domains and may also be useful for testing theories pertaining to the nature and direction of change. Another potentially promising area yet to be explored is participatory action and cooperative inquiry (Reason, 1994) because of their congruence with Rogers' notions of knowing participation in change, continuous mutual process, and integrality. Cowling (1998) proposed that a case-orientated approach is useful in Rogerian research, because case inquiry allows the researcher to attend to the whole and strives to comprehend his or her essence.

Selecting a Focus of Rogerian Inquiry

In selecting a focus of inquiry, concepts that are congruent with the Science of Unitary Human Beings are most relevant. The focus of inquiry flows from the postulates, principles, and concepts relevant to the conceptual system. Noninvasive voluntary patterning modalities such as guided imagery, therapeutic touch, humor, sound, dialogue, affirmations, music, massage, journaling, exercise, nutrition, reminiscence, aroma, light, color, artwork, meditation, storytelling, literature, poetry, movement, and dance provide a rich source for Rogerian science–based research. Creativity, mystical experiences, transcendence, sleeping-beyond-waking experiences, time experience, and paranormal experiences as they relate to human health and well-being are of interest in this science. New concepts that describe unitary phenomena may be developed through research. Dispiritedness (Butcher, 1996), human field image (Johnson, 1994), and power (Barrett, 1983) are just a few examples of concepts developed through research within Rogers' nursing science. Feelings and experiences are a manifestation of human/environmental field patterning and are a manifestation of the whole (Rogers, 1970); thus, feelings and experiences relevant to health and well-being are an unlimited source for potential Rogerian research. Discrete particularistic biophysical phenomena are usually not an appropriate focus for inquiry because Rogerian science focuses on irreducible wholes. Diseases or medical diagnoses are not the focus of Rogerian inquiry. Disease conditions are conceptualized as labels and as manifestations of patterning emerging

> **Measurement tools have been developed within Rogerian science and provide potential for future research.**

acausally from the human/environmental mutual process. However, the researcher needs to ensure that concepts and measurement tools used in the inquiry are defined and conceptualized within a unitary perspective. Several measurement tools have already been developed within Rogerian science, and they provide an abundant potential for future research within this conceptual system.

Measurement of Rogerian Concepts

The Human Field Motion Test (HFMT) is an indicator of the continuously moving position and flow of the human energy field. Two major concepts—"my motor is running" and "my field expansion"—are rated using a semantic differential technique (Ference, 1979). Examples of indicators of higher human field motion include feeling imaginative, visionary, transcendent, strong, sharp, bright, and active. Indicators of relative low human field motion include feeling dull, weak, dragging, dark, pragmatic, and passive. The tool has been widely used in numerous Rogerian studies.

The Power as Knowing Participation in Change Tool (PKPCT) has been used in over 26 major research studies (Caroselli & Barrett, 1998) and is a measure of one's capacity to participate knowingly in change as manifested by awareness, choices, freedom to act intentionally, and involvement in creating changes using semantic differential scales. Statistically significant correlations have been found between power as measured by the PKPCT and the following: human field motion, life satisfaction, spirituality, purpose in life, empathy, transformational leadership style, feminism, imagination, and socioeconomic status. Inverse relations with power have been found with anxiety, chronic pain, personal distress, and hopelessness (Caroselli & Barrett, 1998).

A number of new tools have been developed that are rich sources of measures of concepts congruent with unitary science. The Human Field Image Metaphor Scale (HFMIS) used 25 metaphors that capture feelings of potentiality and integrality rated on a Likert-type scale. For example, the metaphor "I feel at one with the universe" reflects a high degree of awareness of integrality; "I feel like a worn-out shoe" reflects a more restricted perception of one's potential (Johnston, 1994; Watson et al., 1997). Future research may focus on developing an understanding of how human field image changes in a variety of health-related situations or how human field image changes in mutual process with selected patterning strategies.

Diversity is inherent in the evolution of the human/environmental mutual field process. The evolution of the human energy field is characterized by the creation of more diverse patterns reflecting the nature of change. The Diversity of Human Field Pattern Scale (DHFPS) measures the process of diversifying human field pattern and may also be a useful tool to test theoretical propositions derived from the postulates and principles of Rogerian science to examine the extent of selected patterning modalities designed to foster harmony and well-being (Hastings-Tolsma, 1992; Watson et al., 1997). Other measurement tools developed within and unitary science perspective that may be used in a wide variety of research studies and in combination with other Rogerian measurements include Assessment of Dream Experience, which measures the diversity of dream experience as a beyond-waking manifestation using a 20-item Likert scale (Watson, 1993; Watson et al., 1997); Temporal Experience Scale (TES), which measures the subjective experience of temporal awareness (Paletta, 1990); and Leddy's (1995) Person-Environment Participation Scale, which measures expansiveness and ease of participation in the continuous human/environmental mutual field process using semantic differential scales. Another noteworthy tool is the Mutual Exploration of the Healing Human Field–Environmental Field Relationship Creative Measurement Instrument developed by Carboni (1992). It is a creative qualitative measure designed to capture the changing configurations of energy field pattern of the healing human/ environmental field relationship. As a means to reach a better understanding of the healing human/environmental field relationship, the participant and the researcher explore together experiences and expressions related to changing configurations of healing. In part of the instrument, the meaning of such terms as flowing, energy, connectedness, oneness, process, whole, harmony, movement, constant change, no boundaries, and resonating is explored.

New tools to measure unitary constructs need to be developed. In addition, the tools described need further testing for validity and reliability in a variety of nursing situations and populations. Although the quantitative measures provide a rich source for future research, Rogerian researchers are encouraged to use methods developed specific to the Science of Unitary Human Beings. Three methods have been developed: Rogerian Process of Inquiry, the Unitary Field Pattern Portrait Research Method, and Unitary Case Inquiry. Each method was derived from Rogers' unitary ontology and participatory epistemology and is congruent with the criteria for Rogerian inquiry presented earlier in this chapter.

Rogerian Process of Inquiry

Carboni (1995b) developed the Rogerian Process of Inquiry from her characteristics of Rogerian inquiry. The purpose of the method is to investigate the dynamic enfolding-unfolding of the human field–environmental field energy patterns and the evolutionary change of configurations in field patterning of the nurse and participant. Rogerian Process of Inquiry transcends both matter-centered methodologies espoused by empiricists and thought-bound methodologies espoused by phenomenologists and critical theorists (Carboni, 1995b). Rather, this process of inquiry is evolution-centered and focuses on changing configurations of human and environmental field patterning.

The flow of the inquiry starts with a summation of the researcher's purpose, aims, and visionary insights. Visionary insights emerge from the study's purpose and researcher's understanding of Rogerian science. The researcher recognizes the integrality of the researcher-participant and natural setting. The inquiry takes place in a setting where nursing is practiced. The focus of inquiry is on pattern manifestations that are significant to the science of nursing and the emergence of evolutionary change. Dynamic purposive sampling is used to select participants. Participants in the study are viewed as integral to the research process and are included in open discussions and the sharing of ideas. Next, the researcher focuses on becoming familiar with the participants and the setting of the inquiry. Shared descriptions of energy field perspectives are identified through observations and discussions with participants and processed through mutual exploration and discovery. Enfoldment of evolutionary change provides a unitary means of accessing potentialities for change. The researcher uses the Mutual Exploration of the Healing Human Field–Environmental Field Relationship Creative Measurement Instrument (Carboni, 1992) as a way to identify, understand, and creatively measure human and environmental energy field patterns. Together, the researcher and the participants develop a shared understanding and awareness of the human/environmental field patterns manifested in diverse multiple configurations of patterning. Conversations can be taped, and video recordings and any documents and artifacts that may help illuminate configurations of patterning emerging from the human and environmental field mutual process related to the focus of the inquiry may be used. Also, field notes and a reflexive journal are used to record data. All the data are synthesized using inductive and deductive data synthesis. Through the mutual sharing and synthesis of data, unitary constructs are identified. The constructs are interpreted within the perspective of unitary science, and a new unitary theory may emerge from the synthesis of unitary constructs. Carboni (1995b) also developed special criteria of trustworthiness to ensure the scientific rigor of the findings conveyed in the form of a Pandimensional Unitary Process Report. The new unitary theory advances the evolution of Rogers' nursing science and may be used to guide unitary nursing practice. Carboni's research method affords a way of creatively measuring manifestations of field patterning emerging during coparticipation of the researcher and participant's process of change.

The Unitary Field Pattern Portrait Research Method

The Unitary Field Pattern Portrait (UFPP) research method (Butcher, 1994, 1996, 1998b) was developed at the same time Carboni was developing the Unitary Process of Inquiry and was derived directly from the criteria of Rogerian inquiry. The purpose of the UFPP research method is to create a unitary understanding of the dynamic kaleidoscopic and symphonic pattern manifestations emerging from the pandimensional human/environmental field mutual process as a means to enhance the understanding of a significant phenomenon associated with human betterment and well-being. There are eight processes in the method: initial engagement, a priori nursing science, immersion, manifestation knowing and appreciation, unitary field pattern *profile* construction, mutual field pattern *portrait* construction, unitary field pattern portrait construction, and *theoretical* unitary field pattern portrait construction. Each process is briefly described (see Figure 1).

1. Initial engagement is a *passionate* search for a research question of central interest to understanding unitary phenomena associated with human betterment and well-being.
2. *A priori* nursing science identifies the Science of Unitary Human Beings as the researcher's perspective. As in all research, the perspective of the researcher guides all processes of the research method, including the interpretation of findings.
3. Immersion involves becoming steeped in the research topic. The researcher may immerse himself or herself in poetry, art, literature, music, dialogue with self and other, research literature, or any activity that enhances the integrality of the researcher and the research topic.
4. Pattern manifestation knowing and appreciation, formally referred to as "pattern appraisal," includes

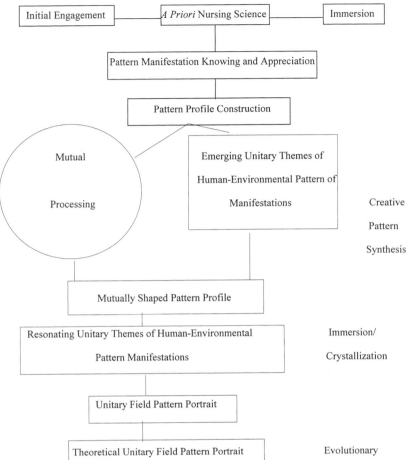

Initial Engagement — *A Priori* Nursing Science — Immersion

Pattern Manifestation Knowing and Appreciation

Pattern Profile Construction

Mutual

Processing

Emerging Unitary Themes of Human-Environmental Pattern of Manifestations

Creative
Pattern
Synthesis

Mutually Shaped Pattern Profile

Resonating Unitary Themes of Human-Environmental Pattern Manifestations

Immersion/
Crystallization

Unitary Field Pattern Portrait

Theoretical Unitary Field Pattern Portrait

Evolutionary
Interpretation

Figure 14–1 *The Unitary Field Pattern Portrait Research Method.*

participant selection, in-depth dialoguing, and recording pattern manifestations. Participant selection is made using intensive purposive sampling. Patterning manifestation knowing and appreciation occurs in a natural setting and involves using pandimensional modes of awareness during in-depth dialoguing. The activities described earlier in the pattern manifestation knowing and appreciation process in the practice method are used in this research method. However, in the UFPP research method the focus of pattern appreciation and knowing is on experiences, perceptions, and expressions associated with the phenomenon of concern. The researcher also maintains an informal conversational style while focusing on revealing the rhythm, flow, and configurations of the pattern manifestations emerging from the human/environmental mutual field process associated with the research topic. The dialogue is taped and transcribed. The researcher maintains observational, methodological, and theoretical field notes, and a reflexive journal. Any artifacts the participant wishes to share that illuminate the meaning of the phenomenon may also be included. Artifacts may include pictures, drawings, poetry, music, logs, diaries, letters, notes, and journals.

5. Pattern profile construction is the process of creating a pattern profile for each participant using creative pattern synthesis. All the information collected for each participant is synthesized into a narrative statement revealing the essence of the participant's description of the phenomenon of concern. The field pattern profile is in the language of the participant, and is then shared with the participant for verification and revision.

6. Mutual unitary field pattern profile construction is the process of mutually sharing an emerging

joint or shared profile with each successive participant at the end of each participant's pattern manifestation knowing and appreciation process. For example, at the end of the interview of the fourth participant, a joint construction of the phenomenon is shared with the participant for comment. The joint construction (mutual unitary field pattern profile) at this phase would consist of a synthesis of the profiles of the first three participants. After verification of the fourth participant's pattern profile, the profile is folded into the emerging mutual unitary field pattern profile. Pattern manifestation knowing and appreciation continues until there are no new pattern manifestations to add to the mutual unitary field pattern profile.

7. Unitary field pattern portrait construction is the process of identifying emerging unitary themes from each participant's field pattern profile, sorting the unitary themes into common categories, creating the resonating unitary themes of human/environmental pattern manifestations through immersion and crystallization, and synthesizing the resonating themes into a descriptive portrait of the phenomenon. The unitary field pattern portrait is expressed in the form of a vivid, rich, thick, and accurate aesthetic rendition of the universal patterns, qualities, features, and themes exemplifying the essence of the dynamic kaleidoscopic and symphonic nature of the phenomenon of concern.

8. Finally, the unitary field pattern portrait is interpreted from the perspective of the Science of Unitary Human Beings, creating a theoretical unitary field pattern portrait of the phenomenon. The purpose of theoretical unitary field pattern portrait construction is to explicate the theoretical structure of the phenomenon from the perspective of Rogers' nursing science. The theoretical unitary field pattern portrait is expressed in the language of Rogerian science, thereby lifting the unitary field pattern portrait from the level of description to the level of unitary science. Scientific rigor is maintained throughout processes by using the criteria of trustworthiness and authenticity. The findings of the study are conveyed in a Unitary Field Pattern Report.

Unitary Case Inquiry

Cowling's Unitary Case Inquiry is very similar to his pattern appreciation practice method (Cowling, 1993b, 1997, 1998): "The approach of pattern appreciation serves both science and practice simultaneously in a scientist/practitioner model" (Cowling, 1997, p. 136). Unitary Case Inquiry is a case-orientated approach guided by the assumptions of Rogerian science. Case-oriented approaches attend to the whole and strive for essence. Essence is pattern (Cowling, 1998). The case-oriented approach fits well with Rogerian science because features in cases can be treated as ensembles rather than as disaggregated variables. An example of a research question within Unitary Case Inquiry may be "What is the patter of a person experiencing pain?" The approach to Unitary Case Inquiry (Cowling, 1997, 1998) includes the following steps.

1. The researcher seeks engagement with a participant who is willing to mutually explore the essence of the phenomenon of interest. Researcher and participant are equal coparticipants in the process of inquiry.

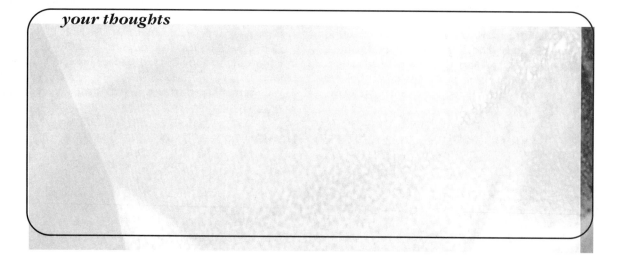

your thoughts

2. Specific intentions of the researcher are made explicit through a mutually derived and negotiated informed consent process.
3. The participant cocreates the form and structure for engagement. Interviewing, observing, and creative expressions or any combination of these may be means for mutually exploring and comprehending essence.
4. Journaling, audiotaping, photographs, drawing, music, and poetry may be used to document the participant's experience, perceptions, and expressions of the phenomenon of concern.
5. The researcher also maintains a journal that may include methodological notes, peer review notes, and general reflections.
6. A pattern appreciation profile is created through a process of synopsis. Features are synthesized into an ensemble that reflects the essence and wholeness of the phenomenon of concern.
7. The pattern appreciation profile of the participant is verified by the participant.
8. A conceptual/theoretical synthesis is developed based on the pattern information collected by interpreting the profile from the perspective of Rogers' postulates and principles.
9. A peer review system may be used to assist the researcher in ensuring logical consistency of the process.
10. To ensure scientific credibility, audit procedures are developed. Both the peer reviewer and the auditor should be an expert on Rogers' conceptual system and the method.

The methods and measurement tools derived from the postulates and principles of Rogerian science are means to answer vital questions related to the well-being and human betterment of unitary human beings. The challenge for students, researchers, and practitioners interested in Rogerian research is to use the methods that have been developed. Furthermore, new methods need to be created and tested. Research conducted consistent with the postulates and principles of Rogerian science advances the evolution of nursing knowledge central to the health and well-being of all.

Summary

Nursing's continued survival rests on its ability to make a *difference* in promoting the health and well-being of people. Making a difference refers to nursing's contribution to the client's desired health goals, and offering care is *distinguishable* from the services of other disciplines. If a discipline has nothing unique and valuable to offer, or offers the same services as another discipline, then that discipline's survival will be in jeopardy.

Every discipline's uniqueness evolves from its philosophical and theoretical perspective. All disciplines are identified and exist because of their uniqueness. The Science of Unitary Human Beings offers nursing a *distinguishable* and new way of conceptualizing health events concerning human well-being congruent with the most contemporary scientific theories. As with all major theories embedded in a new worldview, new terminology is needed to create clarity and precision of understanding and meaning. Rogers' nursing science leads to a new understanding of the experiences, perceptions, and expressions of health events and leads to innovative ways of practicing nursing. There is an ever-growing body of literature demonstrating the application of Rogerian science to practice and research. This chapter included a description of the Rogerian practice model and a set of criteria for Rogerian inquiry. In addition, five mid-level practice theories and three research methods derived from the postulates and principles of Rogerian science were presented. Rogers' nursing science is applicable in all nursing situations. Rather than focusing on disease and cellular biological processes, the Science of Unitary Human Beings focuses on human beings as irreducible wholes inseparable from their environment. People seeking health care want to be more involved in the decision-making process. Mutuality between the nurse and client is inherent to Rogerian practice. For 30 years, Rogers advocated that nurses should become the experts and providers of noninvasive modalities that promote health. Now, the growth of "alternative medicine" and noninvasive practices is outpacing the growth of traditional medicine. If nursing continues to be dominated by biomedical frameworks indistinguishable from medical care, nursing will lose an opportunity to become expert in holistic health-care modalities.

> In the new millennium, Rogerian science will have more relevance as outdated reductionistic models are replaced by those depicting the emerging worldview of wholeness.

In this new millennium, the Science of Unitary Human Beings will have more relevance as outdated reductionistic models are replaced by models depicting the emerging worldview of wholeness. The Science of Unitary Human Beings has even more relevance as nursing moves into more autonomous health-care settings such as communities, homes, and nurse-owned and nurse-run wellness centers. The space age future that Rogers envisioned has arrived. The international space station is under construction. Space-bound human civilizations will follow. Autonomous nurse health patterning centers will be established in space communities. In this new millennium, nurse entrepreneurial opportunities abound for nurses who dare to be creative. Nursing's future is replete with infinite possibilities.

References

American Heritage Dictionary. (1992). (3rd ed.). New York: Houghton Mifflin.

Anderson, M.D., & Hockman, E. M. (1997). Well-being and high-risk drug use among active drug users. In Madrid, M. (Ed.), *Patterns of Rogerian knowing* (pp. 152-166). New York: National League for Nursing.

Anderson, M. D., & Smereck, G. A. D. (1989). Personalized LIGHT model. *Nursing Science Quarterly, 2,* 120-130.

Anderson, M. D., & Smereck, G. A. D. (1992). The consciousness rainbow: An explication of Rogerian field pattern manifestation. *Nursing Science Quarterly, 5,* 72-79.

Anderson, M. D., & Smereck, G. A. D. (1994). Personalized nursing: A science-based model of the art of nursing. In Madrid, M. & Barrett, E. A. M. (Eds.), *Rogers' scientific art of nursing practice* (pp. 261-283). New York: National League for Nursing.

Barrett, E. A. M. (1983). *An empirical investigation of Martha E. Rogers' principle of helicy: The relationship of human field motion and power.* Unpublished dissertation, New York University, New York.

Barrett, E. A. M. (1988). Using Rogers' Science of Unitary Human Beings in nursing practice. *Nursing Science Quarterly, 1,* 50-51.

Barrett, E. A. M. (1989). A nursing theory of power for nursing practice: Derivation from Rogers' paradigm. In Riehl-Sisca, J. (Ed.), *Conceptual models for nursing practice* (3rd ed., pp. 207-217). Norwalk, CT: Appleton & Lange.

Barrett, E. A. M. (1990). Rogers' science-based nursing practice. In Barrett, E. A. M. (Ed.), *Visions of Rogers' science-based Nursing.* New York: National League for Nursing.

Barrett, E. A. M. (1996). Canonical correlation analysis and its use in Rogerian research. *Nursing Science Quarterly, 9,* 50-52.

Barrett, E. A. M. (1998). A Rogerian practice methodology for health patterning. *Nursing Science Quarterly, 11,* 136-138.

Barrett, E. A. M., & Caroselli, C. (1998). Methodological ponderings related to the Power as Knowing Participation in Change Tool. *Nursing Science Quarterly, 11,* 17-22.

Barrett, E. A. M., Cowling, W. R. I., Carboni, J. T., & Butcher, H. K. (1997). Unitary perspectives on

methodological practices. In Madrid, M. (Ed.), *Patterns of Rogerian knowing* (pp. 47-62). New York: National League for Nursing.

Bohm, D. (1980). *Wholeness and the implicate order.* London: Ark Paperbacks.

Briggs, J. P., & Peat, F. D. (1984). *Looking glass universe: The emerging science of wholeness.* New York: Simon & Schuster.

Briggs, J., & Peat, F. D. (1989). *Turbulent mirror: An illustrated guide to chaos theory and the science of wholeness.* New York: Harper & Row.

Bultemeier, K. (1997). Rogers' Science of Unitary Human Beings in nursing practice. In Alligood, M. R. & Marriner-Tomey, A. (Eds.), *Nursing theory: Utilization and application* (pp. 153-174). St. Louis: Mosby.

Butcher, H. K. (1993). Kaleidoscoping in life's turbulence: From Seurat's art to Rogers' nursing science. In Parker, M. E. (Ed.), *Patterns of nursing theories in practice* (pp. 183-198). New York: National League for Nursing.

Butcher, H. K. (1994). The unitary field pattern portrait method: Development of research method within Rogers' Science of Unitary Human Beings. In Madrid, M. & Barrett, E. A. M. (Eds.), *Rogers' scientific art of nursing practice* (pp. 397-425). New York: National League for Nursing.

Butcher, H. K. (1996). A unitary field pattern portrait of dispiritedness in later life. *Visions: The Journal of Rogerian Nursing Science, 4,* 41-58.

Butcher, H. K. (1997). Energy field disturbance. In McFarland, G. K. & McFarlane, E. A. (Eds.), *Nursing diagnosis and intervention* (3rd ed., pp. 22-33). St. Louis: Mosby.

Butcher, H. K. (1998a). Weaving a theoretical tapestry supporting pandimensionality: Deep connectedness in the multiverse. *Visions: The Journal of Rogerian Nursing Science, 6,* 51-55.

Butcher, H. K. (1998b). Crystallizing the processes of the unitary field pattern portrait research method. *Visions: The Journal of Rogerian Nursing Science, 6,* 13-26.

Butcher, H. K. (1999). Rogerian-ethics: An ethical inquiry into Rogers' life and science. *Nursing Science Quarterly, 12,* 111-117.

Capra, F. (1982). *The turning point: Science, society, and the rising culture.* New York: Bantam Books.

Carboni, J. T. (1992). Instrument development and the measurement of unitary constructs. *Nursing Science Quarterly, 5,* 134-142.

Carboni, J. T. (1995a). Enfolding health-as-wholeness-and-harmony: A theory of Rogerian nursing practice. *Nursing Science Quarterly, 8,* 71-78.

Carboni, J. T. (1995b). A Rogerian process of inquiry. *Nursing Science Quarterly, 8,* 22-37.

Caroselli, C., & Barrett, E. A. M. (1998). A review of the Power as Knowing Participation in Change literature. *Nursing Science Quarterly, 11,* 9-16.

Cowling, W. R. I. (1986). The Science of Unitary Human Beings: Theoretical issues, methodological challenges, and research realities. In Malinski, V. M. (Ed.), *Explorations on Martha Rogers' science of unitary human beings* (pp. 65-78). Norwalk, CT: Appleton-Century-Crofts.

Cowling, W. R. I. (1990). A template for unitary pattern-based nursing practice. In Barrett, E. A. M. (Ed.), *Visions of Rogers' science-based nursing* (pp. 45–65). New York: National League for Nursing.

Cowling, W. R. I. (1993a). Unitary knowing in nursing practice. *Nursing Science Quarterly, 6,* 201–207.

Cowling, W. R. I. (1993b). Unitary practice: Revisionary assumptions. In Parker, M. E. (Ed.), *Patterns of nursing theories in practice* (pp. 199–212). New York: National League for Nursing.

Cowling, W. R. I. (1997). Pattern appreciation: The unitary science/practice of reaching essence. In Madrid, M. (Ed.), *Patterns of Rogerian knowing* (pp. 129–142). New York: National League for Nursing.

Cowling, W. R. I. (1998). Unitary case inquiry. *Nursing Science Quarterly, 11,* 139–141.

Csikszentmihalyi, M. (1990). *Flow: The psychology of optimal experience.* New York: Harper & Row.

Dossey, B. (1997). *Core curriculum for holistic nursing.* Gaithersburg, MD: Aspen.

Dossey, B., Keegan, L., Guzzetta, C., & Kolkmeirer, L. (1995). *Holistic nursing: A handbook for practice.* Gaithersburg, MD: Aspen.

Dykeman, M. C., & Loukissa, D. (1993). The science of unitary human beings: An integrative review. *Nursing Science Quarterly, 6,* 179–188.

Fawcett, J. (1995). *Analysis and evaluation of conceptual models of nursing* (3rd ed.). Philadelphia: F. A. Davis.

Ference, H. (1979). *The relationship of time experience, creativity traits, differentiation, and human field motion.* Unpublished doctoral dissertation, New York University, New York.

Guba, E. G., & Lincoln, Y. S. (1989). *Fourth generation evaluation.* Newbury Park, CA: Sage.

Guzzetta, C. E. (Ed.). (1998). *Essential readings in holistic nursing.* Gaithersburg, MD: Aspen.

Hastings-Tolsma, M. T. (1992). *The relationship among diversity and human field pattern, risk taking, and time experience: An investigation of Rogers' principles of homeodynamics.* Unpublished doctoral dissertation, New York University, New York.

Johnston, L. W. (1994). Psychometric analysis of Johnson's Human Field Metaphor Scale. *Visions: The Journal of Rogerian Nursing Science, 2,* 7–11.

Leddy, S. K. (1995). Measuring mutual process: Development and psychometric testing of the person-environment participation scale. *Visions: The Journal of Rogerian Nursing Science, 3,* 20–31.

Lovelock, J. E. (1979). *Gaia: A new look at life on earth.* Oxford, England: Oxford University Press.

Madrid, M. (Ed.). (1997). *Patterns of Rogerian knowing.* New York: National League for Nursing.

Madrid, M., & Barrett, E. A. M. (Eds.). (1994). *Rogers' scientific art of nursing practice.* New York: National League for Nursing.

Madrid, M., & Winstead-Fry, P. (1986). Rogers' conceptual model. In Winstead-Fry, P. (Ed.), *Case studies in nursing theory* (pp. 73–102). New York: National League for Nursing.

Malinski, V. M. (1986). Further ideas from Martha Rogers. In Malinski, V. M. (Ed.), *Explorations on Martha Rogers' Science of Unitary Human Beings* (pp. 9–14). Norwalk, CT: Appleton-Century-Crofts.

Malinski, V. M. (1994). A family of strong-willed women. In Malinski, V. M. & Barrett, E. A. M. (Eds.), *Martha E. Rogers: Her life and her work* (pp. 3–9). Philadelphia: F. A. Davis.

Martin, M.-L., Forchuk, C., Santopinto, N., & Butcher, H. K. (1992). Alternative approaches to nursing practice: Application of Peplau, Rogers, and Parse. *Nursing Science Quarterly, 5,* 80–85.

McCloskey, J. C., & Bulechek, G. M. (Eds.). (1996). *Nursing interventions classification (NIC)* (2nd ed). St. Louis: Mosby.

Paletta, J. L. (1990). The relationship of temporal experience to human time. In Barrett, E. A. M. (Ed.), *Visions of Rogers' science-based nursing* (pp. 239–253). New York: National League for Nursing.

Peat, F. D. (1991). *The philosopher's stone: Chaos, synchronicity, and the hidden world of order.* New York: Bantam.

Phillips, J. (1988). The looking glass of nursing research. *Nursing Science Quarterly, 1,* 96.

Phillips, J. (1989a). Qualitative research: A process of discovery. *Nursing Science Quarterly, 2,* 5–6.

Phillips, J. (1989b). Science of unitary human beings: Changing research perspectives. *Nursing Science Quarterly, 2,* 57–60.

Phillips, J. R. (1990). Research and the riddle of change. *Nursing Science Quarterly, 3,* 55–56.

Rawnsley, M. M. (1994). Multiple field methods in unitary human field science. In Madrid, M. & Barrett, E. A. M. (Eds.), *Rogerian scientific art of nursing practice* (pp. 381–395). New York: National League for Nursing.

Reason, P. (1994). Three approaches to participative inquiry. In Denzin, N. K. & Lincoln, Y. S. (Eds.), *Handbook of qualitative research* (pp. 324–339). Thousand Oaks, CA: Sage.

Reeder, F. (1986). Basic theoretical research in the conceptual system of unitary human beings. In Malinski, V. M. (Ed.), *Explorations on Martha E. Rogers' Science of Unitary Human Beings* (pp. 45–64). Norwalk, CT: Appleton-Century-Crofts.

Rogers, M. E. (1970). *An introduction to the theoretical basis of nursing.* Philadelphia: F. A. Davis.

Rogers, M. E. (1980). Nursing: A science of unitary man. In Riehl, J. P. & Roy, C. (Eds.), *Conceptual models for nursing practice* (2nd ed., pp. 329–337). New York: Appleton-Century-Crofts.

Rogers, M. E. (1988). Nursing science and art: A prospective. *Nursing Science Quarterly, 1,* 99–102.

Rogers, M. E. (1992). Nursing and the space age. *Nursing Science Quarterly, 5,* 27–34.

Rogers, M. E. (1994). Nursing science evolves. In Madrid, M. & Barrett, E. A. M. (Eds.), *Rogers' scientific art of nursing practice* (pp. 3–9). New York: National League for Nursing.

Sheldrake, R. (1988). *The presence of the past: Morphic resonance and the habits of nature.* New York: Times Books.

Smith, M. J. (1988). Perspectives on nursing science. *Nursing Science Quarterly, 1,* 80–85.

Watson, J. (1993). *The relationships of sleep-wake rhythm, dream experience, human field motion, and time experience in older women.* Unpublished doctoral dissertation, New York University, New York.

Watson, J., Barrett, E. A. M., Hastings-Tolsma, M., Johnston, L., & Gueldner, S. (1997). Measurement in Rogerian Science: A review of selected instruments. In Madrid, M. (Ed.), *Patterns of Rogerian knowing* (pp. 87–99). New York: National League for Nursing.

Woodhouse, M. B. (1996). *Paradigm wars: Worldviews for a new age.* Berkeley, CA: Frog, Ltd.

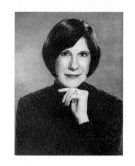

Chapter *15* Part 1

Rosemarie Rizzo Parse
The Human Becoming
School of Thought

Rosemarie Rizzo Parse

INTRODUCING THE THEORIST

Rosemarie Rizzo Parse is professor and Niehoff chair at Loyola University in Chicago. She is founder and editor of *Nursing Science Quarterly;* president of Discovery International, Inc., which sponsors international nursing theory conferences; and founder of the Institute of Human Becoming, where she teaches the ontological, epistemological, and methodological aspects of the human becoming school of thought. Her most recent work is *Hope: An International Human Becoming Perspective* (1999). Previous works include *Nursing Fundamentals* (1974); *Man-Living-Health: A Theory of Nursing* (1981); *Nursing Science: Major Paradigms, Theories, and Critiques* (1987); *Illuminations: The Human Becoming Theory in Practice and Research* (1995); and *The Human Becoming School of Thought* (1998). Her theory is a guide for practice in health-care settings in the United States, Canada, Finland, and Sweden; her research methodology is used as a method of inquiry by nurse scholars in Australia, Canada, Denmark, Finland, Greece, Italy, Japan, South Korea, Sweden, the United Kingdom, and the United States.

Dr. Parse is a graduate of Duquesne University in Pittsburgh and received her master's and doctorate from the University of Pittsburgh. She was on the faculty of the University of Pittsburgh, was dean of the Nursing School at Duquesne University, and from 1983 to 1993 was professor and coordinator of the Center for Nursing Research at Hunter College of the City University of New York. She has been a visiting professor at a number of universities in the United States and around the world. She has consulted with numerous doctoral programs in nursing and with health-care settings that are using her theory as a guide to practice and research.

THE HUMAN BECOMING SCHOOL OF THOUGHT

by Rosemarie Rizzo Parse

As the twenty-first century dawns, nurse leaders in research, administration, education, and practice are focusing attention on expanding the knowledge base of nursing through enhancement of the discipline's frameworks and theories. Nursing is a discipline and a profession. The goal of the *discipline* is to expand knowledge about human experiences through creative conceptualization and research. This knowledge is the scientific guide to living the art of nursing. The discipline-specific knowledge is given birth and fostered in academic settings where research and education move the knowledge to new realms of understanding. The goal of the *profession* is to provide service to humankind through living the art of the science. Members of the nursing profession are responsible for regulation of standards of practice and education based on disciplinary knowledge that reflects safe health service to society in all settings.

> Knowledge of the discipline is the scientific guide to living the art of nursing.

The Discipline of Nursing

The discipline of nursing encompasses at least two paradigmatic perspectives related to the human-universe-health process. One view is of the human as body-mind-spirit (totality paradigm) and the other is of the human as unitary (simultaneity paradigm) (Parse, 1987). The body-mind-spirit perspective is particulate—focusing on the bio-psycho-social-spiritual parts of the whole human as the human interacts with and adapts to the environment. Health is considered a state of biological, psychological, social, and spiritual well-being. This ontology leads to research and practice on phenomena related to preventing disease and maintaining and promoting health according to societal norms. In contrast, the unitary perspective is a view of the human as irreducible in mutual process with the universe. Health is considered a process of changing value priorities. It is not a static state but, rather, ever-changing as the human chooses ways of living. This ontology leads to research and practice on patterns (Rogers, 1992), lived experiences, and quality of life (Parse, 1981, 1992, 1997a, 1998a). Because the ontologies of these paradigmatic perspectives lead to different research and practice modalities, they lead to different professional services to humankind.

The Profession of Nursing

The profession of nursing consists of people educated according to nationally regulated, defined, and monitored standards. The standards and regulations are to preserve the safety of health care for members of society. The nursing regulations and standards are specified predominantly in medical scientific terms. This is according to tradition and largely related to nursing's early subservience to medicine. Recently the nurse leaders in health-care systems and in regulating organizations have been developing standards (Mitchell, 1998) and regulations (Damgaard & Bunkers, 1998) consistent with discipline-specific knowledge as articulated in the theories and frameworks of nursing. This is a very significant development that will fortify the identity of nursing as a discipline with its own body of knowledge—one that specifies the service that society can expect from members of the profession. With the rapidly changing health policies and the general dissatisfaction of consumers with health-care delivery, clearly stated expectations for services from each paradigm are a welcome change.

Just as in other disciplines, the nursing education and practice standards must be broad enough to encompass the possibility of practice within each paradigm. The totality paradigm frameworks and theories are more closely aligned with the medical model tradition. Nurses living the beliefs of this paradigm are concerned with participation of persons in health-care decisions but have specific regimes and goals to bring about change for the people they serve. Nurses living the beliefs of the simultaneity paradigm hold people's perspectives of their health situations and their desires to be primary. Nurses focus on knowing participation (Rogers, 1992) and bearing witness, as persons in their presence choose ways of changing health patterns (Parse, 1981, 1987, 1992, 1995, 1997a, 1998a).

Human Becoming, a school of thought named such because it encompasses an ontology, epistemology, and methodologies, emanates from the simultaneity paradigm (Parse, 1997c). It is this school of thought that is explained and discussed in this chapter.

A Metaperspective of Parse's Human Becoming School of Thought

Parse's (1981) original work was named *Man-Living-Health: A Theory of Nursing*. When the term "mankind" was replaced with "male gender" in the dictionary definition of "man," the name of the theory was changed to "human becoming" (Parse, 1992). No aspect of the principles changed. With the 1998 publication of *The Human Becoming School of Thought*, Parse expanded the original work to include descriptions of three research methodologies and a unique practice methodology, thus classifying the science of Human Becoming as a school of thought (Parse, 1997c). The original work (Parse, 1981) included the ontology and epistemology with general specifications for the research and practice methodologies. In the years following the 1981 publication, the research and practice methodologies

> Human becoming is a basic human science that has cocreated human experiences as its central focus.

were refined, tested, presented, and published in a variety of venues. As a school of thought, the philosophical ideas provide nurses and other health professionals with guides for their research and practice.

Human Becoming is a basic *human science* that has cocreated human experiences as its central focus. The ontology—that is, the assumptions and principles—sets forth beliefs that are clearly different from other nursing frameworks and theories. Discipline-specific knowledge is articulated in unique language specifying a position on the phenomenon of concern for each discipline. The Human Becoming language is unique to nursing. The three Human Becoming principles contain nine concepts written in verbal form with "ing" endings to make clear the importance of the ongoing process of change as basic to human-universe emergence. The fundamental idea that humans are unitary beings, as specified in the ontology, precludes any use of terms such as "physiological," "biological," "psychological," or "spiritual," because these terms describe the human in a particular way.

Philosophical Assumptions

The assumptions of the human becoming school of thought are written at the philosophical level of discourse (Parse, 1998a). There are nine fundamental assumptions: four about the human and five about becoming (Parse, 1998a). Also, three assumptions about human becoming were synthesized from these nine assumptions (Parse, 1998a). The assumptions arose from a synthesis of ideas from Rogers' Science of Unitary Human Beings (Rogers, 1992) and existential phenomenological thought (Parse, 1981, 1992, 1994a, 1995, 1997a, 1998a). In the assumptions, the author sets forth the view that unitary humans, in mutual process with the universe, are cocreating a unique becoming. The mutual process is the all-at-onceness of living freely chosen meanings arising with multidimensional experiences. The chosen meanings are the value priorities cocreated in transcending with the possibles in unitary emergence (see Parse 1998a, pp. 19–30).

Principles of Human Becoming

The principles and the assumptions of the human becoming school of thought make up the ontology. The principles are referred to as the theory. A *theory* is a set of congruent concepts written at the same level of discourse and connected in a unique way to describe the central phenomenon of a discipline. The principles of human becoming, which describe the central phenomenon of nursing (the human-universe-health process), arise from the three major themes of

the assumptions: *meaning*, *rhythmicity*, and *transcendence*. Each principle describes a theme with three concepts. Each of the concepts explicates fundamental paradoxes of human becoming (see Parse, 1998a, p. 58). The paradoxes are dimensions of the same rhythm lived all-at-once. Paradoxes are not opposites or problems to be solved but, rather, ways humans live their chosen meanings. This way of viewing paradox is unique to the human becoming school of thought (Mitchell, 1993; Parse, 1981, 1994b).

With the first principle (see Parse, 1981, 1998a), the author explicates the idea that humans construct personal realities with unique choosings from multidimensional realms of the universe. Reality, the meaning given to the situation, is the individual human's ever-changing seamless symphony of becoming (Parse, 1996). The seamless symphony is the unique story of the human as mystery emerging with the explicit-tacit knowings of *imaging*. The human lives priorities of *valuing* in confirming–not confirming cherished beliefs, while *languaging* with speaking–being silent and moving–being still.

The second principle (see Parse, 1981, 1998a) is a description of the rhythmical patterns of relating human with universe. The paradoxical rhythm is "*revealing–concealing* is disclosing–not disclosing all-at-once" (Parse, 1998a, p. 43). Not all is explicitly known or can be told in the unfolding mystery of human becoming. "*Enabling–limiting* is living the opportunities-restrictions present in all choosings all-at-once" (Parse, 1998a, p. 44). There are opportunities and restrictions no matter what the choice. "*Connecting–separating* is being with and apart from others, ideas, objects and situations all-at-once" (Parse, 1998a, p. 45). It is coming together and moving

apart, and there is closeness in the separation and distance in the closeness.

With the third principle (see Parse, 1981, 1998a), the author explicates the idea that humans are everchanging; that is, moving beyond with the possibilities, which are their intended hopes and dreams. A changing diversity unfolds as humans push and resist with *powering* in creating new ways of living the conformity-nonconformity and certainty–uncertainty of *originating*, while shedding light on the familiar-unfamiliar of *transforming*. "*Powering* is the pushing-resisting process of affirming–not affirming being in light of nonbeing" (Parse, 1998a, p. 47). The being-nonbeing rhythm is all-at-once living the everchanging now moment as it melts with the not-yet. Humans, in *originating*, seek to conform-not conform; that is, to be like others and unique all-at-once, while living the ambiguity of the certainty–uncertainty embedded in all change. The changing diversity arises with *transforming* the familiar–unfamiliar as others, ideas, objects, and situations are viewed in a different light.

The three principles are referred to as the human becoming theory. The concepts, with the paradoxes, describe the human-universe-health process. This ontological base gives rise to the epistemology and methodologies of human becoming. "Epistemology" refers to the focus of inquiry. Consistent with the human becoming school of thought, the focus of inquiry is on humanly lived experiences.

HUMAN BECOMING RESEARCH METHODOLOGIES

Sciencing Human Becoming is the process of coming to know; it is an ongoing inquiry to discover and understand the meaning of lived experiences. The Human Becoming research tradition has three methods; two are basic research methods and the other is an applied research method (Parse, 1998a, pp. 59–68). The methods flow from the ontology of the school of thought. The basic research methods are the Parse Method (Parse, 1987, 1990, 1992, 1995, 1997a, 1998a) and the Human Becoming Hermeneutic Method (Cody, 1995c; Parse, 1995, 1998a). The purpose of these two methods is to advance the science of Human Becoming by studying lived experiences from participants' descriptions (Parse Method) and written texts and art forms (Human Becoming Hermeneutic Method). The phenomena for study with the Parse Method are universal lived experiences such as joy–sorrow, hope, grieving, and courage, among others. Written texts from any literary source or any art form may be the subject of research with the Human Becoming Hermeneutic Method. The processes of both methods call for a unique dialogue, researcher with participant or researcher with text or art form. The researcher in the Parse Method is truly present as the participant moves through an unstructured discussion about the lived experience under study. The researcher in the Human Becoming Hermeneutic Method is truly present to the emerging possibilities in the horizon of meaning arising in dialogue with texts or art forms. True presence is an intense attentiveness to unfolding essences and emergent meanings. The researcher's intent with these research methods is to discover essences (Parse Method) and emergent meanings (Human Becoming Hermeneutic Method). The contributions of the findings from studies using these two methods is "new knowledge and understanding of humanly lived experiences" (Parse, 1998a, p. 62). Many studies have been conducted and some have been published in which nurse scholars used the Parse Method (for example, Allchin-Petardi, 1996; Baumann, 1996; Beauchamp, 1990; Blanchard, 1996; Bunkers, 1998; Cody, 1991, 1995a, 1995b; Daly, 1995; Gouty, 1996; Jonas-Simpson, 1998; Kelley, 1991; Kruse, 1996; Lui, 1993; Milton, 1998; Mitchell, 1990a, 1995b; Mitchell & Heidt, 1994; Northrup, 1995; Parse, 1990, 1994a, 1997b, 1999; Pilkington, 1993, 1997; Smith, 1990a, 1990b; Thornburg, 1993; Wang, 1997, among others). Only one study has been published in which the author

used the Human Becoming Hermeneutic Method (Cody, 1995c).

The applied research method is the descriptive qualitative preproject-process-postproject method. It is used when a researcher wishes to evaluate the changes, satisfactions, and effectiveness of health care when human becoming guides practice. A number of studies have been published in which the authors used this method (Jonas, 1995a; Mitchell, 1995; Northrup & Cody, 1998; Santopinto & Smith, 1995). Details of the processes of these three methods can be found in Parse's 1998 work, *The Human Becoming School of Thought*.

HUMAN BECOMING PRACTICE METHODOLOGY

The goal of the discipline from the human becoming perspective is quality of life. The goal of the nurse living the human becoming beliefs is true presence in bearing witness and being with others in their changing health patterns. True presence is lived through the human becoming dimensions and processes: illuminating meaning, synchronizing rhythms, and mobilizing transcendence (Parse, 1987, 1992, 1994a, 1995, 1997a, 1998a). The nurse with individuals or groups is truly present with the unfolding meanings as persons *explicate*, *dwell with*, and *move on* with changing patterns of diversity.

Living true presence is unique to the art of human becoming. It is sometimes misinterpreted as simply asking persons what they want and respecting their desires. This alone is not true presence. "True presence is an intentional reflective love, an interpersonal art grounded in a strong knowledge base" (Parse, 1998a, p. 71). The knowledge base underpinning true presence is specified in the assumptions and principles of human becoming (see Parse, 1981, 1992, 1995, 1997a, 1998a). True presence is a free-flowing attentiveness that arises from the belief that the human in mutual process with the universe is unitary, freely chooses in situation, structures personal meaning, lives paradoxical rhythms, and moves beyond with changing diversity (Parse, 1998a). Parse states: "To know, understand, and live the beliefs of human becoming requires concentrated study of the ontology, epistemology, and methodologies and a commitment to a different way of being with people. The different way that arises from the human becoming beliefs is true presence" (Parse, 1998b). Many papers are published explicating human becoming practice; for example, Arndt, 1995; Banonis, 1995; Butler, 1988; Butler & Snodgrass, 1991; Chapman, Mitchell, & Forchuk, 1994;

> The goal of the nurse living the human becoming beliefs is true presence in bearing witness and being with others in their changing health patterns.

Jonas, 1994, 1995b; Lee & Pilkington, in press; Liehr, 1989; Mattice, 1991; Mattice & Mitchell, 1990; Mitchell, 1988, 1990b; Mitchell & Copplestone, 1990; Mitchell & Pilkington, 1990; Quiquero, Knights, & Meo, 1991; Rasmusson, 1995; Rasmusson, Jonas, & Mitchell, 1991, among others.

True presence is a powerful human-universe connection experienced in all realms of the universe. It is lived in face-to-face discussions, silent immersions, and lingering presence (Parse, 1998a, pp. 71–80). Nurses may be with persons in discussions, imaginings, or remembrances through stories, films, drawings, photographs, movies, metaphors, poetry, rhythmical movements, and other expressions (Parse, 1998a, p. 72).

HUMAN BECOMING GLOBAL PRESENCE

The human becoming school of thought is a guide for research and practice in settings throughout the world. Scholars from four continents have embraced the belief system and live human becoming in research and practice.

In Toronto, Sunnybrook Health Science Centre's multidisciplinary standards of care arise from the beliefs and values of the human becoming school of thought. There are other health centers throughout the world that have these beliefs and values as guides to health care.

In South Dakota, a parish nursing model was built on the principles of human becoming to guide nursing practice at the First Presbyterian Church in Sioux Falls (Bunkers & Putnam, 1995; Bunkers, Michaels, & Ethridge, 1997). Also, the Board of Nursing of South Dakota has adopted a decisioning model based on the human becoming school of thought (Damgaard & Bunkers, 1998). Augustana College (in Sioux Falls) has human becoming as one central focus of the curricula for the baccalaureate and master's programs. It is the basis of Augustana's Health Action Model for Partnership in Community (Bunkers, Nelson, Leuning, Crane, & Josephson, 1999).

A research project on the lived experience of hope was conducted using the Parse method, with participants from Australia, Canada, Finland, Italy, Japan, Sweden, Taiwan, the United Kingdom, and the United States. The findings from these studies and the stories of the participants are published in the book *Hope: An International Human Becoming Perspective* (Parse, 1999).

Approximately 300 participants subscribe to Parse-L, an E-mail listserv where Parse scholars share ideas. There is a Parse homepage on the World Wide Web that is updated regularly.

Each year most of the 100 or more members of the International Consortium of Parse Scholars meet in Niagara-on-the-Lake, Canada, for a weekend immersion in human becoming research and practice. Members of the consortium have prepared a set of teaching modules (Pilkington & Jonas-Simpson, 1996) and a video recording (International Consortium of Parse Scholars, 1996) of Parse nurses in true presence with persons in different settings. Parse scholars present lectures and symposia regularly at international forums.

The Institute of Human Becoming, founded in 1992, was created to offer interested nurses and others the opportunity to study with the author the on-

your thoughts

> True presence is intentional reflective love, an interpersonal art grounded in a strong knowledge base.

tological, epistemological, and methodological aspects of the human becoming school of thought. Toward that goal, the institute offers regular sessions devoted to the study of the ontology and the research and practice methodologies. All of the sessions have as their goal the understanding of the meaning of the human-universe-health process from a human becoming perspective.

Summary

Through the efforts of Parse scholars the human becoming school of thought will continue to emerge as a force in the twenty-first century evolution of nursing science. Knowledge gained from the basic research studies will be synthesized to explicate further the meaning of lived experiences. The findings from applied research projects related to evaluation of human becoming practice will be synthesized and conclusions drawn. These syntheses will guide decisions in creating the continuing vision for sciencing and living the art of the human becoming school of thought.

References

Allchin-Petardi, L. (1996). *Weathering the storm: Persevering through a difficult time.* Unpublished doctoral dissertation, Loyola University, Chicago.

Arndt, M. J. (1995). Parse's Theory of Human Becoming in practice with hospitalized adolescents. *Nursing Science Quarterly, 8,* 86-90.

Banonis, B. C. (1995). Metaphors in the practice of the human becoming theory. In Parse, R. R. (Ed.), *Illuminations: The human becoming theory in practice and research* (pp. 87-95). New York: National League for Nursing Press.

Baumann, S. L. (1996). Feeling uncomfortable: Children in families with no place of their own. *Nursing Science Quarterly, 9,* 152-159.

Beauchamp, C. (1990). *The lived experience of struggling with making a decision in a critical life situation.* Unpublished doctoral dissertation, University of Miami, FL.

Blanchard, D. (1996). *The lived experience of intimacy: A study using Parse's theory and research methodology.* Unpublished doctoral dissertation, Wayne State University, Detroit, MI.

Bunkers, S. S. (1998). Considering tomorrow: Parse's theory-guided research. *Nursing Science Quarterly, 11,* 56-63.

Bunkers, S. S., Michaels, C., & Ethridge, P. (1997). Advanced practice nursing in community: Nursing's opportunity. *Advanced Practice Nursing Quarterly, 2*(4), 79-84.

Bunkers, S. S., Nelson, M. L., Leuning, C. J., Crane, J. K., & Josephson, D. K. (1999). The Health Action Model: Academia's partnership with the community.

In Cohen, E. L. & DeBack, V. (Eds.), *The outcomes mandate: Case management in health care today* (pp. 92-100). St. Louis: Mosby.

Butler, M. J. (1988). Family transformation: Parse's theory in practice. *Nursing Science Quarterly, 1,* 68-74.

Butler, M. J., & Snodgrass, F. G. (1991). Beyond abuse: Parse's theory in practice. *Nursing Science Quarterly, 4,* 76-82.

Chapman, J. S., Mitchell, G. J., & Forchuk, C. (1994). A glimpse of nursing theory-based practice in Canada. *Nursing Science Quarterly, 7,* 104-112.

Cody, W. K. (1991). Grieving a personal loss. *Nursing Science Quarterly, 4,* 61-68.

Cody, W. K. (1995a). The lived experience of grieving, for families living with AIDS. In Parse, R. R. (Ed.), *Illuminations: The human becoming theory in practice and research* (pp. 197-242). New York: National League for Nursing Press.

Cody, W. K. (1995b). The meaning of grieving for families living with AIDS. *Nursing Science Quarterly, 8,* 104-114.

Cody, W. K. (1995c). Of life immense in passion, pulse, and power: Dialoguing with Whitman and Parse, A hermeneutic study. In Parse, R. R. (Ed.), *Illuminations: The human becoming theory in practice and research* (pp. 269-307). New York: National League for Nursing Press.

Daly, J. (1995). The lived experience of suffering. In Parse, R. R. (Ed.), *Illuminations: The human becoming theory in practice and research* (pp. 243-268). New York: National League for Nursing Press.

Damgaard, G., & Bunkers, S. S. (1998). Nursing science-guided practice and education: A state board of nursing perspective. *Nursing Science Quarterly, 11,* 142-144.

Gouty, C. A. (1996). *Feeling alone while with others.* Unpublished doctoral dissertation, Loyola University, Chicago.

International Consortium of Parse Scholars. (1996). *The human becoming theory: Living true presence in nursing practice.* Available from ICPS, c/o Pat Lyon, The Rehabilitation Institute of Toronto, 550 University Avenue, Toronto, Ontario, Canada M5G 2A2.

Jonas, C. M. (1994). True presence through music. *Nursing Science Quarterly, 7,* 102-103.

Jonas, C. M. (1995a). Evaluation of the human becoming theory in family practice. In Parse, R. R. (Ed.), *Illuminations: The human becoming theory in practice and research* (pp. 347-366). New York: National League for Nursing Press.

Jonas, C. M. (1995b). True presence through music for persons living their dying. In Parse, R. R. (Ed.), *Illuminations: The human becoming theory in practice and research* (pp. 97-104). New York: National League for Nursing Press.

Jonas-Simpson, C. (1998). *Feeling understood: A melody of human becoming.* Unpublished doctoral dissertation, Loyola University, Chicago.

Kelley, L. S. (1991). Struggling to go along when you do not believe. *Nursing Science Quarterly, 4,* 123-129.

Kruse, B. (1996). *The lived experience of serenity: Using Parse's research method.* Unpublished doctoral dissertation, University of South Carolina at Columbia.

Lee, O. J., & Pilkington, F. B. (2000). Practice with persons living their dying: A human becoming perspective. *Nursing Science Quarterly.*

Liehr, P. R. (1989). The core of true presence: A loving center. *Nursing Science Quarterly, 2,* 7-8.

Lui, S. L. (1993). *The meaning of health in hospitalized older women in Taiwan.* Unpublished doctoral dissertation, University of Colorado Health Sciences Center, Denver.

Mattice, M., & Mitchell, G. J. (1990). Caring for confused elders. *The Canadian Nurse, 86*(11), 16-18.

Milton, C. (1998). *Making a promise.* Unpublished doctoral dissertation, Loyola University, Chicago.

Mitchell, G. J. (1988). Man-Living-Health: The theory in practice. *Nursing Science Quarterly, 1,* 120-127.

Mitchell, G. J. (1990a). The lived experience of taking life day-by-day in later life: Research guided by Parse's emergent method. *Nursing Science Quarterly, 3,* 29-36.

Mitchell, G. J. (1990b). Struggling in change: From the traditional approach to Parse's theory-based practice. *Nursing Science Quarterly, 3,* 170-176.

Mitchell, G. J. (1993). Living paradox in Parse's theory. *Nursing Science Quarterly, 6, 44-51.*

Mitchell, G. J. (1995). The lived experience of restriction-freedom in later life. In Parse, R. R. (Ed.), *Illuminations: The human becoming theory in practice and research* (pp. 159-195). New York: National League for Nursing Press.

Mitchell, G. J. (1998). Standards of nursing and the winds of change. *Nursing Science Quarterly, 11,* 97-98.

Mitchell, G. J., & Copplestone, C. (1990). Applying Parse's theory to perioperative nursing: A nontraditional approach. *AORN Journal, 51*(3), 787-798.

Mitchell, G. J., & Heidt, P. (1994). The lived experience of wanting to help another: Research with Parse's method. *Nursing Science Quarterly, 7,* 119-127.

Mitchell, G. J., & Pilkington, B. (1990). Theoretical approaches in nursing practice: A comparison of Roy and Parse. *Nursing Science Quarterly, 3,* 81-87.

Northrup, D. (1995). Exploring the experience of time passing for persons with HIV disease: Parse's theory-guided research. Doctoral dissertation, The University of Austin, 1995. University Microfilms International, 9534912.

Northrup, D., & Cody, W. K. (1998). Evaluation of the human becoming theory in practice in an acute care psychiatric setting. *Nursing Science Quarterly, 11,* 23-30.

Parse, R. R. (1981). *Man-Living-Health: A theory of nursing.* New York: Wiley.

Parse, R. R. (1987). *Nursing science: Major paradigms, theories, and critiques.* Philadelphia: Saunders.

Parse, R. R. (1990). Parse's research methodology with an illustration of the lived experience of hope. *Nursing Science Quarterly, 3,* 9-17.

Parse, R. R. (1992). Human becoming: Parse's theory of nursing. *Nursing Science Quarterly, 5,* 35-42.

Parse, R. R. (1994a). Laughing and health: A study using Parse's research method. *Nursing Science Quarterly, 7,* 55-64.

Parse, R. R. (1994b). Quality of life: Sciencing and living the art of human becoming. *Nursing Science Quarterly, 7,* 16-21.

Parse, R. R. (Ed.). (1995). *Illuminations: The human becoming theory in practice and research.* New York: National League for Nursing Press.

Parse, R. R. (1996). Reality: A seamless symphony of becoming. *Nursing Science Quarterly, 9,* 181-183.

Parse, R. R. (1997a). The human becoming theory: The was, is, and will be. *Nursing Science Quarterly, 10,* 32-38.

Parse, R. R. (1997b). Joy-sorrow: A study using the Parse research method. *Nursing Science Quarterly, 10,* 80-87.

Parse, R. R. (1997c). The language of nursing knowledge: Saying what we mean. In Fawcett, J. & King, I. M. (Eds.), *The language of theory and metatheory* (pp. 73-77). Sigma Theta Tau monograph.

Parse, R. R. (1998a). *The human becoming school of thought.* Thousand Oaks, CA: Sage.

Parse, R. R. (Summer, 1998b). On true presence. *Illuminations, 7*(3), 1.

Parse, R. R. (1999). *Hope: An international human becoming perspective.* Sudbury, MA: Jones & Bartlett.

Pilkington, F. B. (1993). The lived experience of grieving the loss of an important other. *Nursing Science Quarterly, 6,* 130-139.

Pilkington, F. B. (1997). *Persisting while wanting to change: Research guided by Parse's theory.* Unpublished doctoral dissertation, Loyola University, Chicago.

Pilkington, F. B., & Jonas-Simpson, C. (1996). *The human becoming theory: A manual for the teaching-learning process.* The International Consortium of Parse Scholars.

Quiquero, A., Knights, D., & Meo, C. O. (1991). Theory as a guide to practice: Staff nurses choose Parse's theory. *Canadian Journal of Nursing Administration, 4*(1), 14-16.

Rasmusson, D. L. (1995). True presence with homeless persons. In Parse, R. R. (Ed.), *Illuminations: The human becoming theory in practice and research* (pp. 105-113). New York: National League for Nursing Press.

Rasmusson, D. L., Jonas, C. M., & Mitchell, G. J. (1991). The eye of the beholder: Parse's theory with homeless individuals. *Clinical Nurse Specialist, 5*(3), 139-143.

Rogers, M. E. (1992). Nursing science and the space age. *Nursing Science Quarterly, 5, 27-34.*

Santopinto, M. D. A., & Smith, M. C. (1995). Evaluation of the human becoming theory in practice with adults and children. In Parse, R. R. (Ed.), *Illuminations: The human becoming theory in practice and research* (pp. 309-346). New York: National League for Nursing Press.

Smith, M. C. (1990a). *The lived experience of hope in families of critically ill persons.* Paper presented at UCLA National Nursing Theory Conference, Los Angeles, CA.

Smith, M. C. (1990b). Struggling through a difficult time for unemployed persons. *Nursing Science Quarterly, 3,* 18-28.

Thornburg, P. D. (1993). *The meaning of hope in parents whose infants died from Sudden Infant Death Syndrome.* Doctoral dissertation, University of Cincinnati, OH. University Microfilms International No. 9329939.

Wang, C. E. H. (1997). *Mending a torn fishnet: Parse's theory-guided research on the lived experience of hope.* Unpublished doctoral dissertation, Loyola University, Chicago.

Bibliography

Banonis, B. C. (1989). The lived experience of recovering from addiction: A phenomenological study. *Nursing Science Quarterly, 2,* 37-43.

Baumann, S. (1994). No place of their own: An exploratory study. *Nursing Science Quarterly, 7,* 162-169.

Baumann, S. (1995). Two views of children's art: Psychoanalysis and Parse's human becoming theory. *Nursing Science Quarterly, 8,* 65-70.

Baumann, S. (1996). Parse's research methodology and the nurse-researcher-child process. *Nursing Science Quarterly, 2,* 27-32.

Baumann, S. (1997). Contrasting two approaches in a community-based nursing practice with older adults: The medical model and Parse's nursing theory. *Nursing Science Quarterly, 10,* 124-130.

Bernardo, A. (1998). Technology and true presence in nursing. *Holistic Nursing Practice, 12*(4), 40-49.

Bournes, D. A., & Das Gupta, D. (1997). Professional practice leader: A transformational role that addresses human diversity. *Nursing Administration Quarterly, 21*(4), 61-68.

Bunkers, S. S. (1998). A nursing theory-guided model of health ministry: Human becoming in parish nursing. *Nursing Science Quarterly, 11,* 7-8.

Bunkers, S. S. (1999). Emerging discoveries and possibilities in nursing. *Nursing Science Quarterly, 12,* 26-29.

Bunkers, S. S., & Putnam, V. (1995). A nursing theory based model of health ministry: Living Parse's theory of human becoming in the parish community. In *Ninth Annual Westberg Parish Nurse Symposium: Parish nursing: Ministering through the arts.* Northbrook, IL: International Parish Nursing Resource Center—Advocate Health Care.

Cody, W. K. (1991). Multidimensionality: Its meaning and significance. *Nursing Science Quarterly, 4,* 140-141.

Cody, W. K. (1995). True presence with families living with HIV disease. In Parse, R. R. (Ed.), *Illuminations: The human becoming theory in practice and research* (pp. 115-133). New York: National League for Nursing Press.

Cody, W. K. (1995). The view of the family within the human becoming theory. In Parse, R. R. (Ed.), *Illuminations: The human becoming theory in practice and research* (pp. 9-26). New York: National League for Nursing Press.

Cody, W. K. (1996). Drowning in eclecticism. *Nursing Science Quarterly, 9,* 86-88.

Cody, W. K. (1996). Occult reductionism in the discourse of theory development. *Nursing Science Quarterly, 9,* 140-142.

Cody, W. K., Hudepohl, J. H., & Brinkman, K. S. (1995). True presence with a child and his family. In Parse, R. R. (Ed.), *Illuminations: The human becoming theory in practice and research* (pp. 135-146). New York National League for Nursing Press.

Cody, W. K., & Mitchell, G. J. (1992). Parse's theory as a model for practice: The cutting edge. *Advances in Nursing Science, 15*(2), 52-65.

Costello-Nickitas, D. M. (1994). Choosing life goals: A phenomenological study. *Nursing Science Quarterly, 7,* 87-92.

Daly, J. (1995). The view of suffering within the human becoming theory. In Parse, R. R. (Ed.), *Illuminations: The human becoming theory in practice and research* (pp. 45-59). New York: National League for Nursing Press.

Daly, J., Mitchell, G. J., & Jonas-Simpson, C. M. (1996). Quality of life and the human becoming theory: Exploring discipline-specific contributions. *Nursing Science Quarterly, 9,* 170-174.

Davis, C., & Cannava, E. (1995). The meaning of retirement for communally-living retired performing artists. *Nursing Science Quarterly, 8,* 8-16.

Fisher, M. A., & Mitchell, G. J. (1998). Patients' views of quality of life: Transforming the knowledge base of nursing. *Clinical Nurse Specialist, 12*(3), 99-105.

Futrell, M., Wondolowski, C., & Mitchell, G. J. (1994). Aging in the oldest old living in Scotland: A phenomenological study. *Nursing Science Quarterly, 6,* 189-194.

Heine, C. (1991). Development of gerontological nursing theory: Applying Man-Living-Health theory of nursing. *Nursing & Health Care, 12,* 184-188.

Jacono, B. J., & Jacono, J. J. (1996). The benefits of Newman and Parse in helping nurse teachers determine methods to enhance student creativity. *Nursing Education Today, 16,* 356-362.

Janes, N. M., & Wells, D. L. (1997). Elderly patients' experiences with nurses guided by Parse's Theory of Human Becoming. *Clinical Nursing Research, 6,* 205-224.

Jonas, C. M. (1992). The meaning of being an elder in Nepal. *Nursing Science Quarterly, 5,* 171-175.

Jonas, C. M. (1995). Evaluation of the human becoming theory in family practice. In Parse, R. R. (Ed.), *Illuminations: The human becoming theory in practice and research* (pp. 347-366). New York: National League for Nursing Press.

Jonas, C. M. (1995). True presence through music for persons living their dying. In Parse, R. R. (Ed.), *Illuminations: The human becoming theory in practice* (pp. 97-104). New York: National League for Nursing Press.

Jonas-Simpson, C. M. (1996). The patient focused care journey: Where patients and families guide the way. *Nursing Science Quarterly, 9,* 145-146.

Jonas-Simpson, C. (1997). Living the art of the human becoming theory. *Nursing Science Quarterly, 10,* 175-179.

Jonas-Simpson, C. M. (1997). The Parse research method through music. *Nursing Science Quarterly, 10,* 112-114.

Kelley, L. S. (1995). The house-garden-wilderness metaphor: Caring frameworks and the human becoming theory. In Parse, R. R. (Ed.), *Illuminations: The human becoming theory in practice and research* (pp. 61-76). New York: National League for Nursing Press.

Kelley, L. S. (1995). Parse's theory in practice with a group in the community. *Nursing Science Quarterly, 8,* 127-132.

Lui, S. L. (1994). The lived experience of health for hospitalized older women in Taiwan. *Journal of National Taipei College of Nursing, 1,* 1-84.

Mattice, M. (1991). Parse's theory of nursing in practice: A manager's perspective. *Canadian Journal of Nursing Administration, 4*(1), 11-13.

Mitchell, G. J. (1986). Utilizing Parse's theory of Man-Living-Health in Mrs. M's neighborhood. *Perspectives, 10* (4), 5-7.

Mitchell, G. J. (1990). Struggling in change: From the traditional approach to Parse's theory-based practice. *Nursing Science Quarterly, 3,* 170-176.

Mitchell, G. J. (1991). Diagnosis: Clarifying or obscuring the nature of nursing. *Nursing Science Quarterly, 4,* 52-53.

Mitchell, G. J. (1991). Distinguishing practice with Parse's theory. In Goertzen, I. E. (Ed.), *Differentiating nursing practice into the twenty-first century* (pp. 55-58). New York: ANA Publication.

Mitchell, G. J. (1991). Human subjectivity: The co-creation of self. *Nursing Science Quarterly, 4,* 144-145.

Mitchell, G. J. (1991). Nursing diagnosis: An ethical analysis. *IMAGE: Journal of Nursing Scholarship, 23*(2), 99-103.

Mitchell, G. J. (1992). Parse's theory and the multidisciplinary team: Clarifying scientific values. *Nursing Science Quarterly, 5,* 104-106.

Mitchell, G. J. (1993). Parse's theory in practice. In Parker, M. E. (Ed.), *Patterns of nursing theories in practice* (pp. 62-80). New York: National League for Nursing Press.

Mitchell, G. J. (1993). The same-thing-yet-different phenomenon: A way of coming to know—or not? *Nursing Science Quarterly, 6,* 61-62.

Mitchell, G. J. (1993). Time and a waning moon: Seniors describe the meaning to later life. *Canadian Journal of Nursing Research, 25*(1), 51-66.

Mitchell, G. J. (1994). The meaning of being a senior: A phenomenological study and interpretation with Parse's theory of nursing. *Nursing Science Quarterly, 7,* 70-79.

Mitchell, G. J. (1995). Evaluation of the human becoming theory in practice in an acute care setting. In Parse, R. R. (Ed.), *Illuminations: The human becoming theory in practice and research* (pp. 367-399). New York: National League for Nursing Press.

Mitchell, G. J. (1995). The lived experience of restriction-freedom in later life. In Parse, R. R. (Ed.), *Illuminations: The human becoming theory in practice and research* (pp. 159-195). New York: National League for Nursing Press.

Mitchell, G. J. (1995). The view of freedom within the human becoming theory. In Parse, R. R. (Ed.), *Illuminations: The human becoming theory in practice and research* (pp. 27-43). New York: National League for Nursing Press.

Mitchell, G. J. (1996). Clarifying contributions of qualitative research findings. *Nursing Science Quarterly, 9,* 143-144.

Mitchell, G. J. (1996). Pretending: A way to get through the day. *Nursing Science Quarterly, 9,* 92-93.

Mitchell, G. J. (1997). Retrospective and prospective of practice applications: Views in the fog. *Nursing Science Quarterly, 10,* 8-9.

Mitchell, G. J. (1998). Living with diabetes: How understanding expands theory for professional practice. *Canadian Journal of Diabetes Care, 22*(1), 30-37.

Mitchell, G. J., Bernardo, A., & Bournes, D. (1997). Nursing guided by Parse's theory: Patient views at Sunnybrook. *Nursing Science Quarterly, 10,* 55-56.

Mitchell, G. J., & Cody, W. K. (1992). Nursing knowledge and human science: Ontological and epistemological considerations. *Nursing Science Quarterly, 5,* 54-61.

Mitchell, G. J., & Copplestone, C. (1990). Applying Parse's theory to perioperative nursing: A nontraditional approach. *AORN Journal, 51*(3), 787-798.

Mitchell, G. J., & Santopinto, M. D. A. (1988). An alternative to nursing diagnosis. *The Canadian Nurse, 84*(10), 25-28.

Mitchell, G. J., & Santopinto, M. D. A. (1988). The expanded role nurse: A dissenting viewpoint. *Canadian Journal of Nursing Administration, 4*(1), 8-14.

Nokes, K. M., & Carver, K. (1991). The meaning of living with AIDS: A study using Parse's Theory of Man-Living-Health. *Nursing Science Quarterly, 4,* 175-179.

BOOKS

Parse, R. R. (1974). *Nursing fundamentals.* Flushing, NY: Medical Examination.

Parse, R. R. (1985). *Nursing research: Qualitative methods.* Bowie, MD: Brady.

Parse, R. R. (Ed.). (1995). *Illuminations: The human becoming theory in practice and research.* New York: National League for Nursing Press.

Parse, R. R. (1998). *The human becoming school of thought: A perspective for nurses and other health professionals.* Thousand Oaks, CA: Sage.

Parse, R. R. (1999). *Hope: An international human becoming perspective,* Sudbury, MA: Jones & Bartlett Publishers.

BOOK CHAPTERS, ARTICLES, AND EDITORIALS

Parse, R. R. (1978). Rights of medical patients. In Fischer, C. T. & Brodsky, S. L. (Eds.), *Client participation in human services.* New Brunswick, NJ: Transaction.

Parse, R. R. (1981). Caring from a human science perspective. In Leininger, M. M. (Ed.), *Caring: An essential human need.* Thorofare, NJ: Slack.

Parse, R. R. (1988). Beginnings. *Nursing Science Quarterly, 1.*

Parse, R. R. (1988). Creating traditions: The art of putting it together. *Nursing Science Quarterly, 1,* 45.

Parse, R. R. (1988). The mainstream of science: Framing the issue. *Nursing Science Quarterly, 1,* 93.

Parse, R. R. (1988). Scholarly dialogue: The fire of refinement. *Nursing Science Quarterly, 1,* 141.

Parse, R. R. (1989). Essentials for practicing the art of nursing. *Nursing Science Quarterly, 2,* 111.

Parse, R. R. (1989). Making more out of less. *Nursing Science Quarterly, 2,* 155.

Parse, R. R. (1989). Man-Living-Health: A theory of nursing. In J. Riehl-Sisca (Ed.), *Conceptual models for nursing practice* (3rd ed.). Norwalk, CT: Appleton & Lange.

Parse, R. R. (1989). Martha E. Rogers: A birthday celebration. *Nursing Science Quarterly, 2,* 55.

Parse, R. R. (1989). Parse's Man-Living-Health Model and administration of nursing service. In Henry, B., Arndt, C., DiVincenti, M., & Marriner-Tomey, A. (Eds.), *Dimensions of nursing administration: Theory, research, education, and practice.* Cambridge, MA: Blackwell Scientific.

Parse, R. R. (1989). The phenomenological research method: Its value for management science. In Henry, B., Arndt, C., DiVincenti, M., & Marriner-Tomey, A. (Eds.), *Dimensions of nursing administration: Theory, research, education, and practice.* Cambridge, MA: Blackwell Scientific.

Parse, R. R. (1989). Qualitative research: Publishing and funding. *Nursing Science Quarterly, 2,* 1.

Parse, R. R. (1990). Health: A personal commitment. *Nursing Science Quarterly, 3,* 136–140.

Parse, R. R. (1990). Nurse theorist conference comes to Japan. *Japanese Journal of Nursing Research, 23*(3), p. 99.

Parse, R. R. (1990). Nursing theory-based practice: A challenge for the 90s. *Nursing Science Quarterly, 3,* 53.

Parse, R. R. (1990). Promotion and prevention: Two distinct cosmologies. *Nursing Science Quarterly, 3,* 101.

Parse, R. R. (1990). A time for reflection and projection. *Nursing Science Quarterly, 3,* 143.

Parse, R. R. (1991). Electronic publishing: Beyond browsing. *Nursing Science Quarterly, 4,* 1.

Parse, R. R. (1991). Growing the discipline of nursing. *Nursing Science Quarterly, 4,* 139.

Parse, R. R. (1991). Mysteries of health and healing: Two perspectives. *Nursing Science Quarterly, 4,* 93.

Parse, R. R. (1991). Nursing knowledge for the 21st century. *Japanese Journal of Nursing Research 24,* (3), 198–202.

Parse, R. R. (1991). Parse's Theory of Human Becoming. In Goertzen, I. E. (Ed.), *Differentiating nursing practice: Into the twenty-first century* (pp. 51–53). Kansas City: American Academy of Nursing.

Parse, R. R. (1991). Phenomenology and nursing. *Japanese Journal of Nursing, 17*(2), 261–269.

Parse, R. R. (1991). The right soil, the right stuff. *Nursing Science Quarterly, 4,* 47.

Parse, R. R. (1992). Moving beyond the barrier reef. *Nursing Science Quarterly, 5,* 97.

Parse, R. R. (1992). Nursing knowledge for the 21st century: An international commitment. *Nursing Science Quarterly, 5,* 8–12.

Parse, R. R. (1992). The performing art of nursing. *Nursing Science Quarterly, 5,* 147.

Parse, R. R. (1992). The unsung shapers of nursing science. *Nursing Science Quarterly, 5,* 47.

Parse, R. R. (1993). Cartoons: Glimpsing paradoxical moments. *Nursing Science Quarterly, 6,* 1.

Parse, R. R. (1993). Critical appraisal: Risking to challenge. *Nursing Science Quarterly, 6,* 163.

Parse, R. R. (1993). Critique of critical phenomena of nursing science suggested by O'Brien, Reed, and Stevenson. *Proceedings of the 1993 Annual Forum on Doctoral Nursing Education: A Call for Substance: Preparing Leaders for Global Health* (pp. 71–81). St. Paul, MN: University of Minnesota School of Nursing.

Parse, R. R. (1993). The experience of laughter: A phenomenological study. *Nursing Science Quarterly, 6,* 39–43.

Parse, R. R. (1993). Nursing and medicine: Two different disciplines. *Nursing Science Quarterly, 6,* 109.

Parse, R. R. (1993). Parse's human becoming theory: Its research and practice implications. In Parker, M. E. (Ed.), *Patterns of nursing theories in practice* (pp. 49–61). New York: National League for Nursing Press.

Parse, R. R. (1993). Plant now; reap later. *Nursing Science Quarterly, 6,* 55.

Parse, R. R. (1993). Scholarly dialogue: Theory guides research and practice. *Nursing Science Quarterly, 6,* 12.

Parse, R. R. (1994). Charley Potatoes or mashed potatoes? *Nursing Science Quarterly, 7,* 97.

Parse, R. R. (1994). Martha E. Rogers: Her voice will not be silenced. *Nursing Science Quarterly, 7,* 47.

Parse, R. R. (1994). Scholarship: Three essential processes. *Nursing Science Quarterly, 7,* 143.

Parse, R. R. (1995). Again: What is nursing? *Nursing Science Quarterly, 8,* 143.

Parse, R. R. (1995). Building the realm of nursing knowledge. *Nursing Science Quarterly, 8,* 51.

Parse, R. R. (1995). Commentary: Parse's Theory of Human Becoming: An alternative to nursing practice for pediatric oncology nurses. *Journal of Pediatric Oncology Nursing, 12*(3), 128.

Parse, R. R. (1995). Foreword. In Frey, M. A., & Sieloff, C. L. (Eds.), *Advancing King's systems framework and theory of nursing.* Thousand Oaks, CA: Sage.

Parse, R. R. (1995). Man-Living-Health. A theory of nursing. In Mischo-Kelling, M., & Wittneben, K. (Eds.), *Auffassungen von pflege in theorie und praxis* (pp. 114–132). Munchen: Urban & Schwarzenberg.

Parse, R. R. (1995). Nursing theories and frameworks: The essence of advanced practice nursing. *Nursing Science Quarterly, 8,* 1.

Parse, R. R. (1996). Building knowledge through qualitative research: The road less traveled. *Nursing Science Quarterly, 9,* 10–16.

Parse, R. R. (1996). Critical thinking: What is it? *Nursing Science Quarterly, 9,* 138.

Parse, R. R. (1996). Hear ye, Hear ye: Novice and seasoned authors! *Nursing Science Quarterly, 9,* 1.

Parse, R. R. (1996). The human becoming theory: Challenges in practice and research. *Nursing Science Quarterly, 9,* 55–60.

Parse, R. R. (1996). Nursing theories: An original path. *Nursing Science Quarterly, 9,* 85.

Parse, R. R. (1996). Quality of life for persons living with Alzheimer's disease: A human becoming perspective. *Nursing Science Quarterly, 9,* 126–133.

Parse, R. R. (1996). [Review of the book *Martha E. Rogers: Her life and her work.*] *Visions: The Journal of Rogerian Science, 2,* 52–53.

Parse, R. R. (1997). Concept inventing: Unitary creations. *Nursing Science Quarterly, 10,* 63–64.

Parse, R. R. (1997). The human becoming theory and its research and practice methodologies. In Osterbrink, J. (Ed.), *Pflegetheorien—eine Zusammenfassung der 1st International Conference.* Freiburg, Germany: Verlag Hans Huber.

Parse, R. R. (1997). Investing the legacy: Martha E. Rogers' voice will not be silenced. *Visions: The Journal of Rogerian Science, 5,* 7-11.

Parse, R. R. (1997). The language of nursing knowledge: Saying what we mean. In Fawcett, J., & King, I. M. (Eds.), *The Language of theory and metatheory* (pp. 73-77). Sigma Theta Tau monograph.

Parse, R. R. (1997). Leadership: The essentials. *Nursing Science Quarterly, 10,* 109.

Parse, R. R. (1997). New beginnings in a quiet revolution. *Nursing Science Quarterly, 10,* 1.

Parse, R. R. (1997). [Review of the book *Quality of life in behavioral medicine.*] *Women and Health, 25*(3), 83-86.

Parse, R. R. (1997). Transforming research and practice with the human becoming theory. *Nursing Science Quarterly, 10,* 171-174.

Parse, R. R. (1998). The art of criticism. *Nursing Science Quarterly, 11,* 43.

Parse, R. R. (1998). Moving on. *Nursing Science Quarterly, 11,* 135.

Parse, R. R. (1998). Will nursing exist tomorrow? A reprise. *Nursing Science Quarterly, 11,* 1.

Parse, R. R. (1999). Expanding the vision: Tilling the field of nursing knowledge. *Nursing Science Quarterly, 12,* 3.

Pickrell, K. D., Lee, R. E., Schumacher, L. P., & Twigg, P. (1998). Rosemarie Rizzo Parse: Human becoming. In Tomey, A. M., & Alligood, M. R. (Eds.), *Nursing theorists and their work* (4th ed). New York: Mosby.

Pilkington, F. B. (1999). An ethical framework for nursing practice: Parse's human becoming theory. *Nursing Science Quarterly, 12,* 21-25.

Rendon, D. C., Sales, R., Leal, I., & Pique, J. (1995). The lived experience of aging in community-dwelling elders in Valencia, Spain: A phenomenological study. *Nursing Science Quarterly, 8,* 152-157.

Saltmarche, A., Kolodny, V., & Mitchell, G. J. (1998). An educational approach for patient-focused care: Shifting attitudes and practice. *Journal of Nursing Staff Development, 14*(2), 81-86.

Santopinto, M. D. A. (1989). The relentless drive to be ever thinner: A study using the phenomenological method. *Nursing Science Quarterly, 2,* 29-36.

Wondolowski, C., & Davis, D. K. (1988). The lived experience of aging in the oldest old: A phenomenological study. *American Journal of Psychoanalysis, 48,* 261-270.

Wondolowski, C., & Davis, D. K. (1991). The lived experience of health in the oldest old: A phenomenological study. *Nursing Science Quarterly, 4,* 113-118.

Chapter 15 Part 2

The Human Becoming Theory in Practice, Research, Administration, Regulation, and Education

William K. Cody
Sandra Schmidt Bunkers
Gail J. Mitchell

This section of the chapter describes the application of Parse's Theory of Human Becoming in practice, research, administration, education, and regulation. An overview of the application of the theory in each arena is given in each section, followed by more detailed and specific illustrations of actual situations.

FOSTERING THE HUMAN BECOMING PRACTICE METHOD: CREATING A SPACE FOR LIVING THE ART OF TRUE PRESENCE

Living the human becoming practice methodology offers nurses infinite opportunities for unique experiences lovingly coparticipating with people as they explore life options, steer-and-yield with the flow of life events, choose paths, and bear the consequences of choices. In choosing to practice from a human becoming perspective, a nurse commits to an explicit matrix of values and beliefs about humans, health, and nursing. What a nurse believes about humans, health, and nursing finds expression in every dimension of her or his way of being with others.

As Rosemarie Rizzo Parse has shown earlier in the chapter, the Theory of Human Becoming has given rise to a school of thought. The theory's assumptions and principles. comprise the ontology of the school of thought, which describes the person as freely choosing meaning in situation, continuously coexisting and interrelating multidimensionally with others in the universe, and transcending with the possibles in uniquely personal ways. Freely choosing meaning is cocreating reality through one's self-expression in living cherished values. In continuously interrelating with others, one cocreates the rhythmic paradoxes experienced in the bittersweet ups and downs of living. One continuously transcends with the possibles through shifting perspectives of unfolding events and committing to a chosen course of action while never fully knowing the outcome.

The human becoming practice methodology flows from these beliefs and delineates a way of authentically living these beliefs. The essence of the methodology is structured in the written dimensions and process first published by Parse in 1987 but augured by less formal guidance for practice offered in 1981. The dimensions and processes are stated in Table 15–1.

Since Parse's theory was published in 1981 (and before that time, among Parse's students and colleagues from Duquesne University, where she first developed the theory), an increasing number of nurses have cited Parse's theory as the single most

important influence on their practice. Nurses of many backgrounds and many different levels of preparation in varied settings have found Parse's perspective to be closest to their own beliefs about nursing and have therefore chosen to use the theory to guide their practice.

As Parse pointed out in the first section of this chapter, the theory serves as the guide to practice in many settings in several countries and has been described in many publications (Arndt, 1995; Banonis, 1995; Butler, 1988; Butler & Snodgrass, 1991; Chapman, Mitchell, & Forchuk, 1994; Cody, 1995a; Jonas, 1994, 1995; Lee & Pilkington, 2000; Liehr; 1989; Mattice, 1991; Mattice & Mitchell, 1990; Mitchell, 1988, 1990b; Mitchell & Copplestone, 1990; Mitchell & Pilkington, 1990; Northrup & Cody, 1998; Quiquero, Knights, & Meo, 1991; Rasmusson, 1995; Rasmusson, Jonas, & Mitchell, 1991). For example, at Sunnybrook Health Science Centre in Toronto, Canada, the nursing leadership developed standards of care based on the Human Becoming Theory to be applied throughout this 1100-bed health science center. On a much smaller scale, the Center for Human Becoming was established in 1997 in Charlotte, North Carolina, as a milieu for the nurse-person process within a 25-unit housing complex for people living with HIV. In other settings, where the human becoming theory is not the overall guide to nursing practice institutionally, individual nurses also live the values and beliefs of the theory.

Implementing the human becoming theory as the central guide to nursing practice is never easy for individuals or institutions. For individuals, adopting the Human Becoming Theory often means confronting doubts about one's profession, experiencing conflict and confusion in practice, and alienating coworkers committed to the old paradigm. Such individual nurses may gain knowledge and encouragement from available texts and other media (Fitne, 1997; International Consortium of Parse Scholars, 1996), from the regular conferences of the International Consortium of Parse Scholars and its regional chapters, and from the annual conferences led by Parse at Loyola University in Chicago. It is difficult, though not impossible, to implement the theory in practice without the support of others. Small enclaves of Parse nurses exist in a wide variety of workplaces in towns and cities around the globe.

In institutions, a dependable commitment of resources from top-level administration and the ready availability of well-prepared education and practice leaders are minimal essentials for implementing Parse's theory-guided practice. Guiding nursing practice in an institution by the Human Becoming Theory

| | | | **TABLE 15-1** | *Themes, Assumptions, Principles, and Practice Dimensions of Parse's Theory* |

Themes	Assumptions	Principles	Practice Dimensions	Comments
Meaning	Human becoming is freely choosing personal meaning in situations in the intersubjective process of relating value priorities.	Structuring meaning multidimension-ally is cocreating reality through the languaging of valuing and imaging.	Illuminating meaning is shedding light through uncovering the what was, is, and will be, as it is appearing now; it happens in explicating what is.	*People always participate in creating their realities through choosing how to understand and interpret experiences. Expressing oneself clarifies values and furthers under-standing of experiences.*
Rhythmicity	Human becoming is cocreating rhythmical patterns of relating in open interchange with the universe.	Cocreating rhyth-mical patterns of relating is living the paradoxical unity of revealing–concealing, enabling–limiting, while connecting–separating.	Synchronizing rhythms happens in dwelling with the pitch, yaw, and roll of the interhuman cadence.	*People live potentialities with actualities all-at-once; the apparent opposite of what is in the fore of experience is always also present with us. Exploring options in the attentive, loving presence of another is a way of connecting–separating with others in the universe.*
Transcendence	Human becoming is transcending multidimensionally with the unfolding possibles.	Cotranscending with the possibles is powering originating in the process of transforming.	Mobilizing transcen-dence happens in moving beyond the meaning moment to what is not yet.	*People live with change in chosen ways that evolve into patterns of living that also change over time. Coparticipating in change through one's choice affirms self and cocreates with the universe what will be. By exploring options in the presence of another, one moves beyond what is to what is not yet.*

requires a profound paradigm shift within the local nursing culture, far beyond what is often called a paradigm shift in the rhetoric of the health-care in-dustry. To adopt Parse's theory as the guide to prac-tice is to adopt fundamentally different definitions of such key notions as health, family, presence, op-tions, person, freedom, and reality. Parse's Theory of Human Becoming is not a model for nursing practice that can be imposed on unwilling workers. The Parse nurse lives the values and beliefs manifest and struc-tured linguistically in the theory. Clearly, this can only become an actuality through individual choice. However, as shown at Sunnybrook Health Science Centre, the Human Becoming school of thought can serve as the guide to generate standards of practice that reflect the values and beliefs of the theory, which thereby brings practice within an institution closer to that school of thought.

Fostering the art of true presence in nursing prac-tice—which is living the values and beliefs under-pinning Parse's practice methodology in the nurse-person process—requires the creation of a space where nurses' choices to move to a new paradigm of nursing practice are honored, a space where per-sons' individual meanings and choices are profoundly valued, and where resources are dedicated to co-creating quality of life from each person's own per-spective. In this section of the chapter, two detailed examples of practice guided by the Human Becom-ing Theory are presented, illustrating a parish nurs-ing model and a community action model.

Human Becoming as a Guide for Parish Nursing

A Human Becoming parish nursing practice model was developed at the First Presbyterian Church in Sioux Falls, South Dakota (Bunkers & Putnam, 1995). The central focus of this nursing theory–based health model is quality of life for the parish community (see

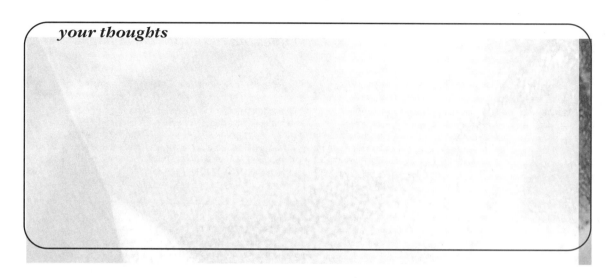
Fig. 15-1). The nurse-person-community health process emphasizes lived experiences of health of individual parishioners and of the entire parish community. The eight beatitudes, being fundamental to the belief system of the parish, are paralleled with concepts of the Human Becoming Theory to guide nursing practice in the parish. For example, true presence is paralleled with the beatitude, "Blessed are those who hunger and thirst for righteousness, for they shall be filled," which expresses the desire for a deep, loving relationship with people and with God (Ward, 1972). True presence, the cornerstone of human becoming nursing practice, is lived with the parish community in a loving, reflective way, bearing witness to others' living health and honoring each person's uniqueness without judging him or her. The nurse, in true presence, respects people as knowing their own way, a chosen personal way of being with the world. A further example of paralleling the beatitudes with the Human Becoming Theory is the beatitude, "Blessed are the pure in heart, for they shall see God," which describes a singleness of purpose for living an ethic of love and care for others (Ward, 1972). This ethic of love and care honors human freedom. The Parse nurse understands that humans are inherently free, and the nurse in parish nursing practice honors this freedom. "The nurse honors how others choose to create their world and seeks to know and understand the wholeness of their lived experiences of

> In practicing from a human becoming perspective, a nurse commits to an explicit matrix of values and beliefs about humans, health, and nursing.

faith and health" (Bunkers, 1998; Bunkers et al., 1999, p. 92).

Living Parse's Theory of Human Becoming in practicing nursing in the parish holds the possibility of transforming community nursing practice and transforming ways of living health in a parish. Bunkers and Putnam (1995) state, "The nurse, in practicing from the human becoming perspective and emphasizing the teachings of the Beatitudes, believes in the endless possibilities present for persons when there is openness, caring, and honoring of justice and human freedom" (p. 210).

Human Becoming as a Guide for Nursing Education-Practice

The Health Action Model for Partnership in Community is a nursing education-practice model originating in the Department of Nursing at Augustana College in Sioux Falls, South Dakota, which addresses "the connections and disconnections existing in human relationship" (Bunkers, Nelson, Leuning, Crane, & Josephson, 1998; Bunkers et al., 1999, p. 92) (see Fig. 15-2). This collaborative community nursing practice model focuses on lived experiences of connection-disconnection "for persons homeless and low income who are challenged with the lack of economic, social and interpersonal resources" (Bunkers et al. 1999, p. 92).

The Health Action Model, based on Parse's human becoming school of thought, focuses on the primacy of the nurse's presence with others. The focus of the nurse-person-community health process is quality of life from the person-community's perspective. Quality of life, the central concept of the model, is elaborated on in the conceptualizations of health as hu-

First Presbyterian Church
Sioux Falls, South Dakota

CONGREGATIONAL HEALTH MODEL
Christ-Centered
Covenant

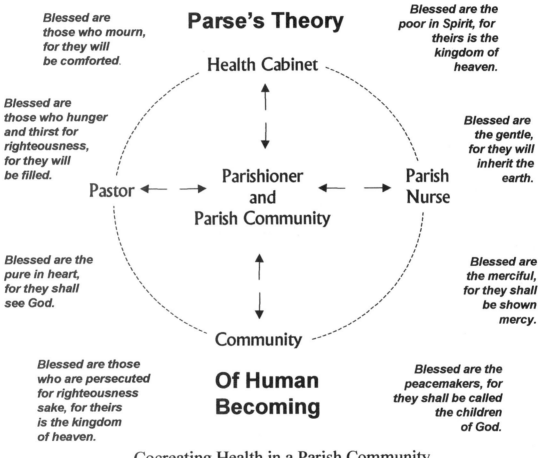

Cocreating Health in a Parish Community

- ❑ "Love one another as I have loved you." *John 13:34*
- ❑ "Health is a personal commitment to a lived value system; cocreating quality of life with the human-universe process." *R.R. Parse, 1992*
- ❑ "Go ye into the world…" *Matthew 25:31-46*
- ❑ "Quality of life is whatever the person living the life says it is." *R.R. Parse, 1994*

© Bunkers, S. & Putnam, V., 1995

Figure 15–1 *Congregational Health Model. Reprinted with permission from the First Presbyterian Church, Sioux Falls, South Dakota.*

The Health Action Model For Partnership In Community

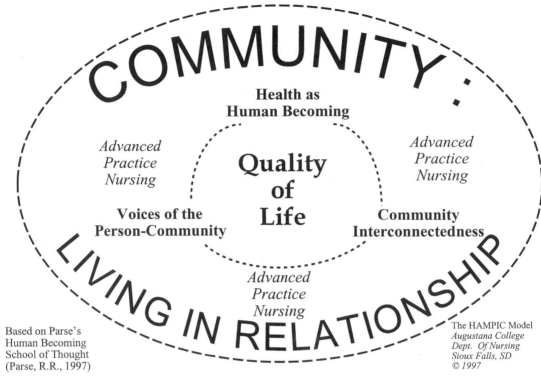

COMMUNITY:

Health as
Human Becoming

*Advanced
Practice
Nursing*

**Quality
of
Life**

*Advanced
Practice
Nursing*

**Voices of the
Person-Community**

**Community
Interconnectedness**

*Advanced
Practice
Nursing*

LIVING IN RELATIONSHIP

Based on Parse's
Human Becoming
School of Thought
(Parse, R.R., 1997)

The HAMPIC Model
*Augustana College
Dept. Of Nursing
Sioux Falls, SD
© 1997*

Figure 15–2   *The Health Action Model for Partnership in Community. Reprinted with permission from Augustana College, Department of Nursing, Sioux Falls, SD © 1997.*

man becoming, community interconnectedness, and voices of the person-community. "The purpose of the model is to respond in a new way to nursing's social mandate to care for the health of society by gaining an understanding of what is wanted from those living these health experiences" (Bunkers et. al, 1999, p. 94). Advanced practice nurses, a steering committee, and six "site communities" are moving together in seeking mutual understanding of human health issues while holding as important the unique perspectives presented by individuals and groups with complex health situations. The community of Sioux Falls, South Dakota, has embraced this theory-based nursing education-practice model by providing funding from community sources, including Augustana College, Sioux Valley Health System Community Fund, Sioux Falls Area

> The Health Action Model, based on Parse's Human Becoming school of thought, focuses on the primacy of the nurse's presence with others.

Foundation, Sioux Falls Public School System Head Start Program, and the Sioux Empire United Way.

In the Health Action Model, "advanced practice nurses work with persons and groups in the 'Site Communities' in creating a prototype of collaboration in addressing issues concerning quality of life" (Bunkers et al., 1999, p. 94). "Site communities" are agencies or places that seek to respond to the health and social-welfare issues of those struggling with lack of resources (see Fig. 15-3). Issues of quality of life are addressed with nurses asking persons, families, and communities what their hopes for the future are and working with them to create personal health descriptions and health action plans. Personal health descriptions are written in the words of the person, family, or community and include: (1) what life is like for me now; (2) my health concerns are—; (3) what's most important to me now; (4) my hopes for the future are—; (5) my plans for the future are—; (6) how I can carry out my plans; and (7) my specific health action plan is— (Bunkers et al., 1999). When a person or community identifies a health pattern they want to develop further or identifies a desire to

THE HEALTH ACTION MODEL
FOR PARTNERSHIP IN COMMUNITY
Connections in Community

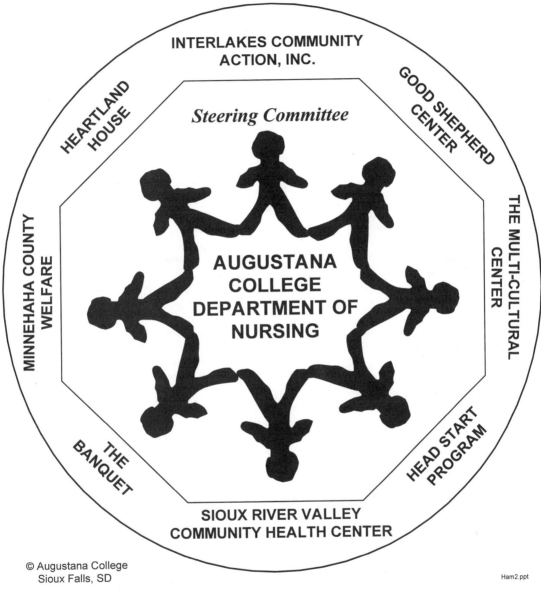

© Augustana College
Sioux Falls, SD

Ham2.ppt

Figure 15–3 *The Health Action Model for Partnership in Community: Connections in Community. Reprinted with permission from © Augustana College, Sioux Falls, SD.*

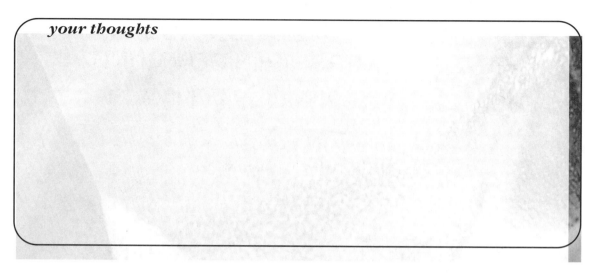

your thoughts

change certain health patterns, the nurse explores how she or he can support that process.

Objectives of the Health Action Model include: (1) creating a nursing practice model to guide provision of health services based on Parse's Human Becoming school of thought for families experiencing economic and social marginalization and/or homelessness; (2) using the Health Action Model to address health issues of "site communities"; (3) providing educational experiences for nursing and other health professional students focusing on diversity; and (4) extending the Health Action Model beyond the local area and sharing it as a prototype for health care regionally, nationally, and internationally (Bunkers et al., 1999).

A steering committee, composed of nursing leaders from health systems in the community, individuals from a variety of social-welfare agencies dedicated to serving society, and people who are experiencing economic marginalization and homelessness, meets quarterly to listen to the emerging health issues of the site communities. The steering committee seeks to create new linkages of care where none exist and to expand sources of funding for the model. These community leaders "have strong beliefs that community interconnectedness occurs when everyone involved has a voice" (Bunkers et al., 1999, p. 94).

Parse's human becoming school of thought serves as the linchpin in this model for developing new ways of connecting person to person, agency to agency, and community to community. Bunkers and colleagues (1999) state:

> The interconnectedness of community involves relationship that transcends *separating differences*. There [is] no lack of spoken and written words about persons experiencing the *separating differences* of living with little or no money and no place to call home. What is missing in community is an intentional listening to the sound of these voices speaking and writing about their own hopes and meanings. To embrace *separating differences* involves listening and understanding others. The nurse-person-community health process involves being truly present with others with a listening receptivity to differing values. Nurses practicing in this model understand that community as process entails moving together in seeking mutual understanding. . . . Moving together in seeking mutual understanding calls for a type of listening to one another where both nurse and person-community engage in contributing to expanding choices for living health. (pp. 94-95)

Parse (1996, p. 4) writes that community in its most abstract sense is "the universe, the galaxy of human connectedness." The Health Action Model for Partnership in Community seeks to cultivate this human connectedness for the betterment of humankind.

RESEARCH ON HUMAN BECOMING

The published research that has been generated, inspired, and guided by the human becoming theory has been of several types. Three research methods have been developed and endorsed by Parse—one by Parse alone, and two others with her collaboration and leadership. The Parse Research Method (Parse, 1987, 1990, 1995, 1999), a phenomenological method in the generic sense, is intended to guide basic research on humanly lived experiences. The Human Becoming Hermeneutic Method (Cody,

1995c) is intended to guide interpretive research on the meanings of texts. The preproject-process-postproject evaluation method is intended to guide applied research on the implementation of Parse's theory-based nursing practice in a given venue.

Parse's Phenomenological Method

The essentials of Parse's phenomenological research methodology were first published in the book *Nursing Science: Major Paradigms, Theories, and Critiques* (Parse, 1987), in Parse's individual chapter on her theory. At the time, no other theorist in nursing had ventured to delineate a particular method congruent with her theory. In 1990, Parse published a more detailed explication of the method, along with an illustration focusing on the lived experience of hope (Parse, 1990). A number of studies using the method have been published over the past 9 years (for examples, see Bunkers, Damgaard, Hohman, & Vander Woude, 1998; Cody, 1991; 1995b; Daly, 1995; Mitchell, 1990a; Parse, 1994, 1997; Pilkington, 1993; Smith, 1990). A previously unpublished example, drawn from a study of the lived experience of bearing witness to suffering, follows. This study focused on the lived experience of bearing witness to suffering, of families and caregivers of persons living with HIV.

Phenomena for study using Parse's research methodology are universal human health experiences—*health* is defined as quality of life from the person's perspective (Parse, 1998, p. 64). Bearing witness to suffering is posited as such an experience. Previous research on the grieving of families living with HIV (Cody, 1995b) suggested that bearing witness to suffering was a common yet profound and life-changing experience of family members and caregivers. Suffering has often been posited as a human universal (Daly, 1995). Bearing witness to suffering is lived in being fully present with others as they live the various dimensions of anguish inherent in humanly lived experience.

> Health is defined as quality of life from the person's perspective. Phenomena for study using Parse's research methodology are universal health experiences.

For this study, family members and occupational caregivers of persons living with AIDS were invited to describe their lived experiences of bearing witness to suffering. The participant group included 13 self-identified family members and 12 occupational caregivers (including nurses, aides, therapists, and others). There were 18 females and 7 males, 23 whites, one Hispanic, and one African-American. Participant ages ranged from 21 to 74. The study was approved by a university review board and all participants read and signed informed consent forms. Confidentiality was maintained throughout the study, and tapes were destroyed when the study was completed.

Data are recorded, in Parse's research methodology, through the process of dialogical engagement. Dialogical engagement is not an interview, but rather is living true presence with participants as they describe their lived experience. In this study, the researcher was personally present in each dialogue. Participants were encouraged to describe their experiences as thoroughly as possible, and the researcher refrained from content-specific prompts while simply encouraging each participant to describe her or his personal experience completely. Dialogues were recorded on audiotape, and on videotape when permitted. Four participants declined to be videotaped. Descriptions were transcribed verbatim.

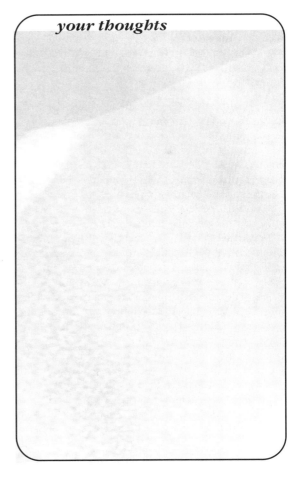

your thoughts

TABLE 15-2 *Extraction-Synthesis Process, Participant 2*

Participant 2

Caregiver: Home Health Aide

Essences in Participant's Language	Essences in Researcher's Language
1. Witnessing the most hideous illness she's ever seen and experiences that would crush her, the participant wants to take the pain away but knows she cannot. She realizes that life is fragile and appreciates the smaller things.	1. Attending to the wretchedness of another prompts a desire to rectify torment and a prizing of the ordinary.
2. The participant wants to be there for the patient as she would want someone to be there for her. Just sitting and talking with a patient means a lot, as each tries to make the other comfortable and she feels at peace while with the patient.	2. Commitment to the other surfaces with the significance of sharing as mutual succor yields to serenity.
3. The closeness makes it hard when the patients get worse or die because the participant goes through it with them. She tries to make a difference in their short time together while admiring the peace and fortitude they achieve.	3. Intimacy intensifies presence with one in calamity, whereas reverence sparks a struggle to enhance the moment.

Proposition

For Participant 2, bearing witness to suffering is attending to the wretchedness of another, which prompts the desire to rectify torment, while reverence sparks a struggle to enhance the moment and commitment to the other surfaces with the significance of sharing as mutual succor yields to serenity.

Data are not "analyzed" in the conventional sense, in Parse's method, as this word implies reductionistic dissection of meaning that is antithetical to the unitary ontology of the theory. "*Extraction-synthesis* is culling the essences from the dialogue in the language of the participant and conceptualizing these essences in the language of science to form a structure of the experience" (Parse, 1998, p. 65). This occurs through long and contemplative dwelling with the dialogues, through reading and listening, while abiding with the meaning of the experience projected by the speaker. Essences are first drawn from the words of participants, then synthesized in the words of the researcher. From the essences generated from one participant's description, a proposition is formulated. From all such propositions, core concepts are extracted and synthesized. From all core concepts, a structure of the lived experience is synthesized. All these processes are illustrated in the presentation of findings found in Tables 15-2 to 15-5.

All of the participants in this study described in some way the first concept, "expressing a commitment sparked by veneration." For example, Participant 10, a group home worker, stated that she

regarded being with the residents as they were suffering as "a sacred experience," and said she was "in awe" that she was the one with the privilege to be with them at that time in their lives. She also gave an example of bearing witness in which she spoke about a resident who, she said, was "so afraid to leave the house [that is, to die]. . . . And he said, 'Could you just hold me?' and so she just climbed in bed with him and held him. This is the idea of "expressing a commitment." It is not simply "expressing" a commitment, but *living* it. Participant 13, who cared for his partner as he died while he himself was also HIV positive, said, "My responsibility as a caregiver was total, complete—mentally, physically, I said, 'I am here for you, you know. My basic life was, you know, sort of put to the side. We needed to concentrate on his health, because at that point, my health was okay."

There was a discernible difference between the descriptions of the families and the caregivers. Whereas family members spoke in very personal details about the person who was suffering, how they valued *that person*, and related very specifically to that individual's suffering, the caregivers described a

TABLE 15-3 *Extraction-Synthesis Process, Participant 25*

Participant 25
Family Member, Spouse

Essences in Participant's Language	Essences in Researcher's Language
1. The participant could see the turmoil in Vinnie as the HIV progressed and he was in constant pain. The participant couldn't stand to see Vinnie like that and Vinnie hated needing help, but he let the participant help.	1. Attentive presence with one in anguish intensifies intimacy, easing limitations.
2. The participant fed and turned Vinnie, knowing he never wanted it to be like that. He tried to carry out Vinnie's wishes, though when Vinnie could no longer talk, there was no way to know. He did it because he loved Vinnie.	2. Endearment inspires persisting in hardship despite doubts.
3. The participant slept with Vinnie every night to be close; those were their special times. Visits with loving family brightened him up. They joked and laughed, knowing that nothing would really help, but holding on to any hope.	3. Prizing the cherished expands the now.
4. Vinnie's suffering got so bad the participant told him to let go. Afterward, they spent time together and said good-byes; it was a good time. The participant thanked God it was over but wondered if he'd done all he could, and loving relatives reassured him.	4. The ending of agony eases loss as sharing joy–sorrow brings contentment and gratitude to the surface.

Proposition

For Participant 25, bearing witness to suffering is attentive presence with one in anguish, which intensifies as intimacy eases limitations while endearment inspires persisting in hardship despite doubts and prizing the cherished expands the now as sharing joy-sorrow surfaces contentment and gratitude.

---

more general veneration of the persons living with AIDS whom they served in the context of a professional or occupational relationship.

The second core concept is "attentive presence with one in anguish." This is basically the essence of the phenomenon of bearing witness to suffering itself. This concept was described very directly by most of the participants. For example, Participant 2 (a home health aide) said, "You can see them one day, and they're up and able to walk and talk. Two days later, you may go in, and they're bedridden. And yet, through it all, they still want you to sit there, hold their hand, and they'll still smile for you." Participant 25, a 35-year-old gay man, described a time near the end of his partner's life, when "he was still in so much *pain*—so we arranged to have IV morphine. . . . And they told me two weeks to two months. And he was such an independent person. . . . So he had a hard time with caregivers. And the primary caregivers were his mother and myself. . . . Mom took care of Vinnie during the day, and

then I would come home in the evening, and I would take care of him during the night." These quotes illustrate the concept of "attentive presence with one in anguish."

The third concept, "expanding the now in light of beliefs and doubts," refers to descriptions given by participants in which they sought to make the most of the time they had with the person living with AIDS in light of the beliefs they held and equally in light of doubts about what was "right" to do, what help or acceptance was available, or indeed what the future held for this relationship in light of the presence of AIDS. For example, Participant 13—who, along with his lover, was HIV positive—said, "We did a lot of things after we were HIV positive that we'd always wanted to do. We did a lot of travelling and, you know, other things that we just new that we needed to get in. . . . And we did a lot of house hunting, things like that . . . but we knew, looking at houses as just a pipe dream, you know?" Participant 25 said about his lover that "the feeling he had about the fu-

TABLE 15-4 *Extracted Core Concepts and Structure of Bearing Witness to Suffering*

Extracted Core Concepts
1. Expressing a commitment sparked by veneration
2. Attentive presence with one in anguish
3. Expanding the now in light of beliefs and doubts
4. A hard-won serenity amidst on-going joy–sorrow

Structure of the Lived Experience
The lived experience of bearing witness to suffering for families and caregivers of persons living with HIV is expressing a commitment sparked by veneration through attentive presence with one in anguish, expanding the now in light of beliefs and doubts, yielding a hard-won serenity amidst ongoing joy–sorrow.

ture was bad. I mean, he would cry about never seeing his nieces and nephews graduate, never seeing them date, and all that. And kinda to ease himself, he made me a promise that I'd always be part of his family. His idea was that he'd be able to see all this happen through me." These are illustrations of the concept of "expanding the now in light of beliefs and doubts."

The fourth core concept, "a hard-won serenity amidst ongoing joy-sorrow," refers to the descriptions that participants gave of a kind of bittersweet peace and contentment that came after witnessing suffering over time. For example, Participant 2 said, "When they are able to feel comfortable enough with me to say, 'I want to share this with you,' it's a feeling of peace with me, and with them. It's just like, like I

TABLE 15-5 *Heuristic Interpretation of the Structure of Bearing Witness to Suffering*

Structure	Heuristic Interpretation	
	Structural Transposition	Conceptual Integration
1. Expressing a commitment sparked by veneration	1. Incarnating devotion	1. Languaging
2. Attentive presence with one in anguish	2. Communion in misery	2. Connecting–separating
3. Expanding the now in light of beliefs and doubts	3. Amplifying possibilities in light of certainty–uncertainty	3. Originating
4. A hard-won serenity amidst ongoing joy–sorrow	4. A bittersweet calm	4. Transforming
Structural Statement	**Structural Statement**	**Structural Statement**
Bearing witness to suffering is expressing a commitment sparked by veneration through attentive presence with one in anguish, expanding the now in light of beliefs and doubts yielding a hard-won serenity amidst ongoing joy–sorrow.	*Bearing witness to suffering is incarnating devotion through communion in misery, amplifying possibilities in light of certainty–uncertainty, yielding a bittersweet calm.*	*Bearing witness to suffering is languaging the paradoxical unity of connecting–separating in originating–transforming.*

said, and old friend." Participant 10 said, "It's a feeling of oneness. . . . There's no conflict, no dissension. She said she has come "to know God better" through the residents, she has "no regrets" because she knows she did what she should in being there, and "it's very comforting."

Through heuristic interpretation, the phenomenological structure is raised to the level of theory. The processes of heuristic interpretation are structural transposition and conceptual integration. The theoretical structure generated through this study is seen in Table 15-5. "Bearing witness to suffering is languaging the paradoxical unity of connecting–separating in originating–transforming." This theoretical structure explicitly interrelated concepts of Parse's theory to represent an emergent conceptualization of the phenomenon. Bearing witness to suffering is *languaging*—expressing who one is—in living the paradoxical unity *of connecting–separating*—intensely being with and apart from the other all-at-once—while *originating–transforming*—choosing a path amid ambiguity, giving rise to a new perspective. The interpretation arises from the phenomenologic-hermeneutic ontology of the Human Becoming Theory.

The implications of this study mainly relate to enhanced understanding of the human experience. Being truly, fully present with one who is suffering un-

> Being truly, fully present with one who is suffering unfolds as an expression of a commitment, living a choice, sparked by veneration—profound respect and genuine fondness.

folds as an expression of a commitment, living a choice, sparked by veneration—profound respect and genuine fondness. This sheds light on family relationships and caregiving relationships and the lived experiences of those who *choose* to be present with the suffering. In contrast, we know that there are those who choose *not* to bear witness to the suffering. Clearly, the value of a loving presence cannot be overestimated. Bearing witness to suffering is also "expanding the now"—or making the most of the time one has—in light of beliefs and doubts. The beliefs and doubts outline the possibilities of what one can become and what one can do in the time remaining. Those who bear witness to suffering report ultimately a sense of a hard-won serenity, a peacefulness that comes from knowing that one was there and one did what one could, even as the joys and sorrows of life continuously unfold.

Hermeneutic Method and Evaluation Method

The Human Becoming Hermeneutic Method (Cody, 1995c; Parse, 1998) was developed in congruence with the assumptions and principles of Parse's theory, drawing on works by Bernstein (1983), Gadamer (1976, 1989), Heidegger (1962), Langer (1967), and Ricoeur (1976). Gadamer's work in particular guided the explication of the method. This method is intended to guide the interpretation of texts in light of the human becoming perspective, possibly giving rise to new understandings of human experiences as manifest in the emergent meanings that are the findings of a hermeneutic study. In Cody's work in developing the method, the herme-

TABLE 15-6	*Explication of the Human Becoming Perspective of the Hermeneutic Processes of Discoursing, Interpreting, and Understanding*
Theme	**Explication**
Meaning	"Discoursing is the interplay of shared and unshared meanings through which beliefs are appropriated and disappropriated. A text, as something written and read, is a form of discourse. Author and reader are discoursing whenever the text is read" (Cody, 1995, p. 275).
Rhythmicity	"Interpreting is expanding the meaning moment through dwelling in situated openness with the disclosed and the hidden. Interpreting a text is constructing meanings with the text through the rhythmic movement between the language of the text and the language of the researcher" (Cody, 1995, p. 275).
Transcendence	"Understanding is choosing from possibilities a unique way of moving beyond the meaning moment. Understanding a text is interweaving the meaning of the text with the pattern of one's life in a chosen way" (Cody, 1995c, p. 276).

neutic processes of *discoursing,* interpreting, and understanding were explicated within a human becoming perspective, informed by important works by the authors above. Each of these key processes is associated with one of the three central themes of the Human Becoming Theory. The processes are described briefly in Table 15-6. Cody (1995c) used the method to interpret a body of poetry by Walt Whitman (1983). A study in progress will examine the concept of mendacity in relation to the refusal to bear witness, in Tennessee Williams's play, *Cat on a Hot Tin Roof.* The possibilities for textual interpretation using the Human Becoming Hermeneutic Method are manifold.

The preproject-process-postproject evaluation method is described in detail in Parse's 1998 work, *The Human Becoming School of Thought.* The purpose of this method is to evaluate the changes that take place when the human becoming theory is adopted in a given venue as the guide to practice.

NURSING LEADERSHIP FROM A HUMAN BECOMING PERSPECTIVE: ONE LEADER'S STORY

The Human Becoming school of thought (Parse, 1981, 1995, 1998) prepares nurses to assume positions of leadership for the purpose of enhancing the quality of human care in all settings. The knowledge base of the theory enables leaders to create and nurture opportunities for staff to change their attitudes, values, and approaches in practice and research. Parse's Theory of Human Becoming helps professionals move toward a more participative, client-centered model of service delivery. Knowledge framed by human becoming constitutes the leader's unique contribution to a community of health-care professionals. The nurse leader's views coexist with multiple other views and beliefs about health care. It is precisely the diversity of ideas and purposes that generate the dynamic culture of comprehensive and compassionate human care.

In the broadest sense, leadership guided by the human becoming theory means working toward creating a particular culture of care. *Culture of care,* as defined here, refers to the assumptions, values, and meanings expressed and shared in the language patterns of a group of people. In general, the changes that are invited include changing from telling and teaching to listening and dialoguing, changing from trying to control patients' decisions to facilitating choices, and changing from judging and labeling differences among people to respecting and representing differences. Like all cultures, the human becoming culture coexists with other cultures of the community. For instance, in hospital settings other cultures include those of medicine and management.

The Human Becoming Theory provides the foundation for leaders to invite others to explore the values, intentions, and desires that shape human care and professional practice. The leading process is not about educating staff—meaning it is not about giving information. Rather, leading is about a process of guided discovery that surfaces insights about self and human becoming—the insights are the windows of change. Personal insights coupled with new knowledge can dramatically change practice and the quality of relationships that staff have with individuals, families, and groups.

your thoughts

Processes of Leading in Change

Leading in a community involves processes of explicating, visioning, discovering, confirming, and disclosing. These processes happen in the context of discussions about human care and meaningful service.

Explicating involves a process of examining the assumptions, values, and meanings embedded in current practices. For example, this includes examination of the assumptions and values of the traditional nursing process multisystem assessments, and prescription. Nurses require opportunities to consider the meanings of words like "dysfunctional," "manipulative," "unrealistic," and "noncompliant." The Human Becoming school of thought offers an alternative framework for all professionals to think about the human-universe process and its connections with practice and human care. The outcome of explicating includes clarification of the values and assumptions of different processes of care and service.

> Leading is about a process of guided discovery that surfaces insights about self and human becoming—the insights are the windows of change.

Visioning is the process whereby staff imagine the forms and patterns that could constitute human care. The predominant questions that invite discourse and insight here are "what if" questions: What if individuals were considered to be the experts about their own health and quality of life? What if nurses were required to listen to individuals' meanings and values in order to know how to care and be helpful? What if people themselves led the healthcare team and selected members of disciplines they wanted involved in their care? What if records were kept at the bedside and patients and families were the ones who monitored access to the record, documented their experiences, and evaluated care? What if there were no assessment tools to evaluate patients' coping styles, degree of compliance, or patterns of decision making? What if nurses considered themselves accountable for their practice to patients and families? These sorts of questions invite staff to think outside of familiar patterns of practice.

Discovering happens as staff see the familiar in a new light. Nurses glimpse contrasting realities and views in discourse with others who discuss alternative ideas. Insights occur in flashes that shed light on how reality in practice could be shaped. The process of discovery can be both exciting and unsettling. There is risk in opening oneself to see things in a new way. Discovery changes everything in a cascading flow of understanding. Leaders can invite and nurture discovery, but ultimately it is a self-directed process that is lived by each person considering and choosing or not choosing to change.

Confirming is a process of seeking personal and organizational coherence with the values clarified in the process of visioning. Nurses seek coherence with cherished values in dialogue with others. Confirming new values is facilitated in standards of practice that specify expectations in the nurse-person process. As members of a self-regulating discipline, nurses have the authority to study and define the knowledge that will guide their practice and research activities. Standards concretize the values chosen to guide practice and clarify the purpose of nursing in any organization.

Disclosing happens through actions taken and words spoken as staff integrate and share their new realities in the context of day-to-day relationships with patients and families. Disclosing is about presenting self to colleagues and to patients and families as a professional with intent and direction. Disclosing also happens through storytelling as members of the staff share their experiences with others. Telling stories of changing realities in practice and research perpetuates the living of new values and is the primary way nurses and other professionals propel the ongoing journey of change.

The way these processes get lived out in any community of professionals will be unique, yet common patterns are recognizable among different groups. In order to demonstrate the complexity of changing a culture of care, the author offers a glimpse of the processes as they are being lived by nurses at a large teaching hospital in Toronto, Canada. Sunnybrook Health Science Centre is an 1100 bed hospital with both acute and long-term care services. There are approximately 1300 nurses. The Aging Program, with approximately 550 beds, employs registered nurses (RNs) and registered practical nurses (RPNs) who work in a primary care model. The acute care programs employ RNs to deliver care in a variety of delivery models.

The First 5 Years

The opportunity began with an invitation and acceptance, by the author, of a leadership role in nursing at Sunnybrook Health Science Centre. The leadership role was newly formed and the expectation was that the chief nurse would participate with staff to embark on a journey to create a new culture of practice consistent with a philosophy of patient-focused care and the Human Becoming school of thought. The leaders of Sunnybrook were committed to the basic tenets of the operational model called "patient-focused" care. These tenets include decentralized program management, simplified processes like charting by exception, multiskilled service workers, and patient empowerment. Additionally, the hospital management team made a commitment to support the principles of shared governance, meaning they endorsed the position that all staff were entitled to a clearly defined scope of responsibility, a meaningful process of accountability, and continuous opportunity for learning and development. The overall intent of the various initiatives was to improve the quality of patient experiences in a compassionate and efficient system that values excellence in all aspects of care.

In addition to efforts to get to know the staff of the organization and their usual practices related to patient care, the first year was characterized by two main activities. The first was to begin explicating the assumptions and values that characterized patient care in the health-care center. The explicating happened in discussions with many different groups and through written documents. A newsletter was published to begin the process of questioning ideas about human health and the way that health-care professionals approached patients. For example, one newsletter focused on explicating "sacred cows"—meaning unexamined practices—in nursing and in health care in general. Another newsletter challenged the assumption that patients were not capable of leading the health-care team. These newsletters prompted discussions of the values and assumptions that guide activities in practice.

A second major activity during the first year was to establish a nursing council that could support and facilitate nursing's mandate to define standards that would guide a new process of care. The nursing council consists of approximately 50 nurses who represent the diverse roles in nursing. Staff nurses were supported in attending a 4-hour council meeting once a month. It was in council that the process of explicating the assumptions and values of traditional nursing practice intensified. Various strategies were used to facilitate discourse, including videos, patient stories, and discussion of journal articles that presented human science views of nursing. The leader's intent during this time was to inspire reflection and introduce creative tension through the presentation of diverging views about patient care. The council was the first group at Sunnybrook to participate in the process of visioning and the clarification of values for guiding the nurse-person process. It is through reflection and openness that nurses discover insights about themselves as professionals and about the process of human becoming.

A critical decision from the beginning was to anchor all discussions of practice and values against the backdrop of patients' lived experiences in health-care systems. The patient's and family's experiences, as presented in videos and in the literature, are critical to sustaining the impetus for change. Valuable video resources on the topic of patient experiences include "Not My Home" (Deveaux & Babin), "Real Stories" (Deveaux & Babin), "Through the Patient's Eyes (Picker), and "The Grief of Miscarriage" (Pilkington), to name a few. Simply stated, people want to be listened to, to be regarded as knowing participants, to be respected for their unique lives and meanings, to have meaningful dialogue, and to have their choices and wishes integrated in plans of care. These basic requests are consistent with what the human becoming theory offers professional staff.

Also critical during this time were discussions to help nurses clarify their shared and unique responsibilities in a multidisciplinary setting. In a hospital, nurses are responsible for many medical and technological activities and these must be carried out with skill and knowledge. But nurses also have a unique practice that happens in the nurse-person process, and it is in this realm that nursing science informs and guides practice. Patterns of thinking and acting, as well as one's attitude and intention in practice, are complex and multidimensional. Nursing practice transcends multiple realms of responsibility, yet there is coherence amid the apparent dissonance of diverging paradigms. Nurses who practice in ways consistent with the Human Becoming Theory are actually more vigilant and attentive to the medical and technological responsibilities, because they are genuinely concerned in a different way about the person as a unitary human being. As a leader in a large system, this author has learned well that instances of serious mishaps in a hospital could often be avoided if professionals truly listened to people and trusted their knowing of potential or impending danger and concern.

The second year at Sunnybrook was marked by the development of a new role and the creation of standards that defined a new process of practice for nurses. The new role, called the Professional Practice Leader (PPL), was created for the purpose of providing the staff with a mentor and guide for changing the culture of care in ways that were consistent with the Human Becoming Theory (Bournes & Das Gupta). The PPL was hired by program directors in order to work directly with staff on patient care units. All disciplines identified PPLs. In nursing there were 12

PPLs selected based on their master's preparation in nursing and a commitment to the human science paradigm and the assumptions and values of the human becoming theory.

The standards of practice developed by members of the council flow from a philosophy that specifies a commitment to view human beings as unitary, irreducible persons who choose unique meanings of health and quality of life. The standards confirm a certain set of values in a coherent nursing process. At Sunnybrook, the standards emphasize dialogue and clarify expectations about how nurses will be with others (Mitchell, 1998a). The standards guide nurses and help them "be with" patients and families for the purposes of clarifying individuals' perspectives, concerns, needs, priorities, and wishes linked to their health care and quality of life. Nurses are responsible for presenting each person's reality in team meetings and in patient records. The standards also specify expectations for actions and evaluation based on the patient's experience and changing medical concerns.

The professional practice leaders created many ways of working with staff in order to facilitate the questioning, reflecting, and learning required for change. Learning modules were developed, as were competencies linked to changing expectations in practice. Perhaps most effective was the ongoing development of an 8-week course in which staff met for 2 to 3 hours a week in small groups to participate in the guided discovery process. More than 300 nurses and other staff, including allied health professionals, managers, and volunteers, have chosen to take the course. Evaluations of the courses indicate that staff find the course changes their ways of thinking about patients, which changes what happens in

their relationships with patients and families. Staff report that patients say they are more satisfied with the care and service at Sunnybrook.

Other structures and systems must also change if staff are to be supported to practice in ways consistent with the human becoming theory. For example, documentation of patient care changes from an observed interpretation of patient behavior to a representation of the patient's experience from the patient/family perpective. This change in documentation is dramatic. For instance, a record in the problem-based, observed behavior model may include a notation like, "Patient refusing to take medications; confused, upset, and occasionally yelling out." In a culture in which patients are respected as leaders of their care, the same occasion might prompt this note: "Mr. B. states he is feeling sick from taking his pills. He would like to speak with the doctor but does not know how to reach him; requests nurse to contact doctor. Mr. B. states that he wants to lie quietly but is too uncomfortable to do so. He plans to call his wife." The nurse guided by standards of practice consistent with Human Becoming records the patient's experiences and the actions taken based on Mr. B.'s concerns and wishes. Follow-up actions with Mr. B. include a discussion to explore and clarify what he is experiencing, an evaluation of Mr. B.'s medical status, notifying the physician of any change, ongoing contact, and helping Mr. B. to lie quietly and contact his wife.

Policies also require evaluation to determine their consistency with the philosophy of patient care. For example, a policy at Sunnybrook for the care of patients who wander was rewritten to be more consistent with the guiding philosophy. The policy changed in the ways patients were approached and

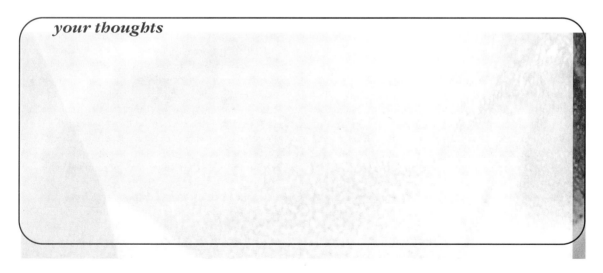

your thoughts

in the attention to the consequences of labeling someone as a wanderer, from the patient's perspective. Hospitals are challenged to find ways to protect patients from harm while simultaneously respecting them as human beings with unique meanings and wishes. Other policies, such as visiting hours and consents, have also been influenced by a change in patient philosophy.

The process of disclosing happens day by day in the practice and research activities that take place across the Sunnybrook campus. A research program guided by the Human Becoming Theory has grown over the years, and researchers are building a knowledge base of lived experiences as described by patients, residents, and families who give of their time to teach us. Multiple studies on quality of life have helped practitioners understand their patients differently, and this has changed practice. For example, a study on quality of life for persons living with diabetes has greatly enhanced understanding about the decisions people make to adhere to strict regimes of care and the relief and help that comes from sometimes breaking those regimes (Mitchell, 1998b). Other studies include the experience of living with persistent pain and quality of life for persons admitted for psychiatric care (Fisher & Mitchell, 1998). Studies in process include quality of life for families living with Alzheimer's disease, the lived experience of waiting, the experience of being listened to, the experience of grieving a loss, and the experience of feeling at home, to name a few. The purpose of all these studies is to enhance understanding so that professionals can change what they know, which changes practice.

Hospital-based practice consistent with the Human Becoming Theory is proving to be a consistent and valuable model for many professionals. Nurses and others are speaking about how their experience of practice is different from before. The outcomes are reflected in patterns of enhanced staff morale and greater patient satisfaction.

Challenges of Change

During the past 2 years, the efforts of the chief nurse and the PPLs, along with the support of managers and other leaders, have continued to support this valued change in how staff relate with patients and families. The change has not been easy, but the outcomes are consistently positive and increasingly desired by staff. The nature of the change with all its obstacles and opportunities requires some additional attention in this brief report.

It became evident early on that the change for many staff was fraught with fear and uncertainty. A commonly expressed fear related to the reality that staff had depended so much on the objective assessment to guide what they said with patients that they did not know how to approach patients just to dialogue and learn from them about their values, meanings, and wishes. Staff did not know how to facilitate dialogue in ways that helped patients describe their realities. Supporting the staff's efforts to learn how to be with others required mentoring about how to ask questions that invite dialogue and that seek depth and clarity without directing and interpreting what people say. Experience with facilitating dialogue was one of the main initiatives in the 8-week patient-focused care course offered to staff.

Additionally, many staff rejected outright the idea that the philosophy and practice model being suggested were possible in a fiscally constrained environment. "No time" was a commonly heard response when staff were first introduced to the change. Initially staff thought that the expectations to listen and to attend to patients' concerns, needs, and wishes were to be "added on" to what was currently being done. The phrase "no time" has not yet prioritized the values of the philosophy. However, what becomes evident to those who decide to change their practice is that it does not take longer to think differently; indeed, staff report that it saves time to work with patients in this way.

Staff begin to see that what happens when the professional-patient relationship is cocreated. They realize that when they think and act differently with patients, different things happen. For instance, in the problem-based model of practice, patients may have been called difficult or manipulative if they did not conform to expectations. But when staff change their expectations, from expecting compliance to facilitating choice, a different dialogue and a different dynamic unfold. Each staff person must experience this change before he or she comes to know the new dynamic. It also helps to realize that difficult situations still happen in a culture of care that respects people as leaders and teachers. People still have some requests that cannot be met, and people still make choices that are different. The thing that changes in this model is the way staff are with patients and families when struggles and differences arise.

Another important obstacle to change is the reality that some staff do not want to relinquish the control they believe they have over patients. This is true despite the reality that patients indicate they have to figure out how to live with new situations and that figuring out comes from their lived experience, not medical directives. That people do not do what experts tell them to do has posed a problem for many providers of health care. Rather than looking at the assumptions and values that guide practice, professionals have spent time and money to continue to study how to increase compliance. Patients have consistently indicated that what they want from professionals is meaningful dialogue and answers to their questions so that they can work through their options and choices. Unsolicited advice is not wanted and effectively closes the door on meaningful dialogue.

A commonly heard answer to the invitation to change is "I already do it." This statement clearly conveys the person is not open to exploring or considering what is being offered. Traditional health care education over the past 3 to 4 decades has ensured a problem-based, holistic, multisystem assessment model of care. This is true even in disciplines that are closely linked to things like recreation and social living. The various health-care disciplines grew up in a model that only knew bio-psycho-social-spiritual-recreational assessments and problems. Indeed, it was the problem-based, reductionistic model that gave birth to the various groups of professionals. When staff say they already practice in a way consistent with the Human Becoming Theory, their assertion usually rests on the reality that they are "caring" within a traditional holistic model. What staff do not realize is that practice consistent with the human becoming perspective is not about being kind and caring while assessing patients to identify problems in bio-psycho-social-spiritual patients. Only staff who are willing to see the difference will change in practice, and this willingness is self-defined and self-directed.

Some professionals who resist change ridicule those who are changing. Others try to instill fear about what the consequences will be if staff do not try to control patients. These forms of resistance represent a rhythm of change. It has helped staff at Sunnybrook to discuss these issues and to hear about the moral courage required to swim against the powerful current of the status quo. It is very difficult to stand out as different and to do so can be isolating. It can also be liberating. The thing that makes it worthwhile is the difference it makes for patients and families who tell staff what it means to have care in the new model. Staff find the strength to go on in the relationships they have with the patients and families and through relationships with others who share their values.

There are many aspects of this journey that cannot be conveyed in this brief account. Staff at Sunnybrook are still on the way to a different place. Some staff report that their practice will always be different because they are different. The learning that happens and the discoveries that come to light with this experience change views of human relating and quality of life.

Practice consistent with the Human Becoming Theory is transformative. Some staff choose to study the theory so that the source of their transforming can continue in more depth and with more clarity. All staff will hopefully have the chance to learn something about their own values and intentions in practice. Whether or not the journey will continue on the current path is not known. Sunnybrook's management team, especially the president and CEO, have provided essential support for this innovation, as have members of the board of the hospital. The professionals and other staff who have accepted the invitation to think and be different are the ones leading the change. The support and courage of the staff at Sunnybrook have created a special opportunity to push the boundaries of what it means to practice when the goal is enhancing the quality of human care from the perspective of those who enter a large hospital system.

From a very personal perspective, the work of being a leader in such an open and innovative system has been a gift. Bearing witness to the joys and the struggles is work worthy of great commitment and energy. There have been some dark days, but I realize this is not my project to control. My work is to try to create the opportunities for others to choose and to try to create new processes that support human science in an environment that has been dominated by natural science. Both sciences must exist if health-care systems hope to achieve compassionate and effective models of care. The work at Sunnybrook has forged meaningful relationships in my life and has melded in my memory the power of human beings to change and transcend in order to serve humankind.

The South Dakota Board of Nursing model, based on Parse's Theory of Human Becoming, focuses on quality of life from the person's/community's perspective, with quality of nursing education, nursing care, and nursing practitioners addressed in the model.

A NURSING REGULATORY DECISIONING MODEL

The South Dakota Board of Nursing has developed a model of decisioning based on the Human Becoming Theory. The board of nursing made explicit in the model its belief that "[n]ursing regulation, as integral to the profession, must establish models for Decisioning which provide a systematic focus on the discipline of nursing as it relates to the mission of public protection" (Bunkers, Damgaard, Hohman, & Vander Woude, 1998, p. 2).

The South Dakota Board of Nursing's Regulatory Decisioning Model's theoretical foundation is based on Parse's human becoming school of thought, values held by the board of nursing, and tenets of public policy making. The decisioning model focuses on quality of life from the person's and/or community's

South Dakota Board of Nursing Regulatory Decisioning Model

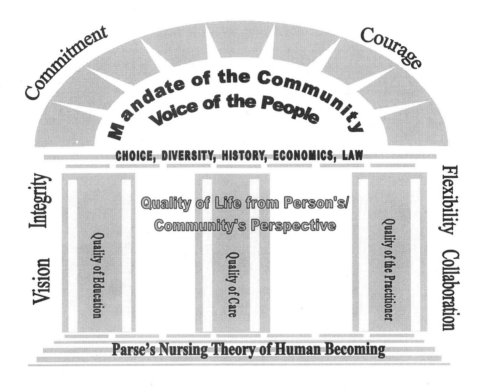

Meaning of Lived Experience
"Each person's reality is the meaning of the situation."
(Parse, 1996)

Paradoxical Patterns of Relating
"Paradox is fundamental to human becoming...."
(Parse, 1995)

Moving Beyond
"The person is co-author of health, free agent and meaning giver, choosing patterns of relating in reaching for hopes and dreams."
(Parse, 1996)

Figure 15–4 *South Dakota Board of Nursing Regulatory Decisioning Model. Reprinted with permission © South Dakota Board of Nursing, 1998, Bunkers, S.S., Damgaard, G., Hohman, M., and Vander Woude, D.*

Section III *Nursing Theory in Nursing Practice, Education, Research, and Administration*

The Teaching-Learning Process and the Theory of Human Becoming

The teaching-learning process confronts the familiar-unfamiliar all-at-once. From a human becoming perspective, teaching-learning is a **process of engaging with others in coming to know.** The **Seeker**, in engaging with others, participates in simultaneous processes of coming to know at an explicit-tacit level. These processes include:

E Expanding Imaginal Margins

N Naming the New

G Going with Content-Process Shifts

A Abiding with Paradox

G Giving Meaning

I Inviting Dialogue

N Noticing the Now

G Growing Story

WITH OTHERS IN THE PROCESS OF COMING TO KNOW

Figure 15–5 *The Teaching-Learning Process and the Theory of Human Becoming. Reprinted with permission from Bunkers, S.S., 1999. The teaching-learning process and the theory of human becoming.* Nursing Science Quarterly, 11, *56–63.*

perspective with quality of nursing education, quality of nursing care, and quality of the nursing practitioner being addressed in the model (see Fig. 15-4).

In operationalizing the decisioning model, the belief system of the board of nursing is lived in its valuing of vision, integrity, commitment, courage, flexibility, and collaboration. These values are defined from a human becoming perspective, are interconnected with the three principles of the Human Becoming Theory, and illuminate the themes of understanding the meaning of lived experience; recognizing paradoxical patterns of relating; and moving beyond to new ways of being. Tenets of public policy making, including choice, diversity, history, economics, and law, are interwoven with these values and themes in framing standards for quality education, quality care, and quality of the practitioner (Bunkers, Damgaard, Hohman, & Vander Woude, 1998).

South Dakota's nursing theory–based Regulatory Decisioning Model is an avenue for developing nursing theory–based education, practice, and research. The model can serve as a vehicle for the advancement of nursing scholarship in developing a nursing science–based profession (Bunkers, Damgaard, Hohman, & Vander Wouden, 1998).

The staff of the board of nursing in South Dakota studied with a Parse scholar for 3 years while creating the decisioning model. The membership of the board of nursing engaged in study of the Human Becoming Theory while implementing the model in their regulatory decisioning process. Nursing theory-based regulatory decisioning based on Parse's Human Becoming school of thought will seek to sculpt a new path for the future of nursing.

THE HUMAN BECOMING THEORY IN TEACHING–LEARNING

A process model of teaching-learning is supported by Parse's Human Becoming school of thought. From a human becoming perspective, Bunkers and colleagues (1998, 1999) defined *teaching-learning* as "an all at once process of engaging with others in coming to know." Eight teaching-learning processes, emphasizing the notion that teaching-learning is a dynamic interactive human encounter with ideas, places, people, and events, are listed in Fig. 15-5. These eight teaching-learning processes include "expanding imaginal margins, naming the new, going with content-process shifts, abiding with paradox, giving meaning, inviting dialogue, noticing the now, and growing story" (Bunkers et al., 1998, 1999).

Bunkers and colleagues (1999) write:

Expanding imaginal margins involves focusing on the imaging process. . . . *Expanding imaginal margins* while engaging with others in coming to know coshapes what one will learn. In imaging valued possibilities one is already moving with those possibilities. . . . *Naming the new* concerns itself with languaging. *Naming the new* in the process of engaging with others in coming to know cocreates the meaning of the moment. . . . *Going with content-process shifts* involves a synthesis of ideas with action. . . . *Going with content-process shifts* while engaging with others in coming to know involves the intentionality of focusing on the unity of idea-action while participating in relationship. . . . *Abiding with paradox* involves recognizing the contradictions in life. . . . *Abiding with paradox* in the process of engaging with others in coming to know involves honoring the tensions of contradiction and living in the questions. . . . *Giving meaning* involves ascribing value to ideas and lived experiences. . . . *Giving meaning* in the process of engaging with others in coming to know involves creating one's personal reality in light of choosing a personal stance toward ideas and experience. *Giving meaning* forms the purpose of one's life. . . . *Inviting dialogue* consists of generating an atmosphere for conversation while being attentive to of-

fered information. . . . *Inviting dialogue* in the process of engaging with others in coming to know involves participating in discerning discourse while focusing on understanding unique patterns of evolving. Such understanding uncovers diverse realities. . . . *Noticing the now* means being present to what was, is, and will be in human evolving. This presence involves an attentive, "being with the other." . . . *Noticing the now* in the process of engaging with others in coming to know involves living an attentive presence with others as possibility becoming actuality. It involves reflecting on how one moves moment to moment in relationship with others as transforming occurs. . . . *Growing story* involves giving meaning to abstract concepts with narrative description. Storytelling reflects the unity and multidimensionality of human experience. . . . *Growing story* in the process of engaging with others in coming to know immerses the community in meaning-making and comprehending personal realities. Meaning-making with storying unveils the wholeness of lived experience.

Bunkers' teaching–learning processes are grounded in the principles of Parse's Theory of Human Becoming. The themes of meaning making, recognizing and participating with shifting paradoxical rhythms, and moving beyond with hopes and dreams manifest themselves in these intuitive-rational processes of coming to know. People who embrace this human becoming perspective of teaching–learning participate in fostering "the unique unfolding of human potential" (Bunkers et al., 1999).

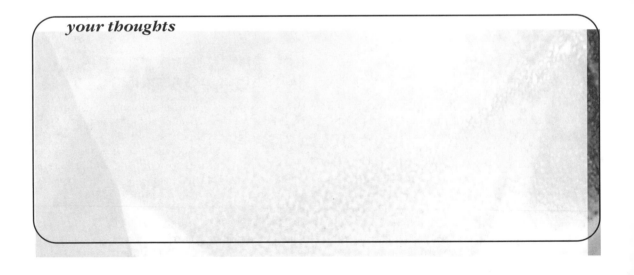

your thoughts

References

Arndt, M. J. (1995). Parse's Theory of Human Becoming in practice with hospitalized adolescents. *Nursing Science Quarterly, 8*, 86-90.

Banonis, B. C. (1995). Metaphors in the practice of the Human Becoming Theory. In Parse, R. R. (Ed.), *Illuminations: The human becoming theory in practice and research* (pp. 87-95). New York: National League for Nursing.

Bernstein, R. J. (1983). *Beyond objectivism and relativism: Science, hermeneutics, and praxis*. Menlo Park, CA: Addison-Wesley.

Bournes, D. A., & Das Gupta, D. (1997). Professional practice leader: A transformational role that addresses human diversity. *Nursing Administration Quarterly, 21*(4), 61-68.

Bunkers, S. S. (1998a). Considering tomorrow: Parse's theory-guided research. *Nursing Science Quarterly, 11*, 56-63.

Bunkers, S. S. (1998b). Translating nursing conceptual frameworks and theory for nursing practice in the parish community. In Solari-Twadell, A., & McDermott, M. (Eds.), *Parish nursing* (pp. 205-214) Thousand Oaks, CA: Sage.

Bunkers, S. S., Damgaard, G., Hohman, M, & Vander Woude, D. (1998). *The South Dakota Nursing Theory-Based Regulatory Decision-Making Model*. Sioux Falls, SD: Unpublished manuscript, Augustana College.

Bunkers, S. S., Nelson, M., Leuning, C. J., Crane, J., & Josephson, D. (1999). The Health Action Model: Academia's alliance with the community. In Cohen, E., & DeBack, V. (Eds.), *The outcomes mandate* (pp. 92-100). St. Louis: Mosby.

Bunkers, S. S., & Putnam, V. (1995). *A nursing theory based model of health ministry: Living Parse's Theory of Human Becoming in the parish community*. In Ninth Annual Westberg Parish Nurse Symposium: Parish Nursing: Ministering through the Arts. Northbrook, Il: International Parish Nurse Resource Center-Advocate Health Care.

Butler, M. J. (1988). Family transformation: Parse's theory in practice. *Nursing Science Quarterly, 1*, 68-74.

Butler, M. J., & Snodgrass, F. G. (1991). Beyond abuse; Parse's theory in practice. *Nursing Science Quarterly, 4*, 76-82.

Chapman, J. S., Mitchell, G. J., & Forchuk, C. (1994). A glimpse of nursing theory-based practice in Canada. *Nursing Science Quarterly, 7*, 104-112.

Cody, W. K. (1991). Grieving a personal loss. *Nursing Science Quarterly, 4*, 61-68.

Cody, W. K. (1995a). True presence with families living with HIV disease. In Parse, R. R. (Ed.), *Illuminations: The human becoming theory in practice and research* (pp. 115-133). New York: National League for Nursing Press.

Cody, W. K. (1995b). The lived experience of grieving for families living with AIDS. In Parse, R. R. (Ed.), *Illuminations: The human becoming theory in practice and research* (pp. 197-242). New York: National League for Nursing Press.

Cody, W. K. (1995c). Of life immense in passion, pulse, and power: Dialoguing with Whitman and Parse—A

hermeneutic study. In Parse, R. R. (Ed.), *Illuminations: The human becoming theory in practice and research* (pp. 269-307). New York: National League for Nursing Press.

Daly, J. (1995). The lived experience of suffering. In Parse, R. R. (Ed.), *Illuminations: The human becoming theory in practice and research* (pp. 243-268). New York: National League for Nursing Press.

Deveaux, B., & Babin, S. (1994). [Review of the Canadian Broadcasting Corporation documentary *Not My Home*.] Deveaux-Babin Productions.

Deveaux, B., & Babin, S. (1996). [Review of the Canadian Ministry of Health video *Real Stories*.] Deveaux-Babin Productions.

Fisher, M. A., & Mitchell, G. J. (1998). Patients' views of quality of life: Transforming the knowledge base of nursing. *Clinical Nurse Specialist, 12*(3), 99-105.

Fitne, Inc. (1997). *The nurse theorists: Portraits of excellence: Rosemarie Rizzo Parse* [CD-ROM]. Athens, OH: Author.

Gadamer, H-G. (1976). *Philosophical hermeneutics* (D. E. Linge, Trans. & Ed.). Berkeley: University of California Press.

Gadamer, H-G. (1989). *Truth and method* (2nd rev. ed.). (Translation revised by J. Weinsheimer & D. G. Marshall.) New York: Crossroad. (Original work published 1960)

Heidegger, M. (1962). *Being and time* (J. Macquarrie & E. Robinson, Trans.). San Francisco: Harper & Row. (Original work published 1927)

International Consortium of Parse Scholars. (1996). *Living true presence in nursing practice* [videotape]. Toronto, Canada: Author.

Jonas, C. M. (1994). True presence through music. *Nursing Science Quarterly, 7*, 102-103.

Jonas, C. M. (1995). True presence through music for persons living their dying. In Parse, R. R. (Ed.), *Illuminations: The human becoming theory in practice and research* (pp. 97-104). New York: National League for Nursing Press.

Langer, S. (1967). *Philosophy in a new key: A study in the symbolism of reason, rite, and art* (3rd ed.). Cambridge, MA: Harvard University Press.

Lee, O. J., & Pilkington, F. B. (2000). Practice with persons living their dying: A human becoming perspective. *Nursing Science Quarterly*.

Liehr, P. R. (1989). The core of true presence: A loving center. *Nursing Science Quarterly, 2*, 7-8.

Mattice, M. (1991). Parse's theory of nursing in practice: A manager's perspective. *Canadian Journal of Nursing Administration, 4*, 11-13.

Mattice, M., & Mitchell, G.J. (1990). Caring for confused elders. *The Canadian Nurse, 86*(11), 16-18.

Mitchell, G. J. (1988). Man-Living-Health: The theory in practice. *Nursing Science Quarterly, 1*, 120-127.

Mitchell, G. J. (1990a). The lived experience of taking life day-by-day in later life: Research guided by Parse's emergent method. *Nursing Science Quarterly, 3*, 29-36.

Mitchell, G. J. (1990b). Struggling in change: From the traditional approach to Parse's theory-based practice. *Nursing Science Quarterly, 3*, 170-176.

Mitchell, G. J. (1998a). Standards of nursing and the winds of change. *Nursing Science Quarterly, 11*, 97-98.

Mitchell, G. J. (1998b). Living with diabetes: How understanding expands theory for professional practice. *Canadian Journal of Diabetes Care, 22*(1), 30–37.

Mitchell, G. J., & Copplestone, C. (1990). Applying Parse's theory to perioperative nursing: A nontraditional approach. *AORN Journal, 51*, 787–798.

Mitchell, G. J., & Pilkington, B. (1990). Theoretical approaches in nursing practice: A comparison of Roy and Parse. *Nursing Science Quarterly, 3*, 81–87.

Northrup, D., & Cody, W. K. (1998). Evaluation of the Human Becoming Theory in practice in an acute care psychiatric setting. *Nursing Science Quarterly, 11*, 23–30.

Parse, R. R. (1981). *Man-Living-Health: A theory of nursing*. New York: Wiley.

Parse, R. R. (1987). *Nursing science: Major paradigms, theories, and critiques*. Philadelphia: Saunders.

Parse, R. R. (1990). Parse's research methodology with an illustration of the lived experience of hope. *Nursing Science Quarterly, 3*, 9–17.

Parse, R. R. (1994). Laughing and health: A study using Parse's research method. *Nursing Science Quarterly, 7*, 55–64.

Parse, R. R. (1995). Man-Living-Health: A theory of nursing. In Mischo-Kelling, M., & Wittneben, K. (Eds.), *Auffassungen von pflege in theorie und praxis* (pp. 114–132). Munchen: Urban & Schwarzenberg.

Parse, R. R. (1996, Spring). Community: A human becoming perspective. *Illuminations: The newsletter of the International Consortium of Parse Scholars*, 4.

Parse, R. R. (1997). Joy-sorrow: A study using the Parse research method. *Nursing Science Quarterly, 10*, 80–87.

Parse, R. R. (1998). *The human becoming school of thought*. Thousand Oaks, CA: Sage.

Parse, R. R. (Ed.). (1999). *Hope: An international human becoing perspective*. Sudbury, MA: Jones & Bartlett.

Pilkington, F. B. (1993). The lived experience of grieving the loss of an important other. *Nursing Science Quarterly, 6*, 130–139.

Quiquero, A., Knights, D., & Meo, C. O. (1991). Theory as a guide to practice: Staff nurses choose Parse's theory. *Canadian Journal of Nursing Administration, 4*(1), 14–16.

Rasmusson, D. L. (1995). True presence with homeless persons. In Parse, R. R. (Ed.), *Illuminations: The human becoming theory in practice and research* (pp. 105–113). New York: National League for Nursing Press.

Rasmusson, D. L., Jonas, C. M., & Mitchell, G. J. (1991). The eye of the beholder: Parse's theory with homeless individuals. *Clinical Nurse Specialist, 5*, 139–143.

Ricoeur, P. (1976). *Interpretation theory: Discourse and the surplus of meaning*. Fort Worth: Texas Christian University Press.

Smith, M. C. (1990). Struggling through a difficult time for unemployed persons. *Nursing Science Quarterly, 3*, 18–28.

Ward, W. (1972). Matthew. In Paschall, H., & Hobbs, H. (Eds.), *The teacher's bible commentary* (pp. 586–616). Nashville, TN: Broadman Press.

Whitman, W. (1983). *Leaves of grass*. New York: Bantam. (Original [7th ed.] published in 1892)

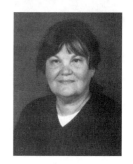

Chapter 16

Margaret A. Newman
Health as Expanding Consciousness

Margaret Dexheimer Pharris

I don't like controlling, manipulating other people.
I don't like deceiving, withholding, or treating
people as subjects or objects.
I don't like acting as an objective non-person.
I do like interacting authentically, listening,
understanding, communicating freely.
I do like knowing and expressing myself in mutual
relationships.

—**Margaret Newman (1985)**

If nursing is to fulfill its social commitment to promote the betterment of the human condition, it must be ready to respond to the ever-increasing complexity of the way people relate to each other and to the environment. Over the past century we've seen a rapid increase in energy interchange around the globe. During the twentieth century the major explanations of morbidity and mortality have moved from microbial agents to behavioral choices, emotional struggles, and environmental stresses; and now they are shifting increasingly back to microbial agents but with behavioral, emotional, and environmental underpinnings. The advent of the atomic bomb has shown all people of the Earth that our fates are intricately intertwined. We've watched TV images projected from outer space of our small, round earthly home, and come to realize that borders are a human construct. The Berlin Wall has come down. Transglobal travel has become commonplace. Some people wake up in Tokyo, Japan, and that very night go to sleep in Kampala, Uganda; whereas others wake up in Bogotá, Colombia, and go to sleep in Paris, France. On the Upper West Side of New York City, a man runs in place on a treadmill to burn excess calories, while the people in Central America who toiled harvesting his coffee and most of the food he ate for lunch try to conserve energy for their lean, hungry bodies. The garbage of New York City is shipped to Guatemala, where it is used to fertilize food, most of which is shipped to the United States. The global economy transfers both nourishment and disease around the world in a matter of hours. Where the resources for computers exist, we have instant Internet communication across the globe with friends, colleagues, family, and people we've never

> There is movement of the life process toward higher consciousness. Each client situation manifests an underlying pattern that is unique and whole; the nurse–client interaction is a mutual process.

met. We stand in amazement as we watch borders and barriers fall away and concepts of space, movement, and time take on new dimensions. These events and relationships have transformed us as a people. Nursing, with its social mandate of caring for people as they strive for health, has also undergone a transformation. Nursing theorist Margaret Newman has been a guiding voice in that process.

Margaret Newman's Theory of Health as Expanding Consciousness (HEC) argues that there is movement of the life process toward higher consciousness, that each client situation manifests an underlying pattern that is unique and whole, and that the nurse–client interaction is a mutual process (Newman, 1994a). Newman's theory emanates from a Rogerian unitary perspective, later termed the "unitary-transformative scientific paradigm," which views the nature of reality as a whole, and the nature of change, as transformative (Newman, Sime, & Corcoran-Perry, 1991).

INTRODUCING THE THEORIST: THE UNFOLDING OF MARGARET NEWMAN'S THEORY OF HEALTH AS EXPANDING CONSCIOUSNESS

The foundation for the Theory of Health as Expanding Consciousness was laid prior to the time Margaret Newman entered nursing school at the University of Tennessee in 1959 (Newman, 1997c). After graduating from Baylor University, she went home to Memphis to work and to care for her mother, who had amyotropic lateral sclerosis (ALS), a degenerative neurological disease that progressively diminishes the ability of all muscles except those of the eyes to move. Caring for her mother was transformative for Margaret Newman. This experience provided her with two profound realizations: that simply having a disease does not make you unhealthy (i.e., health is not the opposite of disease, but rather can be present in the midst of disease), and that time, movement, and space are in some way interrelated. The restrictions of movement that Margaret's mother experienced immobilized her in terms of time and space and effectively did the same to Margaret, whose movement was necessarily restricted because of her commitment to caring for her physically immobilized mother (Newman, 1997c).

Later, when Newman decided to pursue doctoral studies in nursing, she was drawn to New York University (NYU), where she would be able to study with Martha Rogers, whose Science of Unitary Hu-

264   **Section III** *Nursing Theory in Nursing Practice, Education, Research, and Administration*

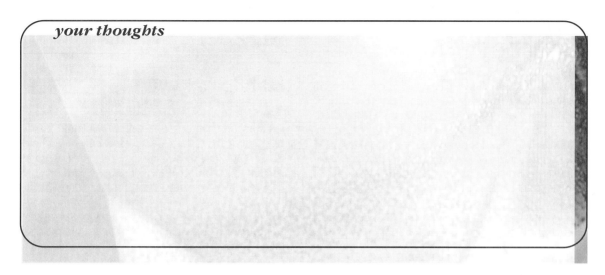

man Beings resonated with Newman's conceptualizations of nursing and health (Newman, 1997b). In her doctoral work at NYU, Newman (1982, 1987) began studying movement, time, and space as parameters of health, but did so out of a logical positivist scientific paradigm. She designed an experimental study that manipulated participants' movement and then measured their perception of time. Her results showed a changing perception of time across the life span, with subjective time increasing with age. Although her results seemed to support what she later would term "health as expanding consciousness," at that time she felt they did little to inform or shape nursing practice (Newman, 1997a).

It soon became evident to Newman that the positivist perspective, which isolated, broke apart, and sought to individually manipulate inextricable aspects of the human health experience, was too simplistic and ineffectual in shedding light on that which she sought to understand. This was a point of transformation for Margaret Newman. It was a time when she realized that the old paradigm was not serving her desire to understand the human experience of health and her commitment to providing a comprehensive guide for nursing practice.

Newman's paradigmatic transformation occurred as she was delving into the works of Martha Rogers and Itzhak Bethov, while at the same time reflecting on her own personal experience (Newman, 1997b). Several of Martha Rogers' assumptions became central in shaping Margaret Newman's theoretical perspective (Newman, 1997b). First, Rogers saw health and illness as a unitary process of the whole, which was congruent with Margaret Newman's earlier experience with her mother and with her patients.

People can experience health when they are physically or mentally ill. Health is not the opposite of illness, but rather health and illness are both manifestations of a greater whole.

Second, Rogers argued that all of reality is a unitary whole and that each human being exhibits a unique pattern. Rogers (1970) saw energy fields to be the fundamental unit of all that is living and non-living, and posited that there is interpenetration between the fields of person, family, and environment. Person, family, and environment are not separate entities, but rather an interconnected, unitary whole. In defining *field,* Rogers wrote: "Field is a unifying concept. Energy signifies the dynamic nature of the field. A field is in continuous motion and is infinite" (Rogers, 1990, p. 29). Rogers defined the *unitary human being* as "[a]n irreducible, indivisible, pandimensional energy field identified by pattern and manifesting characteristics that are specific to the whole and which cannot be predicted from knowledge of the parts" (Rogers, 1990, p. 29). Finally, Rogers saw the life process as showing increasing complexity. This assumption, along with the work of Itzhak Bentov (1978), which viewed life as a process of expanding consciousness, helped to shape Margaret Newman's conceptualization of health and eventually her theory.

> The responsibility of the nurse is not to make people well, or to prevent them from getting sick, but to assist them to recognize the power that is within them to move to higher levels of consciousness.

THE DEBUT OF MARGARET NEWMAN'S THEORY

In 1977, when Margaret Newman was teaching nursing theory development at Penn State, she received an invitation to speak at a nursing theory conference. It was in preparing for that presentation, entitled "Toward a Theory of Health," that the Theory of Health as Expanding Consciousness (HEC) began to take shape. In her address (Newman, 1978) and in a written overview of the address (Newman, 1979), Newman outlined the basic assumptions that were integral to her theory. Drawing on the work of Martha Rogers and Itzhak Bentov and on her own experience and insight, she proposed that:

- health encompasses conditions known as disease as well as states where disease is not present;
- disease, when it manifests itself, can be considered a manifestation of the underlying pattern of the person;
- the pattern of the person manifesting itself as disease was present prior to the structural and functional changes of disease; and
- health is the expansion of consciousness (Newman, 1979).

Her presentation drew thunderous applause as she ended with "[t]he responsibility of the nurse is not to make people well, or to prevent their getting sick, but to assist people to recognize the power that is within them to move to higher levels of consciousness" (Newman, 1978).

Although Margaret Newman never set out to become a nursing theorist, in that 1978 presentation in New York City she articulated a theory that resonated with what was meaningful in the practice of nurses in many countries throughout the world. Nurses wanted to go beyond combating diseases; they wanted to accompany their patients in the process of discovering meaning and wholeness in their lives. Margaret Newman's proposed theory would serve as a guide for them to do so.

After identifying the basic assumptions of the HEC theory, the next step for Margaret Newman was to focus on how to test the theory with nursing research and how the theory could inform nursing practice. Newman began to concentrate on the uniqueness and wholeness of the pattern in each client situation, the sequential configurations of pattern evolving over time, the movement of the life process toward expanded consciousness, insights occurring as choice points of action potential, and the mutuality of the nurse–client interaction in the process of pattern recognition (Newman, 1997a).

UNIQUENESS AND WHOLENESS OF PATTERN

Margaret Newman (1979, 1986, 1994a), like Martha Rogers (1970, 1990), sees human beings as unitary energy fields that are inseparable from the larger unitary field that combines person, family, and community all at once. A nurse operating out of the unitary being perspective does not think of mind, body, spirit, and emotion as separate entities, a conceptualization that focuses on parts rather than on the undivided whole.

Nursing's historical alignment with medicine and social sciences fostered a fragmented, particulate view of reality. In the seventeenth century, medicine was propelled toward treating only the physical aspect of human beings when René Descartes, a philosopher and founding father of modern medicine, made a deal with the Roman Catholic pope so that he could get the human bodies he needed for dissection. Descartes agreed to concentrate only on the physical body and not have anything to do with the soul, the emotions, or the mind, for they were under the jurisdiction of the church. This deal set the tone for two centuries of medical practice, which became aimed at treating diseases and ignoring the wholeness of patients. Nursing, by association, got temporarily caught up in this fragmented perspective.

As nurses moved into research to test nursing theory and improve nursing practice, they drew heavily on research methodologies used by medical and social science, which entailed isolation, quantification, and manipulation of variables aimed at predicting cause and effect. The medical model focused on the body and causal explanations of illness (i.e., A causes B, or atherosclerotic plaque causes heart attacks). The social science model took a systems approach, which looked at the interrelationships between variables and their effect on a specified outcome (i.e., A + B + C + D are interrelated in their effect on E; or diet, exercise, smoking, family history, and lifestyle are interconnected in their effect on heart attacks). Margaret Newman's theory (1979, 1990, 1994a, 1997a, 1997b) proposes that we cannot isolate, manipulate, and control variables in order to understand the whole of a phenomenon. The nurse and client form a mutual partnership to attend to the pattern of meaningful relationships and experiences in the client's life, as well as the meaning of the heart attack, and through the insight gained, the

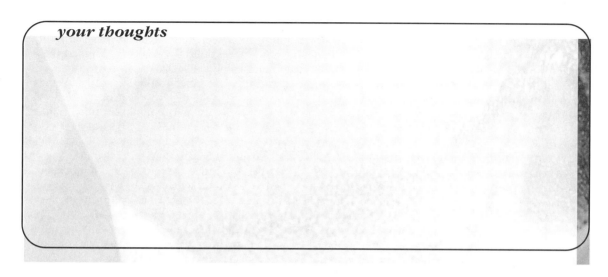
client undergoes an expansion of consciousness. We must use a methodology that does not divide people's lives into fragmented variables, but rather attends to the nature and meaning of the whole (Newman, 1994a, 1997a, 1997b).

Research methodologies must be consistent with our theory and paradigmatic view. The old paradigm proposes methods that are analogous to trying to appreciate a loaf of warm bread by analyzing flour, water, salt, yeast, and oil. No matter how much we come to know these ingredients separately, we will not know the texture, smell, taste, and essence of the loaf of bread that has just come out of the oven. The whole is greater than the sum of its parts and exhibits unique qualities that cannot be fully comprehended by looking at parts. Individual qualities of the whole, however, do give us some understanding of the nature of the whole. For example, the smell of the loaf of bread provides one insight into its nature, the texture provides another, and so on. A nurse practicing out of the HEC theoretical perspective possesses multifaceted levels of awareness and is able to sense how physical signs, emotional conveyances, spiritual insights, physical appearances, and mental insights are all meaningful manifestations of a person's underlying pattern.

A NEW PARADIGM EMERGES

In an attempt to acknowledge and define the various scientific paradigmatic perspectives and to eliminate some of the confusion regarding the nature of the discipline of nursing, Margaret Newman, Marilyn Sime, and Sheila Corcoran-Perry (1991) collaborated on an article to define the overarching focus of the discipline of nursing and its prevailing paradigms.

They defined the focus of the discipline of nursing to be *caring in the human health experience,* which they saw as the common umbrella under which three distinct paradigmatic perspectives fell. The paradigmatic perspectives they defined were the particulate-deterministic, the interactive-integrative, and the unitary-transformative (with the first word indicating the nature of reality and the second word indicating the nature of change in each paradigm).

The particulate-deterministic paradigm holds that phenomena are isolatable, reducible entities with definable, measurable properties. Relationships between entities are seen as orderly, predictable, linear, and causal (i.e., A causes B). In this perspective, health is dichotomized with clearly defined characteristics that are either healthy or unhealthy.

The interactive-integrative perspective, which stems from the particulate-deterministic, views reality as multidimensional and contextual. Multiple antecedents and probabilistic relationships are believed to bring about change in a phenomenon outcome (i.e., A + B + C + D are interrelated in their effect on E). Relationships may be reciprocal, and subjective data are seen as legitimate.

The unitary-transformative perspective is distinct from the other two. Here a phenomenon is seen as a "unitary, self-organizing field embedded in a

> Each person exhibits a distinct pattern, which is constantly unfolding and evolving as it responds to the person-environment interactions. Pattern is information depicting the whole of a person's relationship with the environment.

larger self-organizing field. It is identified by pattern and by interaction with the larger whole" (Newman, Sime, & Corcoran-Perry, 1991, p. 4). Change is unpredictable and unidirectional, always moving toward a higher level of complexity. Knowledge is arrived at through pattern recognition and reflects both the phenomenon viewed and the viewer.

Newman, Sime, and Corcoran-Perry (1991) concluded that the knowledge generated by the particulate-deterministic paradigm and the interactive-integrative was relevant to nursing, but that the knowledge gained by using the unitary-transformative paradigm was *essential* to the discipline of nursing. In a later work, Newman (1997a) asserted that knowledge emanating from the unitary-transformative paradigm is the knowledge of the discipline and that the focus, philosophy, and theory of the discipline must be consistent with each other and therefore cannot flow out of different paradigms. Newman states:

> The paradigm of the discipline is becoming clear. We are moving from attention on the other as object to attention to the we in relationship, from fixing things to attending to the meaning of the whole, from hierarchical one-way intervention to mutual process partnering. It is time to break with a paradigm of health that focuses on power, manipulation, and control and move to one of reflective, compassionate consciousness. The paradigm of nursing embraces wholeness and pattern. It reveals a world that is moving, evolving, transforming—a process. (Newman, 1997a, p. 37)

SEQUENTIAL CONFIGURATIONS OF PATTERN EVOLVING OVER TIME

Essential to Margaret Newman's theory is the belief that each person exhibits a distinct pattern, which is constantly unfolding and evolving as it responds to the person-environment interactions. Pattern is information that depicts the whole of a person's relationship with the environment and gives an understanding of the meaning of the relationships all at once (Endo, 1998; Newman, 1994a). Pattern is a manifestation of consciousness, which Newman (1994a) defines as the informational capacity of the system to interact with its environment.

In explaining the nature of pattern, Newman draws on the work of David Bohm (1980) who said that anything *explicate* (that which we can hear, see, taste, smell, touch) is a manifestation of the *implicate* order (the unseen underlying pattern) (New-

man, 1997b). That which is "explicate" is a manifestation of the underlying "implicate" pattern. In other words, there is information about the underlying pattern of each person in all that we sense about them, such as their movements, tone of voice, interactions with others, activity level, genetic pattern, vital signs. There is also information about their underlying pattern in all that they tell us about their experiences and perceptions, including stories about their life, recounted dreams, and portrayed meanings. An example from this writer's research (Dexheimer Pharris, in progress) involves a 16-year-old young man in an adult correctional facility after a murder conviction. This young man was constantly getting into fights and generally feeling lost. As he and the nurse researcher met over several weeks to look at what was meaningful in his life, the process seemed to be blocked, with the pattern not emerging and little insight being gained. He spoke of how he felt he had lost himself several years back. One week he walked into the room and his movements seemed more controlled and labored; he sat with his arms cradling his abdomen and his chest expanded as though it were about to explode. His palms were glistening with sweat. His face was erupting with acne. He talked as usual in a very detached manner, but his words came out in bursts. The nurse chose to give him feedback about what she was seeing and sensing from his body. She reflected that he seemed to be exerting a great deal of energy keeping in something that was erupting within him. With this insight, he suddenly opened up and began talking about a very painful family history of sexual abuse that had been kept secret for many years. It became obvious that the experience of covering up the abuse had been so all-encompassing that it was suppressing his pattern. This young man had reached a choice point at which he realized his old ways of interacting with others were no longer serving him, and he chose to interact with his environment in a different way. By the next meeting, his movements had become smooth and sure, his complexion had cleared up, he was becoming able to reflect on his insights, and he no longer was involved in the chaos and fighting in his cellblock. In their subsequent work together, this young man and the nurse were able to distinguish between his implicit pattern, which had become clear, and the impact that keeping the abusive experience a secret had had on him and on other members of his family. Since that time, this person has been able to transcend previous limitations and has become involved in several efforts to help others, both in and out of the prison environment, and has achieved great success academically.

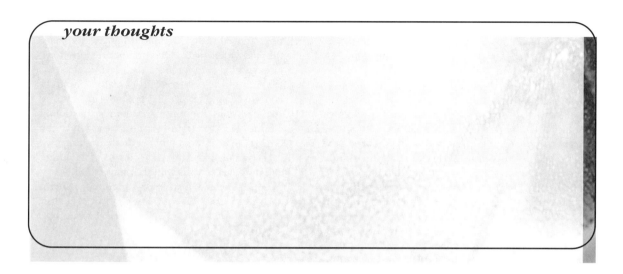
That which is underlying makes itself known in the physical realm, and nurses operating out of the HEC theory are able to sense it and mobilize the insight of their patients into expanded levels of consciousness through pattern recognition. Another example, at the community level, arose out of the work of Frank Lamendola and Margaret Newman (1994) with people with HIV/AIDS. They found that the experience of HIV/AIDS opened the participants to suffering and physical deterioration and at the same time introduced greater sensitivity and openness to themselves and to others. Drawing on the work of cultural historian William Irwin Thompson, systems theorist Will McWhinney, and musician David Dunn, Lamendola and Newman stated:

> They [Thompson, McWhinney, and Dunn] see the loss of membranal integrity as a signal of the loss of autopoetic unity analogous to the breaking down of boundaries at a global level between countries, ideologies, and disparate groups. Thompson views HIV/AIDS not simply as a chance infection but part of a larger cultural phenomenon and sees the pathogen not as an object but as heralding the need for living together characterized by a symbiotic relationship. (Lamendola & Newman, 1994, p. 14)

In making the appeal that AIDS calls us to a reconceptualization of the nature of the self and greater interconnectedness on the interpersonal, community, and global level, Lamendola and Newman quoted Thompson (1989, p. 99), who states we need to "learn to tolerate aliens by seeing the self as a cloud in a clouded sky and not as a lord in a walled-in fortress."

The HEC perspective sees disease as an explication of the underlying implicit pattern of the person, family, or community. Disease can be part of the process of expanding consciousness (Newman 1994a, 1997a, 1997b). To provide a metaphorical illustration of how disease can be an explication of the underlying implicit pattern, Newman (1994a) uses Bohm's image of a fish tank with two video cameras focused on it—one from the narrow side of the tank and the other from the broad side. If two television screens were projecting the two images, they would project very different views of the movements of the fish, but the observer would get a sense of the underlying pattern. So, too, it is with disease and states of health—they are both explicit projections of the underlying pattern of the person or of the community.

INSIGHTS OCCURRING AS CHOICE POINTS OF ACTION POTENTIAL

Disease and other traumatic life events cause a disruption that can help a person, a family, or a community move into an expanded level of consciousness. To explain this phenomenon, Newman draws on the work of Ilya Prigogine (1976), whose Theory of Dissipative Structures asserts that a system fluctuates in an orderly manner until some disruption occurs and the system moves in a seemingly random, chaotic, disorderly way until at some point it chooses to move into a higher level of organization (Newman, 1997b). Nurses see this all the time—the patient who is lost to his work and has no time for his family or himself, and then suddenly has a heart attack, an experience that causes him to reflect on how he is using his energy and as a result his life pattern changes to become more creative, relational, and meaningful; or the person diagnosed with a terminal illness that causes her to reevaluate what is really important, attend to it, and then to state that for the first time she feels as though she is really living. The expansion of consciousness is an innate tendency of human beings; however, some experiences and processes precipitate more rapid transformations. Nurse researchers operating out of the HEC theory have clearly demonstrated how nurses can create a mutual partnership with their patients to reflect on the evolving pattern of their life. The insights gained in this process lead to an awakening and transformation to a higher level of consciousness (Dexheimer Pharris, in progress; Endo, 1998; Jonsdottir, 1998; Lamendola, 1998; Lamendola & Newman, 1994; Litchfield 1993, 1997; Moch, 1990; Newman, 1995; Newman & Moch, 1991; Noveletsky-Rosenthal, 1996; Tommet, 1997).

The disruption brought about by the presence of disease, illness, and traumatic or stressful events creates an opportunity for transformation to a higher, expanded level of consciousness (Newman, 1997b). This disrupted state presents a *choice point* for the person either to continue going on as before, even though the old rules are not working, or to shift into a new way of being. To explain the concept of a *choice point* more clearly, Newman draws on Arthur Young's (1976) Theory of Evolution of Consciousness. Young suggests that there are seven stages of binding and unbinding, which begin with total freedom and unrestricted choice, followed by a series of losses of freedom. After these losses comes a choice point and a reversal of the losses of freedom, ending with total freedom and unrestricted choice. These stages can be conceptualized as seven equidistant points on a V shape. Beginning at the uppermost point on the left is the first stage, *potential freedom.* The next stage is *binding*. In this stage, the individual is sacrificed for the sake of the collective, with no need for initiative because everything is being regulated for the individual. The third stage, *centering*, involves the development of an individual identity, self-consciousness, and self-determination. "Individualism emerges in the self's break with authority" (Newman 1994b). The fourth stage, *choice*, is situated at the base of the V. In this stage the individual learns that the old ways of being are no longer working. It is a stage of self-awareness, inner growth, and transformation. A new way of being becomes necessary. Newman (1994b) describes the fifth stage, *decentering*, as being characterized by a shift

. . . from the development of self (individuation) to dedication to something greater than the individual self. The person experiences outstanding competence; their works have a life of their own beyond the creator. The task is transcendence of the ego. Form is transcended, and the energy becomes the dominant feature—in terms of animation, vitality, a quality that is somehow infinite. Pattern is higher than form; the pattern can manifest itself in different forms. In this stage the person experiences the power of unlimited growth and has learned how to build order against the trend of disorder. (Newman, 1994b, pp. 45–46)

Newman (1994b) goes on to state that few experience the sixth stage, *unbinding*, or the seventh stage, *real freedom*, unless they have had these experiences of transcendence characterized by the fifth stage. Newman proposes a strong corollary between her Theory of Health as Expanding Consciousness and Young's Theory of the Evolution of Consciousness in that we "come into being from a state of potential consciousness, are bound in time, find our identity in space, and through movement we learn 'the law' of the way things work and make choices that ultimately take us beyond space and time to a state of absolute consciousness" (Newman 1994b, p. 46).

HEALTH AS EXPANDING CONSCIOUSNESS

The process of expanding consciousness is characterized by the evolving pattern of the person–environment interaction (Newman, 1994a). Consciousness is much more than just cognitive thought. Margaret Newman defines consciousness as:

. . . the information of the system: The capacity of the system to interact with the environment. In the human system the informational capacity includes not only all the things we normally associate with consciousness, such as thinking and feeling, but also all the information embedded in the nervous system, the immune system, the genetic code, and so on. The information of these and other systems reveals the complexity of the human system and how the information of the system interacts with the information of the environmental system. (Newman, 1994a, p. 33)

To illustrate consciousness as the interactional capacity of the person-environment, Newman (1994a) draws on the work of Bentov (1978), who presents consciousness on a continuum ranging from rocks, on one end of the spectrum (which have little interaction with their environment), to plants (which draw nutrients and provide carbon dioxide), to animals (which can move about and interact freely), to humans (who can reflect and make in-depth plans on how they want to interact with their environment), and ultimately to spiritual beings on the other end of the spectrum. Newman sees death as a transformation point, with a person's consciousness continuing to develop beyond the physical life, becoming a part of a universal consciousness after death (Newman, 1994a).

Nurses and their clients know that there has been an expansion of consciousness when there is a richer, more meaningful quality to their relationships. Relationships that are more open, loving, caring, connected, and peaceful are a manifestation of expanding consciousness. These deeper, more meaningful relationships may be interpersonal, or relationships with the wider community. The nurse and client may also see movement through Young's spectrum of evolving consciousness referred to earlier, where people transcend their own egos, dedicate their energy to something greater than the individual self, and learn to build order against the trend of disorder. In speaking of her experience with cancer, Chris Forth (1999) writes that it "has illuminated for me much of what is good in this world. It has allowed me to experience all that I hold precious in myself and those around me. It has encouraged me to find those things that are truly important and urged me to renew my participation in making our world a better place. It has presented me with a walk between life and death and a chance to see how right it is that they coexist. I will continue to live fully until my soul decides to fly free."

THE MUTUALITY OF THE NURSE–CLIENT INTERACTION IN THE PROCESS OF PATTERN RECOGNITION

We come to the meaning of the whole not by viewing the pattern from the outside, but by entering into the evolving pattern as it unfolds.

—M. A. Newman

Nursing out of the HEC perspective involves being fully present to the client without judgements, goals, or intervention strategies. It involves *being* rather than *doing*. It is caring in its deepest, most respectful sense. It is a mutual process of uncovering for meaning. The nurse-client interaction becomes like a pure reflection pool through which both the nurse and the client get a clear picture of their pattern and come away transformed by the insights gained.

To illustrate the mutually transforming effect of the nurse–client interaction, Newman (1994a) offers the image of a smooth lake into which two stones are thrown. As the stones hit the water, concentric waves circle out until the two patterns reach one another and interpenetrate. The new pattern of their interaction ripples back and transforms the two original circling patterns. Nurses are changed by their interactions with their clients, just as clients are changed by their interactions with nurses. This mutual transformation extends to the surrounding environment and relationships of the nurse and client.

In the process of doing this work, it is important that the nurse sense his or her own pattern. Newman states: "We have come to see nursing as a process of relationship that co-evolves as a function of the interpenetration of the evolving fields of the nurse, client, and the environment in a self-organizing, unpredictable way. We recognize the need for process wisdom, the ability to come from the center of our truth and act in the immediate moment" (Newman, 1994b, p. 155). Sensing one's own pattern is an essential starting point for the nurse. In her book *Health as Expanding Consciousness,* Newman (1994a, pp. 107–109) outlines a process of focusing to aid nurses as they begin working out of the HEC perspective. It is important that the nurse be able to practice from the center of his or her own truth and be fully present to the client. The nurse's consciousness, or pattern, becomes like the vibrations of a tuning fork that resonates at a centering frequency and the client has the opportunity to resonate and tune to that frequency during their interactions (Newman, 1994a; Quinn, 1992). The nurse–client relationship ideally continues until the client finds his or her own rhythmic vibrations without the need of the tuning fork. In other words, in the context of their interaction, the nurse and client get in touch with

> Nursing from the HEC perspective involves being fully present to the client, without judgements, goals, or intervention strategies. It is important that the nurse sense his or her own pattern.

their center, their power; and the interaction continues until the client is able to center by himself or herself.

HERMENEUTIC DIALECTIC METHOD OF RESEARCH

Margaret Newman describes her research methodology as hermeneutic dialectic—*hermeneutic* in that it focuses on meaning, interpretation, and understanding; and *dialectic* in that both the process and content are dialectic (Newman, 1997b). Guba and Lincoln (1989, p. 149) describe the dialectic process as representing "a comparison and contrast of divergent views with a view to achieving a higher synthesis of them all in the Hegelian sense." Hegel proposed that opposite points of view can come together and fuse into a new, synthesized view of reality (Newman, 1994a). It is in the contrast that pattern can be appreciated. For example, one cannot fully comprehend joy unless one has fully comprehended sorrow, and vice versa. Although they seem to be opposites, these two emotions are two manifestations of human connectedness. If you want to see a dark pattern more clearly, you would put it against a light background. The dialectic aspect of this methodology permits a nurse to be present to a client whose life circumstances are very different from those of the nurse. For example, the pattern recognition interaction for a homeless 16-year-old teenage boy from Bordeaux, France, with a female nurse from a very intact, loving family in Nigeria may provide clearer insight than with a young male nurse from Bordeaux, because less will be assumed and taken for granted. The Nigerian nurse will have to ask more clarifying questions and seek to understand that which has not

been her experience. This clarifying process, if done in an open, caring, and nonjudging manner, provides great insight for both participants in the pattern recognition process as they realize their interconnectedness. Because the nurse-client interaction is focused on attending to meaning, it transcends barriers of culture, gender, age, class, race, education, and ethnicity. The nurse is tapping into a way of relating that runs deeper than these barriers. The HEC theory focuses on the interconnectedness and common humanity of all people.

THE HEALTH AS EXPANDING CONSCIOUSNESS RESEARCH PROCESS

The process of pattern recognition for research purposes has been proposed in an appendix of *Health as Expanding Consciousness* (Newman, 1994a, pp. 147–149). It is summarized as follows:

The Interview: After the study has been explained and informed consent obtained, the data collection process begins with the nurse asking the participant a simple, open-ended question such as, "Tell me about the most meaningful people and events in your life." The interview proceeds in a nondirectional manner, with the nurse asking clarifying questions if necessary. The nurse researcher focuses on being fully present and sensing intuitively what to say or ask. Pauses are respected and attended to.

Transcription: Soon after the interview is completed, the nurse researcher transcribes the tape of the interview, including only the information that seems relevant to the participant's life pat-

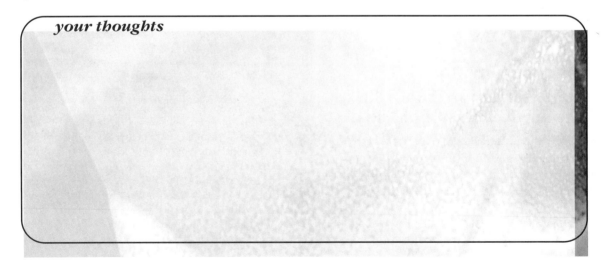

your thoughts

tern, but noting separately any information that was omitted, in case it becomes relevant after subsequent interviews.

The Narrative: The nurse researcher then organizes the transcribed data into a chronological narrative, highlighting the most significant events and persons. Pattern shifts and sequential patterns of significant relationships are noted.

Diagram: A diagram is drawn of the sequential patterns of relationships and transformation points. Although optional, this step has been found to be helpful in visualizing the pattern of the whole.

Follow-up: At the second interview the diagram (or other visual portrayal) is shared with the participant without any causal interpretation. The participant is given the opportunity to comment on what has been portrayed. This dialectic process is repeated in subsequent interviews, with data added to the narrative and the diagram redrawn until no further insight can be reached about the pattern of person–environment interaction. The pattern emerges in terms of the energy flow, for example, blocked, diffused, disorganized, and repetitive. It is important not to force pattern recognition; sometimes no signs of pattern recognition emerge, and if so, that characterizes the pattern for that particular person.

Application of the Theory: The HEC theory is applied throughout the process. It is the theory that guides the interaction. The theory is pervasive in the unfolding and grasping of insights. After completion of the interviews, the data are analyzed more intensely in light of the Theory of Health as Expanding Consciousness. Young's spectrum of consciousness is applied and the quality and complexity of the sequential patterns of interaction are evaluated. Similarities of pattern among participants are identified in terms of themes.

Newman (1994a, 1997a, 1997b) has clearly stated that this research is *research as praxis,* meaning that the researcher is an active participant in the research and helps the participant understand the meaning of his or her situation and its potential for action (Newman, 1997a). In this research, the researcher is also a practitioner. Newman states: "Not only is our science a *human science,* but, within the context of a practice

> **Research as praxis: The researcher is an active participant in the research and helps the participant understand the meaning of his or her situation and its potential for action.**

discipline, it is a science of *praxis*. This kind of theory is *embodied* in the investigator-nurse. It informs the situation being addressed by making a difference in the situation, as well as being informed by the data of the situation" (Newman, 1994b, p. 155).

THEORY AS MOVING INTUITION AND EVOLVING INSIGHTS

In some ways, writing a chapter about Margaret Newman's theory of nursing is like trying to convey the experience of a symphony by presenting only pages of the musical score. Only really well-trained musicians could hear the music in their minds, because they have been immersed in these sounds for many years. They understand the written symbols and are able to bring them to life. So, too, the words on these pages in and of themselves are one-dimensional and present only a glimpse of the spirit of what is trying to be conveyed; however, they represent a multidimensional reality and will become more clearly understood by those willing to immerse themselves in the praxis of the theory. The HEC theory has many dimensions: It is a lived experience, it has transformative power, and it is evolving. Newman states: "Theory for nursing practice is more than the application of single-dimension theories in specific practice situations. It is a matter of *the nurse's being transformed by the theory and thereby becoming a transforming partner in interaction with clients*" (Newman, 1994b, p. 156).

Margaret Newman's Theory of Health as Expanding Consciousness is being used throughout the world, but it has been more quickly embraced and understood by nurses from indigenous and Eastern cultures, who are less bound by linear, three-dimensional thought and physical concepts of health and who are more immersed in the metaphysical, mystical aspect of human existence.

Margaret Newman challenges nurses to take what they've learned from nursing theory as it exists and to go further. She states: "[T]heory is moving intuition, evolving insights" (Newman, 1997d, p. 9). Newman sees the "dialogic nature" of the theory to be (as Bohm, 1980, has suggested): "[I]t is *meaning flowing through* . . . the meaning is fluid and blends with each person's thinking once it has been shared."

Nurses who are interested in practicing and doing research out of the Health as Expanding Consciousness perspective would do well to read the book *Health as Expanding Consciousness* (Newman, 1994a), and to enter into dialogue with other nurses practicing from the Health as Expanding Consciousness theoretical perspective. There is also a web site with current works emanating from the Health as Expanding Consciousness theory. The website address is: www.tc.umnj.edu/~hoym0003/. The theory is being tested by nurses in many countries who are coming into a deeper understanding of the transformative power of Health as Expanding Consciousness research and practice for nurses, their clients, and their communities.

References

Bentov. I. (1978). *Stalking the wild pendulum.* New York: E. P. Dutton.

Bohm, D. (1980). *Wholeness and the implicate order.* London: Routledge & Kegan Paul.

Dexheimer Pharris, M. (in progress). *Life patterns of adolescent males convicted of murder.* Unpublished doctoral thesis, University of Minnesota, Minneapolis.

Endo, E. (1998). Pattern recognition as a nursing intervention with Japanese women with ovarian cancer. *Advances in Nursing Science, 20*(4), 49–61.

Forth, C. (1999, February 28). Illuminated by cancer. *Minneapolis Star Tribune,* p. A25.

Guba. E. G., & Lincoln, Y. S. (1989). *Fourth generation evaluation.* Newbury Park, CA: Sage Publications.

Jonsdottir, H. (1998). Life patterns of people with chronic obstructive pulmonary disease: Isolation and being closed in. *Nursing Science Quarterly, 11*(4), 160–166.

Lamendola, F. (1998). *Patterns of the caregiver experiences of selected nurses in hospice and HIV/AIDS care.* Unpublished doctoral thesis, University of Minnesota, Minneapolis.

Lamendola, F., & Newman, M. A. (1994). The paradox of HIV/AIDS as expanding consciousness. *Advances in Nursing Science, 16*(3), 13–21.

Litchfield, M. C. (1993). *The process of health patterning in families with young children who have been repeatedly hospitalized.* Unpublished master's thesis, University of Minnesota, Minneapolis.

Litchfield, M. C. (1997). *The process of nursing partnership in family health.* Unpublished doctoral thesis, University of Minnesota, Minneapolis.

Moch, S. D. (1990). Health within the experience of breast cancer. *Journal of Advanced Nursing, 15,* 1426–1435.

Newman, M. A. (1978). *Nursing theory.* (Audiotape of an address to the 2nd National Nurse Educator Conference in New York.) Chicago: Teach'em Inc.

Newman, M. A. (1979). *Theory development in nursing.* Philadelphia: F. A. Davis.

Newman, M. A. (1982). Time as an index of expanding consciousness with age. *Nursing Research, 31,* 290–293.

Newman, M. A. (1986). *Health as expanding consciousness.* St. Louis, MO: Mosby.

Newman, M. A. (1987). Aging as increasing complexity. *Journal of Gerontological Nursing, 12,* 16–18.

Newman, M. A. (1990). Newman's theory of health as praxis. *Nursing Science Quarterly, 3,* 37–41.

Newman, M. A. (1994a). *Health as expanding consciousness* (2nd ed.). Boston: Jones & Bartlett (formerly, New York: National League for Nursing Press).

Newman, M. A. (1994b). Theory for nursing practice. *Nursing Science Quarterly, 7*(4), 153–157.

Newman, M. A. (1995). Recognizing a pattern of expanding consciousness in persons with cancer. In *A developing discipline* (pp. 159–171). Boston: Jones & Bartlett (formerly, New York: National League for Nursing Press).

Newman, M. A. (1997a). Experiencing the whole. *Advances in Nursing Science, 20*(1): 34–39.

Newman, M. A. (1997b). Evolution of the theory of health as expanding consciousness. *Nursing Science Quarterly, 10*(1), 22–25.

Newman, M. A. (1997c). Margaret Newman: Health as expanding consciousness. In Fuld Institute for Technology in Nursing Education, *The Nurse Theorists: Portraits of Excellence* [CD-ROM]. Athens, OH: FITNE, Inc.

Newman, M. A. (1997d). A dialogue with Martha Rogers and David Bohm about the science of unitary human beings. In Madrid, M. (Ed.), *Patterns of Rogerian knowing* (pp. 3–10). New York: National League for Nursing Press.

Newman. M. A., & Moch, S. D. (1991). Life patterns of persons with coronary heart disease. *Nursing Science Quarterly, 4,* 161–167.

Newman, M. A., Sime, A. M., & Corcoran-Perry, S. A. (1991). The focus of the discipline of nursing. *Advances in Nursing Science, 14*(1), 1–6.

Noveletsky-Rosenthal, H. T. (1996). *Pattern recognition in older adults living with chronic illness.* Unpublished doctoral thesis, Boston College.

Prigogine, I. (1976). Order through fluctuation: Self-organization and social system. In Jantsch, E. & Waddington, C. H. (Eds.), *Evolution and consciousness* (pp. 93–133). Reading, MA: Addison-Wesley.

Quinn, J. F. (1992). Holding sacred space. The nurse as healing environment. *Holistic Nursing Practice, 6*(4), 26–36.

Rogers, M. E. (1970). *An introduction to the theoretical basis of nursing.* Philadelphia: F. A. Davis.

Rogers, M. E. (1990). Nursing science and the space age. *Nursing Science Quarterly, 5*(1), 27–34.

Thompson, W. I. (1989). *Imaginary landscape: Making worlds of myth and science.* New York: St. Martin's Press.

Tommet, P. A. (1997). *Nurse-parent dialogue: Illuminating the pattern of families with children who are medically fragile.* Unpublished doctoral thesis, University of Minnesota, Minneapolis.

Young, A. M. (1976). *The reflexive universe: Evolution of consciousness.* San Francisco, CA: Robert Briggs Associates.

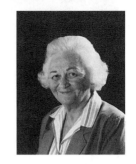

Chapter 17 Part 1

Imogene M. King
Theory of Goal Attainment

- ❖ Introducing the Theorist
- ❖ Worldview: Conceptual System and Middle-Range Theory of Goal Attainment
- ❖ Initial Ideas: The Beginning
- ❖ Philosophy of Science
- ❖ Design of a Conceptual System
- ❖ Theory of Goal Attainment
- ❖ Summary
- ❖ References

Imogene M. King

INTRODUCING THE THEORIST

My beginnings as the youngest of three children started in a small midwestern community in a family filled with love and joy. As children, we learned that honesty and respect for each individual were valued. My parents were always available to support and guide us as we set goals. We learned that goal-setting helped us make positive decisions in our journey through life. We were taught at home to look at the consequences of our decisions before finalizing plans. We learned how to work hard and play hard and to know the difference. Many of these values were reinforced in formal education; the details may be found in a book edited by Thelma Schorr and Ann Zimmerman, entitled *Making Choices, Taking Chances* (1990).

Postsecondary education experiences included a diploma in nursing from St. John's Hospital School of Nursing in St. Louis; the baccalaureate and master's degrees in nursing from St. Louis University; and the doctor of education from Teachers College, Columbia University, New York. Postdoctoral study included work in advanced statistics, systems research, and computers. Continuing education is an ongoing process. My avocation includes nursing history in the context of world history, and philosophy with emphasis on science and ethics. To this day, I enjoy life that includes music, the theater, golf, and swimming. In addition, I am an artist and work in oils and acrylics.

The majority of nursing experience, which spans over 50 years, included clinical practice of nursing adults in hospitals. While working my way through college, I worked in a physician's office, as a school nurse, and as an occupational health nurse. I have always believed that as a teacher one must also be an excellent practitioner so my experience as a teacher of nursing at undergraduate and graduate levels included practice. I taught at Loyola University, Chicago; the Ohio State University; and the University of South Florida, advancing from assistant professor to full professor and now as professor emeritus.

Multiple honors and awards have been given to me and can be reviewed in *Who's Who in America, American Women,* and *Who's Who in Nursing.* The most recent are the Jessie Scott Award for Leadership, presented by the American Nurses Association at the 100th anniversary convention in 1996, and an honorary doctor of science degree in 1998. My peers at the house of delegates at the Florida Nurses Association voted in 1996 to give me lifetime membership. The University of Tampa Department of Nursing named the annual research award given to students the Imogene M. King Research Award. I was honored at the 75th anniversary convention of Sigma Theta Tau International with a research grant named for me and with a program that presented a description of me as a caring individual.

A question that continues to be asked is: What contribution do you think you have made to the nursing profession? My response is: I have taught thousands of students who have become leaders and practitioners, teachers and researchers. In addition, I have been involved in the scientific movement in nursing and have developed a conceptual system from which a theory of goal attainment has been derived, including a transaction process model leading to outcomes. These ideas are useful for measuring practice-based outcomes.

WORLDVIEW: CONCEPTUAL SYSTEM AND MIDDLE-RANGE THEORY OF GOAL ATTAINMENT
by Imogene M. King

Continuous discoveries in telecommunications and technology, and a daily bombardment of information about world events bring complexity to one's life that is unprecedented in history. Instant communication reminds us that we live in an information processing world of systems: "A system is defined as a series of functional components connected by communication links exhibiting purposeful goal-directed behavior" (King, 1996). As individuals, we are born, grow, and develop within each nation. Nations make up the world society. A sense of a global community can be understood as we view the interactions of individuals and groups with linguistic, ethnic, and religious differences. The commonality in this worldview is the human being. How is this global community and health care related to theory construction and testing in research in nursing?

The commonality in my worldview is human beings who communicate and interact in their small groups within their nations' social systems, that is, human environments as well as physical environments. Three dynamic interacting systems, shown in Figure 17-1, represent individuals as personal systems, groups as interpersonal systems, and large groups as social systems that make up most societies in the world (King, 1981). These systems represent interconnected links for information processing in a high-tech world of health care and nursing. This conceptual system provides one approach to structure a world community of human beings. Human beings are the recipients of nursing care.

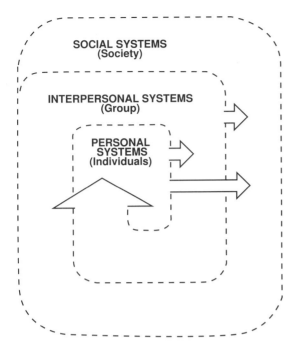

Figure 17–1 *King's conceptual system.*

A review of my ideas about developing theoretical knowledge for nursing is presented in this chapter. A process for developing a conceptual system is explained. The method used to derive a theory of goal attainment from my conceptual system is demonstrated. The use of this conceptual system and Theory of Goal Attainment in practice, education, research, and administration is described in many nurses' publications. The application of this theory is also discussed in the second part of this chapter.

INITIAL IDEAS: THE BEGINNING

My first theory publication made pronouncements about the problems and prospect of knowledge development in nursing (King, 1964). Over 30 years ago, the problems were identified as: (1) lack of a professional nursing language; (2) nursing phenomena appeared to be atheoretical; and (3) concept development was limited. The nursing informatics movement continues to identify a professional nursing language system (King, 1998). Theories and conceptual frameworks have identified theoretical approaches to knowledge development and utilization of knowledge in practice. Concept development is a continuous process in the nursing science movement (King, 1988).

My rationale for developing a schematic representation of nursing phenomena was influenced by the

Howland Systems Model (Howland, 1976) and the Howland and McDowell conceptual framework (Howland & McDowell, 1964). The levels of interaction in these authors' work influenced my ideas relative to organizing a conceptual frame of reference for nursing, as shown in Figure 17–1. Because concepts offer one approach to structure knowledge for nursing, a comprehensive review of nursing literature provided ideas for me to identify five comprehensive concepts as a basis for a conceptual system for nursing. The overall concept is a human being, commonly referred to as an "individual" or a "person." Initially, I selected abstract concepts of perception, communication, interpersonal relations, health, and social institutions (King, 1968). These ideas forced me to review my knowledge of philosophy relative to the nature of human beings (ontology) and the nature of knowledge (epistemology).

> The goal of nursing is to help individuals and groups attain, maintain, and regain a healthy state.

PHILOSOPHY OF SCIENCE

In the late 1960s, while auditing a series of courses in systems research, I was introduced to a philosophy of science called General System Theory (Von Bertalanffy, 1968). This philosophy of science gained momentum in the 1950s, although its roots date to an earlier period. This philosophy refuted logical positivism and reductionism and proposed the idea of isophomorphism and perspectivism in knowledge development. Von Bertalanffy, credited with originating the idea of General System Theory, defined this philosophy of science movement as a "general science of wholeness: systems of elements in mutual interaction" (Von Bertalanffy, 1968, p. 37).

My philosophical position is rooted in General System Theory, which guides the study of organized complexity as whole systems. This philosophy gave me the impetus to focus on knowledge development as an information-processing, goal-seeking, and decision-making system. General System Theory provides a holistic approach to study nursing phenomena as an open system and frees one's thinking from the parts versus whole dilemma. In any discussion of the nature of nursing, the central ideas revolve around the nature of human beings and their interaction with internal and external environments. During this journey through a wilderness of ideas, I began to conceptualize a theory for nursing. However, because a manuscript was due in the publisher's office,

I organized my ideas into a conceptual system (formerly called a "conceptual framework") and the result was the publication of a book entitled *Toward a Theory of Nursing* (King, 1971).

DESIGN OF A CONCEPTUAL SYSTEM

A conceptual system provides structure for organizing multiple ideas into meaningful wholes. From my initial set of ideas in 1968 and 1971, my conceptual framework was refined to show some unity and relationships among the concepts. In addition, the next step in this process was to review the research literature in the discipline in which the concepts had been studied. For example, the concept of perception has been studied in psychology for many years. The literature indicated that most of the early studies dealt with sensory perception. Around the 1950s, psychologists began to study interpersonal perception, which related to my ideas about interactions. From this research literature, I identified the characteristics of perception and defined the concept for my framework. I continued this search of literature for knowledge of each of the concepts in my framework. An update on my conceptual system was published in 1995 (King, 1995).

Process for Developing a Concept

"Searching for scientific knowledge in nursing is an ongoing dynamic process of continuous identification, development, and validation of relevant concepts" (King, 1975). What is a concept? A *concept* is an organization of reference points. Words are the verbal symbols used to explain events and things in our environment and relationships to past experiences. Northrop (1969) noted: "[C]oncepts fall into different types according to the different sources of their meaning. . . . A concept is a term to which meaning has been assigned." Concepts are the categories in a theory.

> King's theory uses concepts of self, perception, communication, interaction, transaction, role, and decision making.

The concept development and validation process used by me to develop knowledge and taught to more than 1000 graduate students in the past 30 years is as follows:

1. Review, analyze, and synthesize research literature related to the concept.

2. From the above review, identify the characteristics (attributes) of the concept.

3. From the characteristics, write a conceptual definition.

4. Review literature to select an instrument or develop an instrument.

5. Design a study to measure the characteristics of the concept.

6. Decisions are made on selection of the population to be sampled.

7. Collect data.

8. Analyze and interpret data.

9. Write results of findings and conclusions.

10. State implications for adding to nursing knowledge.

Concepts that represent phenomena in nursing are structured within a framework and a theory to show relationships.

King's Conceptual System

Twelve concepts—self, body image, role, perception, communication, interaction, transaction, growth and development, power, authority, organization, and decision making—were identified from my analysis of nursing literature (King, 1981). The concepts that provided substantive knowledge about human beings were placed within the personal system, those related to groups were placed within the interpersonal system, and those related to large groups that make up a society were placed within the social system. However, knowledge from all of the concepts is used in nurses' interactions with individuals and groups within social organizations, such as the family, the educational system, and the political system. Knowledge of these concepts came from my synthesis of research in many disciplines. These concepts are abstract. It is difficult to apply a conceptual system, which is someone's abstraction of reality. Concepts, when defined from research literature, give nurses knowledge that can be applied in the concrete world of nursing. The concepts represent basic knowledge that nurses use in their role and functions either in practice, or education, or administration. In addition, the concepts provide ideas for research in nursing.

One of my goals was to identify what I call the essence of nursing. That brought me back to the question: What is the nature of human beings? A vicious circle? Not really! Because nurses are first and foremost other human beings and give nursing care to human beings, my philosophy of the nature of human beings has been presented along with assumptions I have made about individuals (King, 1989a). Recognizing that a conceptual system represents structure for a discipline, the next step in the process of knowledge development was to derive one or more theories from this structure. Lo and behold, a theory of goal attainment was developed (King, 1981, 1992). More recently, several dissertations, by Frey (1995), Sieloff (1995), and Killeen (1996), have derived theories from my conceptual system.

THEORY OF GOAL ATTAINMENT

Generally speaking, the goal of nursing care is to help individuals maintain health or regain health (King, 1990). Concepts are essential elements in theories. When a theory is derived from a conceptual system, concepts are selected from that system. Remember my question: What is the essence of nursing? The concepts of self, perception, communication, interaction, transaction, role, and decision making were selected. Self is an individual whose perception and role influence that person's communication, interaction, and decision making in small and large groups. So, what is the health-care system within which nurses function? Is it a social system of individuals and groups interacting to achieve goals related to health? A transaction model, shown in Figure 17–2, was developed that represented the process whereby individuals interact to mutually set goals that result in goal attainment (King, 1981).

As the twenty-first century begins, cost containment appears to be the primary goal of health-care administrators and insurance companies. If the goals and the means to achieve them are mutually agreed upon by nurses and patients, 99% of the time, goals will be achieved (King, 1989b). Goal attainment represents outcomes. Outcomes indicate effective nursing care. Nursing care is a critical element to provide quality care that is also cost-effective. Using the transaction process model is one way to achieve this goal.

Transaction Process Model

The model shown in Figure 17–2 is a human process than can be observed in many situations when two or more people interact, such as in the family and in social events (King, 1996). As nurses, we bring knowledge and skills that influence our perceptions, communications, and interactions in performing the functions of the role. Stop reading now and engage someone in conversation. Then analyze your behavior to determine whether you used this process. In your role as a nurse, after interacting with a patient,

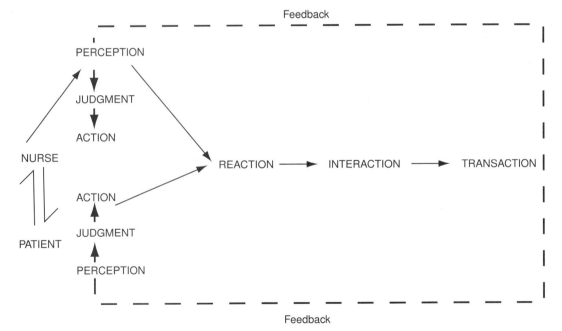

Figure 17–2 *Transaction process model. From King, I. M. (1981).* A Theory for Nursing: Systems, Concepts, Process. *New York: John Wiley & Sons, Inc., p. 145.*

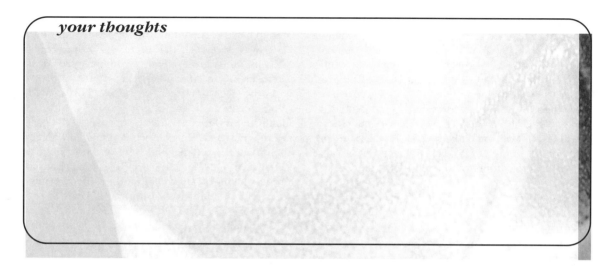

your thoughts

sit down and write down your behavior and that of the patient. It is my belief that you can identify your perceptions, mental judgments, mental action, and reaction (negative or positive). Did you make a transaction? That is, did you exchange information and set a goal with the patient? Did you explore the means for the patient to use to achieve the goal? Was the goal achieved? If not, why not? It is my opinion that most nurses use this process but are not aware that it is based in a nursing theory. With knowledge of the concepts and the process, nurses have a scientific base for practice that can be articulated clearly and documented to show quality care. How can a nurse document this transaction model in practice?

Documentation System

A documentation system was designed to implement the transaction process that leads to goal attainment (King, 1984a). Most nurses use the nursing process of assess, diagnose, plan, implement, and evaluate, which I call a method. My transaction process provides the theoretical knowledge base to implement this method. For example, as one assesses the patient and the environment and makes a nursing diagnosis, the concepts of perception, communication, and interaction represent knowledge the nurse uses to gather information and make a judgment. A transaction is made when the nurse and patient decide mutually on the goals to be attained, agree on the means to attain goals that represent the plan of care, and then implement the plan. Evaluation determines whether or not goals were attained. If not, you ask why not, and the process begins again. The documentation is recorded directly in the patient's chart. The patient's record indicates the process used to achieve goals. On discharge, the summary indicates goals set and goals achieved. One does not need multiple forms to complete when this documentation system is in place and the quality of nursing care is recorded. Why do nurses insist on designing critical paths, various care plans, and other types of forms when, with knowledge of this system, the nurse documents nursing care directly on the patient's chart? Why do we use multiple forms to complicate a process that is knowledge-based and also provides essential data to demonstrate outcomes and to evaluate quality nursing care?

Federal laws have been passed that indicate that patients must be involved in decisions about their care and about dying. This transaction process provides a scientifically based process to help nurses implement federal laws such as the Patient Self-Determination Act. It is my humble opinion that every student should be taught this transaction process as we move into the twenty-first century. In addition, every practicing nurse should be taught this process. This is what is meant when nurses say we must articulate the scientific basis for our practice. This process is also useful in education in the student-teacher relationship. In addition, the process is very useful in staff-administrator relationships. How can one measure goal attainment?

Goal Attainment Scale

Analysis of nursing research literature in the 1970s revealed that very few instruments were designed for nursing research. In the late 1980s, the faculty at the University of Maryland, experts in measurement and evaluation, applied for and received a grant to conduct conferences to teach nurses to design reliable and valid instruments. I had the privilege of participating in this 2-year continuing education conference, where I developed a Goal Attainment Scale (King, 1989b). This instrument may be used to measure goal attainment. It may also be used as an assessment tool to provide patient data to plan and implement nursing care.

In summary, a systematic approach to develop a conceptual system from which a theory was derived has been explained. This has provided one approach to structure scientific knowledge and use a process that leads to outcomes. The Transaction Process Model in the Theory of Goal Attainment indicates a way in which goal attainment may be predicted. A documentation system and goal attainment scale were constructed to implement the nursing process as method and the transaction process as theoretical knowledge to accompany the method.

Use of King's Conceptual System and Theory

There has been no change in the conceptual system or theory except to add the concept of coping in the personal system. The word "spiritual" was added to my assumptions about human beings. This was in my original manuscript in 1971 but was accidentally omitted in the publication (King, 1995).

Over the years of presenting my ideas at theory conferences throughout the world, nurses have asked many excellent questions, which I have tried to answer. Initially, the questions pertained to "How do I implement this in practice?" This motivated me to design the documentation system to show the relationship between the nursing process as method and my nursing process as theory. Prior to presenting this at a national meeting, several staff nurses tested this and suggested this system be implemented in practice. I reminded the nurses that they were not applying a theory, but were applying the knowledge of the concepts of the theory. This has become a repetitive statement of mine; that is, one cannot apply an abstraction, which is what conceptual frameworks, models, and theories represent. What one applies is the knowledge of the concepts of the structure and process proposed in the abstractions. The last thing I had to do before retiring from a full-time teaching position was to design an instrument to measure goal attainment. The use of my ideas in practice, education, administration, and research is shown in articles in a variety of nursing journals.

Nursing Education

My first faculty position following completion of a doctor of education degree at Teachers College, Columbia University, New York, in 1961, was appoint-

ment as an assistant professor at Loyola University, Chicago. Because my area of study was curriculum and instruction, I was selected to chair a faculty committee to develop a curriculum leading to a master of science degree in nursing. This was one of the first master's programs that used a nursing framework to design a curriculum. The theoretical model was designed by a nurse as part of a dissertation from the University of California (Kaufman, 1958). The model was composed of three concepts—time, stress, and perception. Needless to say, this approach to develop a new graduate program appeared to be revolutionary in 1961. This activity provided the impetus for me to reflect on my knowledge of curriculum and instruction, and also to think about structure for organizing undergraduate and graduate nursing programs. The rest is history and is recorded in my books and articles over the past 30 years (King, 1986a).

In the 1970s the professional nursing staff at the National League for Nursing conducted conferences to disseminate information about the curriculum process for developing or revising a baccalaureate nursing program (King, 1978). The major components in a curriculum discussed at these conferences were "a philosophy, conceptual framework, course objectives, and evaluation of the curriculum" (National League for Nursing, 1978).

The scope of knowledge is so vast that it is impossible to teach students everything they need to learn to begin to practice nursing today and tomorrow. It is imperative that nursing curricula be based on a conceptual framework. Such curricula must be structured to provide students with the essential concepts, skills, and values that serve as foundations and as catalysts to continue to learn after graduation (National League for Nursing, 1978).

As a participant observer who provided administrative support for a faculty engaged in constructing a new undergraduate curriculum, I witnessed the development of a curriculum that moved nursing education into the future (Daubenmire & King, 1973). This baccalaureate nursing curriculum, based on my conceptual framework, was published in 1989. According to Daubenmire (1989, p. 167), "[T]he curriculum model and conceptual framework implemented in 1970 based on King's theory have remained essentially the same for about 15 years except for updating knowledge from year to year. King's framework, continues to provide a viable curriculum strategy. A curriculum model which is conceptually based allows for updating content and skills without the necessity for major curriculum change."

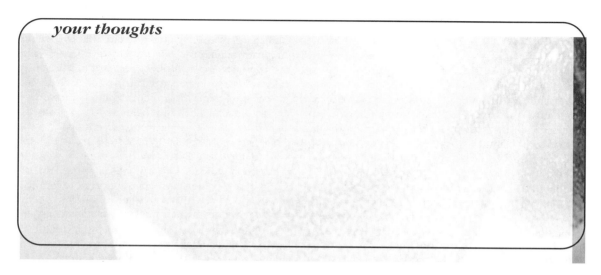

One of the criteria used to develop nursing curricula in colleges and universities is a clear statement of a philosophy consistent with the institution offering the nursing program. The philosophy is essential for faculty to identify a conceptual framework and program objectives. A study was conducted in order to identify the major terms used in stated philosophies in nursing programs to attempt to describe the philosophical foundations of nursing. A random sample of schools of nursing, stratified by type of program and by region of the country, was selected from the National League for Nursing's published list of accredited baccalaureate, associate degree, and diploma nursing programs. A pilot study was conducted from which a classification resulted in the formation of 12 categories (King, 1984b). A table of random numbers was used to select 20% of the schools within each category, distributed according to region and type of program. The conclusion reported differences in use of the terms "man," "health," "perception," "role," "social systems," and "God" by type of program. Use of the terms "man," "role," "social systems," and "God" differed by location of the program in a university, community college, and hospital. The findings of this national survey provided some information about similarities and differences in major terms used in statements of philosophy. The terms "nursing," "environment," and "interpersonal relations" did not differ significantly, which indicated a few commonalities in those three programs. However, differences in statements of philosophy imply differences in curricula, which in turn provide different kinds of education for different kinds of nursing practice. This study, done over 15 years ago, raised the questions: What is the philosophy of nursing education? Has a philosophy of nursing education changed historically?

A publishing company asked me to write a curriculum book. In the 1980s, articulation between associate degree nursing programs and baccalaureate programs seemed to be a problem. Using my conceptual framework, I designed a hypothetical baccalaureate degree program and an associate degree program to begin to identify differences and commonalities, because the same structure was used. My idea was to show clear and reasonable articulation between the two programs when the same conceptual framework is used. It would be interesting for a faculty group to design a curriculum in a university today that offers both a baccalaureate and an associate degree program to test out this hypothetical curriculum (King, 1986b).

In 1988 a colleague discussed with me the complexity and variety in health care and nursing, and we agreed that a conceptualization of substantive knowledge for curriculum development was essential in order to move into the twenty-first century. We explored ideas about a philosophy of nursing education, a conceptual framework that identified interacting systems, individuals, groups, and social systems and the concepts that identified substantive knowledge. Examples of objectives were cited that reflected our philosophy and conceptual framework. A process of interactions that leads to transactions and goal attainment was explored. We agreed that the use of my conceptual framework and Theory of Goal Attainment provided an approach to develop a curriculum that is an open system based on a general system framework and theory. When curricula are developed that identify common concepts (knowledge), skills, and professional values, the practice of professional nursing will be the center of health care in the twenty-first century. Increased technology and knowledge require a conceptually based curriculum for the future (Gulitz & King, 1988).

Practice

In the past 10 years, nurses have published their use of my conceptual system and Theory of Goal Attainment in practice. Some nurses have used knowledge of the concepts to implement theory-based practice (Coker & Schreiber, 1989; Hanna, 1995; Messmer, 1995; Smith, 1988).

The goal of nursing is to help individuals and groups attain, maintain, and regain a healthy state: "In nursing situations where the goal of life and health cannot be achieved, as in a terminal illness, nurses give care and help individuals die with dignity" (King, 1971). My systems framework has described a holistic view of the complexity in nursing within various groups, in different types of health care systems. This framework differs from other conceptual schema in that it is concerned not with fragmenting human beings and the environment but with human transactions in different types of environments (King, 1995). A few examples from the literature are given.

Family Health

The use of my conceptual system and Theory of Goal Attainment in family health was suggested (King, 1983). The family is usually the immediate social environment in which individuals grow and develop and learn through interactions to set goals. Nurses work with families and with individual members of families. The family is seen as a social system, a group of interacting individuals. The family is also viewed as an interpersonal system. For example, nurses' perception of family members and family members' perception of the nurse influence their responses in situations and their openness in giving information. Congruence in perceptions of nurse and family members helps in assessing a situation to identify concerns and/or problems in the interpersonal system. Knowledge of a concept of role is essential and related to growth and development, and to stress in family environments. Two cases were presented and the use of the Theory of Goal Attainment was described in each situation.

Community Health

At the Eighth Annual Community Health Nursing Conference (1984) in North Carolina (King, 1984b), I presented the use of my conceptual system and Theory of Goal Attainment in community health nursing. Community health nursing involves a variety of populations within a variety of social systems.

For example, school nurses must understand the education system. Occupational health nurses must understand the political system, the economic system, and the belief system in a community. Some nurses have used the Transaction Process Model in the Theory of Goal Attainment in community health programs as they interact and set goals with interdisciplinary teams to manage health care (Hampton, 1994; Sowell & Fuszard, 1989; Sowell & Lowenstein, 1994). Nurses in community health focus on different populations. In this sense, they are relating to the interpersonal systems in the framework. This is done within a variety of social systems in the community. Although the focus is groups, nurses work with individuals for whom they provide services. My conceptual system (Fig. 17-1) shows the interactions of the three systems in community health.

Use in Hospitals

Two case studies were presented to demonstrate nurses' use of the transaction process and knowledge of the concepts of perception, communication, interaction, and role (King, 1986b). Nurses in a Canadian hospital used the framework to structure the delivery of nursing care. They determined that nurses could identify the published nursing diagnoses in 1990 with the concepts in the framework (Coker et al., 1990). Nurses in Canada in which two hospitals were involved at a distance from each other used the conceptual framework to design a system for delivery of nursing care (Fawcett, Vaillancourt, & Watson, 1995). A director of nursing research and education in a large municipal hospital in the United States reported the implementation of theory-based nursing practice using my conceptual system (Messmer, 1995). Theory-based practice in an emergency department used my framework and Theory of Goal Attainment (Benedict & Frey, 1995). The Theory of Goal Attainment was used in adult orthopedic nursing (Alligood, Evans, & Wilt, 1995).

The transaction process was used in short-term group psychotherapy settings. Laben and colleagues (Laben, Dodd, & Sneed, 1991) stated that my interactive systems approach of goal attainment is an ideal basis for short-term group psychotherapy. This group used my theory with inpatient juvenile sexual offenders, offenders in maximum security, and community parolees.

Research

A sample of studies that have been published that test the Theory of Goal Attainment is cited. In addition, several dissertations have derived theories from my conceptual system.

Several nurses have tested the theory in research in aging, parenting, psychiatric-mental health, and ambulatory care (Alligood et al., 1995; Benedict & Frey, 1995; Norris & Hoyer, 1993; Woods, 1994). Nurses in Japan, Sweden, and Canada have conducted studies in their cultures to test the Theory of Goal Attainment (Coker et al., 1990; Kameoka, 1995; Rooke, 1995).

A theory of power for nursing administration was developed by Sieloff (1995). Frey (1995) proposed a theory of family, children, and chronic illness and continues to test it in research. Killeen's dissertation (1996) studied patient-consumer perceptions and responses to professional nursing care resulted in an instrument that measures patient satisfaction.

Continuous Quality Improvement

Continuous quality improvement in nursing and health care is a reality. Three major categories have been suggested as a way to develop a program. These elements are: (1) structure, (2) process, and (3) outcomes. *Structure* provides an overall organization of the program. *Process* relates to nursing activities. *Outcomes* are separate from but related to performance criteria for evaluation of nursing care and nurses' performance. My conceptual system provides structure for a continuous quality improvement program (King, 1994). The Transaction Process Model in my Theory of Goal Attainment gives a process that leads to goal attainment that represents outcomes. Outcomes indicate effective nursing care. An example was given to document effectiveness of nursing care if one uses a goal-oriented nursing record (King, 1984a). The record system is an information system based on my Theory of Goal Attainment. The record system can be designed and adapted to most health-care systems. For nurses, it was designed to gather data from assessments of the patient, make a nursing diagnosis, construct a goal list, write orders for nursing care, and write mutually agreed-upon goals and means to attain them. Goals that are achieved are outcomes and represent effective nursing care. Elements in the goal-oriented nursing record are: (1) data base, (2) goal list, (3) nursing orders, (4) flow sheets, (5) progress notes, and (6) discharge summary. This information system can be designed for any patient population and for current and future computerization of records in a health-care system.

Summary

The health-care system in the United States is in constant flux in an attempt to restructure health-care delivery. How can a conceptual system and the Theory of Goal Attainment provide the structure, process, and outcomes that represent a way to manage and deliver quality health care for all citizens? My conceptual system and transaction process in the Theory of Goal Attainment provides one approach to accomplish the goal of access and quality in the following ways:

1. For interaction between nurses and health-care professionals and between health-care agencies for continuity of care, respect for roles and responsibilities of each health profession; for case management, and collaborative and integrated practice.
2. Essential knowledge to assess, diagnose, plan, implement, and evaluate care.
3. For common discourse among health professionals and between nurses and nursing personnel.
4. A framework within health-care systems and between health care providers and agencies.
5. Direct measure of outcomes resulting in quality care and cost-effective care; that is, goals are set and goals are attained.
6. A systematic and efficient documentation system.
7. One valid and reliable assessment instrument to assess activities of daily living as a basis for goal-setting.
8. For continuity of care within and between health-care agencies.
9. Results in satisfaction for patients, families, physicians, and administrators.

When knowledge of the concepts and the transaction process has been used in hospitals, homes, nursing homes, and community health agencies, nurses have been motivated to seek additional knowledge in formal educational programs.

Vision for the Future

My vision for the future of nursing is that nursing will provide access to health care for all citizens. The United States health-care system will be structured using my conceptual system. Entry into the system will be via nurses' assessment so individuals are directed to the right place in the system for nursing care, medical care, social services information, health teaching, or rehabilitation. My transaction process will be used by every practicing nurse so that goals can be achieved to demonstrate quality care that is cost-effective. My conceptual system, Theory of Goal Attainment, and Transaction Process Model will continue to serve a useful purpose in delivering professional nursing care. The ideas have been tested in research and in practice, and knowledge of the concepts has been used by nurses in education and practice. The relevance of evidence theory–based practice, using my theory, has been shown to join the art of nursing of the twentieth century to the science of nursing in the twenty-first century.

References

Alligood, M., Evans, G. W., & Wilt, D. L. (1995). King's interacting system and empathy. In Frey, M. A., & Sieloff, C. L. (Eds.), *Advancing King's systems framework and theory of nursing* (p. 64). Thousand Oaks, CA: Sage.

Benedict, M., & Frey, M. A. (1995). Theory-based practice in the emergency department. In Frey, M. A., & Sieloff, C. L. (Eds.), *Advancing King's systems framework and theory of nursing* (p. 327). Thousand Oaks, CA: Sage.

Coker, E. A., & Schreiber, R. (1989). King at the bedside. *The Canadian Nurse*, 24.

Coker, E., Fradley, T., Harris, J., Tomarchio, D., Chan, V., & Caron, C. (1990). Implementing nursing diagnoses within the context of King's conceptual framework. *Nursing Diagnosis, 1*, 107.

Daubenmire, M. J. (1989). A baccalaureate nursing curriculum based on King's conceptual framework. In Riehl-Sisca, J. (Ed.), *Conceptual models for nursing practice* (p. 167). New York: Appleton & Lange.

Daubenmire, M. J., & King, I. M. (1973). Nursing process models: A systems approach. *Nursing Outlook, 21,* 512.

Fawcett, J. M., Vaillancourt, V. M., & Watson, C. A. (1995). Integration of King's framework into nursing practice. In Frey, M. A., & Sieloff, C. L. (Eds.), *Advancing King's systems framework and theory of goal attainment* (p. 176). Thousand Oaks, CA: Sage.

Frey, M. A. (1995). Toward a theory of families, children, and chronic illness. In Frey, M. A., & Sieloff, C. L. (Eds.), *Advancing King's systems framework and theory of nursing* (p. 109). Thousand Oaks, CA: Sage.

Gulitz, E. A., & King, I. M. (1988). King's general system model: Application to curriculum development. *Nursing Science Quarterly, 1,* 128.

Hampton, D. C. (1994). King's theory of goal attainment as a framework for managed care implementation in a hospice setting. *Nursing Science Quarterly, 7,* 170.

Hanna, U. M. (1995). Use of King's Theory of Goal Attainment to promote adolescents' health behavior. In Frey, M. A., & Sieloff, C. L. (Eds.), *Advancing King's system framework and theory of goal attainment* (p. 239). Thousand Oaks, CA: Sage.

Howland, D. (1976). An adaptive health system model. In Werley, H. H., et al. (Ed.), *Health systems research: The systems approach* (p. 109). New York: Springer Publishing.

Howland, D., & McDowell, W. (1964). A measurement of patient care: A conceptual framework. *Nursing Research, 13*(4), 320–324.

Kameoka, T. (1995). Analyzing nurse-patient interactions in Japan. In Frey, M. A., & Sieloff, C. L. (Eds.), *Advancing King's system framework and Theory of Goal Attainment* (p. 251). Thousand Oaks, CA: Sage.

Kaufman, M. (1958). *Identification of a theoretical basis for nursing practice.* Unpublished doctoral dissertation, University of California, Los Angeles.

Killeen, M. (1996). *Patient-consumer perceptions and responses to professional nursing care: Instrument development.* Unpublished doctoral dissertation, University of Michigan, Detroit.

King, I. M. (1964). Nursing theory: Problems and propect. *Nursing Science Quarterly, 2,* 294.

King, I. M. (1968). A conceptual frame of reference for nursing. *Nursing Research, 17,* 27–31.

King, I. M. (1971). *Toward a theory of nursing.* New York: John Wiley.

King, I. M. (1975). A process for developing concepts for nursing through research. In. Verhonick, P. J., (Ed.), *Nursing Research* (p. 25). Boston: Little, Brown.

King, I. M. (1978). How does the conceptual framework provide structure for the curriculum? In *Curriculum process for developing or revising a baccalaureate nursing program.* New York: National League for Nursing, pp. 23–34.

King, I. M. (1981). *A theory of goal attainment: Systems, concepts, process.* New York: Wiley.

King, I. M. (1983). King's Theory of Goal Attainment. In Clements, I. W., & Roberts, F. B. (Eds.), *Family health: A theoretical approach to nursing care* (p. 177). New York: Wiley.

King, I. M. (1984b). A theory for nursing: King's conceptual model applied to community health nursing. In *Conceptual models of nursing applications in community health nursing* (p. 14). Chapel Hill, NC: Department of Public Health Nursing.

King, I. M. (1984a). Effectiveness of nursing care: Use of a goal oriented nursing record in end stage renal disease. *American Association of Nephrology Nursing and Technology, 11*(11), 60.

King, I. M. (1984c). Philosophy of nursing education: A national survey. *Western Journal of Nursing Research, 6,* 387.

King, I. M. (1986a). *Curriculum and instruction in nursing.* Norwalk, CT: Appleton-Century-Crofts.

King, I. M. (1986b). King's Theory of Goal Attainment. In Fry, P. (Ed.), *Case studies in nursing theory* (p. 197). New York: National League for Nursing.

King, I. M. (1988). Concepts: Essential elements of theories. *Nursing Science Quarterly, 1*(1), 22–24.

King, I. M. (1989a). King's general systems framework and theory. In Riehl-Sisca, J. P. (Ed.), *Conceptual models for nursing practice* (p. 149). Norwalk, CT: Appleton & Lang.

King, I. M. (1989b). King's systems framework for nursing administration. In Henry, B., et al. (Eds.), *Dimensions of nursing administration: Theory, research, education* (p. 35). Cambridge, England: Blackwell Scientific.

King, I. M. (1989c). Measuring health goal attainment in patients. In Waltz, C. F., & Strickland, O. L. (Eds.), *Measurment of nursing outcomes* (p. 108). New York: Springer Publishing.

King, I. M. (1990). Health the goal for nursing. *Nursing Science Quarterly, 3,* 123.

King, I. M. (1992). King's Theory of Goal Attainment. *Nursing Science Quarterly, 5,* 19.

King, I. M. (1994). Quality of life and goal attainment. *Nursing Science Quarterly, 7,* 29.

King, I. M. (1995). The theory of goal attainment. In M. Frey & C. Sieloff (Eds.), *Advancing King's systems framework and Theory of Goal Attainment* (p. 23). Thousand Oaks, CA: Sage.

King, I. M. (1996). The Theory of Goal Attainment in research and practice. *Nursing Science Quarterly, 9,* 61.

King, I. M. (1998). Nursing informatics: A universal nursing language. *The Florida Nurse, 46,* 1.

Laben, J., Dodd, D., & Sneed, L. (1991). King's Theory of Goal Attainment applied in group therapy for inpatient juvenile sexual offenders, maximum security state offenders and community parolees. *Issues in Mental Health Nursing, 12,* 52.

Messmer, P. (1995). Implementation of theory-based nursing practice. In Frey, M. A., & Sieloff, C. L. (Eds.), *Advances in King's systems framework and Theory of Goal Attainment* (p. 294). Thousand Oaks, CA: Sage.

National League for Nursing. (1978). *Curriculum process for developing or revising a baccalaureate nursing program.* New York: National League for Nursing.

Norris, D. M., & Hoyer, P. J. (1993). Dynamism in practice: Parenting within King's framework. *Nursing Science Quarterly, 6,* 79.

Northrop, F. C. S. (1969). *The logic of the sciences and the humanities.* Cleveland: Meridian.

Rooke, L. (1995). Focusing on King's theory and systems framework in education by using an experiential learning model: A challenge to improve the quality of nursing care. In Frey, M., & Sieloff, C. L. (Eds.), *Advancing King's systems framework and Theory of Goal Attainment* (p. 178). Thousand Oaks, CA: Sage.

Schorr, T. M., & Zimmerman, A. (1990). *Making Choices, Taking Chances.* St. Louis: Mosby-Year Book, Inc.

Sieloff, C. L. (1995). Development of a theory of departmental power. In Frey, M. A. & Sieloff, C. L. (Eds.), *Advancing King's systems framework and Theory of Goal Attainment* (p. 35). Thousand Oaks, CA: Sage.

Smith, M. C. (1988). King's theory in practice. *Nursing Science Quarterly, 1,* 145.

Sowell, R. L., & Fuszard, A. H. (1989). Inpatient nursing care management as a strategy for rural hospitals: A case study. *Journal of Rural Health, 5,* 201.

Sowell, R. L., & Lowenstein, A. (1994). King's theory as a framework for quality: Linking theory to practice. *Nursing Connections, 7*(2), 19-31.

Von Bertalanffy, L. (1968). *General system theory.* New York: Braziller.

Woods, B. C. (1994). King's theory in practice with elders. *Nursing Science Quarterly, 7,* 5-8.

Chapter *17*

Application of King's Work to Nursing Practice

❖ Review of the Literature

❖ Summary

❖ References

Christina Leibold Sieloff
Maureen Frey
Mary Killeen

Since the first publication of Dr. Imogene King's work, nursing's interest in the application of her work to practice has grown. The fact that she was one of the few theorists who generated both a framework and a theory further expanded her work. Although there were few publications in the 1970s and 1980s, today new publications are a continuous occurrence. In 1995, Frey and Sieloff collected a sample of the ongoing work related to King's systems framework and theory.

Although this chapter summarizes the application of Dr. King's work within nursing, it is limited to published applications. This eliminates current works in progress or planned applications. In addition, in reviewing the literature, it has been noted that many publications apply concepts or ideas from King's work, such as the achievement of goals or perceptions, without referencing Dr. King. Therefore, it is believed that the application of King's work is far more extensive than the literature would lead the reader to believe. Thus, the authors suggest that the application of Dr. King's work is currently pervasive throughout nursing in the United States. In today's practice environment, the concepts of "cultural diversity" and "cultural competence" are identified as critical to the delivery of client-focused or -centered care. Hence, it is particularly relevant to identify the application of Dr. King's work as documented in several different countries in addition to the United States: namely, Canada, Japan, and Sweden. Again, these countries, with their variety of cultures, are the only countries being identified in publications that specifically reference Dr. King's work. It is expected that many other cultures would find Dr. King's work equally valuable in improving the quality of patient care.

This section of the chapter will not analyze or evaluate the work of Dr. King or its application. The purpose is to describe the state of the art in terms of the work being done in relation to the application of King's conceptual framework and theory in a variety of areas: practice, administration, education, and research. Frey and Sieloff's (1995) work, as well as nursing knowledge development from a review of the literature, will be summarized and briefly discussed. Finally, recommendations will be made for future knowledge development in relation to King's systems framework and theory, particularly in relation

> The literature reviewed reports use of King's interacting systems framework as a guide to nursing practice.

to the importance of application within an evidence-based practice environment.

REVIEW OF THE LITERATURE
Application of Interacting Systems Framework

In conducting the literature review, the authors began with the broadest category of application—application within the interacting systems framework. All other application could be discussed within the interacting systems framework because the framework provides the basis for concept development and theory development and testing. However, this section will address only those applications that apply King's interacting systems framework to nursing care situations. Other applications will be discussed in the remainder of the chapter. Because a conceptual framework is, by nature, very broad and abstract, it can only serve to guide, rather than prescriptively direct, nursing practice. Hence, the literature discussed here used King's interacting systems framework in order to guide nursing practice. Coker et al. (1995) used the framework to guide the implementation of nursing diagnosis in a large community hospital. Fawcett, Vaillancourt, and Watson (1995) used the framework to guide nursing practice in a large tertiary care hospital.

In contrast, several authors used the framework to guide nursing practice with specific patient populations. Doornbos (1995) explored family health in families with chronically mentally ill family members. Hobdell (1995, p. 132) examined the "relationship between chronic sorrow and accuracy of perception of a child's cognitive development in parents of children with neural tube defects." Sharts-Hopko (1995) used concepts within King's framework to study health status as perceived by women during the menopause transition. Table 17–1 delineates applications related to King's interacting systems framework.

Concept Development within the Framework

Concept development within a conceptual framework is particularly valuable, as it often explicates concepts more clearly than a theorist may have done in his or her original work. Such explication further assists the development of nursing knowledge as it enables the practicing nurse to understand more easily the application of the concept within specific practice situations. Examples of concepts developed

TABLE 17-1	Application of the Interacting Systems Framework	
Topic	**Author(s)**	**Year**
Anxiety	LaFontaine	1989
Autonomy	Glenn*	1989
Change	DeFeo	1990
Child health	Steele	1981
Chronic mental illness	Doornbos	1995
Communication	Daubenmire, Searles, and Ashton	1978
Community assessment	Hanchett	1988
Community	Hanchett	1990
	Myks Babb, Fouladbakhsh, and Hanchett	1988
	King	1984
	Asay and Ossler	1984
Continuing education	Brown and Lee	1980
Education	Daubenmire	1989
	King	1989
	Gulitz and King	1988
	King	1986
	Froman and Sanderson	1985
	Daubenmire and King	1973
Family therapy	Gonot	1986
Menopause	Sharts-Hopko	1995
	Heggie and Gangar	1992
Neural tube defect	Hobdell	1995
Nursing administration	Elberson	1989
	Sieloff	1995
Nursing diagnosis	Byrne-Coker, Fradley, Harris, Tomarchio, and Caron	1990
Operating room	Gill, Hopwood-Jones, Tyndall, Gregoroff, LeBlance, Lovett, Rasco, and Ross	1995
Patient education	Spees	1991
	Martin	1990
	King and Tarsitano	1982
Perception	Bunting	1988
Reproductive health	Davis and Dearman	1991
Smoking	Kneeshaw	1990
Social support	Frey	1989
Theory-based practice	Messmer	1995
		1992
	West	1991
	Byrne and Schreiber	1990

*Indicates thesis or dissertation

TABLE 17-2	*Concept Development within the Framework*	
Topic	**Author(s)**	**Year**
Advocacy	Bramlett, Gueldner, and Sowell	1990
Autonomy	Glenn*	1989
Coping	King	1983
Empathy	Alligood, Evans, and Wilt	1995
Health	King	1990
Health (social system)	Sieloff	1995
Health (systems)	Winker	1995
Power	Hawkes	1991
Quality of life	King	1993
Social support	Frey	1989
Space	Rooke	1995
Transaction	Binder*	1992

*Indicates thesis or dissertation

from within King's work include the following: empathy (Alligood, Evans, & Wilt, 1995), health of a social system (Sieloff, 1995b), health of systems (Winker, 1995), and space (Rooke, 1995b). Table 17-2 further details applications related to concept development within King's framework (1981).

Theory of Goal Attainment

Dr. King's work is unique in that, in addition to the interacting systems framework, she developed the Theory of Goal Attainment, in 1981. This theory has found great application to nursing practice. One of the reasons for such a broad application is the fact that the theory focuses on a concept relevant throughout all nursing situations—the attainment of client goals. From a review of the literature, it can be demonstrated that the application of the Theory of Goal Attainment (King, 1981) is documented in several categories: (1) general application of the theory, (2) exploring a particular concept within the context of the Theory of Goal Attainment, (3) exploring a particular concept related to the Theory of Goal Attainment, and (4) application of the theory in nonclinical nursing situations. The Theory of Goal Attainment has been generally applied in a variety of nursing practice areas. Alligood (1995) applied the theory

to orthopedic nursing with adults, whereas Hanna (1995) used the theory in the promotion of the health behaviors of adolescent clients. Short-term group psychotherapy was the focus of theory application for Laben, Sneed, and Seidel (1995). In contrast, Benedict and Frey (1995) examined the use of the theory within the delivery of emergency care.

The Theory of Goal Attainment (King, 1981) is also used when nurses wish to explore a particular concept within a theoretical context. Perceptual congruency between nurses and clients was explored by Froman (1995).

Nurses also use the Theory of Goal Attainment (King, 1981) to examine concepts related to the theory. This application was demonstrated by Kameoka (1995) as she analyzed nurse-patient interactions in Japan.

Finally, the theory has been applied in nonclinical nursing situations. Rooke (1995b) applied the theory and framework in nursing education. Messmer (1995) used the theory in implementing theory-based nursing practice. And Jolly and Winker (1995) applied the theory to organizations. In summary, Table 17–3 chronicles applications of King's Theory of Goal Attainment.

TABLE 17-3	Application of the Theory of Goal Attainment	
Topic	**Author(s)**	**Year**
Adolescent health behavior	Hanna	1995
	Hanna	1993
Anxiety	La Fontaine	1989
	Swindale	1989
Birth	Smith	1988
Cardiac rehabilitation	McGirr, Rukhorm, Salmoni, O'Sullivan, and Koren	1990
Case management	Sowell and Lowenstein	1994
Coma	Ackerman, Brink, Clanton, Jones, Moody, Pirlech, Price, and Prusinsky	1989
Diabetes	Husband	1988
Emergency room	Benedict and Frey	1995
	Hughes	1983
Family	Rawlins, Rawlins, and Horner	1990
	King	1989
		1986
		1983
Group psychotherapy	Laben, Sneed, and Seidel	1995
	Laben, Dodd, and Sneed	1991
Health promotion	Calladine	1996
Hospitals	Messmer	1995
HIV	Kemppainen	1990
Interactions	Kameoka	1995
Managed care	Hampton	1993
Neurofibromatosis	Messmer and Neff Smith	1986
Nursing care effectiveness	King	1984
Nursing situations	Nagano and Funashima	1995
	Rooke and Norberg	1988
Oncology	Lockhart*	1992
	Porter	1991
Organ donation	Richard-Hughes	1997
Organizations	Jolly and Winker	1995
Parenting	Norris and Hoyer	1994
Perceptual congruence	Froman	1995

*Indicates thesis or dissertation

TABLE 17-3   *Continued*

Topic	Author(s)	Year
Psychosis	Kemppainen	1990
Psychotherapy	DeHowitt	1992
Quality of life	King	1993
Recovery	Hanucharurnkui and Vinya-nguag	1991
Reproductive health	Hanna	1993
Role strain	Temple and Fawdrey	1992
Senior adults	Woods Jonas	1994 1987
Theory-based practice	Messmer West	1992 1991
Transactions	Monti*	1992
Transcultural critique	Husting	1997

*Indicates thesis or dissertation

Development of Middle-Range Theories within the Framework

Development of middle-range theories is a part of the natural growth in application of a conceptual framework. Middle-range theories, clearly developed from within a conceptual framework, accomplish several goals:

1. Such theories can be directly applied to nursing situations, whereas a conceptual framework is usually too abstract for such direct application.
2. Validation of middle-range theories, clearly developed within a particular conceptual framework, lends validation to the conceptual framework itself.

In addition to the Theory of Goal Attainment (King, 1981), several middle-range theories have been developed from ideas within King's interacting systems framework, using each of the systems defined within that framework. In terms of the personal system, Brooks and Thomas (1997) used King's framework to derive a theory of perceptual awareness. The focus was to

> Several middle-range theories have been developed from King's interacting systems framework.

develop the concepts of judgement and action as core concepts in the personal system. Other concepts in the theory included communication, perception, and decision making.

In relation to the interpersonal system, several middle-range theories have been developed regarding families. Doornbos (1995) addressed family health in terms of families with young chronic mentally ill individuals. Frey (1995) developed a middle-range theory regarding families, children, and chronic illness, and Wicks (1995) delineated a middle-range theory regarding the broader concept of family health.

In relation to social systems, Sieloff (1995a) developed the Theory of Departmental Power to assist in explaining the power of groups within organizations. This theory reformulated selected concepts from the Strategic Contingencies Theory of Departmental Power (Hickson, Hinings, Lee, Schneck, & Pennings, 1971) within King's framework to propose concepts that contribute to a department's power capacity and its actualized power. Table 17–4 lists middle-range theories developed within King's framework (1981).

Instrument Development

Instrument development is needed through nursing knowledge in order to assist nurses and researchers in measuring concepts relevant to nursing phenom-

TABLE 17-4	Development of Middle-Range Theories within the Framework		
Topic		**Author(s)**	**Year**
Departmental power (revised to group power)		Sieloff	1998* 1996* 1995
Families, children, and chronic Illness		Frey	1995 1993
Family health		Wicks	1995
Family health (families with young chronic mentally ill individuals)		Doornbos	1995
Perceptual awareness		Brooks and Thomas	1997
Satisfaction, client		Killeen*	1996

*Indicates thesis or dissertation or research in progress

ena. However, instruments are frequently developed as part of an overall research study rather than serving as the main focus of the study. Within the context of a larger study, rather than as the outcome of a research project, reports regarding these instruments are often not as extensive as they should be in order to facilitate the further growth of nursing knowledge. Hence, review of the literature identified only two instruments specifically designed within King's framework. King (1988) developed the Health Goal Attainment instrument designed to detail the level of attainment of health goals by individual clients. The Family Needs Assessment Tool was developed by Rawlins, Rawlins, and Horner (1990). Table 17–5 provides a listing of instruments that were developed in relation to King's work.

Clients Across the Life Span

Additional evidence of the scope and usefulness of King's framework and theory is its use across a broad range of patient populations. When reviewing the literature in terms of whether King's work has been applied to clients across the life span, the following categories were used: (1) infants; (2) children; (3) adolescents; (4) adults, young; (5) adults; and (6) adults, mature. The application of King's work was evident in all categories. Several applications have targeted high-risk infants (Frey & Norris, 1997; Norris & Hoyer, 1993; Syzmanski, 1991). Interestingly, these each considered personal systems (infants), interpersonal systems (parents, families), and social systems (the nursing staff and hospital environment). Clearly, a strength of King's framework and theory is their utility in encompassing complex settings and situations.

Frey (1993, 1995, 1996) developed and tested relationships among multiple systems with children and youth with insulin-dependent diabetes and asthma. Ongoing testing is being done with children and adolescents with HIV/AIDS and adolescents in

TABLE 17-5	Instrument Development Related to King's Work		
Topic		**Author(s)**	**Year**
Family Needs Assessment Tool		Rawlins, Rawlins, and Horner	1990
Health goal attainment		King	1988
Nursing Care Survey (client-consumer perceptions and responses to professional nursing care)		Killeen	1996
Sieloff-King assessment of group power within organizations		Sieloff	1998

primary care settings (Frey, personal communication, 1998). In addition, Hobdell (1995) applied the framework to children with neural tube defects.

Hanna (1993, 1995) applied King's work in nursing situations with adolescent client populations. Hanna (1993) investigated the effect of nurse-client interactions on oral contraceptive adherence in adolescent females and worked with adolescents in primary-care settings in order to better understand health actions (1995).

The systems framework and Theory of Goal Attainment have been used to guide practice with adults with a broad range of illness conditions. In relation to adult clients, the literature is divided into: (1) young adults, (2) adults, and (3) mature adults. Doornbos (1995) used King's work in her study of young adults experiencing chronic mental illness.

Examples of applications focusing on adults include cardiac disease (McGirr, Rukholm, Salmoni, O'Sullivan, & Koren, 1990; Sirles & Selleck, 1989), diabetes (Husband, 1988), renal procedures (Hanucharurnkui & Vinya-nguag, 1990), elective minor surgery (Swindale, 1989), and orthopedic surgery (Alligood, 1995). Gender-specific work included Sharts-Hopko's (1995) use of concepts within the systems framework to study the health status of women during menopause transition, and Martin's (1990) application of the framework to cancer awareness among males.

Several of the applications with adults have targeted the mature adult, thus demonstrating considerable contribution to the nursing specialty of gerontology. Kohler (1988) used the framework to increase elderly clients' sense of shared control over health and health behaviors. Kenny (1990) also addressed the role of the elderly in their care. Despite using similar populations and a similar focus, these applications were quite different, with Kohler using the nursing process and Kenny using concepts from the Theory of Goal Attainment. Both approaches and foci are likely to lead to better health outcomes for the clinical group. In addition, Woods (1994) proposed the Theory of Goal Attainment in order to decrease chronic health problems among nursing home residents. Clearly, these applications show how the complexity of King's framework and theory increases its usefulness for nursing (refer to Table 17–6).

Client Systems

A major strength of King's work is that it can be used with virtually all client populations. In addition to discussing client populations across the life span, client populations can be identified by focus of care (client system) and/or focus of health problem (phenomenon of concern). The focus of care or interest can be an individual (personal system) or group (interpersonal or social system). Application of King's work across client systems would then logically be divided into the three systems identified within King's interacting systems framework (1981): personal (the individual), interpersonal (small groups), and social (large groups/society). Use with personal systems has included both patients and nurses. Patients as personal systems were the focus of applications by DeHowitt (1992), Frey and Norris (1997), Hanucharurnkui and Vinya-ngaug (1990), Husband (1988), Kemppainen (1990), Kenny (1990), and McGirr, Rukholm, Salmoni, O'Sullivan, and Koren (1990). Levine, Wilson, and Guido (1988) considered critical care nurses as the personal system of interest, as did Brooks and Thomas (1997).

When the focus of interest moves from an individual to include interaction between two people, an interpersonal system is involved. Interpersonal systems often, but not always, include clients and nurses. Examples of applications to nurse-client dyads and larger groups include Messmer and Neff Smith's (1986) approach to nursing with clients with neurofibromatosis, Swindale's (1989) exploration of nurses' role in reducing anxiety in hospitalized clients, and Kohler's (1988) application to nurses and elderly clients. Martin (1990) used the systems framework to develop and test an educational intervention about cancer with males in the work setting. Laben, Dodd, and Sneed (1991) applied the Theory of Goal Attainment to group psychotherapy with inpatient juvenile offenders. Temple and Fawdry (1992) used the Theory of Goal Attainment to examine role strain when the caregiver of an elderly patient is also a nurse.

In relation to interpersonal systems, or small groups, many publications focus on the family, such as Davis (1987), Frey and Norris (1997), Gonot (1986), Hobdell (1995), Norris and Hoyer (1993), Sirles and Selleck (1989), Syzmanski (1991), and Wicks (1995). Gonot proposed the systems framework as a model for family therapy. Davis considered individuals, parent dyads, and families when addressing the problem of infertility. Sirles and Selleck used the systems framework to examine the impact of cardiac disease on the family. Syzmanski (1991) focused on the Theory of Goal Attainment in planning care with families of premature infants. Frey and Norris used both the systems framework and Theory of Goal Attainment in planning care with a similar population and setting.

King's systems framework and Theory of Goal Attainment have a long history of application, and use,

TABLE 17-6 · *Application to Clients across the Life Span*

Topic	Author(s)	Year
Infants	Frey and Norris	1997
	Norris and Hoyer	1993
	Syzmanski	1991
Children	Scott	1998
	Frey	1996
		1995
	Hobdell	1995
	Frey	1993
		1989
	Steele	1981
Adolescents	Hanna	1995
		1993
	Binder*	1992
	Laben, Dodd, and Sneed	1991
	Hughes	1983
	Daubenmire, Searles, and Ashton	1978
Adults, young	Doornbos	1995
Adults	Ollsson and Forsdahl	1996
	Alligood	1995
	Froman	1995
	Jones, Clark, Merker, and Palau	1995
	Kameoka	1995
	Nagano and Funashima	1995
	Rooke	1995
	Sharts-Hopko	1995
	Norris and Hoyer	1994
	Hanna	1993
	DeHowitt	1992
	Heggie and Gangar	1992
	Hobdell	1992
	Lockhart*	1992
	Laben, Dodd, and Sneed	1991
	Hanucharurnkui and Vinya-nguag	1990
	Kemppainen	1990
	McGirr, Rukholm, Salmoni, O'Sullivan, and Koren	1990
	Martin	1990
	Glenn*	1989
	O'Shall*	1989
	Sirles and Selleck	1989
	Swindale	1989
	Husband	1988
	Smith	1988
	Laben, Sneed, and Seidel	1986
	Jonas	1987
	Pearson and Vaughan	1986
	King and Tarsitano	1982
	King	1984
	Strauss	1981
	Brown and Lee	1980
	Daubenmire, Searles, and Ashton	1978

*Indicates thesis or dissertation

| TABLE 17-6 | *Continued* |

Topic	Author(s)	Year
Adults, mature	Allan*	1995
	Jones, Clark, Merker, and Palau	1995
	Rooke	1995
	Woods	1994
	Tawil*	1993
	Temple and Fawdry	1992
	Zurakowski*	1991
	Kenny	1990
	Miller	1990
	Kohler	1988
	Jonas	1987
	King	1983
	Rosendahl and Ross	1982

*Indicates thesis or dissertation

with large groups or social systems (organizations, communities). One of the earliest applications was the use of the framework and theory to guide continuing education (Brown & Lee, 1980) and nursing curricula (Daubenmire, 1989; Gulitz & King, 1988). More contemporary applications address models of care. For example, the framework and Theory of Goal Attainment serve as the basis for practice in several acute-care settings (Byrne & Schreiber, 1989; Fawcett, Vaillancourt, & Watson, 1995). Several applications proposed the Theory of Goal Attainment as the practice model for case management (Hampton, 1994; Tritsch, 1996). These latter applications are especially important, as they may be the first use of the framework by other disciplines.

Within organizations, Jolly and Winker (1995) applied the Theory of Goal Attainment in the context of an organizational structure. A theory of departmental power has been developed (Sieloff, 1995a). Messmer (1995) implemented theory-based nursing practice, based on King's work, in a large, urban public hospital. Educational settings, also considered as social systems, have also been the focus of application of King's work (Brown & Lee, 1980; Daubenmire, 1989; Daubenmire & King, 1973; Froman & Sanderson, 1985; Gulitz & King, 1988). Table 17–7 consolidates applications of King's work to various client systems.

Phenomena of Concern to Clients

Within King's work, it is obviously critically important for the nurse to focus on, and address, the phenomenon of concern to the client. Without this emphasis on the client's perspective, mutual goal-

your thoughts

TABLE 17-7 *Application to Various Client Systems*

Topic	Author(s)	Year
Personal systems	Brooks and Thomas	1997
	Frey and Norris	1997
	Hanna	1993
	Jackson, Pokorny, and Vincent	1993
	DeHowitt	1992
	Hanucharurnkui and Vinya-nguag	1990
	Kemppainen	1990
	Kenny	1990
	McGirr, Rukholm, Salmoni, O'Sullivan, and Koren	1990
	Husband	1988
	Kohler	1988
	Levine, Wilson, and Guido	1988
	Smith	1988
	Jonas	1987
	Pearson and Vaughan	1986
	King	1984
	Hughes	1983
	King and Tarsitano	1982
Interpersonal systems	O'Shall*	1989
Interpersonal systems (families)	Frey and Norris	1997
	Norris and Hoyer	1994
	Frey	1993
	Temple and Fawdry	1992
	Spees	1991
	Syzmanski	1991
	Dispenza*	1990
	Rawlins, Rawlins, and Horner	1990
	Sirles and Selleck	1989
	Frey	1989
	Davis	1987
	Gonot	1986
	Messmer and Neff Smith	1986
	King	1983
	Strauss	1981
Interpersonal systems (groups)	Woods	1994
	Monti*	1992
	Laben, Dodd, and Sneed	1991
Interpersonal systems (nurse-client)	Nagano and Funashima	1995
	DeHowitt	1992
	Houfek	1992
	Temple and Fawdry	1992
	Rundell	1991
	Martin	1990
	Swindale	1989
	Kohler	1988
	Messmer and Smith	1986
	Daubenmire, Searles, and Ashton	1978
Interpersonal systems (stepfamilies)	Omar*	1990
Social systems	Brown and Lee	1980

*Indicates thesis or dissertation

TABLE 17-7	*Continued*	
Topic	**Author(s)**	**Year**
Social systems (aggregates)	Norgan, Ettipio, and Lasome	1995
Social systems (communities)	Temple and Fawdry	1992
	Hanchett	1990
	Hanchett	1988
	Myks Babb, Fouladbakhsh, and Hanchett	1988
	Asay and Ossler	1984
	King	1984
Social system (education)	Daubenmire	1989
	Gulitz and King	1988
	Froman and Sanderson	1985
	Brown and Lee	1980
	Daubenmire and King	1973
Social system (nursing unit)	Rundell	1991
Social systems (organizations)	Tritsch	1996
	Fawcett, Vaillancourt, and Watson	1995
	Jolly and Winker	1995
	Messmer	1995
	Sieloff	1995
	Fitch, Rogers, Ross, Shea, Smith, and Tucker	1991
	Schreiber	1991
	West	1991
	Byrne-Coker, Fradley, Harris, Tomarchio, and Caron	1990
	Kenny	1990
	Byrne and Schreiber	1989
	Elberson	1989
	Hampton	1989
	LaFontaine	1989

*Indicates thesis or dissertation

setting could not occur. Clients will not work toward goals that they do not value. King noted (1981) that nurses and clients may not always have the same goals, or agree with clients on ways to achieve goals.

In the literature, information regarding client phenomena of concern has been categorized by disease classification or client complaint or problem. Such categorization could often be perceived as having either a negative focus, or a medical rather than a nursing focus. In addition, this type of categorization could hinder nurses working within a health promotion or health education model. Therefore, for the purpose of this section of the chapter, client phenomena of concern was selected as a more neutral terminology that would enable nurses in all settings to see clearly the broad application of King's work to their practice situations. Table 17-8 summarizes applications related to client phenomena of concern, and groups these applications, primarily identified

by disease or medical diagnosis, as illness management.

One area that certainly binds clients and nurses is health. Improved health is clearly the desired end point or outcome of nursing care and something to which clients aspire. Review of the focus, or outcome, of nursing care as addressed in published applications tends to support the goal of improved health directly and/or indirectly. Health status is explicitly the outcome of concern in research and practice applications by Doornbos (1995), Frey (1995, 1996), Smith (1988), and Woods (1994). Several applications used health-related terms or limited dimensions of health. For example, Kohler (1988) focused on increased morale and satisfaction. Swindale (1989) focused on reducing anxiety, and DeHowitt (1992) focused on well-being.

Health promotion has also been an emphasis for the application of King's ideas. Health behaviors

TABLE 17-8	*Application to Client Concerns*	
Topic	**Author(s)**	**Year**
Care of self	Hanucharurnkui and Vinya-nguag	1991
Autonomy	Glenn*	1989
	Husband	1988
Birth	Smith	1988
Goal-setting	Tritsch	1996
Health promotion	Calladine	1996
	Hanna	1995
Body weight	Sharts-Hopko	1995
Menopause	Hanna	1993
	Heggie and Gangar	1992
Morale	Kohler	1988
Parenting	Norris and Hoyer	1993
Reproductive health	Hanna	1993
Role	O'Shall*	1989
Sexual counseling	Villeneuve and Ozolins*	1991
Stress	DeHowitt	1992
	Dispenza*	1990
Health status	Frey	1996
		1995
	Doornbos	1995
	Woods	1994
	Smith	1988
Illness management		
Asthma	Frey	1995
Anxiety	Swindale	1989
Bronchopneumonia	Pearson and Vaughan	1986
Cardiac rehabilitation	McGirr, Rukhorm, Salmoni, O'Sullivan, and Koren	1990
Cardiovascular	Sirles and Selleck	1989
Carpal tunnel syndrome	Norgan, Ettipio, and Lasome	1995
Chronic illness	Wicks	1995
Chronic obstructive pulmonary disorder	Wicks	1995
Coma	Ackerman, Brink, Clanton, Jones, Moody, Pirlech, Price, and Prusensky	1989
Diabetes	Frey	1995
		1988
	White-Linn*	1994
	Husband	1988
	Jonas	1987
End-stage renal disease	King	1984
HIV	Kemppainen	1990
	Syzmanski	1991
High-risk infants	Woods	1994
Hypertension	Hanucharurnkui and Vinya-nguag	1991
Nephrology	Hobdell	1995
	Messmer and Neff Smith	1986
Neural tube defects	Nagano and Funashima	1995
Neurofibromatosis	Lockhart*	1992
Oncology	Temple and Fawdry	1992
	Porter	1991
	Martin	1990
	Alligood	1995

*Indicates thesis or dissertation

Topic	Author(s)	Year
TABLE 17-8 *Continued*		
Illness management, continued		
Orthopedic	Kameoka	1995
	Jackson, Pokorny, and Vincent	1993
Ostomy	Temple and Fawdry	1992
Pain management	Hanucharurnkui and Vinya-nguag	1991
	Murray and Baier	1996
	Doornbos	1995
Psychiatric	Laben, Sneed, and Seidel	1995
	DeHowitt	1991
	Gonot	1990
	Schreiber	1990
	Kemppainen	1982
	Rosendahl and Ross	1982
Terminal illness	Woods	1994
Risky health behaviors	Frey	1996
Smoking	Kneeshaw	1990
Well-being	DeHowitt	1992

*Indicates thesis or dissertation

were Hanna's (1995) focus of study. The health status of clients experiencing menopause was explored by Sharts-Hopko (1995). The experience of parenting was studied by Norris and Hoyer (1993). Sexual counseling was the focus of work by Villeneuve and Ozolins (1991).

King (1981) stated that individuals act to maintain their own health. Although not explicitly stated, the converse is probably true as well: individuals often do things that are not good for their health. Accordingly, it is not surprising that the systems framework and theory are often directed toward patient and group behaviors that influence health. Several authors have directly or indirectly focused on patients caring for themselves (Hanucharurnkui & Vinya-nguag, 1991; Husband, 1988). Hanna (1993, 1995) focused on health behaviors with the intent of health promotion with adolescents. Tritsch (1996) focused on goal-setting behaviors. Frey (1995, 1997), Frey and Denyes (1989), and Frey and Fox (1990) looked at both health behaviors and illness management behaviors in several groups of children with chronic conditions. In addition, Frey (1996) expanded her research to include risky behaviors.

As stated previously, in relation to illness management, diseases or diagnoses are often identified as the focus of the nursing application. Asthma was the client concern addressed by Frey (1995). Diabetes, another chronic illness affecting clients across the life span, has been studied by Frey (1995) and Hus-

band (1988). Chronic illness in general was the focus of Wicks in 1995. Clients with HIV infections were involved in work by Kemppainen (1990).

Several additional areas demonstrate a cluster of application of King's work. Infants and children were populations of focus for several practice applications of King's work. Syzmanski (1991) used King's work to explore nursing situations with high-risk infants. Hobdell (1995) worked with parents of children with neural tube defects. Frey (1995) explored the experience of chronic illness of children within families.

Clients experiencing a variety of psychiatric concerns have also been the focus of work, using King's conceptualizations (DeHowitt, 1992; Doornbos, 1995; Kemppainen, 1990; Laben, Sneed, & Seidel, 1995; Murray & Baier, 1996; Schreiber, 1991). Clients' concerns ranged from psychotic symptoms (Kemppainen, 1990) to families experiencing chronic mental illness (Doornbos, 1995) and clients in short-term group psychotherapy (Laben, Sneed, & Seidel, 1995). Table 17–8 delineates applications related to clients' phenomena of concern.

Nursing Specialties

An area that frequently divides nurses is their area of specialty. However, by using a consistent framework across specialties, nurses would be able to focus more clearly on their commonalities, rather than highlighting their differences. A review of the litera-

TABLE 17-9	Application within Nursing Specialties	
Topic	**Author(s)**	**Year**
Administration	Olsson and Forsdahl	1996
	Winker*	1996
	Sieloff	1995
	Batchelor*	1994
	Hampton	1994
	Elberson	1989
	Glenn*	1989
	King	1989
	O'Shall*	1989
Cardiovascular	Woods	1994
Case management	Sowell and Lowenstein	1994
Chronic illness	White-Linn*	1994
Continuing education	Brown and Lee	1980
Critical care	Scott	1998
	Norris and Hoyer	1994
Education	Brooks*	1995
	Rooke	1995
	Daubenmire	1989
	King	1986
	Froman and Sanderson	1985
	Asay and Ossler	1984
	Brown and Lee	1980
	Daubenmire and King	1973
Education, client	King and Tarsitano	1982
Endocrinology	Frey	1989
	Husband	1988
	Jonas	1987
Forensic	Laben, Dodd, and Sneed	1991
Genetics	Messmer and Neff Smith	1988
Gerontology	Rooke	1995
	Woods	1994
	Temple and Fawdry	1992
	Kenny	1990
	Jonas	1987
Hospice	Woods	1994
Medical-surgical	Froman	1995
	Rooke	1995
Mother-child	Dawson*	1996
	Omar*	1990
Nephrology	King	1984

*Indicates thesis or dissertation

TABLE 17-9	*Continued*	
Topic	**Author(s)**	**Year**
Oncology	Nagano and Funashima	1995
	Lockhart*	1992
	Porter	1991
Orthopedics	Alligood	1995
	Kameoka	1995
Neurology	Messmer and Neff Smith	1986
Nurses	Olsson and Forsdahl	1996
	Kneeshaw	1990
Political action	Krassa*	1994
Psychiatric/Mental health	Murray and Baier	1996
	Doornbos	1995
	Laben, Sneed, and Seidel	1995
	DeHowitt	1992
	Schreiber	1991
	Kemppainen	1990
	Gonot	1986
Quality improvement	Killeen* (client satisfaction)	1996
	O'Connor* (client satisfaction)	1990
Respiratory	Davis and Dearman	1991
	Pearson and Vaughan	1986
Reproductive health	Hanna	1993
Surgery	Gill, Hopwood-Jones, Tyndall, Gregoroff, LeBlanc, Lovett, Rasco, and Ross	1995
	Rooke	1995
	Porteous and Tyndall	1994
	King and Tarsitano	1982
	Daubenmire, Searles, and Ashton	1978

*Indicates thesis or dissertation

ture clearly demonstrates that Dr. King's framework and related theories have application within nursing specialties (see Table 17–9). This application is evident whether one is reviewing "traditional" specialties of medical-surgical (Froman, 1995; Gill et al., 1995; King & Tarsitano, 1982; Porteous & Tyndall, 1994; Rooke, 1995b) or psychiatric nursing (De-Howitt, 1992; Doornbos, 1995; Laben, Sneed, & Seidel, 1995; Murray & Baier, 1996). The application of King's work is also evident in the nontraditional specialties of forensic nursing (Laben, Dodd, & Sneed, 1991) and/or nursing administration (Elberson, 1989; Hampton, 1994).

Work Settings

An additional source of division within the nursing profession is the work sites where nursing is practiced and care is delivered. As the delivery of health care moves from the more traditional site of the acute care hospital to community-based agencies and clients' homes, it is ever more important to highlight commonalities across these settings rather than emphasize their differences, and important to identify that King's framework and Theory of Goal Attainment continue to be applicable. Although many applications tend to be with nurses and clients in traditional settings, successful application has been shown across other, including newer and nontraditional, settings. From hospitals (Jacono, Hicks, Antonioni, O'Brien, & Rasi, 1990; Levine, Wilson, & Guido, 1988; Messmer, 1995) to nursing homes (Woods, 1994), and clinics (Frey, 1995; Gonot, 1986), King's framework and related theories provide a foundation on which nurses can build their practice interven-

TABLE 17-10	*Application within Nursing Work Settings*	
Topic	**Author(s)**	**Year**
Clinics	Hanna	1993
	DeHowitt	1992
	Porter	1991
	Kemppainen	1990
	Frey	1989
	Husband	1988
	Gonot	1986
Community	Sowell and Lowenstein	1994
	Temple and Fawdry	1992
	King	1984
Home health	Rosendahl and Ross	1982
Hospitals	Frey and Norris	1997
	Olsson and Forsdahl	1996
	Tritsch	1996
	Gill, Hopwood-Jones, Tyndall, Gregoroff, LeBlanc, Lovett, Rasco, and Ross	1995
	Jones, Clark, Merker, and Palau	1995
	Nagano and Funashima	1994
	Sowell and Lowenstein	1993
	Hampton	1993
	Jackson, Pokorny, and Vincent	1993
	Norris and Hoyer	1993
	Messmer	1992
	Fitch, Rogers, Ross, Shea, Smith, and Tucker	1991
	West	1991
	Kemppainen	1990
	Kenny	1990
	LaFontaine	1989
	Levine, Wilson, and Guido	1988
	Jonas	1987
	Pearson and Vaughan	1986
	King	1984
	Rosendahl and Ross	1982
	Daubenmire, Searles, and Ashton	1978
Hospitals, community	Coker, Fradley, Harris, Tomarchio, Chan, and Caron	1995
	Byrne-Coker, Fradley, Harris, Tomarchio, Chan, and Caron	1990
	Byrne and Schreiber	1989
	Schreiber	1991
Hospitals, public	Messmer	1995
Hospitals, urban	Messmer	1995
	King and Tarsitano	1982
Intensive care units	Scott	1998
	Rooke	1995
	Norris and Hoyer	1994
	Jacono, Hicks, Antontoni, O'Brien, and Rasi	1990
Nursing homes	Woods	1994
	Zurakowski*	1991
Step-down units	Rundell	1991

*Indicates thesis or dissertation

tions. Table 17–10 lists applications within a variety of nursing work settings.

Nursing Process and Related Languages

Within the nursing profession, the nursing process has consistently been used as the basis for nursing practice. King's framework and Theory of Goal Attainment have been tied to the process of nursing. Although many published applications have broad reference to the nursing process, several deserve special recognition. First, Dr. King herself (1981) clearly linked the Theory of Goal Attainment to nursing process and theory and nursing process as method.

> King's work has been applied with nurses and clients in traditional settings as well as in newer, nontraditional settings.

Application of King's work to nursing curricula further strengthened this link. Other explicit examples of integration with the nursing process are those by Woods (1994) and Frey and Norris (1997). Additionally, Frey and Norris drew parallels between the transaction process, nursing process, and critical thinking process.

In addition, over time, nursing has developed standardized nursing language (SNL) that is being used to assist the profession to improve communication both within and external to the profession. These languages include the Nursing Diagnoses, Nursing Interventions, and Nursing Outcomes. Although these languages were developed after many of the original nursing theorists had completed their original works, nursing frameworks such as King's interacting systems framework (1981) can still find application and use in the SNLs. And it is this type of application that further demonstrates the framework's utility across time. For example, Coker et al.

(1995) implemented nursing diagnoses within the context of King's framework. Table 17–11 provides a listing of applications of King's work in relation to the nursing process and nursing languages.

Application to Health Care Beyond Nursing

When originally developing the interacting systems framework, King borrowed from knowledge external to nursing, and used a systems framework perspective to assist in explaining nursing phenomena. This use of knowledge across disciplines occurs frequently and can be very appropriate if both disciplines' perspectives are similar and reformulation occurs. Because of King's emphasis on the attainment of goals and the relevancy of goal attainment to many disciplines, both within and external to health care, it is reasonable to expect that King's work could find application beyond situations that are nursing-specific. Two specific examples of the above include the application of King's work to case management (Hampton, 1994; Sowell & Lowenstein, 1994; Tritsch, 1996) and managed care (Hampton, 1994). Both case management and managed care incorporate multiple disciplines as they work to improve the overall quality and cost efficiency of the health care provided. These applications also address the continuum of care, a priority in today's health-care environment. Table 17–12 details applications of King's work beyond nursing.

Multicultural Applications

Multicultural applications of King's interacting systems framework and related theories are many. Such applications are particularly critical as a frequent limitation expressed regarding theoretical formulations are their culture-bound nature. Theoretical formulations originating in the United States, such as those

TABLE 17-11	*Application within the Nursing Process and Related Languages*	
Topic	Author(s)	Year
Documentation	King	1984
Nursing diagnoses	Gill, Hopwood-Jones, Tyndall, Gregoroff, LeBlanc, Lovett, Rasco, and Ross	1995
	Byrne-Coker, Fradley, Harris, Tomarchio, Chan, and Caron	1990
Nursing process	Frey and Norris	1997
	Calladine	1996
	Woods	1992
	Schreiber	1991

TABLE 17-12	*Application to Health Care beyond Nursing*	
Topic	**Author(s)**	**Year**
Advocacy	Bramlett, Gueldner, and Sowell	1990
Case management	Tritsch	1996
	Hampton	1994
	Sowell and Lowenstein	1994
Managed care	Hampton	1994

of Dr. King, may not be perceived as readily applicable to non-Western cultures. In the case of the interacting systems framework and related theories, this is not the case. Several authors specifically addressed the utility of King's framework and theory for transcultural nursing. Spratlen (1976) drew heavily from King's framework and theory to integrate ethnic cultural factors into nursing curricula and develop a culturally oriented model for mental health care. Key elements derived from King's work were the focus on perceptions and communication patterns that motivate action, reaction, interaction, and transaction. Rooda (1992) derived propositions from the Theory of Goal Attainment as the framework for a conceptual model for multicultural nursing. Again, perception and the influence of culture on perception were identified as strengths of King's theory.

Cultural relevance has also been demonstrated in reviews by Frey, Rooke, Sieloff, Messmer, and Kameoka (1995), and Husting (1997). Although Husting identified that cultural issues were implicit variables throughout King's framework, particular attention was given to the concept of health, which, according to King (1990), acquires meaning from cultural values and social norms.

Undoubtedly the strongest evidence for the cultural utility of King's conceptual framework and Theory of Goal Attainment (1981) is the extent of work that has been done in other cultures. Applications of the framework and related theories have been documented in the following countries beyond the United States: Canada (Coker et al., 1995), Japan (Funashima, 1990; Kameoka, 1995; Kameoka & Sugimori, 1992), and Sweden (Rooke, 1995a, 1995b). In Japan, a culture very different from the United States with regard to communication style, Kameoka (1995) used the classification system of nurse–patient interactions, identified within the Theory of Goal Attainment (King, 1981), to analyze nurse–patient interactions. In addition to research and publications regarding the application of King's work to nursing

practice internationally, publications by and about Dr. King have been translated into Japanese (King, 1976, 1985; Kobayashi, 1970).

The variety of countries, including both Western and Eastern cultures, where the theory has been applied clearly demonstrates not only the current multicultural application of King's work, but also future potential applications in other countries around the world. Dr. King has traveled extensively to many countries around the world to speak and consult with nurses regarding their application of her work. This multicultural interest also led to the establishment of the King International Nursing Group (K. I. N. G.), based at Oakland University, Rochester, Michigan. The K. I. N. G. is an international nursing group, the primary mission of which is the improvement of nursing care and contribution to the science of nursing through the advancement of King's interacting systems framework for nursing and related theories. Table 17–13 lists applications of King's work in countries outside the United States.

Recommendations for Knowledge Development Related to King's Framework and Theory

Obviously, nursing knowledge development has resulted from applications of King's framework and theory. However, nursing, as all sciences, is evolving. Additional work continues to be needed. Based on a review of the applications discussed above, recommendations for future knowledge development focus on: (1) the need for evidenced-based nursing practice that is theoretically derived; (2) the role of the research based on King's work in evidence-based nursing practice; (3) King's concepts in the nursing process within standardized nursing language; and (4) the future impact of managed care, continuous quality improvement, and technology on King's concepts. From this discussion, specific research questions for the future can be derived.

TABLE 17-13	*Multicultural Application*	
Topic	**Author(s)**	**Year**
Documentation	King	1984
African-American	Richard-Hughes	1997
Canada	Gill, Hopwood-Jones, Tyndall, Gregoroff, LeBlanc, Lovett, Rasco, and Ross	1995
	Porteous and Tyndall	1994
	Byrne-Coker, Fradley, Harris, Tomarchio, Chan, and Caron	1990
	Fitch, Rogers, Ross, Shea, Smith, and Tucker	1991
	Porter	1991
	Schreiber	1991
	Byrne and Schreiber	1989
England	Pearson and Vaughan	1986
Japan	Kameoka	1995
	Nagano and Funashima	1995
	Kusaka	1991
Norway	Olsson and Forsdahl	1996
Sweden	Rooke	1995
		1995
	Rooke and Norberg	1988
Multicultural approach	Frey, Rooke, Sieloff, Messmer, and Kameoka	1995
	Rooda	1992
	King	1990
	Spratlen	1976

Evidence-based Practice Derived from Theory

What is evidence-based practice and how will evidence-based nursing practice evolve? Even though Florence Nightingale realized the importance of using evidence to guide practice 135 years ago, the field of medicine takes credit for the current trend to evidence-based practice. Evidence-based medicine (EBM) means that practicing physicians are expected to base their clinical decisions on "the evidence" from all the best studies rather than expert opinion and past practice (Davidoff, 1995). Standards for gathering the evidence, the tools for analyzing evidence, and the role of client preferences in clinical decision making have become more important than in the past. Rules for evaluating the scientific merit of studies evolved from the concept of rules of evidence in the legal profession. Evidence-based health care, evolving at lightning speed since the establishment of the Cochran Collaboration (Jadadd & Haynes, 1998) in 1993, compares to the Human Genome Project in its impact on modern medicine, according to Naylor (1995).

Nursing as a discipline also continues to evolve in the use of scientific evidence. Titler (1998, p. 1), a nurse, defines evidence-based practice as "the conscientious and judicious use of current best evidence to guide health care decisions." Similar to evidence-based medicine, nursing must attend to what is important for nursing. The questions practicing nurses address and the types of research that provide these answers are likely to be different from the questions of our physician colleagues and the randomized controlled trials (RCT) research design that is the "gold standard" for medicine.

Another factor that distinguishes nursing from medicine is the use of nursing theory to guide research. Theoretically based nursing problems, nursing interventions, and nursing outcomes are the sources of research questions that generate clinical evidence with usefulness for nursing practice. Theory invention is the work of King and other nurses interested in expanding the quality of nursing practice. The purpose of theory-informed research applied to practice is ultimately to improve the quality of practice. Fawcett (1978, p. 56) made the link between research and theory explicit in discussing the development of the body of nursing knowledge as a science and the need to advance the discipline of nursing: "Theory should guide all phases of the research process, from choice of a research issue to dissemination of results."

Though the direct application of theory to practice is often implied, theory cannot be directly applied to practice. King (1971, p. 157) succinctly stated: "[T]heory, because it is abstract, cannot be immediately applied to nursing practice or to concrete nursing education programs. When empirical referents are identified, defined, and described, theory is useful and can be applied in concrete situations." Theory can influence nurses' outlooks and philosophies, but it cannot be used directly in practice. For theory to be ultimately applied to practice, theory needs to guide nursing research. Subsequent research findings, informed by a theory perspective, can be directly applied to practice.

Nurses often wonder why they should include a theory component when formulating research. Is this really necessary? they ask. The answer is, emphatically, yes! Nursing research, providing the underpinning for evidence-based nursing practice, needs to be theory-related research. "Evidence-based" demands more rigorous standards for research. Nursing might add theory as a necessary criterion based on the added critical thought process required. Theory building or theory testing using King's systems framework and related theories makes repeated investigations of theoretically based problems more fruitful as research results accumulate. Science is built stronger and better when questions and answers build upon each other. Evidence-based nursing practice that is based on theoretically derived research findings has improved the potential for closing the gap between nursing research and practice.

Readers of this chapter are interested in the applicability of nursing research, specifically using King's systems framework and related theories toward practice. From an evidence-based practice and King's perspective, the profession must implement three strategies to apply theory-based research findings effectively. First, nursing as a discipline must develop rules of evidence in evaluation of quality research that reflect the unique contribution of nursing to health care. For example, qualitative methods uniquely reflect nursing's paradigm (Leininger, 1985) and can be conducted as rigorously as quantitative research. Second, the nursing rules of evidence must include heavier weight for research that is derived from, or adds to, nursing theory, for the reasons discussed previously. Third, the nursing rules of evidence must reflect higher scores when nursing's

central beliefs are affirmed in the choice of variables. Nursing science as a unique body of knowledge is largely dependent on discovery or verification of key concepts. King's work on the concepts of client and nurse perceptions and the achievement of mutual goals has been assimilated and accepted as core beliefs of the discipline. This third strategy of use of concepts central to nursing has clear relevance for evidence-based practice when using King's concepts such as perception.

Perceptions, according to King (1981), reflect each person's representation of reality. Observers of medical and nursing practice would no doubt agree that perceptions are emphasized in the nursing paradigm rather than the medical paradigm. Perceptions are not routinely valued in the medical quantitative paradigm of research, which relies on objective reality independent of the researcher. Rather, perceptions fit more with the nursing naturalism paradigm concerned with understanding situations. Therefore, acceptable research evidence in nursing requires a research philosophy and designs that answer different research questions than medicine. Research guided by King on client and nurse perceptions in achieving nursing-sensitive client outcomes generates particularly relevant research questions for nursing. For example, What are clients' perceptions and experiences in out-client versus in-patient surgery? Furthermore, the nature of health- and disease-related events and client exposure to those events needs to be studied using nursing-specific concepts like King's so nurses may effectively influence nursing situations. Likewise, research with theory-based concepts associated with nursing interventions (communication, interactions, transactions) should weigh higher in merit when judging nursing effectiveness research.

One definition of evidence-based medicine (Cook, 1998, pp. 24–25) includes the caregivers' and consumers' points of view: "Evidence-based medicine is a style of practice and teaching that seeks to explicitly integrate knowledge of pathophysiology, caregiver experience, and client preferences with clinical research evidence within the restraints of local health care systems." However, this idealistic view of medicine is everyday reality for nursing practice. Research conducted with a King theoretical base is well positioned to apply to nurse caregivers and nurse administrators (Sieloff, 1996) and client-consumers (Killeen, 1996) as part of an evolving definition of evidence-based nursing practice. For example, King (1971) addressed client preference, a possible part of an evidence-based nursing definition, as satisfaction. In an update of the concept of satisfaction, King submits that satisfaction is a subset of her central concept of perceptions (Killeen, 1996). A nursing perspective for evidence-based health care will, no doubt, include many concepts initially defined by King that now are well integrated into nursing's belief system and culture.

King's Concepts, the Nursing Process, and Standardized Nursing Languages

The steps of the nursing process have long been integrated within King's systems framework and Theory of Goal Attainment (Daubenmire & King, 1973; Gulitz & King, 1988; Husband, 1988; Jonas, 1987; Pearson & Vaughan, 1986; Woods, 1994). In these process applications, based in King, assessment, diagnosis, and goal-setting occur, followed by actions based on the nurse-client goals. The evaluation component of the nursing process refers back to the original goal statement(s). With the use of standardized nursing language, the nursing process will be further refined; standardized terms for diagnoses, interventions, outcomes, and so on should potentially improve communication among nurses internally and externally. (Note: "standardized nursing language" refers to the six ANA-recognized languages: nursing diagnosis as defined by the North American Nursing Diagnosis Association [NANDA], Nursing Interventions Classification [NIC], Nursing Outcomes Classification [NOC], Home Health Care Classification Client Care Data Set, the Omaha System, and the Ozbolt System.)

Whatever the setting, client population, or specialty, a common language of nursing diagnosis, interventions, and outcomes streamlines written and verbal nursing communication. The use of a nationally standardized language and classification system, with accepted coding, would allow for the aggregation of data internally for organization reports and nursing administration research. Externally, nursing would be in a strong position to add more comprehensive data to community and national databases.

Using SNLs allows middle-range theory development to build on concepts unique to nursing, such as those concepts of King directly applied to the nursing process: action, reaction, interaction, transaction, goal-setting, and goal attainment. Beigen and Tripp-Reimer (1997) suggested middle-range theories be constructed from the concepts in the taxonomies in the nursing languages focusing on outcomes. However, it is not necessary to build sterile new theories based on taxonomies of nursing languages focusing on phenomena of diagnoses, interventions, and client outcomes, as suggested by Biegen and Tripp-Reimer (1997). Alternatively, King's framework and theory could be used as a theoretical basis for these phenomena and assist in knowledge development in nursing in the next millennium.

The use of SNLs will also standardize how the nursing process is taught and used. No universal agreement has been evident in the number of components or the labels for the steps of the nursing process. With the advent of SNLs, recent terminology includes "outcome identification" as a step following assessment and diagnosis (McFarland & McFarland, 1997, p. 3). Baseline outcomes identification, with measurable indicators, is essential to describe nursing-sensitive client outcomes (Johnson & Maas, 1997). King's concept of mutual goal-setting is analogous to the outcomes identification step, because

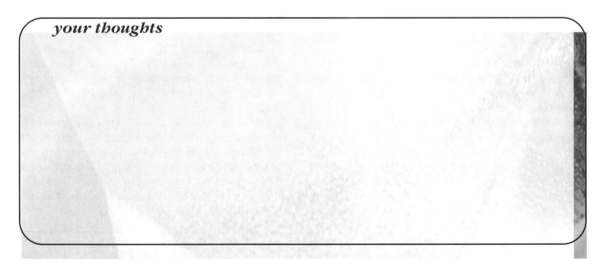

your thoughts

King's concept of goal attainment fits with the evaluation of client outcomes in the nursing process. King (1981, p. 177) states: "[O]utcomes are identified as goals attained."

In addition, King's concept of perception (1981) lends itself well to the definition of client outcomes. Johnson and Maas (1997, p. 22) define a nursing-sensitive client outcome as "a measurable client or family caregiver state, behavior, or perception that is conceptualized as a variable and is largely influenced and sensitive to nursing interventions." This is fortuitous because the development of nursing knowledge requires the use of client outcome measurement. The use of standardized client outcomes as study variables increases the ease with which findings could be compared across settings, and contributes to knowledge development. Therefore, King's concept of mutually set goals could be studied as "expected outcomes" and King's Theory of Goal Attainment could be conceptualized as "attainment of expected outcomes" in the application of the nursing process using SNLs.

Impact of Managed Care, Performance Improvement, and Technology on King's Concepts

As previously discussed, research on health care beyond nursing is evolving. With managed care, nursing is increasingly involved with developing care planning tools and critical pathways protocols and guidelines collaboratively with other disciplines. King has always promoted cooperation and collaboration among disciplines (1981). In the managed-care environment, personal, interpersonal, and social systems need to include an expanded conceptualization of King's concept of goal-setting. Personal and professional goal-setting, nurse-client/consumer dyad goal-setting, nurse task force goal-setting, and nurse leader-organization goal-setting are examples of broader applications common in nursing situations for today and tomorrow.

Multidisciplinary care conferences are examples of situations where goal-setting among professionals occurs, with "multidisciplinary care conference" as a label for an indirect nursing intervention within the Nursing Interventions Classification. Some of the activities listed under this label reflect King's concepts: "establish mutually agreeable goals" [mutual goal-setting]; "solicit input for client care planning, revise client care plan, as necessary, discuss progress toward goals" [explore means to achieve goal, agree on means to achieve goal]; and "provide data to facilitate evaluation of client care plan" [evaluation of goal attainment]. The products of multidisciplinary care conferences are guidelines to assist in clinical decision making. Many times guidelines have agendas of cost-saving, decreasing malpractice exposure, or other combinations of purposes. In contrast, if guidelines were based on a single overall purpose of client goal attainment, a surer path to quality care might ensue.

The continuous quality improvement movement as developed by Deming (Walton, 1986) is rooted in the scientific method and used for improving a system's performance in providing care. In the years to come, a framework that binds methods together within the continuous improvement effort in organizations is essential. One possible framework could be derived from King. In 1971 (p. 177), King stated that "effectiveness of health care can be evaluated." King's contribution to quality improvement is "the Theory of Goal Attainment that provides knowledge of process and outcomes" (1971, p. 157). In continuous quality improvement, alternatives to the status quo are sought. Many of the better practices in nursing are not in common use. Furthermore, wide variations in nursing practice exist within hospitals and across the country (Jacox, 1993). The success of nurses and others in improving care within systems is dependent on how we approach improvement (Kilo, Kabcenell, & Berwick, 1998). The gap between what we know and how we practice calls us to use the practice-ready reservoirs of scientific evidence and nursing knowledge, related to King as summarized in this chapter, in nursing's approach to continuous improvement.

King (1997) is keeping pace with the world of technology in the form of health-care informatics and exploring the impact of nursing knowledge and positing that her conceptual system provides the structure of health-care informatics. Specifically, she recommends using her concepts of self, role, power, authority, decisions, time, space, communication, and interaction, with an emphasis on goal-setting and goal attainment as the theoretical basis for nursing informatics. With this forward-looking direction set by the theorist, nurse scholars need to further evaluate the use of King's concepts and possibly redefine them in future contexts. For example, the concepts of interactions and transactions occur without visual perceptions in the emerging area of telenursing. Expansion of these and other concepts is potentially possible from examining other ways of knowing clients—for example, enhanced intuitive skills.

Summary

An essential component in the analysis of conceptual frameworks and theories is the consideration of adequacy (Ellis, 1968). Adequacy depends on the three interrelated characteristics of scope, usefulness, and complexity. Conceptual frameworks are broad in scope and sufficiently complex to be useful for many situations. Theories, on the other hand, are narrower in scope, usually addressing less abstract concepts, and are more specific in terms of the nature and direction of relationships and focus. King fully intended her conceptual system for nursing to be useful in all nursing situations. Likewise, the Theory of Goal Attainment has broad scope since interaction is a part of every nursing encounter. Although evaluation of the scope of King's framework and theory has resulted in mixed reviews (Austin & Champion, 1983; Carter & Dufour, 1994; Frey, 1996; Jonas, 1987; Meleis, 1985), the nursing profession has clearly recognized its scope and usefulness. In addition, the varity of practice applications evident in the literature clearly attest to the complexity of King's work. As researchers continue to integrate King's theory and framework with the dynamic health-care environment, future applications will further demonstrate the adequacy of King's work in terms of nursing practice.

References

Alligood, M. R. (1995). Theory of Goal Attainment: Application to adult orthopedic nursing. In Frey, M. A., & Sieloff, C. L. (Eds.), *Advancing King's systems framework and theory of nursing* (pp. 209–222). Thousand Oaks, CA: Sage Publications.

Alligood, M. R., Evans, G. W., & Wilt, D. L. (1995). King's interacting systems and empathy. In Frey, M. A., & Sieloff, C. L., (Eds.), *Advancing King's systems framework and theory of nursing* (pp. 66–78). Thousand Oaks, CA: Sage Publications.

Austin, J. K., & Champion, V. L. (1983). King's theory for nursing: Explication and evaluation. In Chinn, P. L. (Ed.), *Advances in nursing theory development* (pp. 49–61). Rockville, MD: Aspen.

Benedict, M., & Frey, M. A. (1995). Theory-based practice in the emergency department. In Frey, M. A., & Sieloff, C. L. (Eds.), *Advancing King's systems framework and theory of nursing* (pp. 317–324). Thousand Oaks, CA: Sage Publications.

Biegen, M. A., & Tripp-Reimer, T. (1997). Implications of nursing taxonomies for middle-range theory development. *Advances in Nursing Science, 19*(3), 37–49.

Brooks, E. M., & Thomas, S. (1997). The perception and judgement of senior baccalaureate student nurses in clinical decision making. *Advances in Nursing Science, 19*(3), 50–69.

Brown, S. T., & Lee, B. T. (1980). Imogene King's conceptual framework: A proposed model for continuing nursing education. *Journal of Advanced Nursing, 5,* 467–473.

Byrne, E., & Schreiber, R. (1989). Concept of the month: Implementing King's conceptual framework at the bedside. *Journal of Nursing Administration, 19*(2), 28–32.

Carter, K. F., & Dufour, L. T. (1994). King's theory: A critique of the critiques. *Nursing Science Quarterly, 7*(3), 128–133.

Coker, E., Fradley, T., Harris, J., Tomarchio, D., Chan, V., & Caron, C. (1995). Implementing nursing diagnoses within the context of King's conceptual framework. In Frey, M. A., & Sieloff, C. L. (Eds.), *Advancing King's systems framework and theory of nursing* (pp. 161–176). Thousand Oaks, CA: Sage Publications.

Cook, D. (1998). Evidence-based critical care medicine: A potential tool for change. *New Horizons 6*(1), 20–25.

Daubenmire, M. J. (1989). A baccalaureate nursing curriculum based on King's conceptual framework. In Riehl-Sisca, J. P. (Ed.), *Conceptual models for nursing practice* (3rd ed., pp. 167–178). Norwalk, CT: Appleton & Lange.

Daubenmire, M. J., & King, I. M. (1973). Nursing process models: A systems approach. *Nursing Outlook, 21,* 512–517.

Davidoff, F., Haynes, B., Sackett, D., & Smith, R. (April 1995) Evidence-based medicine [editorial comment]. *British Medical Journal 310*(6987), 1085–1086.

Davis, D. C. (1987). A conceptual framework for infertility. *Journal of Obstetric, Gynecologic, and Neonatal Nursing, 16,* 30–35.

DeHowitt, M. C. (1992). King's conceptual model and individual psychotherapy. *Perspectives in Psychiatric Care, 28*(4), 11–14.

Doornbos, M. M. (1995). Using King's systems framework to explore family health in the families of the young chronically mentally ill. In Frey, M. A., & Sieloff, C. L. (Eds.), *Advancing King's systems framework and theory of nursing* (pp. 192–205). Thousand Oaks, CA: Sage Publications.

Elberson, K. (1989). Applying King's model to nursing administration. In Henry, B., DiVicenti, M., Arndt, C., & Marriner, A. (Eds.), *Dimensions of nursing administration: Theory, research, education and practice* (pp. 47–53). Boston: Blackwell Scientific Publications.

Ellis, R. (1968). Characteristics of significant theories. *Nursing Research, 17,* 217–222.

Fawcett, J. (1978). The relationship between theory and research: A double helix. *Advances in Nursing Science, 1*(1), 49–62.

Fawcett, J. M., Vaillancourt, V. M., & Watson, C. A. (1995). Integration of King's framework into nursing practice. In Frey, M. A., & Sieloff, C. L. (Eds.), *Advancing King's systems framework and theory of nursing* (pp. 176–191). Thousand Oaks, CA: Sage Publications.

Frey, M. A. (1993). A theoretical perspective of family and child health derived from King's conceptual framework of nursing: A deductive approach to theory building. In Feetham, S. L., Meister, S. B., Bell, J. M., & Gillis, C. L. (Eds.), *The nursing of fam-*

ilies: Theory/research/education/practice (pp. 30-37). Newbury Park, CA: Sage Publications.

Frey, M. A. (1995). Toward a theory of families, children, and chronic illness. In Frey, M. A., & Sieloff, C. L. (Eds.), *Advancing King's systems framework and theory of nursing* (pp. 109-125). Thousand Oaks, CA: Sage Publications.

Frey, M. A. (1996). Behavioral correlates of health and illness in youths with chronic illness. *Advanced Nursing Research, 9*(4), 167-176.

Frey, M. A. (1997). Health promotion in youth with chronic illness: Are we on the right track? *Quality Nursing, 3*(5), 13-18.

Frey, M. A., & Denyes, M. J. (1989). Health and illness self-care in adolescents with IDDM: A test of Orem's theory. *Advances in Nursing Science, 12*(1), 67-75.

Frey, M. A., & Fox, M. A. (1990). Assessing and teaching self-care to youths with diabetes mellitus. *Pediatric Nursing, 16*, 597-599.

Frey, M. A., & Norris, D. M. (1997). King's systems framework and theory in nursing practice. In Marriner-Tomey, A. (Ed.), *Nursing theory utilization and application* (pp. 71-88). St. Louis: Mosby.

Frey, M. A., Rooke, L., Sieloff, C. L., Messmer, P., & Kameoka, T. (1995). King's framework and theory in Japan, Sweden, and the United States. *Image: Journal of Nursing Scholarship, 27*(2), 127-130.

Frey, M. A., & Sieloff, C. L. (1995). *Advancing King's systems framework and theory of nursing.* Thousand Oaks, CA: Sage Publications.

Froman, D. (1995). Perceptual congruency between clients and nurses: Testing King's Theory of Goal Attainment. In Frey, M. A., & Sieloff, C. L. (Eds.), *Advancing King's systems framework and theory of nursing* (pp. 223-238). Thousand Oaks, CA: Sage Publications.

Froman, D., & Sanderson, H. (1985). *Application of Imogene King's framework.* Paper presented at the Nursing Theory in Action Conference, Edmonton, Alberta, Canada.

Funashima, N. (1990). King's goal attainment theory. *Knago MOOK, 35,* 56-62.

Gill, J., Hopwood-Jones, L., Tyndall, J., Gregoroff, S., LeBlanc, P., Lovett, C., Rasco, L., & Ross, A. (1995). Incorporating nursing diagnosis and King's theory in the O. R. documentation. *Canadian Operating Room Nursing Journal, 13*(1), 10-14.

Gonot, P. J. (1986). Family therapy as derived from King's conceptual model. In Whall, A. L. (Ed.), *Family therapy for nursing: Four approaches* (pp. 33-48). Norwalk, CT: Appleton-Century-Crofts.

Gulitz, E. A., & King, I. M. (1988). King's general systems model: Application to curriculum development. *Nursing Science Quarterly, 1,* 128-132.

Hampton, D. C. (1994). King's Theory of Goal Attainment as a framework for managed care implementation in a hospital setting. *Nursing Science Quarterly, 7*(4), 170-173.

Hanna, K. (1993). Effect of nurse-client transaction on female adolescents' oral contraceptive use. *Image, 25*(4), 285-290.

Hanna, K. M. (1995). Use of King's Theory of Goal Attainment to promote adolescents' health behavior. In Frey, M. A., & Sieloff, C. L. (Eds.), *Advancing King's systems framework and theory of nursing*

(pp. 239-250). Thousand Oaks, CA: Sage Publications.

Hanucharurnkui, S., & Vinya-nguag, P. (1991). Effects of promoting patients' participation in self-care on postoperative recovery and satisfaction with care. *Nursing Science Quarterly, 4,* 14-20.

Hickson, D. J., Hinings, C. R., Lee, C. A., Schneck, R. E., & Pennings, J. M. (1971). A strategic contingencies' theory of intraorganizational power. *Administrative Science Quarterly, 16,* 216-229.

Hobdell, E. F. (1995). Using King's interacting systems framework for research on parents of children with neural tube defects. In Frey, M. A., & Sieloff, C. L. (Eds.), *Advancing King's systems framework and theory of nursing* (pp. 126-136). Thousand Oaks, CA: Sage Publications.

Husband, A. (1988). Application of King's theory of nursing to the care of the adult with diabetes. *Journal of Advanced Nursing, 13,* 484-488.

Husting, P. M. (1997). A transcultural critique of Imogene King's Theory of Goal Attainment. *Journal of Multicultural Nursing & Health, 3*(3), 15-20.

Jacono, J., Hicks, G., Antonioni, C., O'Brien, K., & Rasi, M. (1990). Comparison of perceived needs of family members between registered nurses and family members of critically ill patients in intensive care and neonatal intensive care units. *Heart and Lung: Journal of Critical Care, 19*(1), 72-78.

Jacox, A. (1993). Addressing variations in nursing practice/technology through clinical practice guidelines methods. *Nursing Economics, 11*(3), 170-172.

Jadadd, A. R., & Haynes, R. B. (1998). Cochrane collaboration: Advances and challenges in improving evidence-based decision making. *Medical Decision Making: An International Journal of the Society for Medical Decision Making, 18*(1), 2-9.

Johnson, M., & Maas, M. (1997). *Nursing outcomes classification (NOC).* St. Louis: Mosby-Year Book.

Jolly, M. L., & Winker, C. K. (1995). Theory of Goal Attainment in the context of organizational structure. In Frey, M. A., & Sieloff, C. L. (Eds.), *Advancing King's systems framework and theory of nursing* (pp. 305-316). Thousand Oaks, CA: Sage Publications.

Jonas, C. M. (1987). King's goal attainment theory: Use in gerontological nursing practice. *Perspectives: Journal of the Gerontological Nursing Association, 11*(4), 9-12.

Kameoka, T. (1995). Analyzing nurse-patient interactions in Japan. In In Frey, M. A., & Sieloff, C. L. (Eds.), *Advancing King's Systems framework and Theory of Goal Attainment* (pp. 251-260). Thousand Oaks, CA: Sage Publications.

Kameoka, T., & Sugimori, M. (1992). *Application to King's goal attainment theory in Japanese clinical setting: Part 2.* Paper presented at the First International Nursing Research Conference, Japan.

Kemppainen, J. K. (1990). Imogene King's theory: A nursing case study of a psychotic client with human immunodeficiency virus infection. *Archives of Psychiatric Nursing, 4*(6), 384-388.

Kenny, T. (1990). Erosion of individuality in care of elderly people in hospital—an alternative approach. *Journal of Advanced Nursing, 15,* 571-576.

Killeen, M. B. (1996). *Patient-consumer perceptions and responses to professional nursing care: Instru-*

ment development. Unpublished doctoral dissertation, Wayne State University, Detroit, Michigan.

Kilo, C. M., Kabcenell, A., & Berwick, D. (1998). Beyond survival: Toward continuous improvement in medical care. *New Horizons, 61*(1), 3-11.

King, I. M. (1971). *Toward a theory for nursing: General concepts of human behavior.* New York: Wiley.

King, I. M. (1976). *Toward a theory of nursing: General concepts of human behavior* (Sugimori, M., Trans.). Tokyo: Igaku-Shoin.

King, I. M. (1981). *A theory for nursing: Systems, concepts, process.* New York: Wiley.

King, I. M. (1985). *A theory for nursing: Systems, concepts, process* (Sugimori, M., Trans.). Tokyo: Igaku-Shoin.

King, I. M. (1988). Measuring health goal attainment in patients. In Waltz, C. F., & Strickland, O. L. (Eds.), *Measurement of nursing outcomes* (Vol. 1, pp. 108-127). New York: Springer.

King, I. M. (1990). Health as a goal for nursing. *Nursing Science Quarterly, 3,* 123-128.

King, I. M. (1997). King's Theory of Goal Attainment in practice. *Nursing Science Quarterly, 10*(4), 180-185.

King, I. M., & Tarsitano, B. (1982). The effect of structured and unstructured pre-operative teaching: A replication. *Nursing Research, 31*(6), 324-329.

Kobayashi, F. T. (1970). A conceptual frame of reference for nursing. *Japanese Journal of Nursing Research, 3*(3), 199-204.

Kohler, P. (1988). Model of shared control. *Journal of Gerontological Nursing, 14*(7), 21-25.

Laben, J. K., Dodd, D., & Sneed, L. (1991). King's Theory of Goal Attainment applied in group therapy for inpatient juvenile offenders, maximum security state offenders, and community parolees, using visual aids. *Issues in Mental Health Nursing, 12*(1), 51-64.

Laben, J. K., Sneed, L. D., & Seidel, S. L. (1995). Goal attainment in short-term group psychotherapy settings: Clinical implications for practice. In Frey, M. A., & Sieloff, C. L. (Eds.), *Advancing King's systems framework and theory of nursing* (pp. 261-277). Thousand Oaks, CA: Sage Publications.

Leininger, M. M. (1985). *Qualitative research methods in nursing.* New York: Grune & Stratton.

Levine, C. D., Wilson, S. F., & Guido, G. W. (1988). Personality factors of critical nurses. *Heart and Lung, 17*(4), 392-398.

Martin, J. P. (1990). Male cancer awareness: Impact of an employee education program. *Oncology Nursing Forum, 17,* 59-64.

McFarland, G. K., & McFarland, E. A. (1997). *Nursing diagnosis and intervention: Planning for patient care.* St. Louis: Mosby-Year Book.

McGirr, M., Rukholm, E., Salmoni, A., O'Sullivan, P., & Koren, I. (1990). Perceived mood and exercise behaviors of cardiac rehabilitation program referrals. *Canadian Journal of Cardiovascular Nursing, 1*(4), 14-19.

Meleis, A. (1985). *Theoretical nursing: Developments and progress* (2nd ed.). Philadelphia: J. B. Lippincott.

Messmer, P. R. (1995). Implementation of theory-based nursing practice. In Frey, M. A., & Sieloff, C. L. (Eds.), *Advancing King's systems framework and theory of nursing* (pp. 294-304). Thousand Oaks, CA: Sage Publications.

Messmer, R., & Neff Smith, M. N. (1986). Neurofibromatosis: Relinquishing the masks: A quest for quality of life. *Journal of Advanced Nursing, 11,* 459-464.

Murray, R. L. E., & Baier, M. (1996). King's conceptual framework applied to a transitional living program. *Perspectives in Psychiatric Care, 32*(1), 15-19.

Naylor, C. D. (1995). Grey zones of clinical practice: Some limits to evidence-based medicine. *Lancet, 335,* 840-842.

Norris, D. M., & Hoyer, P. J. (1993). Dynamism in practice: Parenting within King's framework. *Nursing Science Quarterly, 6*(2), 79-85.

Pearson, A., & Vaughan, B. (1986). *Nursing models for practice.* London: William Heinemann Medical Books.

Porteous, A., & Tyndall, J. (1994). Yes, I want to talk to the OR. *Candian Operating Room Nursing, 12*(2), 15-16, 18-19.

Rawlins, P. S., Rawlins, T. D., & Horner, M. (1990). Development of the family needs assessment tool. *Western Journal of Nursing Research, 12,* 201-214.

Rooda, L. A. (1992). The development of a conceptual model for multicultural nursing. *Journal of Holistic Nursing, 10*(4), 337-347.

Rooke, L. (1995a). The concept of space in King's systems framework: Its implications for nursing. In Frey, M. A., & Sieloff, C. L. (Eds.), *Advancing King's systems framework and theory of nursing* (pp. 79-96). Thousand Oaks, CA: Sage Publications.

Rooke, L. (1995b). Focusing on King's theory and systems framework in education by using an experiential learning model: A challenge to improve the quality of nursing care. In Frey, M. A., & Sieloff, C. L. (Eds.), *Advancing King's systems framework and theory of nursing* (pp. 278-293). Thousand Oaks, CA: Sage Publications.

Schreiber, R. (1991). Psychiatric assessment—"A la King." *Nursing Management, 22*(5), 90, 92, 94.

Sharts-Hopko, N. C. (1995). Using health, personal, and interpersonal system concepts within the King's systems framework to explore perceived health status during the menopause transition. In Frey, M. A., & Sieloff, C. L. (Eds.), *Advancing King's system framework and theory of nursing* (pp. 147-160). Thousand Oaks, CA: Sage Publications.

Sieloff, C. L. (1995a). Development of a theory of departmental power. In Frey, M. A., & Sieloff, C. L. (Eds.), *Advancing King's systems framework and theory of nursing* (pp. 46-65). Thousand Oaks, CA: Sage Publications.

Sieloff, C. L. (1995b). Defining the health of a social system within Imogene King's framework. In Frey, M. A., & Sieloff, C. L. (Eds.), *Advancing King's systems framework and theory of nursing* (pp. 137-146). Thousand Oaks, CA: Sage Publications.

Sieloff, C. L. (1996). *Development of an instrument to estimate the actualized power of a nursing department.* Unpublished doctoral dissertation, Wayne State University, Detroit.

Sirles, A. T., & Selleck, C. S. (1989). Cardiac disease and the family: Impact, assessment, and implications. *Journal of Cardiovascular Nursing, 3*(2), 23-32.

Smith, M. C. (1988). King's theory in practice. *Nursing Science Quarterly, 1,* 145-146.

Sowell, R. L., & Lowenstein, A. (1994). King's theory: A framework for quality; linking theory to practice. *Nursing Connections, 7*(2), 19–31.

Spratlen, L. P. (1976). Introducing ethnic-cultural factors in models of nursing: Some mental health care applications. *Journal of Nursing Education, 15*(2), 23–29.

Swindale, J. E. (1989). The nurse's role in giving pre-operative information to reduce anxiety in patients admitted to hospital for elective minor surgery. *Journal of Advanced Nursing, 14,* 899–905.

Syzmanski, M. E. (1991). Use of nursing theories in the care of families with high-risk infants: Challenges for the future. *Journal of Perinatal and Neonatal Nursing, 4*(4), 71–77.

Temple, A. F., & Fawdry, M. K. (1992). King's Theory of Goal Attainment: Resolving filial caregiver role strain. *Journal of Geronotological Nursing, 18*(3), 11–15.

Titler, M. G. (1998, June). Evidence-based practice and research utilization: One and the same? Paper presented at the ANA Council for Nursing Research's 1998 Pre-Convention Research Utilization Conference, Evidence-based Practice, San Diego, CA.

Tritsch, J. M. (1996). Application of King's Theory of Goal Attainment and the Carondelet St. Mary's case management model. *Nursing Science Quarterly, 11*(2), 69–73.

Villeneuve, M. J., & Ozolins, P. H. (1991). Sexual counselling in the neuroscience setting: Theory and practical tips for nurses. *AXON, 12*(3), 63–67.

Walton, M. (1986). *The Deming management method.* New York: Putnam.

Wicks, M. N. (1995). Family health as derived from King's framework. In Frey, M. A., & Sieloff, C. L. (Eds.), *Advancing King's systems framework and theory of nursing* (pp. 97–108). Thousand Oaks, CA: Sage Publications.

Winker, C. K. (1995). A systems view of health. In Frey, M. A., & Sieloff, C. L. (Eds.), *Advancing King's systems framework and theory of nursing* (pp. 35–45). Thousand Oaks, CA: Sage Publications.

Woods, E. C. (1994). King's theory in practice with elders. *Nursing Science Quarterly, 7*(2), 65–69.

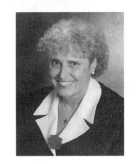

Chapter *18*

Sister Callista Roy
The Roy Adaptation Model

Sister Callista Roy and Lin Zhan

INTRODUCING THE THEORIST

Sister Callista Roy is a highly respected nurse theorist, writer, lecturer, researcher, and teacher who currently holds the position of professor and nurse theorist at the Boston College School of Nursing. It is often said that her name is the most recognized name in the field of nursing today worldwide, and she is one of our greatest living thinkers. Dr. Roy shakes her head on hearing these premature epitaphs and notes that her best work is yet to come. As a theorist, Dr. Roy often emphasizes her primary commitment to define and develop nursing knowledge and regards her work with the Roy Adaptation Model as one rich source of knowledge for clinical nursing. At the beginning of a new century, Dr. Roy has provided an expanded, values-based concept of adaptation based on insights related to the place of the person in the universe. She hopes her redefinition of adaptation, with its cosmic philosophical and scientific assumptions, will become the basis for developing knowledge that will make nursing a major social force in the century to come.

Dr. Roy credits her major influences in personal and professional growth as her family, her religious commitment, and her teachers and mentors. Dr. Roy was born in Los Angeles, California, on October 14, 1939. Her middle name, Callista, is the feminine form of Callistus, the Saint of the Day from the Roman Catholic calendar, who was a pope and martyr. She was the oldest daughter of a family of seven boys and seven girls. A deep spirit of faith, hope, love, and commitment to God and service to others was central in the family. Her mother was a licensed vocational nurse and instilled the values of always seeking to know more about people and their care and of selfless giving as a nurse. Dr. Roy notes that she also had excellent teachers in parochial schools, high school, and college. At age 14 she began working at a large general hospital, first as a pantry girl, then as a maid, and finally as a nurse's aid. After a soul-searching process of discernment, she entered the Sisters of Saint Joseph of Carondelet, of which she has been a member for 40 years. Her college education began with a bachelor of arts degree with a major in nursing at Mount St. Mary's College, Los Angeles; followed by master's degrees in pediatric nursing and sociology at the University of California, Los Angeles, and a Ph.D. in sociology at the same school. Later, Dr. Roy had the opportunity to be a clinical nurse scholar in a 2-year postdoctoral program in neuroscience nursing at the University of California at San Francisco. Important mentors in her life have included Dorothy E. Johnson, Ruth Wu, Connie Robinson, and Barbara Smith Moran.

Dr. Roy is still best known for developing and continually updating the Roy Adaptation Model as a framework for theory, practice, and research in nursing. Books on the model have been translated into many languages, including French, Italian, Spanish, Finnish, Chinese, Korean, and Japanese. Two recent publications that Dr. Roy considers of great significance are *The Roy Adaptation Model* (2nd edition), written with Heather Andrews (Appleton & Lange); and *The Roy Adaptation Model-based Research: Twenty-five Years of Contributions to Nursing Science,* published as a research monograph by Sigma Theta Tau. The latter is a critical analysis of the 25 years of model-based literature, which includes 163 studies published in 46 English-speaking journals, and dissertations and theses. This project was completed by the Boston-Based Adaptation Research Society in Nursing (BBARNS), a group of scholars founded by Dr. Roy in the interest of advancing nursing practice by developing basic and clinical nursing knowledge based on the Roy Adaptation Model.

One of Dr. Roy's major activities includes cochairing the annual Knowledge Conferences hosted by the Boston College School of Nursing in 1996, 1997, 1998 and the major International Knowledge Conference scheduled for October 2000, with cohosts from around the world. Dr. Roy has been a major speaker throughout North America and around 25 other countries over the past 30 years on topics related to nursing theory, research, curriculum, clinical practice, and professional trends for the future. She received a Fulbright Senior Scholar Award from the Australian-American Educational Foundation for travel to Australia, where she gave speeches and talked with colleagues in several regions. She has played a major role in at least 30 research projects. Results of research and papers on nursing knowledge have appeared in *Image: Journal of Nursing Scholarship, Nursing Science Quarterly, Scholarly Inquiry for Nursing Practice,* and other journals. Her current clinical research continues her long-time interest in neuroscience. Since her days as a nursing student in the 1960s, Dr. Roy has been fascinated by the neurosciences, which she calls "the frontier of knowledge development." She is currently continuing her research on cognitive adaptation and nursing interventions with patients who have sustained head injuries, as well as promoting adaptation of patients with chronic neurologic conditions.

Dr. Roy has been the recipient of many awards, including the National League for Nursing Martha

Rogers Award for advancing nursing science; the Sigma Theta Tau International Founders Award for contributions to professional practice; and honorary doctorates from Eastern Michigan University, Alverno College in Milwaukee, and St. Joseph's College in Standish, Maine. The Sister Callista Roy Lectureship was established at the Department of Nursing at Mount St. Mary's College in Los Angeles and has been an annual event. Dr. Roy has also received the outstanding Alumna Award and Carondelet Medal from Mount St. Mary's, where she holds a concurrent position as research professor in nursing at her alma mater.

The Roy Adaptation Model has been in use for about 30 years, providing direction for nursing practice, education, and research. Extensive implementation efforts around the world, and continuing philosophical and scientific developments by the theorist, have contributed to model-based knowledge for nursing practice. The purpose of this chapter is to describe the use of the model in developing knowledge for practice, with particular emphasis on research with the elderly. A study of cognitive adaptation and self-consistency in the elderly with hearing impairment provides an exemplar of both some of the key concepts of the model and a research design to test the relationships among the concepts. Specifically, the study provides a test of a generic proposition derived from the Roy Adaptation Model. A brief review of the Roy Adaptation Model is provided, with emphasis on recent developments of the theoretical work and its use in nursing research. Then the theoretical and empirical concepts of cognitive adaptation processing and self-consistency are described in greater detail. Finally, the problem, design, and findings of an exemplar research project with the elderly are discussed.

THE ROY MODEL AS A FRAMEWORK FOR RESEARCH

The Roy Adaptation Model (Roy, 1984, 1988a, 1988b; Roy & Andrews, 1991, 1999; Roy & Roberts, 1981) provides the framework for programs of nursing research, particularly the constructs for the research exemplar involving elderly patients with hearing impairment.

Assumptions

The model's philosophical assumptions are rooted in the general principles of humanism, and in what Roy has termed "veritivity and cosmic unity" (Roy & Andrews, 1999). Scientific assumptions for the model

have been based on general systems theory and adaptation-level theory (Roy & Corliss, 1993). More recently, the assumptions have been extended to include Roy's redefinition of adaptation for the twenty-first century (Roy & Andrews, 1999). The cosmic unity stressed in Roy's vision for the future emphasizes the principle that people and the earth have common patterns and integral relationships. Rather than the system acting to maintain itself, the emphasis shifts to the purposefulness of human existence in a universe that is creative.

Major Concepts

Humans, both individually and in groups, are viewed as holistic adaptive systems, with coping processes acting to maintain adaptation, and to promote person and environment transformations. The coping processes are broadly described within the regulator and cognator subsystems for the individual, and the stabilizer and innovator subsystems for groups. Through these coping processes, persons as holistic adaptive systems interact with the internal and external environment, transform the environment, and are transformed by it. A particular aspect of the internal environment is the adaptation level. This is the name given to the three possible conditions of the human life processes of the human adaptive system: integrated, compensatory, and compromised (Roy & Andrews, 1999). Processing of the internal and external environment by the coping subsystems results in human behavior. Four categories for assessing behaviors are termed "adaptive modes." Initially developed to describe human systems as individuals (Roy, 1971), the modes have been expanded to include groups, and are termed physiologic-physical, self-concept-group identity, role function, and interdependence (Roy & Andrews, 1999). Central to Roy's theoretical model is the belief that adaptive responses support *health,* which is defined as a state and a process of being and becoming integrated and whole.

Uses in Research

Roy has described strategies for knowledge development based on the model and a structure of knowledge to guide research (Roy & Andrews, 1999). Knowledge development strategies that she has integrated through decades of work include model construction; theory development (including concept analysis, synthesis, and derivation of propositional statements); philosophic explication; and research, qualitative, quantitative, and instrument development. The structure for knowledge includes the broad categories of the basic and clinical science of nursing.

Basic nursing science discovers knowledge about persons and groups from a nursing perspective that can provide understandings for practice. The clinical science of nursing investigates specifically the role of the nurse in promoting adaptation and human and environment transformations. Within the basic science, the investigator studies the person or group as an adaptive system, including: (1) the adaptive processes; that is, cognator and regulator activity, stabilizer and innovator activity, stability of adaptation level patterns, and dynamics of evolving adaptive patterns; (2) the adaptive modes; that is, their development, interrelatedness, and cultural and other influences; and (3) adaptation related to health, particularly person and environment interaction and integration of the adaptive modes. Topics for research in the clinical science of nursing include: (1) changes in cognator-regulator or stabilizer-innovator effectiveness; (2) changes within and among the adaptive modes; and (3) nursing care to promote adaptive processes, particularly in times of transition, during environmental changes, and during acute and chronic illness, injury, treatment, and technologic threats.

In a recent text (Roy & Andrews, 1999), Roy summarized her own research within the structure of knowledge. In her earlier work, Roy (1975, 1977) used three methods to explore how the cognator coping processes act to promote adaptation and how they relate to the adaptive modes. Two inductive processes involved content analysis of patient interviews before diagnostic tests and recordings of the nursing process done by students in 10 schools where the Roy Adaptation Model was the basis of their curricula. A total of 41 different coping processes were inferred from the two sets of data and refined with literature review. Samples of the cognator processes include selective attention—differential focus on a good outcome and affective isolation. The second major research effort, again within the basic science of nursing, used a systematic controlled comparison of survey data collected in six hospitals across the United States. One purpose within the larger study aims was to examine levels of wellness in relation to levels of adaptation. For the 208 patients of the sample, some of the measures of physio-

> Adaptive responses support *health*, which is defined as a state and a process of being and becoming integrated and whole.

logic adaptation were related to levels of wellness, but no evidence was found of a relationship between psychosocial adaptation and measures of levels of wellness. There was, however, such a relationship in the least acute care setting and for patients with longer hospital stays. Thus, it was suggested that adaptation is a process that takes place over time. Further, Roy (1977) noted that the measures of levels of wellness were limited and not entirely consistent with the dynamic and holistic concept of health as defined by the model.

Roy's more recent research is related to clinical nursing science. A model of cognitive information processing was developed (Roy, 1988b) and a program of research initiated to contribute to further understanding of cognitive processes; that is, how people take in and process environmental interactions and how nurses can help people use these processes to affect their health status positively. Cognitive recovery from head injury was the focus of the research. The first study used a repeated measures design to describe changes in cognitive performance over 6 months of recovery for 50 patients (Roy, 1985). Nursing intervention protocols were then developed for use during the first month, which is considered the critical period for recovery. The initial pilot study of nine matched pairs shows some promising trends. Graphs of recovery curves on all nine measures showed earlier improvement of performance in the treated group as compared with the matched group that did not receive the planned nursing interventions to promote cognitive recovery from head injury (Roy & Hanna, 1999). Another aspect of Roy's current clinical research focuses on relating cognitive abilities and adapting to chronic illness. This work has included development of an instrument, the Cognitive Adaptation Processing Scale (CAPS), which is described later in this chapter.

The use of the Roy Adaptation Model for nursing research is strikingly demonstrated by a research synthesis project conducted by The Boston-Based Adaptation Research Society in Nursing (BBARNS). Roy worked with seven other scholars for about four years to develop a method to conduct a review and synthesis of research based on the Roy Adaptation Model, to identify and locate the literature from a 25-year period, to conduct the critical analysis, and present the findings in a research monograph (Roy et al., 1999). From 1970 through 1994, a total of 163 studies met the inclusion criteria. Only English-language publications were included. The sample included 94 articles in 44 different research and specialty journals from five continents. In addition, there were 77 dissertations and theses from a total of

35 universities and colleges in the United States and Canada that were retrieved and included in the synthesis review. The major concepts of the model were used to organize the presentation of the review of this extensive use of the Roy Adaptation Model in nursing research. Although studies focused on more than one model concept, it was possible to group the studies by their major topic, as follows: multiple adaptive modes and processes ($n = 36$); physiologic ($n = 21$), self-concept ($n = 18$), role function ($n = 21$), and interdependence ($n = 20$) modes; stimuli ($n = 19$); and intervention ($n = 28$).

The critical analysis involved evaluating each study according to predetermined criteria for the quality of the research and for the linkages of the research to the model. The studies that met the established criteria for adequacy of the quality of the research and links to the model ($n = 116$ of the total 163) were used to test propositions derived from the model. They were based on 12 generic propositions from Roy's published work. As the studies were analyzed, the findings were used to state ancillary and practice propositions. "Ancillary propositions" are special instances of the general propositions and sometimes are stated in terms directly relevant to practice and thus referred to as "practice propositions." Significant research support for the ancillary propositions lent support to the theoretical statements of the generic propositions. This process is demonstrated in the exemplar study reported below.

The BBARNS reviewers also examined the application of findings to nursing practice. They used three categories to assess the potential of research findings for use in practice: Category 1—high potential for implementation based on positive findings with methodologic adequacy and without risk to pa-

tients; Category 2—need further clinical evaluation before implementation, for example, by teams of advanced practice nurses in the practice area to evaluate potential effectiveness relative to risk; and Category 3—further research warranted before implementation, designation used in cases where findings were negative or equivocal, or that were promising, but posed a risk to patients and thus needed replication and clarification before being recommended for practice. This review showed the breadth and depth of the use of the Roy model in nursing research in qualitative and quantitative research, and in instrument development studies, using populations of individuals and groups, of all ages, both in health and illness, in all areas of nursing practice.

COGNITIVE ADAPTATION PROCESSING

Two concepts of the model—cognitive adaptation processing and self-consistency—are discussed in greater detail as a basis for applying the model in the research exemplar with the elderly. The Roy Adaptation Model focuses on enhancing the basic life processes of the individual and group. The cognator and regulator of the individual, and innovator and stabilizer of the group, have basic abilities to promote adaptation; that is, the process and outcome whereby thinking and feeling are used in conscious awareness and choice to create human and environmental integration (Roy & Andrews, 1999). A major concentration of nursing activity is to assist people in using their cognitive abilities to handle their internal and external environment effectively. Given the priority of this notion, Roy focused efforts on further con-

> **The Roy Adaptation Model focuses on enhancing basic life processes of the individual and group.**

ceptual and empirical work to understand this human ability and nursing practice based on that understanding. "Cognitive adaptation processing" is the specialized term used for a significant coping strategy that the nurse promotes using the adaptation model.

Conceptual Development

The conceptual basis for cognitive adaptation processing lies in Roy's work on understanding the cognator and regulator as processors of adaptation (Roy & Andrews, 1999), on the development of a nursing model for cognitive processing (Roy, 1988a, 1988b), and on understanding of Das and Luria's model of simultaneous and successive information processing (Das, 1984; Luria, 1980). Drawing from knowledge in the neurosciences, her early theory development and research on the model, and observations in neuroscience nursing practice, Roy proposed a nursing model for cognitive processing (Roy, 1988b). Cognitive processes in human adaptation are described as follows: input processes (arousal and attention, sensation and perception), central processes (coding, concept formation, memory, language), output processes (planning and motor responses), and emotion. Through these cognitive processes, adaptive responses occur.

Taylor (1983), in a study of cancer patients, proposed a related theory of cognitive adaptation. According to Taylor, cognitive adaptation is centered on three themes: a search for a meaning in the experience, an attempt to regain mastery over the event, and an effort to restore self-esteem through self-enhancing evaluation. Taylor's propositions are in concert with Roy's assumptions of cognitive adaptation, in which individuals make cognitive efforts to understand the purpose of their lives, maintain their sense of self, and enhance their well-being.

Instrument Development

To identify a typology of adaptation strategies, Roy conducted two qualitative interview studies, content analysis of nursing process care plans, and clinical research in patient information processing (Roy, 1988a, 1988b), as noted above. The 41 items of inferred coping mechanisms identified in the early qualitative studies were compared with the later conceptual development of cognitive adaptation processing. In this way, Roy organized and completed the scheme to create a 72-item Cognitive Adaptation Process Scale (CAPS) (Roy & Kazanowski, 1999).

The number of items was reduced by content experts to a 48-item CAPS for the elderly in a Likert-format scale, and this version of the scale was used in the research exemplar described in this chapter. The items retained were inclusive of the inferred coping mechanisms and the categories of the nursing model for cognitive processing. Content-validity of the CAPS was based on both the strong theoretical-empirical basis for its development and the review by content experts. Internal consistency reliability for the total scale was .85 (Zhan, 1993a). The conceptual clarification of the CAPS was further examined by using a principal component factor extraction with a varimax rotation, resulting in five factors that accounted for 48% of variances among the scores (Zhan, 1993b). Roy termed these five factors (1) cognitive processing of self-perception, (2) clear focus and method, (3) knowing awareness, (4) sensory regulation, and (5) selective focus. The scores on this version of the CAPS can range from 48 to 192, and a total high score represents a greater use of cognitive adaptation strategies.

Cognitive processing of self-perception refers to self-awareness, self-analysis, emotion, and consciousness (Carver & Scheier, 1991). It serves to signal needs for cognitive efforts, to help the person to attend, and to interfere with cognition. Examples of items were "keep in touch with emotions," "put things into perspective," "rechannel feelings," and "be aware of self-limits." Cognitive processing of clear focus and method refers to programming, attention, thinking, reasoning, problem solving, concept formation, and cognitive coding. It involves systematic thinking. The real process of systematic thinking lacks full understanding. However, it can be viewed in part as a process in which people classify the problem, organize information to accomplish some desired end, and weigh the benefits and risks of their efforts to their self-structure (Das, 1984; Luria, 1980; Roy, 1988b). The thinking process requires knowledge of the adaptation encounter, perceptions of one's thoughts, action tendencies, and bodily changes. Items included: "give self time to grasp situations," "be objective about what happened," "identify the situation," and "follow directions." Cognitive processing of knowing awareness involves retrieving information from one's mind and recognizing what has worked for the person in the past. It can be viewed as a self-regulating process (Carver & Scheier, 1991). The overall function of such cognitive processing is to minimize discrepancies between a desirable sense of self and a present perception of self. It includes cognitive input processing of receiving, analyzing, storing, memory, successive processing, and arousal-attention (Roy, 1988b). Example items were "gather information," "recall past strategies," "keep eyes and ears open," "get more resources," "learn from others," "feel alert and active," and "be creative."

Cognitive processing of sensory regulation involves immediate sensory experience, output processing, motor response, movement, and regulating tone (Roy & Hanna, 1999). Example of items include "try to maintain balance," "change physical activity," "picture actions," and "share concerns with others." Cognitive processing of selective focus refers to one's cognitive efforts to select attention and focus in coping with stressful encounters. Some examples of items were "useful to focus," "tend not to blame self," "get away by self," and "put the events out of mind." These five cognitive processes form subscales of the CAPS. Internal consistency reliability of these five subscales ranged from .56 to .89 (Zhan, 1993). Further development of the tool continues to improve the reliability of the subscales (Roy & Kazanowski, 1999).

SELF-CONSISTENCY

Roy (Roy & Andrews, 1999) describes "self-concept" as one adaptive mode of the individual within an adaptive system. The self-concept mode for the individual has two subareas: the physical self and the personal self. The physical self includes two components: body sensation and body image; and the personal self has three components: self-consistency, self-ideal, and moral-ethical-spiritual self.

Conceptual Development

Self-consistency was introduced during the development of the Roy Adaptation Model based on the work of Coombs and Snyggs (1959). These authors noted that people strive to maintain a consistent self-organization and thus avoid disequilibrium (Coombs & Snyggs, 1959; Lecky, 1961; Roy & Andrews, 1991). Lecky (1961) proposed the Theory of Self-Consistency to conceptualize a person as a holistic and consistent structure. Central to Lecky's Self-Consistency Theory is that people are motivated to act in a way that is congruent with their sense of self and thereby maintain intactness when facing potentially challenging situations. To maintain self-consistency in the transaction between the person and the environment (Elliot, 1986, 1988; Lecky, 1961; Rogers, 1961; Roy & Roberts, 1981), one initiates cognitive and emotional responses (Roy & Andrews, 1991).

An individual's sense of self may influence the person's ability to heal and to do what is necessary to maintain health. In particular, related to the application exemplar in this chapter, previous studies (Atchley, 1988; Kaufman, 1987; Klarkowska & Klarkowska, 1987; Zhan, 1994) report that older persons with greater self-consistency had more positive levels of well-being. Further, they coped better with physical and psychosocial changes in aging than did those who had less consistency of self-perceptions. Being old does not necessarily mean one forms a new self-concept. Instead, older people carry their sense of self and personality with them into the later stage of their lives and adapt to a given situation as best as they can (Gove, Ortage, & Style, 1989). Lieberman and Tobin (1988) examined how older people coped with certain stressful life events such as the loss of loved ones, relocation, the experience of chronic conditions, and the approach of death. Their findings suggested that the older people who had a stability of self-concept coped well in stressful encounters. Therefore, the critical task for older people is to maintain self-consistency by transcending internal and external losses in the aging process. They further assert that central to understanding how well a person can cope with any stressful condition in aging is understanding how one maintains consistency of self and whether one is able to achieve that goal.

> The individual's sense of self may influence the person's ability to heal and to do what is necessary to maintain health.

Instrument Development

Based on extensive literature review on theories of self-concept and self-consistency (Andrews, 1990; Beck, 1976; Elliot, 1986; Goffman, 1959; Lecky, 1961; Mead, 1934; Rogers, 1961; Rosenberg, 1979; Roy & Andrews, 1991; Wylie, 1989), Zhan developed the Self-Consistency Scale (SCS). A measure of self-consistency is based on the assumption that an individual has the capacity for self-examination and evaluation. Therefore, self-perception and self-evaluation are consciously available and can be reported by the individual. Twenty-seven items in the SCS reflect the concepts of self-esteem, private consciousness, social anxiety, and stability of self-concept.

Self-esteem was measured by a global index containing six items that were originally developed by Rosenberg (1979, 1989). Elliott (1986, 1988), in examining the relationship between self-esteem and self-consistency among a sample of 2625 young people (ages 8 to 19), found that self-esteem was highly correlated with self-consistency. An example item reflecting the concept of self-esteem in the SCS was "I feel that I am a person of worth, at least on an equal with others." Private self-consciousness measures how preoccupied the individual is with his or her personal characteristics, or the individual's tendency to be the focus of his or her own attention. Being excessively focused on one's own characteristics is likely to lead to negative affect, as the individual becomes increasingly aware that he or she does not meet those "standards of correctness" set for the self (Elliot, 1986). Therefore, excessive private consciousness leads to less self-consistency. A sample item in the SCS was: "I spend a lot of time thinking about what I am like."

> The critical task for older people is to maintain self-consistency by transcending internal and external losses in the aging process.

Stability of self-concept refers to the sameness of self-concept across time and space (Elliot, 1988). It measures the continuity of self-concept. A sample item in the SCS was: "I feel I know just who I am." Social anxiety is viewed as one's reaction to social stimuli. It measures one's worry about others' appraisals in social settings. High social anxiety leads to less self-consistency (Elliot, 1986). A sample item in the SCS was: "I think about how others are looking at me when I am talking to someone." Private self-consciousness and social anxiety could be viewed as mediating factors in self-consistency.

Each item of the SCS was scored on an ordinal scale from 1 to 4, with 1 indicating "never" and 4 indicating "always." Positive and negative items were ordered in a way to reduce the responsive set. For analysis, all negative items were reverse scored, so that a higher score would indicate a greater self-consistency. An example of a reverse-scored item was: "I feel mixed up about what I am really like." The SCS was administered to a sample of 130 older people. Psychometric evaluations of the SCS revealed an internal consistency reliability of .89, with a score range from 51 to 104, a mean total score of 85.10, and standard deviations of 11.04 (Zhan & Shen, 1994). Content validity was supported by extensive and concurrent literature research in the field of self-consistency and self-theory, and an expert panel consisting of four university faculty members who validated each item in the SCS. Convergent validity was supported by a significantly positive correlation between a Visual Analog Scale, "A Sense of Self," and the SCS, $r = .60$, $p < .01$. Divergent validity was supported by a significantly negative correlation between the SCS and the Geriatric Depression Scale (GDS), $r = -.57$, $p < .01$. Using the GDS was based on the theoretical proposition that a lack of self-consistency leads to certain affective disorders, including depression (Beck, 1976; Lecky, 1961; Rosenberg, 1979, 1989). Therefore, the effects of its absence can perhaps best assess the strength of self-consistency.

APPLICATION OF THE MODEL (RESEARCH EXEMPLAR): ELDERLY PATIENTS WITH HEARING IMPAIRMENT

It has been noted that the Roy Adaptation Model is useful in all areas of nursing practice and has been the basis of research questions to develop basic and clinical nursing science for people of all ages in health and illness (Roy & Andrews, 1999). Several authors have noted the model's particular relevance to assessment and intervention during the changes that occur across the life span. Particular changes within human development are the physical changes experienced in aging. Thus, research with elderly adults who are adapting to physical changes can provide an exemplar of use of the Roy Adaptation Model in nursing research.

Problem and Significance

Hearing impairment, a common but neglected physical change in old age, affects approximately 24 million older Americans (National Institute of Aging, 1990). The degree and types of hearing loss in older persons vary, ranging from decreased sensitivity to high frequency tones, to peripheral loss, sensorineural loss, presbycusis, or tinnitus (Maguire, 1985; Ritter, 1991). Older persons with presbycusis, for example, have more difficulty filtering out background noises (Von Wedel, Von Wedel, & Streppel, 1990). Tinnitus, a common hearing problem, is characterized by the symptoms of ringing, buzzing, hissing, whistling, or swishing sounds arising in the ear, and it affects nearly 11% of the elderly population ("Information about Tinnitus," 1996).

Hearing serves as a sensory input necessary for one's interaction with the changing environment and for a number of critical adaptive functions. It provides the individual with cues of oncoming threats that can be heard only. The sense of hearing augments visual cues for orienting individuals in space and for locating other people and objects. Loss of hearing can have profound psychological effects on

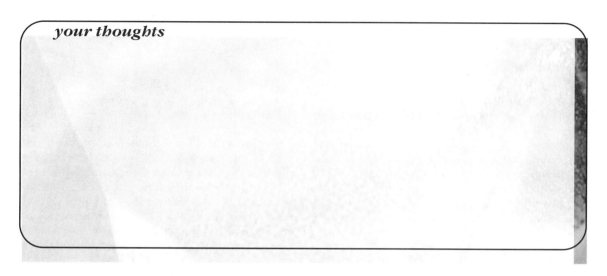
one's life, including feeling insecure, rejected, and depressed; family stress; social isolation; and a decline in one's overall self-concept (Chen, 1994; Salomon, 1986; Whitbourne, 1985; Zhan, 1993b). One elderly man described that "the greatest annoyance of hearing loss is in the subtle aspect of daily living with a partner who also has a hearing loss. You have to constantly repeat what you said; you have to raise your voice since your partner cannot hear well; after all, you are in your own silent world" (Zhan, 1992).

The core problem of hearing loss lies in communication failures and relationship stress, which in turn affects one's self-concept and well-being. Older people with hearing loss therefore face a major task that involves coping with and adapting to hearing impairment so as to maintain their senses of self. Roy (1991) indicates that either sensory deprivation or overload can initiate one's cognitive efforts or cognator subsystem. It is through cognitive efforts that effective adaptation takes place. One effective adaptive response, as described by Roy, is the maintenance of self-consistency. Roy's basic theoretical premises are that individuals are rarely passive in the face of what happens to them. They are adaptive, self-protective, and functional in the face of setbacks, and seek higher levels of adaptation by enhancing person and environment interactions. People seek to change things if they can, and when they cannot, they may use cognitive adaptation processes to change the meaning of the situation in order to protect themselves and enhance their selves and their world (Lazarus, 1991; Roy & Andrews, 1999; Taylor, 1983). To empirically validate Roy's generic theoretical proposition relating the cognator processes to adaptation, the author conducted a quantitative study to examine the relationship between cognitive adaptation processes and the maintenance of self-consistency in older persons with impaired hearing.

Study Design

Based on Roy's Adaptation Model—specifically, on the cognator subsystem of the individual—hearing loss in this study was viewed as a focal stimulus. In the elderly person, hearing loss during aging initiates cognitive coping efforts to bring about the effective adaptation: the maintenance of self-consistency. Personal characteristics and social, cultural, and environmental factors influence maintenance of self-consistency through cognitive adaptation processes.

Research Hypotheses

The usefulness of a model for research depends on the ability of the model to generate testable hypotheses. Within a larger study, the following hypothesis was tested: There will be a positive correlation between cognitive adaptation processes and self-consistency in older persons with hearing impairment.

Sample

The nonprobability sample consisted of 130 subjects who were age 64 or older, manifested hearing loss (defined for this study as an elevated threshold equal to or larger than 26 dB in the speech frequencies of 1000, 2000, and 3000 Hertz), with the onset at age 40 or older, had no cognitive impairment, and resided in the northeastern part of the United States. Subjects were drawn from two nonprofit organizations for hard-of-hearing people, and from several community senior centers. Informed consents were obtained and the study was approved by the appropriate institutional review board. The mean age of this sample was 74, with a range from 64 to 94.

Forty-five percent of the sample were men, and 55 percent were women.

Major Variables

Cognitive adaptation processes referred to cognitive and emotional efforts made by individuals to cope with hearing loss. These efforts were operationalized by the Cognitive Adaptation Processing Scale (form for elders) (Roy & Kazanowski, 1999). *Self-consistency* was defined as an organized set of congruent self-perceptions, including stability of self-concept, self-esteem, private consciousness, and social anxiety. It was operationalized by the Self-Consistency Scale (Zhan & Shen, 1994).

Data Collection and Analysis

Data were collected through mailed and hand-delivered survey questionnaires, and for the entire study, included the Cognitive Adaptation Processing Scale (CAPS) (Roy & Kazanowski, 1999); Self-Consistency Scale (SCS), Geriatric Depression Scale (Sheikh & Yesavage, 1986), Visual Analog Scale, Demographic Profile, and Health Status Questionnaire (SF–36) (Interstudy Outcome Management System, 1991). The research hypothesis of interest here was analyzed via a Pearson product moment correlation.

Findings

The research hypothesis examined whether a positive relationship existed between cognitive adaptation processes and self-consistency. This relationship was tested via Pearson's product moment correlation on the total scores of the CAPS and the SCS, resulting in a positive, moderately strong correlation of .65, $p < .01$. The research hypothesis was supported. To describe the effect of cognitive adaptation processes on self-consistency, a liner regression equation using the least square criterion was performed. The result of $R^2 = .48$ indicated that cognitive adaptation processes accounted for 48 percent of the variance in self-consistency, suggesting that the cognitive adaptation processing be a significant predictor for self-consistency.

Empirical evidence of this study supports the generic proposition of the Roy Adaptation Model that the adequacy of cognator and regulator processes affects adaptive responses (Roy & Andrews, 1999, p. 547). Further, the following ancillary proposition is derived: Patterns of unique cognator processing identified in a given patient group are related to effective adaptation. In particular, a practice proposition derived for elderly persons with hearing impairment states that the cognitive adaptation processes of self-perception, clear focus and method, and knowing awareness are related to the maintenance of self-consistency.

NURSING PRACTICE IMPLICATIONS OF THE RESEARCH

Because in this sample, cognitive adaptation processes explained 48 percent of the variances in self-consistency, it is suggested that cognitive adaptation processes play an active role in keeping one's self system in balance in the face of physical changes such as hearing loss. Further, cognitive processing of clear focus and method, knowing awareness, and self-perception contributed most to the maintenance of self-consistency in this sample. Understanding these cognitive processes can help nurses to promote individuals' coping and adaptation in the context of health and illness, particularly with elderly patients.

Cognitive processing of clear focus and method has to do with the internal restructuring of the person in challenging encounters. It involves mental construction of concept formation (Roy, 1988a, 1988b). Concepts allow the person to organize information into manageable units or related data. For example, an understanding of the relationships among the concepts of hearing loss, aging, and self guides the person's behavior in a given situation. In the situation of hearing loss, the person may modify or change the meaning of the term "hearing loss," which may in turn reduce the threat to the person and his or her sense of self. Realistic concept formation results in effective coping. Therefore, to promote this adaptive process, nursing interventions need to identify how the person represents the problem, what meaning and concepts are attached to the person's experience, and what strategies can be used for effective adaptation.

Cognitive processing of knowing awareness involves individuals' efforts in searching for coping resources and strategies, retrieving information, recognizing workable methods or experience in the past, and learning from or comparing with others who have experienced similar or different encounters. Taylor (1983) viewed downward and upward social comparison as one effort of cognitive adaptation. In using an upward comparison, the person may select a physically disadvantaged person who

> Understanding cognitive processes can help the nurse promote coping and adaptation in health and illness, particularly with elderly patients.

adapts effectively as a role model for the purpose of self-enhancement. Cognitively, a person may use downward comparison to compare his or her hearing problem to the more serious problems of other individuals, so as to reduce the threat of hearing loss and to enhance a sense of self. Such cognitive comparisons may serve the purpose of preventing discrepancies between a desired sense of self and the current self-perception. Another source of the knowing-awareness dimension of cognitive adaptation processing in older persons is how they address and integrate their historical self into their current life. This cognitive strategy provides a source of pride for older persons. Nurses can facilitate older people's adaptation to chronic conditions by encouraging them to review the course of their lives in perspective, to draw on sources of positive life experiences, and to identify relevant information that promotes effective coping.

Cognitive processing of self-perception refers to self-awareness, self-analysis, emotion, and consciousness (Zhan, 1993a). This cognitive processing serves three functions in adaptation. First, self-awareness signals the need for adaptive efforts. A case in point is the inability to discriminate pain. In such cases, in order to survive, the person must be trained to recognize and react to strong stimuli, such as the danger of handling sharp objects. Maintenance of self-consistency involves efforts of self-adjustment as the person interacts with the environment. If a discrepancy is sensed, cognitive processes of self-awareness, analysis, and emotions are activated to reduce that discrepancy.

Second, self-analysis and emotions interrupt ongoing behavior patterns, so that the person can attend to a more salient danger in order to deal with it. For example, keeping in touch with emotion directs the person's attention and efforts toward goals imperative and important for the person in a given situation. In a study of coping strategies, Folkman and Lazarus (1988) found that stressful health events elicited greater use of emotion-focused coping responses than use of problem-focused coping strategies. Keeping in touch with emotions creates a sense of the emergency, without which adaptive reactions would be too pallid.

Third, self-consciousness and self-analysis involve a person's efforts to restore a sense of self through self-enhancing evaluation (Taylor, 1983). Self-enhancing evaluation may involve how an individual perceives the encounter. If older people view hearing loss as a challenge rather than as a threat, the anxiety associated with hearing loss may be minimized. Emotionally, older people with hearing loss

may be less overwhelmed, and their self-structure hence would be protected. However, the relationship between perceiving the encounter as a threat or as a challenge can shift as an encounter unfolds (Lazarus & Folkman, 1984). The individual's coping resources and personality may influence how he or she views the encounter. Therefore, nursing intervention needs first to assess how the person affected perceives the stressful encounter and then to develop strategies that encourage perceptions of being challenged rather than being threatened. It is critical to keep in mind that the relationship between the threat and challenge is recursive, in part depending on the individual's interaction with the external environment. As the environment is altered, cognitive perception may be changed. For example, as a supportive environment is given and a person searches for more resources, the perceived encounter can be changed from negative to positive.

APPLICATION OF EXEMPLAR

This empirical study provided support for the Roy Adaptation Model and the theoretical proposition that cognitive processing brings about adaptive responses such as the maintenance of self-consistency. Cognitive adaptation theory asserts that cognitive processing is an essential feature of a complete analysis of human responses to stressful conditions of life (Lazarus, 1991; Roy & Andrews, 1999; Taylor, 1983). Cognitive adaptation processing is not just information processing per se, although it partakes of such a process. Rather, it is largely evaluative, focusing on meaning and significance attached to each individual's lived experience. Further, cognitive adaptation processing takes place continuously in the transaction between the person and the environment.

Cognitive adaptation processing is dynamic, evolving, and complex. Cognitive processes that were effective in this sample of older adults may not necessarily work in other populations and situations. In addition, cognitive processing of selective focus and sensory regulation did not contribute significantly to the maintenance of self-consistency in this sample; however, it may serve effective coping purposes in different situations. Equally important is the fact that there are potentially both effective and ineffective cognitive adaptation processes. It may be adaptive for a person to be cognitively selective in a stressful situation in order to preserve his or her self-regard. However, this cognitive effort may alter reality and result in improbable hopes. This is a real challenge for nurses in research and in practice, because the conditions under which a particular method of cognitive adaptation processing is beneficial or deleterious have yet to be elaborated. Self-concept is cognitive presentation of self. Cognitive efforts are necessary to protect one's positive self-image and maintain self-consistency. Understanding cognitive adaptation processing helps nurses assess how individuals perceive themselves in a stressful situation; that is, what their levels of self-awareness are, what kinds of emotional responses they manifest, and what meanings and significance they attach to their experience in the context of health and illness.

This study, though limited by the sample size and representation, provided knowledge related to the cognator conceptualization of the Roy Adaptation Model. Maintenance of self-consistency is a task that engages older persons. It can be achieved through cognitive processes and influenced by multiple factors. It can be viewed as a health indicator of how well a person copes with stress in the aging process. Self-consistency is a complex multidimensional construct. Maintenance of self-consistency is not necessarily a rigid, never-changing self-concept. Modifications of the self-concept are expected. Maturation and social learning provide the instance of a naturally changing self-concept. However, these changes need not imply inconsistency of self (Elliot, 1986, 1988; Roy & Andrews, 1999).

To further understand the complex human phenomenon—cognitive adaptation processing and self-consistency—future studies are needed with larger and diverse samples within and across populations. Because the relationship between cognitive adaptation processing and self-consistency is embedded in human experiences that are shaped by history, culture, politics, and social structure, a grounded theory approach may help to illuminate the meaning attached by each individual and identify multiple functions in cognitive adaptation processing. A longitudinal study may be necessary to identify patterns of cognitive adaptation processing in human coping with health-related problems and to examine dynamic changes that take place in individuals and groups over time.

The Roy Adaptation Model provides a useful framework for research inquiry. The theoretical and empirical study of cognitive adaptation processing is still in the early stages. The processes used to maintain self-consistency may be highly variable. Specific cognitive processes may be functionally overlapping. Understanding cognitive adaptation processes, though often challenging, can help nurses in their efforts to restore hope for patients in sometimes hopeless situations, and to help them find new meaning in their lives, to empower themselves, and to promote their well-being.

Summary

This chapter focused on the Roy Adaptation Model as a basis for developing knowledge for clinical practice. There is an extensive literature on both the theoretical development of the model and the use of the model in research. A brief review of the model focused on recent developments in theory and research. Two major concepts of the model were elaborated: cognitive adaptation processing and self-consistency. The introduction on the model and two key concepts provided the basis for an application of the model in a research exemplar with elderly patients. The exemplar research project served to demonstrate support for a generic theoretical proposition based on the model. Further, the study illustrates how a hypothesis based on the model, with adequate conceptual and empirical development of the variables, can be used to derive clinical knowledge for a given patient population.

References

Andrews, J. D. W. (1990). Interpersonal self-confirmation and challenge in psychotherapy. *Psychotherapy, 27*(4), 485–504.

Atchley, R. C. (1988). *Social forces and aging: An introduction to social gerontology* (5th ed.). Belmont, CA: Wadsworth.

Beck, T. (1976). *Cognitive therapy and the emotional disorder.* New York: International Psychiatry.

Carver, C. S., & Scheier, M. F. (1991). Self-regulation and the self. In Strauss, J., & Goethals, G. R. (Eds.), *The self: Interdisciplinary approaches* (pp. 172–207). New York: Springer-Verlag.

Chen, H. L. (1994). Relation of hearing loss, loneliness and self esteem. *Journal of Gerontological Nursing, 20*(6), 22.

Coombs, A., & Snyggs, D. (1959). *Individual behavior—A perceptual approach to behavior.* New York: Harper Brothers.

Das, P. (1984). Intelligence and information integration. In Kirby, J. (Ed.), *Cognitive strategies and education: Performance* (pp. 13–31). New York: Academic Press.

Elliot, G. C. (1986). Self-esteem and self-consistency: A theoretical and empirical link between two primary motivations. *Social Psychology Quarterly, 49*(3), 207–218.

Elliot, G. C. (1988). Gender differences in self-consistency: Evidence from an investigation of self-concept structure. *Journal of Youth and Adolescence, 17*(1), 41–57.

Folkman, S., & Lazarus, R. (1988). *Manual for the ways of coping questionnaire*. Palo Alto, CA: Consulting Psychologists Press.

Goffman, E. (1959). *The presentation of self in everyday life*. New York: Anchor.

Gove, W. R., Ortage, S. T., & Style, C. B. (1989). The maturation and role perspective on aging and self through the adult years: An empirical evaluation. *American Journal of Sociology, 94*, 1117–1145.

Information about tinnitus. (1996). Portland, OR: American Tinnitus Association.

InterStudy outcome management system: The health status questionnaire (SF-36). (1991). *Interstudy quality edge, 1*(1).

Kaufman, S. (1987). *The ageless self*. Madison: University of Wisconsin Press.

Klarkowska, G. H., & Klarkowska, A. (1987). Perceived self-concept discontinuity as a determinant of defensive information processing in conditions of threat to self. *Psychological Bulletin, 19*, 21–29.

Lazarus, R. S. (1991). *Emotion and adaptation*. New York: Oxford University Press.

Lazarus, R. S., & Folkman, S. (1984). *Stress, appraisal, and coping*. New York: Springer Publishing Co.

Lecky, P. (1961). *Self-consistency: A theory of personality*. Frederisk, CT: Shoe String Press.

Lieberman, M. A., & Tobin, S. S. (1988). *The experience of old age: Stress, coping and survival*. New York: Basic Books.

Luria, A. R. (1980). *The working brain: An introduction to neuropsychology*. New York: Basic Books.

Maguire, G. (1985). The changing realm of senses. In Lewis, C. (Ed.), *Aging: The health care challenge*, (pp. 101–116). Philadelphia: F. A. Davis.

Mead, G. (1934). *Mind, self, and society*. Chicago: University of Chicago Press.

National Institute of Aging. (1990). *Hearing problems common in older people studied*. National Institute on Deafness and Other Communication Disorders. U.S. Department of Health and Human Services. Washington, DC: U.S. Government Printing Office.

Ritter, M. (1991, November 26). Study suggested men losing hearing earlier. *Erie Daily Times*, p. 2.

Rogers, C. (1961). *On becoming a person*. Boston: Houghton Mifflin.

Rosenberg, M. (1979). *Conceiving self*. New York: Basic Books.

Rosenberg, M. (1989). *Society and adolescent self-image*. Princeton, NJ: Princeton University Press.

Roy, C. (1971). Adaptation: A basis for nursing practice. *Nursing Outlook, 19*(4), 254–257.

Roy, C. (1975). *Psycho-social adaptation and the coping mechanisms*. Unpublished manuscript.

Roy, C. (1977). Decision-making by the physically ill and adaptation during illness. Doctoral dissertation, University of California, Los Angeles. University Microfilms International.

Roy, C. (1984). *Introduction to nursing: An adaptation model* (2nd ed.). Englewood Cliffs, NJ: Prentice-Hall.

Roy, C. (1985). *Cognitive processing in patients with closed head injury*. Poster session, 18th Annual Communicating Nursing Research Conference. Seattle, Washington. Western Society for Research in Nursing.

Roy, C. (1988a). Altered cognition: An information processing approach. In Mitchell, P. H., Hodges, L. C., Muwaswes, M., & Walleck, C. A., (Eds.), *AANN's neuroscience nursing: Phenomenon and practice: Human responses to neurological health problems* (pp. 185–211). Norwalk, CT: Appleton & Lange.

Roy, C. (1988b). Human information processing. In Fitzpatrick, J. J., Taunton, R. L., & Benoliel, J. Q. (Eds.), *Annual review of nursing research* (pp. 237–261). New York: Springer Publishing.

Roy, C., & Andrews, H. (1991). *The Roy Adaptation Model: The definitive statement*. Norwalk, CT: Appleton & Lange.

Roy, C., & Andrews, H. (1999). *The Roy Adaptation Model* (2nd ed.). Norwalk, CT: Appleton & Lange.

Roy, C., & Corliss, P. (1993). The Roy Adaptation Model: Theoretical update and knowledge for practice. In Parker, M. E. (Ed.), *Patterns for nursing theories in practice* (pp. 215–229). New York: National League for Nursing Press.

Roy, C., & Hanna, D. (1999, April 9–11). *Acute phase nursing interventions for improving cognitive functional status in patients with closed head injury*. 11th Annual ENRS scientific sessions. New York.

Roy, C., & Kazanowski, M. *Cognitive adaptation processing scale: Instrument development* (in press).

Roy, C., Pollock, S., Massey, V., Lauchner, K., Whetsel, V., Frederickson, K., Barone, S., & Carson, M. (1999). *The Roy Adaptation Model-based research: Twenty-five years of contributions to nursing science*. Indianapolis: Sigma Theta Tau International.

Roy, C., & Roberts, S. (1981). *Theory construction in nursing: An adaptation model*. Englewood Cliffs, NJ: Prentice-Hall.

Salomon, C. (1986). Hearing problems and the elderly. *Danish Medical Bulletin, 33*(Suppl. 3), 1–21.

Sheikh, J. L., & Yesavage, J. A. (1986). A geriatric depression scale: Recent evidence and development of a shorter version. *Clinical Gerontologist, 5*(1/2), 165–173.

Taylor, C. (1983, November). Adjustment to threatening events: A theory of cognitive adaptation. *American Psychologists*, 1611–1173.

Whitbourne, S. (1985). *The aging body: Physiological changes and psychological consequences*. New York: Springer-Verlag.

Wylie, R. (1989). *Measures of self-concept*. Lincoln: University of Nebraska Press.

Von Wedel, H., Von Wedel, U. C., & Streppel, M. (1990). Selective hearing in the aged in regard to speech perception in quiet and in noise. *Acta Otolaryngol, 476* (Suppl.), 131.

Zhan, L. (1992). Interviewing with hearing impaired older persons. Unpublished paper, Boston College, Chestnut Hill, MA.

Zhan, L. (1993a). *Coping with hearing loss*. Unpublished paper, Boston College, Chestnut Hill, MA.

Zhan, L. (1993b). *Cognitive adaptation process in hearing impaired elderly*. Doctoral dissertation, Boston College, Chestnut Hill, MA.

Zhan, L., & Shen, C. (1994). The development of an instrument to measure self-consistency. *Journal of Advanced Nursing, 20*, 509–516.

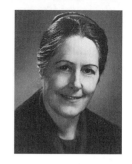

Chapter *19*

Betty Neuman
The Neuman Systems Model
and Global Applications

- ❖ Introducing the Theorist
- ❖ The Neuman Systems Model
- ❖ Global Applications of the Model
- ❖ Projections for Use of the Model in the Twenty-first Century
- ❖ Summary
- ❖ References

Patricia Deal Aylward

INTRODUCING THE THEORIST

Betty Neuman developed the Neuman Systems Model in 1970 to "provide unity, or a focal point, for student learning" at the School of Nursing, University of California, in Los Angeles (Neuman, 1995, p. 674). Neuman recognized the need for educators and practitioners to have a framework to view nursing comprehensively within various contexts. She developed the model strictly as a teaching aid. The model is now highly recognized and used globally as a conceptual model for nursing. Dr. Neuman has been a pioneer in several areas within and outside of nursing. One example of her pioneer work is that she was one of the first nurses licensed as a marriage, family, and child counselor in the state of California, in 1970. She is an author, lecturer, and independent nursing curriculum consultant. Neuman has published numerous books and journal articles in response to requests for support in applying the model to education, practice, research, and administration. Dr. Neuman received two honorary doctorates—one in science in 1998 from Grand Valley State University in Allendale, Michigan, and the other in letters in 1992 from Neuman College in Aston, Pennsylvania. In 1993, Dr. Neuman became an honorary member of the Fellowship of the American Academy of Nursing.

THE NEUMAN SYSTEMS MODEL

The Neuman Systems Model provides a comprehensive, flexible, holistic, and systems-based perspective for nursing. This conceptual model of nursing focuses attention on the response of the client system to actual or potential environmental stressors, and the use of primary, secondary, and tertiary nursing prevention interventions for retention, attainment, and maintenance of optimal client system wellness.

—**Betty Neuman (1996)**

As its name suggests, the Neuman Systems Model is classified as a systems model or a systems category of knowledge. Neuman (1995) defined *system* as a pervasive order that holds together its parts. With this definition in mind, she writes that nursing can be readily conceptualized as a complete whole, with identifiable smaller wholes or parts. The complete whole structure is maintained by interrelationships among identifiable smaller wholes or parts through regulations that evolve out of the dynamics of the open system. In the system there is dynamic energy exchange, moving either toward or away from stability. Energy moves toward negentropy or evolution as a system absorbs energy to increase its organization, complexity, and development when it moves toward a steady or wellness state. An open system of energy exchange is never at rest. The open system tends to move cyclically toward differentiation and elaboration for further growth and survival of the organism. With the dynamic energy exchange, the system also can move away from stability. Energy can move toward extinction (entropy) by gradual disorganization, increasing randomness, and energy dissipation.

> Neuman described system as a pervasive order that holds together its parts.

The Neuman Systems Model illustrates a client-client system and presents nursing as a field primarily concerned with defining appropriate nursing actions in stressor-related situations or in possible reactions of the client-client system. The client and environment may be positively or negatively affected by each other. There is a tendency within any system to maintain a steady state or balance among the various disruptive forces operating within or upon it. Neuman has identified these forces as stressors, and suggests that possible reactions and actual reactions with identifiable signs or symptoms may be mitigated through appropriate early interventions (Neuman, 1995).

Propositions

Neuman has identified 10 propositions inherent within her model. Fawcett (1995a, p. 2) defined *propositions* as "statements that describe or link concepts." She provided additional clarity to the term "proposition" by adding that some propositions are general descriptions or definitions of the conceptual model concepts, whereas other propositions state the relationships between conceptual model concepts in a general manner. In Fawcett's analysis of the Neuman Systems Model, she acknowledged that Neuman's propositions that link person, environment, health, and nursing leave no gaps between these concepts. Fawcett believes that Neuman's primary, secondary, and tertiary preventions provide the required linkages among the concepts of the model (1995a). The following propositions describe, define, and connect concepts essential to understanding the conceptual model that is presented in the next section of this chapter.

1. Although each individual client or group as a client system is unique, each system is a composite of common known factors or innate char-

acteristics within a normal, given range of response contained within a basic structure.

2. Many known, unknown, and universal environmental stressors exist. Each differs in its potential for disturbing a client's usual stability level or normal line of defense. The particular interrelationships of client variables—physiological, psychological, sociocultural, developmental, and spiritual—at any point in time can affect the degree to which a client is protected by the flexible line of defense against possible reaction to a single stressor or a combination of stressors.

3. Each individual client-client system has evolved a normal range of response to the environment that is referred to as a normal line of defense, or usual wellness/stability state. It represents change over time through coping with diverse stress encounters. The normal line of defense can be used as a standard from which to measure health deviation.

4. When the cushioning, accordionlike effect of the flexible line of defense is no longer capable of protecting the client-client system against an environmental stressor, the stressor breaks through the normal line of defense. The interrelationships of variables—physiological, psychological, sociocultural, developmental, and spiritual—determine the nature and degree of system reaction or possible reaction to the stressor.

5. The client, whether in a state of wellness or illness, is a dynamic composite of the interrelationships of variables—physiological, psychological, sociocultural, developmental, and spiritual. Wellness is on a continuum of available energy to support the system in an optimal state of system stability.

6. Implicit within each client system are internal resistance factors know as lines of resistance, which function to stabilize and return the client to the usual wellness state (normal line of defense) or possibly to a higher level of stability following an environmental stressor reaction.

7. Primary prevention relates to general knowledge that is applied in client assessment and intervention in identification and reduction or mitigation of possible or actual risk factors associated with environmental stressors to prevent possible reaction. The goal of health promotion is included in primary prevention.

8. Secondary prevention relates to symptomatology following a reaction to stressors, appropriate ranking of intervention priorities, and treatment to reduce their noxious effects.

9. Tertiary prevention relates to the adaptive processes taking place as reconstitution begins and maintenance factors move the client back in a circular manner toward primary prevention.

10. The client as a system is in a dynamic, constant energy exchange with the environment. (Neuman, 1995, pp. 20–21, with permission)

The Conceptual Model

Neuman's original diagram of her model is illustrated in Figure 19-1. The conceptual model was developed to explain the client-client system as an individual person for the discipline of nursing. Neuman chose the terms "client" or "client system" instead of "human" to show respect for collaborative relationships that exist between the client and caregiver in Neuman's model. Neuman now believes the model can be equally well applied to a group, larger com-

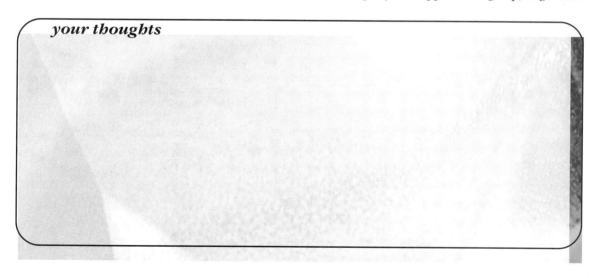

your thoughts

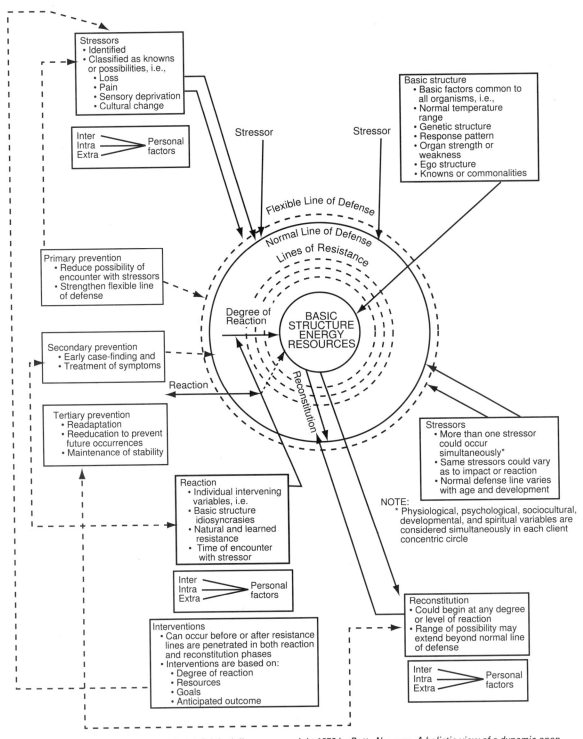

Figure 19–1 *The Neuman Systems Model. Original diagram copyright 1970 by Betty Neuman. A holistic view of a dynamic open client-client system interacting with environmental stressors, along with client and caregiver collaborative participation in promoting an optimum state of wellness. From Neuman, 1995, p. 17, with permission.*

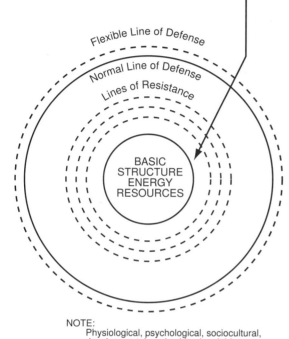

Basic structure
• Basic factors common to all organisms, i.e.,
• Normal temperature range
• Genetic structure
• Response pattern
• Organ strength or weakness
• Ego structure
• Knowns or commonalities

Flexible Line of Defense
Normal Line of Defense
Lines of Resistance

BASIC STRUCTURE ENERGY RESOURCES

NOTE:
Physiological, psychological, sociocultural, developmental, and spiritual variables occur and are considered simultaneously in each client concentric circle

Figure 19–2 *Client-client system. The structure of the client-client system, including the five variables that are occurring simultaneously in each client concentric circle. From Neuman, 1995, p. 26, with permission.*

munity, or social issue, and is appropriate for nursing and other health disciplines (Neuman, 1995).

The Neuman Systems Model provides a way of looking at the domain of nursing: humans, environment, health, and nursing. Figures 19–2, 19–3, and 19–4 are included to help focus on the client-client system, environment, and nursing aspects of the nursing domain.

Client-Client System

The structure of the client-client system is illustrated in Figure 19-2. The client-client system consists of the flexible line of defense, the normal line of de-

fense, lines of resistance, and the basic structure energy resources (shown at the core of the concentreic circles in Figure 19-2). Five client variables—physiological, psychological, sociocultural, developmental, and spiritual—occur and are considered simultaneously in each concentric circle that makes up the client-client system (Neuman, 1995).

Flexible Line of Defense

Stressors must penetrate the flexible line of defense before they are capable of penetrating the rest of the client system. Neuman described this line of defense as an accordionlike mechanism that acts like a protective buffer system to help prevent stressor invasion of the client system. The flexible line of defense protects the normal line of defense. The client has more protection from stressors when the flexible line expands away from the normal line of defense. The opposite is true when the flexible line moves closer to the normal line of defense. The effectiveness of the buffer system can be reduced by single or multiple stressors. The flexible line of defense can be rapidly altered over a relatively short time period. States of emergency, or short-term conditions such as loss of sleep, poor nutrition, or dehydration, are examples of what the client is like in the temporary state that is represented by the flexible line of defense (Neuman, 1995). Consider the latter examples. What are the effects of short-term loss of sleep, poor nutrition, or dehydration, on a client's normal state of wellness? Will these situations increase the possibility for stressor penetration? The answer is that the possibility for stressor penetration may be increased. The actual response depends upon the accordionlike mechanism described above, along with the other components of the client system.

Normal Line of Defense

The normal line of defense represents what the client has become over time, or the usual state of wellness. The nurse should determine the client's usual level of wellness in order to recognize a change in the level of wellness. The normal line of defense is considered dynamic by Neuman, because it can expand or contract over time. She demonstrated this dynamic state by giving an example in which the usual wellness level or system stability decreases, remains the same, or improves following treatment of a stressor reaction. Neuman also considers the normal line of defense dynamic because of its ability to become and remain stabilized with life stresses over time. The basic structure and system integrity are protected (Neuman, 1995).

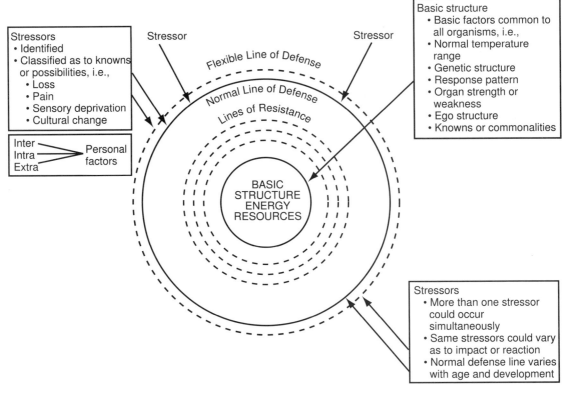

Stressors
• Identified
• Classified as to knowns
  or possibilities, i.e.,
  • Loss
  • Pain
  • Sensory deprivation
  • Cultural change

Inter ──┐
Intra ──┼──► Personal
Extra ──┘   factors

Stressor

Stressor

Flexible Line of Defense

Normal Line of Defense

Lines of Resistance

BASIC
STRUCTURE
ENERGY
RESOURCES

Basic structure
• Basic factors common to
  all organisms, i.e.,
• Normal temperature
  range
• Genetic structure
• Response pattern
• Organ strength or
  weakness
• Ego structure
• Knowns or commonalities

Stressors
• More than one stressor
  could occur
  simultaneously
• Same stressors could vary
  as to impact or reaction
• Normal defense line varies
  with age and development

Figure 19–3 *Environment. Internal and external factors surrounding the client-client system. From Neuman, 1995, p. 27, with permission.*

Primary prevention
• Reduce possibility of
  encounter with stressors
• Strengthen flexible line
  of defense

Secondary prevention
• Early case-finding and
• Treatment of symptoms

Tertiary prevention
• Readaptation
• Reeducation to prevent
  future occurrences
• Maintenance of stability

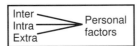

Inter ──┐
Intra ──┼──► Personal
Extra ──┘   factors

Interventions
• Can occur before or after resistance
  lines are penetrated in both reaction
  and reconstitution phases
• Interventions are based on:
  • Degree of reaction
  • Resources
  • Goals
  • Anticipated outcome

Figure 19–4 *Nursing. Accurately assessing the effects and possible effects of environmental stressors (inter-, intra-, and extrapersonal factors) and using appropriate prevention by interventions to assist with client adjustments for an optimal level of wellness. From Neuman, 1995, p. 29, with permission.*

Lines of Resistance

Neuman identified the series of concentric circles that surround the basic structure as lines of resistance for the client. When the normal line of defense is penetrated by stressors, a degree of reaction, or signs and/or symptoms, will occur. Lines of resistance are activated following invasion of the normal line of defense by environmental stressors. Each line of resistance contains known and unknown internal and external resource factors. These factors support the client's basic structure and the normal line of defense, resulting in protection of system integrity. Examples of the factors that support the basic structure and normal line of defense include the body's mobilization of white blood cells and activation of the immune system mechanisms. There is a decrease in the signs or symptoms, or a reversal of the reaction to stressors, when the lines of resistance are effective. The system reconstitutes itself or system stability is returned. The level of wellness may be higher or lower than it was prior to the stressor penetration. When the lines of resistance are ineffective, energy depletion and death occur (Neuman, 1995).

> The normal line of defense represents the dynamic state of wellness that the client has developed over time.

Basic Structure

The basic structure or central core structure consists of basic factors that are common to all organisms. Neuman offered the following examples of basic survival factors: normal temperature range, genetic structure, response pattern, organ strength or weakness, ego structure, and knowns or commonalities (Neuman, 1995).

Five Client Variables

Neuman has identified five variables that are contained in all client systems: physiological, psychological, sociocultural, developmental, and spiritual. These variables are present in varying degrees of development, and a wide range of interactive styles and potential. Neuman offers the following definitions for each variable:

Physiological—refers to bodily structure and function.
Psychological—refers to mental processes and relationships.
Sociocultural—refers to combined social and cultural functions.
Developmental—refers to life developmental processes.
Spiritual—refers to spiritual belief influence. (Neuman, 1995, p. 28)

Neuman elaborated on the spiritual variable in order to assist readers in understanding the variable by presenting that variable as an innate component of the basic structure. This variable may or may not be acknowledged or developed by the client or client system. Neuman views the spiritual variable as being on a continuum of development that penetrates all other client system variables. The client-client system can have a complete unawareness of the spiritual variable's presence and potential, deny its presence, or have a conscious and highly developed spiritual understanding that supports the client's optimal wellness.

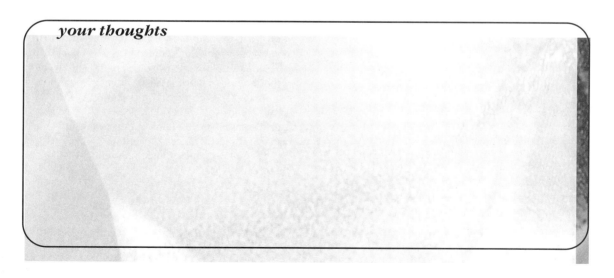

your thoughts

Neuman explained that the spirit controls the mind, and the mind consciously or unconsciously controls the body. The spiritual variable affects or is affected by a condition, and interacts with other variables in a positive or negative way. She gave the example of grief or loss (psychological state), which may inactivate, decrease, initiate, or increase spirituality. There can be movement in either direction of a continuum (Neuman, 1995). Neuman believes that spiritual variable considerations are necessary for a truly holistic perspective and truly caring concern for the client-client system.

Fulton (1995) has studied the spiritual variable in depth. She elaborated on research studies that extend our understanding of the following aspects of spirituality: spiritual well-being, spiritual needs, spiritual distress, and spiritual care. She suggested that spiritual needs include (1) the need for meaning and purpose in life; (2) the need to receive love and give love; (3) the need for hope and creativity; and (4) the need for forgiving, trusting relationships with self, others, and God, or a deity, or a guiding philosophy.

Environment

The second concept identified by Neuman is the environment. Figure 19-3 illustrates this. Neuman defined *environment* broadly as "all internal and external factors or influences surrounding the identified client or client system" (Neuman, 1995, p. 30). Neuman has identified and defined the following environmental typology or classification of types for her model:

Internal environment—intrapersonal in nature.
External environment—inter- and extrapersonal in nature.
Created environment—intra-, inter-, and extrapersonal in nature. (Neuman, 1995, p. 31)

The internal environment consists of all forces or interactive influences contained within the boundaries of the client-client system. Examples of intrapersonal forces are presented for each variable.

Physiological variable—degree of mobility, range of body function.
Psychological and sociocultural variables—attitudes, values, expectations, behavior patterns, coping patterns.
Developmental variable—age, degree of normalcy, factors related to the present situation.
Spiritual variable—hope, sustaining forces. (Neuman, 1995)

The external environment consists of all forces or interactive influences existing outside the client system. Interpersonal factors in the environment are forces between people or client systems. These factors include the relationships and resources of family, friends, or caregivers. Extrapersonal factors include education, finances, employment, and other resources (Neuman, 1995).

Neuman (1995) has identified a third environment as the "created environment." The client unconsciously mobilizes all system variables including the basic structure energy factors toward system integration, stability, and integrity to create a safe environment. This safe, created environment offers a protective coping shield that helps the client to function. A major objective of the created environment is to stimulate the client's health. Neuman pointed out that what was originally created to safeguard the health of the system may have a negative outcome effect because of the binding of available energy. This environment represents an open system exchanging energy with the internal and external environments. The created environment supersedes or goes beyond the internal and external environments, while encompassing both. The created environment provides an insulating effect to change the response or possible response of the client to environmental stressors. Neuman (1995) gave the following examples of responses: use of denial or envy (psychological), physical rigidity or muscle constraint (physiological), life cycle continuation of survival patterns (developmental), required social space range (sociocultural), and sustaining hope (spiritual).

Neuman believes the caregiver, through assessment, will need to determine (1) what has been created (nature of the created environment), (2) the outcome of the created environment (extent of its use and client value), and (3) the ideal that has yet to be created (the protection that is needed or possible, to a lesser or greater degree). This assessment is necessary to best understand and support the client's created environment (Neuman, 1995). Neuman suggested that nursing may wish to pursue and develop further an understanding of the client's awareness of the created environment and its relationship to health. Neuman believes that as the caregiver recognizes the value of the client-created environment and purposefully intervenes, the interpersonal relationship can become one of important mutual exchange (Neuman, 1995).

Health

Health is the third concept in Neuman's model. Neuman believes that wellness and illness are on opposite ends of the continuum. *Health* is the best possible wellness at any given time. Wellness exists when more energy is built and stored than expended, whereas death occurs when more energy is needed than is available to support life. Neuman views health as a manifestation of living energy available to preserve and enhance system integrity. Health is seen as varying levels within a normal range, rising and falling throughout the life span. These changes are in response to basic structure factors, and reflect satisfactory and unsatisfactory adjustment by the client system to environmental stressors (Neuman, 1995).

> Nursing's major concern is to keep the client system stable through nursing actions, or prevention by intervention.

Nursing

Nursing is the fourth concept in Neuman's model and is depicted in Figure 19-4. Nursing's major concern is to keep the client system stable by (1) accurately assessing the effects and possible effects of environmental stressors and (2) assisting client adjustments required for optimal wellness. Neuman defined *optimal* as the best possible health state achievable at a given point in time. Nursing actions, which she labels as prevention by intervention, are initiated to keep the system stable. Neuman has created a typology for her prevention by intervention nursing actions. They include primary prevention by intervention, secondary prevention by intervention, and tertiary prevention by intervention. All of these actions are initiated to best retain, attain, and maintain optimal client health or wellness. Neuman (1995) believes the nurse creates a linkage among the client, the environment, health, and nursing in the process of keeping the system stable.

Prevention as Intervention

Primary prevention as intervention involves the nurse's use of interventions that promote client wellness by stressor prevention and reduction of risk factors. These interventions can begin at any point a stressor is suspected or identified, before a reaction has occurred. They protect the normal line of defense and strengthen the flexible lines of defense. Health promotion is a significant intervention. The goal of these interventions is to "retain" optimal stability or wellness. The nurse should consider primary prevention along with secondary and tertiary preventions as interventions. Once a reaction occurs from a stressor, the nurse can use secondary prevention as intervention to protect the basic structure by strengthening the internal lines of resistance. The

goal of these interventions is to "attain" optimal client-system stability, or wellness, and energy conservation. The nurse should use as much of the client's existing internal and external resources to stabilize the system by strengthening the internal lines of resistance and reducing the degree of reaction to the stressors. Neuman suggested the nurse should collaborate with the client to establish relevant goals. The goals are derived only after synthesizing comprehensive client data and relevant theory in order to determine an appropriate nursing diagnostic statement. With the nursing diagnostic statement and goals in mind, appropriate interventions can be planned and implemented (Neuman, 1995).

Reconstitution represents the return and maintenance of system stability following nursing intervention for stressor reaction. The state of wellness may be higher, the same, or lower than the state of wellness before the system was stabilized. Death occurs when secondary prevention as intervention fails to protect the basic structure and thus fails to reconstitute the client (Neuman, 1995).

Tertiary prevention as intervention can begin at any point in the client's reconstitution. These actions are designed to "maintain" an optimal wellness level by supporting existing strengths and conserving client system energy. Tertiary prevention tends to lead back toward primary prevention in a circular fashion. Neuman pointed out that one or all three of these prevention modalities give direction to or may be used for nursing action with possible synergistic benefits (Neuman, 1995).

Nursing Tools for Model Implementation

Neuman has designed the Neuman Nursing Process format and the Format for Prevention as Intervention to facilitate implementation of the Neuman model. These formats are presented in the third edition of Neuman's book (1995, pp. 18-20). The format demonstrates a process that guides information processing and goal-directed activities. Neuman used the nursing process within three categories: nursing diagnosis, nursing goals, and nursing outcomes. Comprehensive data are collected prior to formulating a nursing diagnosis. This process is facilitated using guides such as the Assessment and Intervention Tool mentioned in Neuman's book (1995). Nursing goals are determined mutually with the caregiver-client-client system, along with mutually agreed upon prevention as intervention strategies. Nursing outcomes are determined by the accomplishment of the interventions and evaluation of goals following intervention. The Neuman Nursing Process format was validated in 1982 by doctoral students. The format's validity and social utility have been proven in a wide variety of nursing education and practice areas. Using the Neuman Systems Model, the nurse acquires significant and comprehensive client data to determine the impact or possible impact of environmental stressors upon the client system. Selected information is prioritized and related to relevant social science and nursing theories. Neuman suggested that the Neuman Nursing Process format has a unique component. This specific uniqueness is that the client and caregiver perceptions are determined for relevant goal-setting. The nurse and the client mutually determine the client intervention goals. Neuman pointed out that mutually agreed-upon goals and interventions are consistent with current mandates within the health-care system for client rights in health-care issues.

Neuman designed the Format for Prevention as Intervention to convey appropriate nursing actions with each typology of prevention. Primary, secondary, and tertiary prevention nursing actions are listed in a table format in Neuman's book (1995, p. 20), to assist with model implementation. The nature of stressors and their threat to the client-client system are first determined for each type of prevention before any other nursing actions are initiated.

GLOBAL APPLICATIONS OF THE MODEL

Because the model is flexible and adaptable to a wide range of groups and situations, people have used the model globally, and for more than two decades. Neuman's first book, *The Neuman Systems Model: Application to Nursing Education and Practice,* was published in 1982 as a response to requests for data and support in applying the model. Neuman published two additional editions of the book, with the third edition published in 1995 in response to expanded use of the model globally. The third edition includes applications of the Neuman Systems Model to nursing education, practice, administration, and research. This edition is used as a primary resource for global applications highlighted in this chapter (Neuman, 1995).

Application of the Neuman Systems Model to Nursing Education

Lowry, Walker, and Mirenda (1995) pointed out that in the 1980s exploration and use of the model greatly accelerated in education at all levels of practice in varied settings. These settings include the United States and locations such as Canada, Europe, Australia, and the Far East.

There are many schools of nursing in the United States that have chosen to use the Neuman Systems Model as a curriculum framework or for selected courses. Most schools surveyed indicated reasons they chose the Neuman model. Generally, the reason for choosing the model was consistency with the school in one or more of the following areas: the school's beliefs; philosophy; and concepts of humans, health, nursing, and environment. Associate degree nursing programs that have used the model include Athens Area Technical Institute, Athens, Georgia; Cecil Community College, North East, Maryland; Central Florida Community College, Ocala, Florida; Los Angeles County Medical Center School of Nursing, Los Angeles Valley College, Van Nuys, California; Santa Fe Community College, Gainesville, Florida; and Yakima Valley Community College, Yakima, Washington. Baccalaureate nursing programs that have used the model include California State University, Fresno; Indiana University; Indianapolis; Purdue University, Fort Wayne, Indiana; University of Tennessee; and the University of Texas, Tyler. Gustavus Adolphus College, and St. Peter and St. Olaf College, Northfield, Minnesota, also have used the model. (Glazebrook, 1995; Hilton & Grafton, 1995; Klotz, 1995; Lowry & Newsome, 1995; Stittich, Flores, & Nuttall, 1995; Strickland-Seng, 1995).

Educational programs in the United States reported benefits with using the model. The model (1) facilitated cultural considerations in the curriculum related to the populations the schools and graduates served (Stittich, Flores, & Nuttall, 1995), (2) provided a nursing focus as opposed to medical focus (Lowry & Newsome, 1995), (3) included the concept of clients as holistic beings (Lowry & Newsome, 1995), (4) allowed flexibility in arrangement of content and conceptualization of program needs (Lowry & Newsome, 1995), (5) was comprehensive and facilitated seeing the person as composites of the five variables, (6) provided a framework to study individual illness and reaction to stressors, (7) was broad enough to allow educational programs to consider family as the context within which individuals live or as the unit of care, and (8) considered the created environment.

Education programs have developed evaluation instruments to determine the effects of using the model as a framework for nursing knowledge. The primary instrument that is cited in the nursing literature is the Lowry-Jopp Neuman Model Evaluation Instrument. This instrument was developed and used

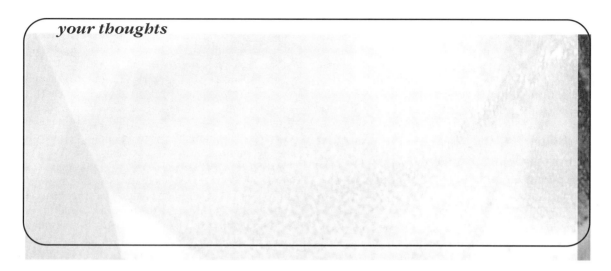
your thoughts

to evaluate the efficacy of using the model at Cecil Community College (Lowry & Newsome, 1995). The results of a five-year longitudinal study showed that the graduates used the model most of the time when fulfilling roles of care provider and teacher. All classes in the study claimed colleagues rarely knew, accepted, or encouraged model use. Therefore, colleagues in work settings tended to have a negative effect on the use of models.

The model is also being used internationally. Craig (1995b) reported on the experiences of 10 educational institutions in Canada that represent six Canadian provinces. These institutions include the University of Saskatchewan, University of Prince Edward Island, University of Calgary, Brandon University of New Brunswick, Université de Moncton, University of Western Ontario, University of Windsor, Okanagan College, University of Toronto, and University of Ottawa. Model strengths were reported by educational institutions in Canada. The holistic approach that addressed levels of prevention guided the student to focus on the client in his or her own environment. The model also assisted the student to carry out in-depth assessments, to categorize comprehensive data, and to plan specific interventions with the client. The students did report some difficulty in understanding the complexity of the model, and the developmental and spiritual variables. The students reported that it was not always easy to differentiate between the lines of defense and resistance, or to assess the degree of stressor penetration.

The Neuman Model is also being used in educational institutions in South Australia, the United Kingdom, and Sweden (Engberg, 1995; McCulloch, 1995; Vaughan & Gough, 1995). McCulloch (1995) reported that a survey of all Australian university pro-

grams showed that four undergraduate programs used the model as the major organizational curriculum framework, and another 16 programs introduced undergraduate and postgraduate students to the Neuman Model as one of several models. Vaughan and Gough (1995) found that many nursing and midwifery students chose to use the model in their own practice in the United Kingdom. They also reported that Avon and Gloucestershire College of Health used the model as the guiding principle behind curriculum development for child care. Engberg (1995) reported that most colleges throughout Sweden use the Neuman Systems Model as the theoretical framework in the module of primary health in nursing education.

Application of the Neuman Systems Model to Nursing Practice

The Neuman Systems Model is being used in diverse practice settings. In the United States, the model is used to guide practice with clients with cognitive impairment, meeting family needs of clients in critical care; to provide stable support groups for parents with infants in neonatal intensive care units; and to meet the needs of home caregivers, with emphasis on clients with cancer, HIV/AIDS, and head traumas. The model is used in psychiatric nursing, gerontological nursing, perinatal nursing, and occupational health nursing (Bueno & Sengin, 1995; Chiverton & Flannery, 1995; McGee, 1995; Peirce & Fulmer, 1995; Russell, Hileman, & Grant, 1995; Stuart & Wright, 1995; Trepanier, Dunn, & Sprague, 1995; Ware & Shannahan, 1995).

Internationally, the model is being used in Canada, the United Kingdom, Sweden, the Netherlands, New Zealand, Australia, Jordan, Israel, Slovenia, and several East Asian countries (e.g., Japan, Korea, and Taiwan). Practice areas include community/public health care (Betty Neuman, personal communication, January 10, 1999; Beddome, 1995; Beynon, 1995; Craig, 1995a; Damant, 1995; Davis & Proctor, 1995; Engberg, Bjalming, & Bertilson, 1995; Felix, Hinds, Wolfe, & Martin, 1995; Vaughan & Gough, 1995; Verberk, 1995).

Nursing Administration and the Neuman Systems Model

The Neuman Systems Model has been used in diverse nursing administration settings in the United States. These settings include a community nursing center, psychiatric hospital, a continuing care retirement community, and Oklahoma State Public Health Nursing (Frioux, Roberts, & Butler, 1995; Rodriguez, 1995; Scicchitani, Cox, Heyduk, Maglicco, & Sargent, 1995; Walker, 1995a).

Poole and Flowers (1995) demonstrated how the model is used in case management of pregnant substance abusers. Kelley and Sanders (1995) presented an assessment tool that intertwines the management process, the Neuman Systems Model, and environmental dimensions. Walker (1995b) demonstrated how the model and total quality management are used to prepare health-care administrators for the future.

Nursing Research and the Neuman Systems Model

Gigliotti (1997) acknowledged that the Neuman Model's use as a guide in directing nursing education and clinical practice has received much national and international attention. However, the model's use as a guide to nursing research and the generation of nursing theory based on the research is in the early stages of development, although growing. In order to facilitate the use of nursing research with the Neuman Systems Model, Meleis (1995) has elaborated on principles and approaches that may be used to develop a futuristic agenda to validate the Neuman Systems Theory.

Fawcett (1995c) has offered guidelines for constructing Neuman Systems Model–based studies. Neuman revisited these guidelines in her 1996 article in *Nursing Science Quarterly.* She acknowledged that the Neuman model has guided a range of study designs, from qualitative descriptions of relevant phenomena to quantitative experiments that tested the effects of prevention interventions on a variety of client-system outcomes. She provided numerous ex-amples of descriptive studies, correlational research, and experimental and quasiexperimental studies. Neuman elaborated on how to construct Neuman Model–based research.

Smith and Edgil (1995) have proposed a plan for testing middle-range theories with the model. Their plan involved the creation of an Institute for the Study of the Model to formulate and test theories through collaboration, including interdisciplinary as well as multisite efforts. They suggested directions for the work to be done, an organizing structure, and a task analysis of what and who would be appropriate to participate in task completion. Breckenridge (1995) has actually used the Neuman model to develop a middle-range theory based on nephrology practice. Gigliotti (1997) has identified conceptual and empirical concerns imposed upon her when she operationalized Neuman's lines of defense and resistance in her research. She concluded that the Neuman Model offers an excellent and comprehensive framework from which to view the metaconcepts relevant to the discipline of nursing: person, environment, health, and nursing. Gigliotti says it is time to institute the comprehensive research program proposed by Smith and Edgil (1995).

PROJECTIONS FOR USE OF THE MODEL IN THE TWENTY-FIRST CENTURY

Neuman believes her model is "both concept and process relevant as a directive toward nursing and other health care activities in the challenging 21st Century" (Betty Neuman, personal communication, January 10, 1999). This model has been used to make projections about the future of nursing and health care. Procter and Cheek (1995) and Tomlinson and Anderson (1995) provided two examples of this use. Procter and Cheek used the model to project the role of the nurse in world catastrophic events, and Tomlinson and Anderson used the model to project family health as a system. Procter and Cheek studied experiences of Serbian Australians at the time of the civil war in the former Yugoslavia using the Neuman Systems Model to understand the experiences. As a result of the study, the researchers came up with implications for the role of nursing in world catastrophic events. The researchers suggested the goal of nursing in such worldwide events should be to assist individuals and communities to retain maximum wellness and system stability as they strive for a sense of inner peace and contentment against impossible odds.

Tomlinson and Anderson (1995) recognized that there is an increasing focus on the family system as a health entity. They acknowledged, however, that there is not a universally accepted definition of "family health" as a systems phenomenon. Tomlinson and Anderson proposed that the nurse who uses the broad concepts of the Neuman Model along with a shared family health systems perspective, in which the whole family is the client in the health promotion enterprise, will be well prepared to meet future nursing challenges.

Summary

The Neuman Systems Model has been used for over 2 decades; first as a teaching tool and later as a conceptual model to observe and interpret the phenomena of nursing and health care globally. Dr. Neuman (1997, p. 20) wrote: "[T]he future of the Neuman Systems Model looks bright." She believes her model can readily accommodate future changes in health care delivery. The reader has been introduced to the model and some of the global applications of the model. The reader is also referred to additional citations compiled by Dr. Jacqueline Fawcett (1995a; 1995b).

References

Beddome, G. (1995). Community-as-client assessment. A Neuman-based guide for education and practice. In Neuman, B., *The Neuman Systems Model* (3rd ed., pp. 567–579). Norwalk, CT: Appleton & Lange.

Beynon, C. E. (1995). Neuman-based experiences of the Middlesex-London Health Unit. In Neuman, B., *The Neuman Systems Model* (3rd ed., pp. 537–547). Norwalk, CT: Appleton & Lange.

Breckenridge, D. M. (1995). Nephrology practice and directions for nursing research. In Neuman, B., *The Neuman Systems Model* (3rd ed., pp. 499–507). Norwalk, CT: Appleton & Lange.

Bueno, M. M., & Sengin, K. K. (1995). The Neuman Systems Model for critical care nursing. A framework for practice. In Neuman, B., *The Neuman Systems Model* (3rd ed., pp. 275–291). Norwalk, CT: Appleton & Lange.

Chiverton, P., & Flannery J. C. (1995). Cognitive impairment. Use of the Neuman Systems Model. In Neuman, B., *The Neuman Systems Model* (3rd ed., pp. 249–259). Norwalk, CT: Appleton & Lange.

Craig, D. M. (1995a). Community/public health nursing in Canada. Use of the Neuman Systems Model in a new paradigm. In Neuman, B., *The Neuman Systems Model* (3rd ed., pp. 529–535). Norwalk, CT: Appleton & Lange.

Craig, D. M. (1995b). The Neuman Systems Model. Examples of its use in Canadian educational programs. In Neuman, B., *The Neuman Systems Model* (3rd ed., pp. 521–527). Norwalk, CT: Appleton & Lange.

Damant, M. (1995). Community nursing in the United Kingdom. A case for reconciliation using the Neuman Systems Model. In Neuman, B., *The Neuman Systems Model* (3rd ed., pp. 607–620). Norwalk, CT: Appleton & Lange.

Davies, P., & Proctor, H. (1995). In Wales: Using the model in community mental health. In Neuman, B., *The Neuman Systems Model* (3rd ed., pp. 621–627). Norwalk, CT: Appleton & Lange.

Engberg, I. B. (1995). Brief abstracts. Use of the Neuman Systems Model in Sweden. In Neuman, B., *The Neuman Systems Model* (3rd ed., pp. 653–656). Norwalk, CT: Appleton & Lange.

Engberg, I. B., Bjalming, E., & Bertilson, B. (1995). A structure for documenting primary health care in Sweden using the Neuman Systems Model. In Neuman, B., *The Neuman Systems Model* (3rd ed., pp. 637–651). Norwalk, CT: Appleton & Lange.

Fawcett, J. (1995a). *Analysis and evaluation of conceptual models of nursing.* Philadelphia: F. A. Davis.

Fawcett, J. (1995b). Bibliography. Citations compiled by Jacqueline Fawcett. In Neuman, B., *The Neuman Systems Model* (3rd ed., pp. 704–718). Norwalk, CT: Appleton & Lange.

Fawcett, J. (1995c). Constructing conceptual-theoretical-empirical structures for research. Future implications for use of the Neuman Systems Model. In Neuman, B., *The Neuman Systems Model* (3rd ed., pp. 459–471). Norwalk, CT: Appleton & Lange.

Felix, M., Hinds, C., Wolfe, C., & Martin, A. (1995). The Neuman Systems Model in a chronic care facility: A Canadian experience. In Neuman, B., *The Neuman Systems Model* (3rd ed., pp. 549–566). Norwalk, CT: Appleton & Lange.

Frioux, T. D., Roberts, A. G., & Butler, S. J. (1995). Oklahoma State public health nursing. In Neuman, B., *The Neuman Systems Model* (3rd ed., pp. 407–414). Norwalk, CT: Appleton & Lange.

Fulton, R. A. (1995). The spiritual variable. In Neuman, B., *The Neuman Systems Model* (3rd ed., pp. 77–91). Norwalk, CT: Appleton & Lange.

Glazebrook, R. S. (1995). The Neuman Systems Model in cooperative baccalaureate nursing education: The Minnesota Intercollegiate Nursing Consortium Experience. In Neuman, B., *The Neuman Systems Model* (3rd ed., pp. 227–230). Norwalk, CT: Appleton & Lange.

Gigliotti, E. (1997). Use of Neuman's lines of defense and resistance in nursing research: Conceptual and empirical considerations. *Nursing Science Quarterly, 10,* 136–143.

Hilton, S. A., & Grafton, M. D. (1995). Curriculum transition based on the Neuman Systems Model. Los Angeles County Medical Center School of Nursing. In Neuman, B., *The Neuman Systems Model* (3rd ed., pp. 163–174). Norwalk, CT: Appleton & Lange.

Kelley, J. A., & Sanders, N. F. (1995). A systems approach to the health of nursing and health care organizations. In Neuman, B., *The Neuman Systems Model* (3rd ed., pp. 347–364). Norwalk, CT: Appleton & Lange.

Klotz, L. C. (1995). Integration of the Neuman Systems Model into the BSN curriculum at the University of Texas at Tyler. In Neuman, B., *The Neuman Systems Model* (3rd ed., pp. 183-195). Norwalk, CT: Appleton & Lange.

Lowry, L. W., & Newsome, G. G. (1995). Neuman-based associate degree programs: Past, present, and future. In Neuman, B., *The Neuman Systems Model* (3rd ed., pp. 197-214). Norwalk, CT: Appleton & Lange.

Lowry, L. W., Walker, P. H, & Mirenda, R. (1995). Through the looking glass: Back to the future. In Neuman, B., *The Neuman Systems Model* (3rd ed., pp. 63-76). Norwalk, CT: Appleton & Lange.

McCulloch, S. J. (1995). Utilization of the Neuman Systems Model: University of South Australia. In Neuman, B., *The Neuman Systems Model* (3rd ed., pp. 591-597). Norwalk, CT: Appleton & Lange.

McGee, M. (1995). Implications for use of the Neuman Systems Model in occupational health nursing. In Neuman, B., *The Neuman Systems Model* (3rd ed., pp. 657-667). Norwalk, CT: Appleton & Lange.

Meleis, A. I. (1995). Theory testing and theory support: Principles, challenges, and a sojourn into the future. In Neuman, B., *The Neuman Systems Model* (3rd ed., pp. 447-457). Norwalk, CT: Appleton & Lange.

Neuman, B. (1982). *The Neuman Systems Model: Application to nursing education and practice.* Norwalk, CT: Appleton-Century-Crofts.

Neuman, B. (1995). *The Neuman Systems Model* (3rd ed.). Norwalk, CT: Appleton & Lange.

Neuman, B. (1996). The Neuman Systems Model in research and practice. *Nursing Science Quarterly, 9,* 67-70.

Neuman, B. (1997). The Neuman Systems Model: Reflections and projections. *Nursing Science Quarterly, 10,* 18-21.

Peirce, A. G., & Fulmer, T. T. (1995). Application of the Neuman Systems Model to gerontological nursing. In Neuman, B., *The Neuman Systems Model* (3rd ed., pp. 293-308). Norwalk, CT: Appleton & Lange.

Poole, V. L., & Flowers, J. S. (1995). Care management of pregnant substance abusers using the Neuman Systems Model. In Neuman, B., *The Neuman Systems Model* (3rd ed., pp. 377-386). Norwalk, CT: Appleton & Lange.

Procter, N. G., & Cheek, J. (1995). Nurses' role in world catastrophic events: War dislocation effects on Serbian Australians. In Neuman, B., *The Neuman Systems Model* (3rd ed., pp. 119-131). Norwalk, CT: Appleton & Lange.

Rodriguez, M. L. (1995). The Neuman Systems Model adapted to a continuing care retirement community. In Neuman, B., *The Neuman Systems Model* (3rd ed., pp. 431-442). Norwalk, CT: Appleton & Lange.

Russell, J., Hileman, J. W., & Grant, J. S. (1995). Assessing and meeting the needs of home caregivers using the Neuman Systems Model. In Neuman, B., *The Neuman Systems Model* (3rd ed., pp. 331-341). Norwalk, CT: Appleton & Lange.

Scicchitani, B., Cox, J. G., Heyduk, L. J., Maglicco, P. A., & Sargent, N. A. (1995). Implementing the Neuman Model in a psychiatric hospital. In Neuman, B., *The Neuman Systems Model* (3rd ed., pp. 387-395). Norwalk, CT: Appleton & Lange.

Smith, M. C., & Edgil, A. E. (1995). Future directions for research with the Neuman Systems Model. In Neuman, B., *The Neuman Systems Model* (3rd ed., pp. 509-517). Norwalk, CT: Appleton & Lange.

Stittich, E. M, Flores, F. C., & Nuttall, P. (1995). Cultural considerations in a Neuman-based curriculum. In Neuman, B., *The Neuman Systems Model* (3rd ed., pp. 147-162). Norwalk, CT: Appleton & Lange.

Strickland-Seng, V. (1995). The Neuman Systems Model in clinical evaluation of students. In Neuman, B., *The Neuman Systems Model* (3rd ed., pp. 215-225). Norwalk, CT: Appleton & Lange.

Stuart, G. W., & Wright, L. K. (1995). Applying the Neuman Systems Model to psychiatric nursing practice. In Neuman, B., *The Neuman Systems Model* (3rd ed., pp. 263-273). Norwalk, CT: Appleton & Lange.

Tomlinson, P. S., & Anderson, K. H. (1995). Family health and the Neuman Systems Model. In Neuman, B., *The Neuman Systems Model* (3rd ed., pp. 133-144). Norwalk, CT: Appleton & Lange.

Trepanier, M., Dunn, S. I., & Sprague, A. E. (1995). Application of the Neuman Systems Model to perinatal nursing. In Neuman, B., *The Neuman Systems Model* (3rd ed., pp. 309-320). Norwalk, CT: Appleton & Lange.

Vaughan, B., & Gough, P. (1995). Use of the Neuman Systems Model in England. In Neuman, B., *The Neuman Systems Model* (3rd ed., pp. 599-605). Norwalk, CT: Appleton & Lange.

Verberk, F. (1995). In Holland: Application of the Neuman Model in psychiatric nursing. In Neuman, B., *The Neuman Systems Model* (3rd ed., pp. 629-636). Norwalk, CT: Appleton & Lange.

Walker, P. H. (1995a). Neuman-based education, practice, and research in a community nursing center. In Neuman, B., *The Neuman Systems Model* (3rd ed., pp. 415-430). Norwalk, CT: Appleton & Lange.

Walker, P. H. (1995b). TQM and the Neuman Systems Model: Education for health care administration. In Neuman, B., *The Neuman Systems Model* (3rd ed., pp. 365-376). Norwalk, CT: Appleton & Lange.

Ware, L. A., & Shannahan, M. K. (1995). Using Neuman for a stable parent support group in neonatal intensive care. In Neuman, B., *The Neuman Systems Model* (3rd ed., pp. 321-330). Norwalk, CT: Appleton & Lange.

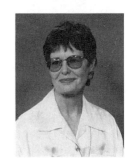

Chapter 20 Part 1

Jean Watson
Theory of Human Caring

Jean Watson

INTRODUCING THE THEORIST

Dr. Jean Watson is distinguished professor of nursing and former dean of the School of Nursing at the University of Colorado. She is the founder of the Center for Human Caring in Colorado. She is also a member of the American Academy of Nursing and has served as president of the National League for Nursing.

Dr. Watson has earned undergraduate and graduate degrees in nursing and psychiatric-mental health nursing and holds a doctorate in educational psychology and counseling. She is a widely published author and recipient of several awards and honors, including an international Kellogg Fellowship in Australia; a Fulbright Research Award in Sweden; and four honorary doctoral degrees, including an international Honorary Doctor of Science from Goteborg University in Sweden.

She has been distinguished lecturer and endowed lecturer at universities throughout the United States and many foreign countries. Her international nursing experiences have taken her around the globe several times. While director of the Center for Human Caring, she established international affiliate relations with colleagues in several countries, including the United Kingdom, Canada, New Zealand, Australia, Scandinavia, Brazil, Thailand, and Korea, among others.

Dr. Watson's published works on the philosophy and theory of human caring and the art and science of nursing are used by clinical nurses and academic programs throughout the world. Her caring philosophy is used to guide new models of caring and healing practices in diverse settings and in several different countries. Dr. Watson has been featured in numerous national videos on nursing theory and the art of nursing. She was the 1993 recipient of the National League for Nursing's Martha E. Rogers Award, "recognizing a nurse scholar who has made significant contributions to nursing knowledge that advances the science of caring in nursing and health sciences." In 1998, she was recognized as distinguished nurse scholar by New York University.

At the University of Colorado, Dr. Watson holds the title of distinguished professor of nursing, the highest honor accorded University of Colorado faculty for scholarly work. In the 1998 to 1999 school year, she assumed the first endowed chair in caring science. Her latest book, *Postmodern Nursing and Beyond,* reflects her most recent work on caring theory and nursing healing practices (Watson, 1999).

THEORY OF HUMAN CARING
by Jean Watson

The Theory of Human Caring was developed between 1975 and 1979, while I was engaged in teaching at the University of Colorado; it emerged from my own views of nursing, combined and informed by my doctoral studies in educational-clinical and social psychology. It was my initial attempt to bring meaning and focus to nursing as an emerging discipline and distinct health profession with its own unique values, knowledge, and practices, with its own ethic and mission to society. The work was also influenced by my involvement with an integrated academic nursing curriculum and efforts to find common meaning and order to nursing that transcended settings, populations, specialty, subspecialty areas, and so forth.

your thoughts

From my emerging perspective, I tried to make explicit that nursing's values, knowledge, and practices of human caring were geared toward subjective inner healing processes and the life world of the experiencing person, requiring unique caring-healing arts and a framework called "carative factors," which complemented conventional medicine but stood in stark contrast to "curative factors." At the same time, this emerging philosophy and theory of human caring sought to balance the cure orientation of medicine, giving nursing its unique disciplinary, scientific, and professional standing with itself and its public.

OVERVIEW OF THE THEORY

The major conceptual elements of the original (and emergent) theory are:

carative factors (evolving toward "clinical caritas processes")
transpersonal caring relationship
caring moment/caring occasion

Other dynamic aspects of the theory which have/ are emerging as more explicit components include:

expanded views of self and person (transpersonal mindbodyspirit unity of being; embodied spirit)
caring-healing consciousness and intentionality to care and promote healing
caring consciousness as energy within the human environment field of a caring moment
phenomenal field/unitary consciousness: unbroken wholeness and connectedness of all
advanced caring-healing modalities/nursing arts as future model for advanced practice of nursing qua nursing (consciously guided by one's nursing theoretical-philosophical orientation)

ORIGINAL AND EVOLVING 10 CARATIVE FACTORS

The original (1979) work was organized around 10 carative factors as a framework for providing a format and focus for nursing phenomena. Although "carative factors" is still the current terminology for the "core" of nursing, providing a structure for the initial work, the term "factor" is too stagnant for my sensibilities today; I offer another concept today that is more in keeping with my own evolution and future directions for the "theory." I offer now the concept of "clinical caritas" and "caritas processes" as consistent with a more fluid and contemporary movement with these ideas and my expanding directions.

Clinical Caritas and Caritas Processes

Caritas comes from the Greek word meaning "to cherish, to appreciate, to give special attention, if not loving, attention to"; it connotes something that is very fine, that indeed is precious. Katie Eriksson in Finland has used the word "caritas" in her theory of caring to convey similar meanings.

The word "caritas" also is closely related to the original word "carative" from my 1979 book. At this time, I now make new connections between carative and caritas, and without hesitation compare them to invoke the "L" word, which caritas conveys—that is, love. This allows love and caring to come together for a new form of deep transpersonal caring. This relationship between love and caring connotes inner healing for self and others, extending to nature and the larger universe, unfolding and evolving within a cosmology that is both metaphysical and transcendent with the coevolving human in the universe. This emerging model of transpersonal caring moves from carative to caritas. This integrative expanded perspective is postmodern, in that it transcends conventional industrial, static models of nursing; while simultaneously evoking both the past and the future. For example, the future of nursing is ironically tied to Nightingale's sense of "calling," guided by a deep sense of commitment and a covenantal ethic of human service; cherishing our phenomena, our subject matter, and those we serve. It is when we include caring and love in our work and our life that we discover and affirm that nursing, like teaching, is more than just a job; it is also a life-giving and life-receiving career for a lifetime of growth and learning. Such maturity and integration of past with present and future now require transforming self and those we serve, including our institutions and the profession itself. As we more publicly and professionally assert these positions for our theories, our ethics, and our practices—even for our science—we also locate ourselves and our profession and discipline within a new, emerging cosmology. Such thinking calls for a sense of reverence and sacredness with regard to life and all living things. It incorporates both art and science, as they are also being redefined, acknowledging a convergence between art, science, and spirituality. As we enter into the transpersonal caring theory and philosophy,

> It is when we include caring and love in our work and our life that we discover and affirm that nursing is . . . for a lifetime of growth and learning.

we simultaneously are challenged to relocate our-selves in these emerging ideas and question for our-selves how the theory speaks to us, which invites us into a new relationship with ourselves and our ideas about life, nursing, and theory. In this framework each one of us is also asked, if not enticed, to examine and explore the critical intersection between the per-sonal and the professional; to translate our unique tal-ents, interests, and gifts into the human service of car-ing and healing, for self and others, and even for the planet Earth itself.

Original Carative Factors

The original carative factors served as a guide to what was referred to as the "core of nursing," in con-trast to nursing's "trim." *Core* pointed to those aspects of nursing that potentiate therapeutic healing pro-cesses and relationships; they affect the one caring and the one-being-cared for. Further, the basic core was grounded in what I referred to as the philoso-phy, science, and even art of caring. Carative is that deeper and larger dimension of nursing that goes be-yond the "trim" of changing times, setting, proce-dures, functional tasks, specialized focus around dis-ease, and treatment and technology. Although the "trim" is important and not expendable, the point is that nursing cannot be defined around its trim and what it does, in a given setting, at a given point in time. Nor can nursing's trim define and clarify its larger professional ethic and mission to society—its raison d'être for the public. That is where nursing theory comes into play and transpersonal caring theory offers another way that both differs from and complements that which has come to be known as "modern" nursing and conventional medical-nursing frameworks.

The 10 carative factors included in the original work are the following:

1. Formation of a humanistic-altruistic system of values.
2. Instillation of faith-hope.
3. Cultivation of sensitivity to one's self and to others.
4. Development of a helping-trusting, human car-ing relationship.
5. Promotion and acceptance of the expression of positive and negative feelings.
6. Systematic use of a creative problem-solving car-ing process.
7. Promotion of transpersonal teaching-learning.
8. Provision for a supportive, protective, and/or corrective mental, physical, societal, and spiri-tual environment.
9. Assistance with gratification of human needs.
10. Allowance for existential-phenomenological-spiritual forces. (Watson, 1979/1985)

Although some of the basic tenets of the original carative factors still hold, and indeed are used as the basis for some theory-guided practice models and re-search, what I am proposing here, as part of my evo-lution and the evolution of these ideas and the theory itself, is to transpose the "carative factors" into "clinical caritas processes." For example, consider the following within the context of clinical caritas and emerging transpersonal caring theory.

From Carative Factors to Clinical Caritas Processes

As carative factors evolve within an expanding per-spective, and as my ideas and values evolve, I now of-fer the following translation of the original carative factors into clinical caritas processes, suggesting more open ways in which they can be considered. For example:

1. Formation of humanistic-altruistic system of values becomes practice of loving kindness and equanimity within the context of caring consciousness.
2. Instillation of faith-hope becomes being authentically present, and enabling and sustaining the deep belief system and subjective life world of self and one-being-cared-for.
3. Cultivation of sensitivity to one's self and to others becomes cultivation of one's own spiritual practices and transpersonal self, going beyond ego self, opening to others with sensitivity and compassion.
4. Development of a helping-trusting, human caring relationship becomes developing and sustaining a helping-trusting, authentic caring relationship.
5. Promotion and acceptance of the expression of positive and negative feelings becomes being present to, and supportive of, the expression of positive and negative feelings as a connection with deeper spirit of self and the one-being-cared-for.
6. Systematic use of a creative problem-solving caring process becomes creative use of self and all ways of knowing as part of the caring process; to engage in artistry of caring-healing practices.
7. Promotion of transpersonal teaching-learning becomes engaging in genuine teaching-learning experience that attends to unity of being and meaning, attempting to stay within others' frames of reference.
8. Provision for a supportive, protective, and/or corrective mental, physical, societal, and spiritual environment becomes creating healing environment at all levels (physical as well as non-physical, subtle environment of energy and consciousness, whereby wholeness, beauty, comfort, dignity, and peace are potentiated).
9. Assistance with gratification of human needs becomes assisting with basic needs, with an intentional caring consciousness, administering "human care essentials," which potentiate alignment of mindbodyspirit, wholeness, and unity of being in all aspects of care, tending to both embodied spirit and evolving spiritual emergence.
10. Allowance for existential-phenomenological-spiritual forces becomes opening and attending to spiritual-mysterious, and existential dimensions of one's own life-death; soul care for self and the one-being-cared-for.

What differs in the clinical caritas framework is that a decidedly spiritual dimension and an overt evocation of love and caring are merged for a new paradigm for the new millennium. Such a perspective ironically places nursing within its most mature framework, consistent with the Nightingale model of nursing—yet to be actualized, but awaiting its evolution within a caring-healing theory. This direction, ironically while embedded in theory, goes beyond theory, but becomes a converging paradigm for nursing's future.

Thus, I consider my work more a philosophical, ethical, intellectual blueprint for nursing's evolving disciplinary/professional matrix, rather than a specific theory per se. Nevertheless, others interact with the original work at levels of concreteness or abstractness; the caring theory has been, and is still being used as a guide for educational curricula, clinical practice models, methods for research and inquiry, and administrative directions for nursing and health care delivery.

This work posits a value's explicit moral foundation and takes a specific position with respect to the centrality of human caring, "caritas" and love as now an ethic and ontology as well as a critical starting point for nursing's existence, broad societal mission, and the basis for further advancement for caring-healing practices. Nevertheless, its use and evolution is dependent upon "critical, reflective practices that must be continuously questioned and critiqued in order to remain dynamic, flexible, and endlessly self-revising and emergent" (Watson, 1996, p. 143).

TRANSPERSONAL CARING RELATIONSHIP

The terms *transpersonal* and *a transpersonal caring relationship* are foundational to the work; "transpersonal" conveys a concern for the inner life world and subjective meaning of another who is fully embodied, but transpersonal also goes beyond the ego self and beyond the given moment, reaching to the deeper connections to spirit and with the broader universe. Thus, a transpersonal caring relationship moves beyond ego self and radiates to spiritual, even cosmic, concerns and connections that tap into healing possibilities and potentials. Transpersonal caring seeks to connect with and embrace the spirit or soul of the other, through the processes of caring and healing and being in authentic relation, in the moment.

Such a transpersonal relation is influenced by the caring consciousness and intentionality of the nurse as she or he enters into the life space or phenomenal field of another person, and is able to detect the other person's condition of being (at the soul, or spirit level). It implies a focus on the uniqueness of self and other and the uniqueness of the moment, wherein the coming together is mutual and reciprocal, each fully embodied in the moment, while paradoxically capable of transcending the moment, open to new possibilities.

Transpersonal caring calls for an authenticity of being and becoming, an ability to be present to self and other in a reflective frame; the transpersonal nurse has the ability to center consciousness and intentionality on caring, healing, and wholeness, rather than on disease, illness, and pathology.

Transpersonal caring competencies are related to ontological development of the nurse's human competencies and ways of being and becoming; thus, "ontological caring competencies" become as critical in this model as "technological curing competencies" were in the conventional modern, Western nursing-medicine model, which is now coming to an end.

Within the model of transpersonal caring, clinical caritas consciousness is engaged at a foundational ethical level for entry into this framework. The nurse attempts to enter into and stay within the other's frame of reference for connecting with the inner life world of meaning and spirit of the other; together they join in a mutual search for meaning and wholeness of being and becoming, to potentiate comfort measures, pain control, a sense of well-being, wholeness, or even a spiritual transcendence of suffering. The person is viewed as whole and complete, regardless of illness or disease (Watson, 1996, p. 153).

Assumptions of Transpersonal Caring Relationship

The nurse's moral commitment, intentionality, and caritas consciousness is to protect, enhance, promote, and potentiate human dignity, wholeness, and healing, wherein a person creates or cocreates his or her own meaning for existence, healing, wholeness, and living and dying.

The nurse's will and consciousness affirm the subjective-spiritual significance of the person while seeking to sustain caring in the midst of threat and despair—biological, institutional, or otherwise. This honors the I-Thou relationship versus an I-It relationship.

The nurse seeks to recognize, accurately detect, and connect with the inner condition of spirit of another through genuine presencing and being centered in the caring moment; actions, words, behaviors, cognition, body language, feelings, intuition, thought, senses, the energy field, and so on, all contribute to transpersonal caring connection.

> Transpersonal caring seeks to connect in the moment.

The nurse's ability to connect with another at this transpersonal spirit-to-spirit level is translated via movements, gestures, facial expressions, procedures, information, touch, sound, verbal expressions, and other scientific, technical, aesthetic, and human means of communication, into nursing human art/acts or intentional caring-healing modalities.

The caring-healing modalities within the context of transpersonal caring/caritas consciousness potentiate harmony, wholeness, and unity of being by releasing some of the disharmony, the blocked energy that interferes with the natural healing processes; thus the nurse helps another through this process to access the healer within, in the fullest sense of Nightingale's view of nursing.

Ongoing personal-professional development and spiritual growth and personal spiritual practice assist the nurse in entering into this deeper level of professional healing practice, allowing the nurse to awaken to the transpersonal condition of the world and to actualize more fully "ontological competencies" necessary for this level of advanced practice of nursing. Valuable teachers for this work include the nurse's own life history and previous experiences, which provide opportunities for focused studies, the nurse having lived through or experienced various human conditions and having imagined others' feelings in various circumstances. To some degree, the necessary knowledge and consciousness can be gained through work with other cultures and study of the humanities (art, drama, literature, personal story, narratives of illness journeys, etc.), along with an exploration of one's own values, deep beliefs, relationship with self and others, and one's world. Other facilitators are personal growth experiences such as psychotherapy, transpersonal psychology, meditation, bioenergetics work, and other models for spiritual awakening. Continuous growth is ongoing for developing and maturing within a transpersonal caring model. The notion of health professionals as wounded healers is acknowledged as part of the necessary growth and compassion called forth within this theory/philosophy.

CARING MOMENT/
CARING OCCASION

A caring occasion occurs whenever the nurse and another come together with their unique life histories and phenomenal fields in a human-to-human transaction. The coming together in a given moment becomes a focal point in space and time. It becomes transcendent, whereby experience and perception take place, but the actual caring occasion has a greater field of its own, in a given moment. The process goes beyond itself yet arises from aspects of itself that become part of the life history of each person, as well as part of some larger, more complex pattern of life (Watson, 1985, p. 59; 1996, p. 157).

A caring moment involves an action and choice by both the nurse and other. The moment of coming together presents the two with the opportunity to decide how to *be in the moment*, in the relationship—what to do with and in the moment. If the caring moment is *transpersonal*, each feels a connection with the other at the spirit level; thus, the moment transcends time and space, opening up new possibilities for healing and human connection at a deeper level than that of physical interaction. For example:

> [W]e learn from one another how to be human by identifying ourselves with others, finding their dilemmas in ourselves. What we all learn from it is self-knowledge. The self we learn about . . . is every self. IT is universal—the human self. We learn to recognize ourselves in others . . . [it] keeps alive our common humanity and avoids reducing self or other to the moral status of object. (Watson, 1985, pp. 59–60)

CARING (HEALING)
CONSCIOUSNESS

The dynamic of transpersonal caring (healing) within a caring moment is manifest in a field of consciousness. The transpersonal dimensions of a caring moment are affected by the nurse's consciousness in the caring moment, which in turn affects the field of the whole. The role of consciousness with respect to a holographic view of science has been discussed in earlier writings (Watson, 1992, p. 148) and include the following points:

- The whole caring-healing-loving consciousness is contained within a single caring moment.

- The one caring and the one-being-cared-for are interconnected; the caring-healing process is connected with the other human(s) and the higher energy of the universe.
- The caring-healing-loving consciousness of the nurse is communicated to the one-being-cared-for.
- Caring-healing-loving consciousness exists through and transcends time and space and can be dominant over physical dimensions.

Within this context, it is acknowledged that the process is relational and connected; it transcends time, space, and physicality. The process is intersubjective with transcendent possibilities that go beyond the given caring moment.

IMPLICATIONS OF
THE CARING MODEL

The Caring Model or Theory can also be considered a philosophical and moral/ethical foundation for professional nursing and part of the central focus for nursing at the disciplinary level. A model of caring includes a call for both art and science; it offers a framework that embraces and intersects with art, science, humanities, spirituality, and new dimensions of mindbodyspirit medicine and nursing evolving openly as central to human phenomena of nursing practice.

I emphasize that it is possible to read, study, learn about, even teach and research the Caring Theory. However, to truly "get it," one has to experience it personally; thus, the model is both an invitation and an opportunity to interact with the ideas, experiment with and grow within the philosophy, and to live it out in one's personal/professional life.

> A caring moment involves an action and choice by both the nurse and other.

The ideas as originally developed, as well as in the current evolving phase (see Watson, 1999), provide us with a chance to assess, critique, and see where or how, or even if, we may locate ourselves within the framework or the emerging ideas in relation to our own "theories and philosophies of professional nursing and/or caring practice."

If one chooses to use the caring perspective as theory, model, philosophy, ethic, or ethos for transforming self and practice, or self and system, the following questions may help (Watson, 1996, p. 161):

- Is there congruence between the values and major concepts and beliefs in the model and the given nurse, group, system, organization, curriculum, population needs, clinical administrative setting, or other entity that is considering interacting with the caring model to transform and/or improve practice?

- What is one's view of "human"? And what does it mean to be human, caring, healing, becoming, growing, transforming, and so on? For example, in the words of Teilhard de Chardin: "Are we humans having a spiritual experience, or are we spiritual beings having a human experience?" Such thinking in regard to this philosophical question can guide one's worldview and help to clarify where one may locate self within the caring framework.

- Are those interacting and engaging in the model interested in their own personal evolution: Are they committed to seeking authentic connections and caring-healing relationships with self and others?

- Are those involved "conscious" of their caring caritas or noncaring consciousness and intentionally in a given moment, at individual and system level? Are they interested and committed to expanding their caring consciousness and actions to self, other, environment, nature, and wider universe?

- Are those working within the model interested in shifting their focus from a modern medical science-technocure orientation to a true caring-healing-loving model?

This work, in both its original and evolving forms, seeks to develop caring as an ontolgoical and theoretical-philosophical-ethical framework for the profession and discipline of nursing and to clarify its mature relationship and distinct intersection with other health sciences. Nursing caring theory-based activities as guides to practice, education, and research have developed throughout the United States and other parts of the world. The Caring Model is consistently one of the nursing caring theories used as a guide. Nurses' reflective-critical practice models are increasingly adhering to a caring ethic and ethos.

Because the nature of the use of the Caring Theory is fluid, dynamic, and undergoing constant change in various settings around the world and locally, I am not able to offer updated summaries of activities. Earlier publications seek to provide examples of how the work is used, or has been used, in specific settings.

Summary

Nursing's future and nursing in the future will depend on nursing maturing as the distinct health, healing, and caring profession that it has always represented across time, but has yet to actualize. Nursing thus ironically is now challenged to stand and mature within its own paradigm, while simultaneously having to transcend it and share with others. The future already reveals that all health-care practitioners will need to work within a shared framework of caring relationships, mindbodyspirit medicine, embracing healing arts and caring practices and processes and the spiritual dimensions of care much more completely. Thus, nursing is at its own crossroad of possibilities, between worldviews and paradigms, between centuries and eras, invited and required to build upon its heritage and latest evolution in science and technology, but to transcend itself for a postmodern future yet to be known. However, nursing's future holds promises of caring and healing mysteries, and models yet to unfold, as opportunities for offering compassionate caritas service await, at individual, system, societal, national, and global levels for self, for profession, and for the broader world community.

References

Watson, J. (1979). *Nursing: The philosophy and science of caring.* Boston: Little, Brown.
Watson J. (1985). *Nursing: Human science and human care.* Norwalk, CT: Appleton-Century-Crofts.
Watson, J. (1992). *Notes on nursing. Guidelines for caring then and now.* In Nightingale, F., *Notes on nursing: What it is, and what it is not.* (Commemorative edition, pp. 80–85.) Philadelphia: J. B. Lippincott. (Original work published in 1859.)
Watson, M. J. (1996). Watson's theory of transpersonal caring. In Hinton-Walker, P., & Neuman, B. (Eds.), *Blueprint for use of nursing models* (pp. 141–194). New York: National League for Nursing.
Watson, J. (1999). *Postmodern nursing and Beyond.* London: Churchill Livingstone.

Bibliography

Allan, H. (1996). Developing nursing knowledge and language. *Nursing Standard, 10*(50), 42–22.
Anderson, A., Borger, F., Smalarz, M., Hays, A., & McGrory, A. (1995). Unsung heroes. *Home Healthcare Nurse, 13*(6), 17–18.
Aucoin-Gallant, G. (1990). La theorie du caring de Watson. Une approache existentielle phenome-

nologique et spirituelle des soins infirmiers. (English abstract.) *The Canadian Nurse, 86*(11), 32-35.

Astorino, G., Hecomovich, K., Jacobs, T., Laxson, L., Mauro, P., Neil, R. M., & Talley, S. (1994). The Denver Nursing Project in Human Caring. In Watson, J. (Ed.), *Applying the art and science of human caring* (pp. 19-39). New York: National League for Nursing.

Audet, M. C. (1995). Caring in nursing education: Reducing anxiety in the clinical setting. *Nursing Connections, 8*(3), 21-29.

Barker, P., & Reynolds, B. (1994). A critique: Watson's caring ideology, the proper focus of psychiatric nursing? *Journal of Psychosocial Nursing and Mental Health Services, 32*(5), 17-22.

Baker, P., Reynolds, B., & Ward, T. (1995). The proper focus of nursing: A critique of the "caring" ideology. *International Journal of Nursing Studies, 32,* 386-397.

Beauchamp, C. J. (1993). The centrality of caring: A case study. In Munhall, P. L., & Boyd, C. O. (Eds.), *Nursing research: A qualitative perspective* (2nd ed., pp. 338-358). New York: National League for Nursing.

Bernick, L., & Avery, L. (1994). Clinical decision-making: The art and science of inquiry in caring for elders. *Perspectives, 18*(1), 2-6.

Bishop, M. E. (1996). Nurses, knowledge, attitude may influence organ donation. *Michigan Nurse, 69*(5), 14.

Brandman, W. (1996). Intersubjectivity, social microcosm, and the here-and-now in a support group for nurses. *Archives of Psychiatric Nursing 10,* 374-378.

Brenner, P. (1986). Disseminating care research literature. *Journal of Nursing Administration, 16*(1), 26-27.

Brooks, B. A., & Rosenberg, S. (1995). Incorporating nursing theory into a nursing department strategic plan. *Nursing Administration Quarterly, 20*(1), 81-86.

Bunkers, S. S., Brendtro, M., Holmes, P. K., Howell, J., Johnson, S., Koerner, J., Larson, J., Nelson, J., & Weaver, R. (1992). The healing web. A transformative model for nursing. *Nursing and Health Care, 13,* 68-73.

Burchiel, R. N. (1995). Does perioperative nursing include caring? *Association of Operating Room Nurses Journal, 62,* 257-289.

Burns, P. (1991). Elements of spirituality and Watson's theory of transpersonal caring: Expansion of focus. In Chinn, P. L. (Ed.), *Anthology on caring* (pp. 141-153). New York: National League of Nursing.

Capik, L. K. (1997). The Watson theory of human care applied to ASPO/Lamaze perinatal education. *Journal of Perinatal Education, 6*(1), 43-47.

Cappell, E. (1994). A step-by-step guide on how to implement caring theory. In J. Watson (Ed.), *Applying the art and science of human caring* (pp. 11-17). New York: National League for Nursing.

Cappell, E., & Leggat, S. (1993). Implementation of theory-based nursing practice: Laying the groundwork for total quality management within a nursing department. *Canadian Journal of Nursing Administration, 7,* 31-41.

Carson, M. G. (1992). An application of Watson's theory to group work with the elderly. *Perspectives, 16*(4), 7-13.

Chipman, Y. (1991). Caring: Its meaning and place in the practice of nursing. *Journal of Nursing Education, 30,* 171-175.

Clayton, G. M. (1989). Research testing Watson's theory: The phenomena of caring in an elderly population. In Riehl-Sisca, J. P. (Ed.), *Conceptual models for nursing practice* (3rd ed., pp. 245-252). Norwalk, CT: Appleton & Lange.

Coates, C. J. (1997). The Caring Efficacy Scale: Nurses, self-reports of caring in practice settings. *Advanced Practice Nursing Quarterly, 3*(1), 53-59.

Cody, W. K. (1995). Intersubjectivity: Nursing's contribution to the explication of its postmodern meaning. *Nursing Science Quarterly, 8,* 52-54.

Cohen, J. A. (1991). Two portraits of caring: A comparison of the artists, Leininger and Watson. *Journal of Advanced Nursing, 16,* 899-909.

Cronin, S. N., & Harrison, B. (1988). Importance of nurse caring behaviors as perceived by patients after myocardial infarction. *Heart and Lung, 17,* 374-380.

Daniel, L. E. (1998). Vulnerability as a key to authenticity. *Image: Journal of Nursing Scholarship, 30,* 191-192.

Dennis, P. M. (1991). Components of spiritual nursing care from the nurse's perspective. *Journal of Holistic Nursing, 9,* 2742.

Duffy, J. T. (1992). The impact of nursing caring on patient outcomes. In Gaut, D. (Ed.), *The presence of caring in nursing* (pp. 113-136). New York: National League for Nursing.

Eddins, B. B., & Riley-Eddins, E. A. (1997). Watson's Theory of Human Caring: The twentieth century and beyond. *Journal of Multicultural Nursing and Health, 3*(3), 30-35.

Eriksson, K. (1987). Vårdandets idé (The idea of caring). Stockholm: Almquist & Wiksell.

Forsyth, D., Delaney, C., Maloney, N., Kubesh, D., & Story, D. (1989). Can caring behavior be taught? *Nursing Outlook, 37,* 164-166.

From, M. A. (1995). Utilizing the home setting to teach Watson's Theory of Human Caring. *Nursing Forum, 30*(4), 5-11.

Gramling, L., & Nugent, K. (1998). Teaching caring within the context of health. *Nurse Educator, 23*(2), 47-51.

Gray, D. P. (1992). A feminist critique of Jean Watson's theory of caring. In Thompson, J. L., Allen, D. G., & Rodrigues-Fisher, L. (Eds.), *Critique, resistance, and action: Working papers in the politics of nursing* (pp. 85-96). New York: National League for Nursing.

Gullo, S. (1997). Oncology nurses: Masters in the art of caring. *Oncology Nursing Forum, 24,* 971-978.

Hagell, E. I. (1989). Nursing knowledge: Women's knowledge. A sociological perspective. *Journal of Advanced Nursing, 14,* 226-233.

Harrison, R. L. (1997). Spirituality and hope: Nursing implications for people with human immunodeficiency virus disease. *Holistic Nursing Practice, 12*(1), 9-16.

Hegyvary, S. T. (1987). Collaboration in nursing research: Advancing the science of human care. *Communicating Nursing Research, 20,* 17-22.

Hogg, K. (1994). Don't let cure be at the expense of care: Is the increased technicality of ICU nursing reducing the care given? *Professional Nurse, 9,* 465-466, 468-470.

Holmes, C. A. (1990). Alternatives to natural science foundations for nursing. *International Journal of Nursing Studies, 27,* 187-198.

Hummelvoll, J. K. (1996). The nurse-client alliance model. *Perspectives in Psychiatric Care, 32*(4), 12-21.

Jensen, K. P., Beck-Petterson, S. R., & Segesten, K. M. (1993). The caring moment and the green-thumb phenomenon among Swedish nurses. *Nursing Science Quarterly, 6,* 98-104.

Jensen, K. P., Beck-Petterson, S. R., & Segesten, K. M. (1996). "Catching my wavelength": Perceptions of the excellent nurse. *Nursing Science Quarterly, 9,* 115-120.

Jones, S. B. (1991). A caring-based AIDS educational model for pre-adolescents: Global health human caring perspective. *Journal of Advanced Nursing, 16,* 591-596.

Joseph, L. (1991). The energetics of conscious caring for the compassionate healer. In Gaut, D. A., & Leininger, M. M. (Eds.), *Caring: The compassionate healer* (pp. 51-60). New York: National League for Nursing.

Karns, P. S. (1991). Building a foundation for spiritual care. *Journal of Christian Nursing, 8*(3), 10-13.

Kennedy, D., & Barloon, L. F. (1997). Managing burnout in pediatric critical care: The human care commitment. *Critical Care Nursing Quarterly, 20,* 63-71, 81-82.

Kerouac, S., & Rouillier, L. (1993). Reflections on the promotion of caring with head nurses. In Gaut, D. (Ed.), *The presence of caring in nursing* (pp. 89-102). New York: National League for Nursing.

Krysl, M., & Watson, J. (1988). Existential moments of caring: Facets of nursing and social support. *Advances in Nursing Science, 10*(2), 12-17.

Leenerts, M. H., Koehler, J. A., & Neil, R. M. (1996). Nursing care models increase care quality while reducing costs. *Journal of the Association of Nursing in AIDS Care, 7*(4), 37-49.

Lemmer, C. M. (1991). Parental Perceptions of caring following perinatal bereavement. *Western Journal of Nursing Research, 13,* 475-494.

Leininger, M., & Watson, J. (Eds.). (1990). *The caring imperative in education.* New York: National League for Nursing.

Lyne, B. A. & Waller, P. R. (1990). The Denver Nursing Project in Human Caring: A model for AIDS nursing and professional education. *Family and Community Health, 13,* 78-84.

Marckx, B. B. (1995). Watson's theory of caring: A model for implementation in practice. *Journal of Nursing Care Quality, 9*(4), 43-54.

Martsolf, D. S. & Mickley, J. R. (1998). The concept of spirituality in nursing theories: Differing world views and extent of focus. *Journal of Advanced Nursing, 27,* 294-303.

McNamara, S. A. (1995). Perioperative nurses' perceptions of caring practices. *Association of Operating Room Nurses Journal, 61,* 377-388.

Mendyka, B. E. (1993). The dying patient in the intensive care unit: Assisting the family in crisis. *AACN Clinical Issues in Critical Care Nursing, 4,* 550-557.

Miller, B. K., Haber, J., & Byrne, M. W. (1992). The experience of caring in the acute care setting: Patient and nurse perspectives. In Gaut, D. (Ed.), *The presence of caring in nursing* (pp. 137-155). New York: National League for Nursing.

Montgomery, C. (1994). The caring/healing relationship of "maintaining authentic caring." In Watson, J. (Ed.), *Applying the art and science of human caring* (pp. 39-45). New York: National League for Nursing.

Morris, L. E. H. (1996). A spiritual well-being model: Use with older women who experience depression. *Issues in Mental Health Nursing, 17,* 439-455.

Morse, J. M., Bottorff, J., Neander, W., & Solberg, S. (1991). Comparative analysis of conceptualizations and theories of caring. *Image: Journal of Nursing Scholarship, 23,* 119-126.

Morse, J. M., Solberg, S. M., Neander, W. L., Bottorff, J. L., & Johnson, J. L. (1990). Concepts of caring and caring as a concept. *Advances in Nursing Science, 13*(1), 1-14.

Neil, R. M. (1990). Watson's theory of caring in nursing: The rainbow of and for people living with AIDS. In Parker, M. E. (Ed.), *Nursing theories in practice* (pp. 289-301). New York: National League for Nursing.

Neil, R. M. (1994). Authentic caring: The sensible answer for clients and staff dealing with HIV/AIDS. *Nursing Administration Quarterly, 18*(2), 36-40.

Neil, R. M. (1995). Evidence in support of basing a nursing center on nursing theory: The Denver Nursing Project in Human Caring. In Murphy, B. (Ed.), *Nursing centers: The time is now* (pp. 33-46). New York: National League for Nursing.

Neil, R. M., & Schroeder, C. A. (1993). Evaluation research within the human caring framework. In Gaut, D. (Ed.), *The presence of caring in nursing* (pp. 103-111). New York: National League for Nursing.

Neil, R. M., & Watts, R. (Eds.). (1991). *Caring and nursing: Explorations in feminist perspectives.* New York: National League for Nursing.

Nyberg, J. (1994). Implementing Watson's theory of caring. In Watson, J. (Ed.), *Applying the art and science of human caring* (pp. 53-61). New York: National League for Nursing.

Parsons, E. C., Kee, C. C., & Gray, D. P. (1993). Perioperative nurse caring behaviors: Perceptions of surgical patients. *Association of Operating Room Nurses Journal, 57,* 1106-1107, 1110-1114.

Percy, M. S. (1995). Children from homeless families describe what is special in their lives. *Holistic Nursing Practice, 9*(4), 24-33.

Piccinato, J. M., & Rosenbaum, J. N. (1997). Caregiver hardiness explored within Watson's Theory of Human Caring in Nursing. *Journal of Gerontological Nursing, 23*(10), 32-39.

Podolak, I. (1995). A comprehensive philosophy for nursing: The total approach. *Canadian Journal of Nursing Administration, 8*(4), 23-41.

Price, N. (1995). The role of the consultation-liaison nurse: Caring for patients with AIDS dementia complex. *Journal of Psychosocial Nursing and Mental Health Services, 33*(12), 31-34, 40-41.

Propst, M. G., Schenk, L. K., & Clairain, S. (1994). Caring as perceived during the birth experience. In Gaut, D. A., & Boykin, A. (Eds.), *Caring as healing: Renewal through hope* (pp. 252-264). New York: National League for Nursing.

Quinn, J. F. (1994). Caring for the caregiver. In Watson, J. (Ed.), *Applying the art and science of human caring* (pp. 63-71). New York: National League for Nursing.

Ray, M. A. (1997). Consciousness and the moral ideal: A transcultural analysis of Watson's theory of transpersonal caring. *Advanced Practice Nursing Quarterly, 3*(1), 25-31.

Reed, P. G. (1996). Transcendence: Formulating nursing perspectives. *Nursing Science Quarterly, 9,* 2-4.

Roberts, J. E. (1990). Uncovering hidden caring. *Nursing Outlook, 38,* 67-69.

Running, A. (1997). Snapshots of experience: Vignettes from a nursing home. *Journal of Advanced Nursing, 25,* 117-122.

Ryan, P. Y. (1992). Perceptions of the most helpful nursing behaviors in a home-care hospice setting: Caregivers and nurses. *American Journal of Hospice and Palliative Care, 9*(5), 22-31.

Sakalys, J. A., & Watson, J. (1985). New directions in higher education: A review of trends. *Journal of Professional Nursing, 1,* 293-299.

Sakalys, J. A., & Watson, J. (1986). Professional education: Postbaccalaureate education for professional nursing . . . Reintegration of the classical liberal arts model. *Journal of Professional Nursing, 2,* 91-97.

Sanford, S., & Lamb, C. R. (1997). Nurse partners: Going beyond the delivery room. *Mother Baby Journal, 2*(6), 8-12.

Sarter, B. (1988). Philosophical sources of nursing theory. *Nursing Science Quarterly, 1,* 52-59.

Saxton, M. (1994). How could theory affect practice? *Nursing Praxis in New Zealand, 9*(1), 13-17.

Schindel-Martin, L. (1991). Using Watson's theory to explore the dimensions of adult polycystic kidney disease. *American Nephrology Nurses' Association Journal, 18,* 493-496.

Schroeder, C., & Neil, R. M. (1992). Focus groups: A humanistic means of evaluating an HIV/AIDS programme based on caring theory. *Journal of Clinical Nursing, 1,* 265-274.

Schroeder, C. (1993). Cost effectiveness of a theory-based nurse-managed center for persons living with HIV/AIDS. In Parker, M. E. (Ed.), *Patterns of nursing theories in practice* (pp. 159-179). New York: National League for Nursing.

Schroeder, C. (1993). Nursing's response to the crisis of access, costs, and quality in health care. *Advances in Nursing Science, 16*(1), 1-20.

Schroeder, C., & Astorino, G. (1996). The Denver Nursing Education Project: Promoting the health of persons living with HIV/AIDS. In Cohen, E. L. (Ed.), *Nurse case management in the 21st century* (pp. 63-67). St. Louis: Mosby-Year Book.

Schroeder, C., & Maeve, M. K. (1992). Nursing care partnerships at the Denver Nursing Project in Human Caring: An application and extension of caring theory in practice. *Advances in Nursing Science, 15*(2), 25-38.

Sithichoke-Rattan, N. (1989). A clinical application of Watson's theory. *Pediatric Nursing, 15,* 458-462.

Smerke, J. M. (1989). *Interdisciplinary guide to the literature for human caring.* New York: National League for Nursing.

Smerke, J. M. (1990). Ethical components of caring. *Critical Care Nursing Clinics of North America, 2,* 509-513.

Smith, M. C. (1991). Existential-phenomenological foundation nursing: A discussion of differences. *Nursing Science Quarterly, 4,* 5-6.

Smith, M. C. (1994). Case management in the caring-healing paradigm. In Watson, J. (Ed.), *Applying the art and science of human caring* (pp. 47-52). New York: National League for Nursing.

Smith, M. C. (1997). Nursing theory-guided practice: Practice guided by Watson's theory—The Denver Nursing Project in Human Caring. *Nursing Science Quarterly, 10,* 56-58.

Sourial, S. (1996). An analysis and evaluation of Watson's Theory of Human Caring. *Journal of Advanced Nursing, 24,* 400.

Stember, M., & Hester, N. K. (1990). Research strategies for developing nursing as the science of human care. In Chaska, N. L. (Ed.), *The nursing profession: Turning points* (pp. 165-172). St. Louis: Mosby.

Sterritt, P. F., & Pokorney, M. E. (1994). Art activities for patients with Alzheimer's and related disorders. *Geriatric Nursing, 15,* 155-159.

Tanner, C. A. (1990). Caring as a value in nursing education. *Nursing Outlook, 38,* 70-72.

Taylor, R. L., & Watson, J. (Eds.). (1989). *They shall not hurt: Human suffering and human caring.* Boulder, CO: Colorado Associated University Press.

Vezeau, T. M., & Schroeder, C. (1991). Caring approaches: A critical examination of origin, balance of power, embodiment, time and space, and intended outcome. In Chinn, P. L. (Ed.), *Anthology on caring* (pp. 1-16). New York: National League for Nursing.

Wadas, T. M. (1993). Case management and caring behavior. *Nursing Management, 4*(9), 40-42, 44-46.

Ward, S. L. (1998). Caring and healing in the 21st century. *MCN, American Journal of Maternal Child Nursing, 23,* 210-215.

Watson, D. S. (1994). Technology in the perioperative environment. *Association of Operating Room Nurses Journal, S9*(1), 268, 270-271, 274-277.

Watson, J. (1981). Some issues related to a science of caring for nursing practice. In Leininger, M. (Ed.), *Caring: An essential human need* (pp. 61-67). Thorofare, NJ: Charles B. Slack.

Watson, J. (1983). Commentary on "The IDIR model for faculty research with students." *Western Journal of Nursing Research, 5,* 310-311.

Watson, J. (1985). *Nursing: Human science and human care.* Norwalk, CT: Appleton Century-Crofts. [Second printing, 1988. Boulder, CO: Colorado Associated University Press. Third printing, 1988. New York: National League for Nursing.]

Watson, J. (1985). Reflections on different methodologies for the future of nursing. In Leininger, M. M. (Ed.), *Qualitative research methods in nursing* (pp. 343-349). New York: Grune & Stratton.

Watson, J. (1996). Watson's theory of transpersonal caring. In Hinton-Walker, P., & Neuman, B. (Eds.), *Blueprint for use of nursing models* (pp. 141-184; see especially pp. 166-1731). New York: National League for Nursing.

Watson, J. (1987). Academic and clinical collaboration: Advancing the art and science of human caring. *Communicating Nursing Research, 20,* 1-16.

Watson, J. (1987). Nursing on the caring edge. Metaphorical vignettes. *Advances in Nursing Science, 10*(1), 10-18.

Watson, J. (1988). A case study: Curriculum in transition. In *Curriculum revolution: Mandate for change* (pp. 1-8). New York: National League for Nursing.

Watson, J. (1988). Human caring as moral context for nursing education. *Nursing and Health Care, 9,* 422-425.

Watson, J. (1988). The professional doctorate in nursing. In *Perspectives in nursing—1987-1989* (pp. 41-47). New York: National League for Nursing.

Watson, J. (1988). Response to "Caring and practice: Construction of the nurse's world." *Scholarly Inquiry for Nursing Practice, 2,* 217-221.

Watson, J. (1990). Caring knowledge and informed moral passion. *Advances in Nursing Science, 13*(1), 15-24.

Watson, J. (1990). Human caring: A public agenda. In Stevenson, J. S., & Tripp-Reimer, T. (Eds.), *Knowledge about care and caring: State of the art and future developments* (pp. 41-48). Kansas City, MO: American Academy of Nursing.

Watson, J. (1990). The moral failure of the patriarchy. *Nursing Outlook, 38,* 62-66.

Watson, J. (1990). Transformation in nursing: Bringing care back to health care. In *Curriculum revolution: Redefining the student-teacher relationship* (pp. 15-20). New York: National League for Nursing.

Watson, J. (1990). Transpersonal caring: A transcendent view of person, health, and nursing. In Parker, M. E. (Ed.), *Nursing theories in practice* (pp. 277-288). New York: National League for Nursing.

Watson, J. (1992). Response to "Caring, virtue theory, and a foundation for nursing ethics." *Scholarly Inquiry for Nursing Practice, 6,* 169-171.

Watson, J. (1993). Rediscovering caring and healing arts. *Nursing Standard, 9*(7), 18-19.

Watson, J. (Ed.). (1994). *Applying the art and science of human caring.* New York: National League for Nursing.

Watson, J. (1995). A Fulbright in Sweden: Runes, academics, archetypal motifs, and other things. *Image: Journal of Nursing Scholarship, 27,* 71-75.

Watson, J. (1995). Nursing's caring-healing paradigm as exemplar for alternative medicine? *Alternative Therapies in Health and Medicine, 1*(3), 64-69.

Watson, J. (1996). The wait, the wonder, the watch: Caring in a transplant unit. *Journal of Clinical Nursing, 5,* 199-200.

Watson, J. (1997). The Theory of Human Caring: Retrospective and prospective. *Nursing Science Quarterly, 10,* 49-52.

Watson, J., & Bevis, E. O. (1990). Nursing education: Coming of age for a new age. In N. L. Chaska (Ed.), *The nursing profession: Turning points* (pp. 100-106). St. Louis: Mosby.

Watson, J., & Phillips, S. (1992). A call for educational reform: Colorado nursing doctorate model as exemplar. *Nursing Outlook, 40,* 20-26.

Watson, J., & Ray, M. A. (1988). *The ethics of care and the ethics of cure: Synthesis in chronicity.* New York: National League for Nursing.

Watson, M. J. (1988). New dimensions of human caring theory. *Nursing Science Quarterly, 1,* 175-181.

Watson, J., Burckhardt, C., Brown, L., Bloch, D., & Hester, N. (1979). A model of caring: An alternative health care model for nursing practice and research. In *American Nurses' Association clinical and scientific sessions* (pp. 32-44). Kansas City, MO: American Nurses' Association.

Weeks, S. K. (1995). What are the educational needs of prospective family caregivers of newly disabled adults? *Rehabilitation Nursing, 20,* 256-260, 272, 298.

Wilson, C. (1994). Care: Superior ideal for nursing? *Nursing Praxis in New Zealand, 9*(3), 4-11.

Wolf, Z. R., Giardino, E. R., Osborne, P. A., & Ambrose, M. S. (1994). Dimensions of nurse care. *Image: Journal of Nursing Scholarship, 26,* 107-111.

Chapter 20 Part 2

Caring for the Human Spirit
in the Workplace

Ruth M. Neil

APPLYING WATSON'S CARING THEORY IN NEW CONTEXTS

During an era when organizational change is rampant—exemplified by reengineering, downsizing, work redesign, and so on—numerous authors are writing about the human element in the workplace (Belanger, 1996; Morris, 1997; Seaward, 1995; Whyte, 1994). The purpose of this chapter is to demonstrate the relevance of the philosophy and science of human caring (Watson, 1979/1985) in an exemplary nurse-directed facility serving HIV/AIDS clients, and, concurrently, to all interpersonal human enterprise—not just to those relationships socially defined as being for the purpose of supporting health and healing. Attention will be given to the attributes and behaviors characteristic of caring leaders.

Providing caring leadership for an organization, a business, or a work group within a larger entity requires an individual to examine the same questions that a nurse seeking to provide authentic caring in the nurse-patient situation needs to ask. These include:

What is the nature of the human being and what does he or she need to experience fulfillment?
What is the basis for harmonious and productive human relationships?
What is the nature of health/healing?
What is the purpose/mission of this organization or work team?

Examining these questions is a reflective activity central to developing not only greater awareness of others, but deepened understanding of ourselves. The following discussion addresses these questions and is presented with the purpose of sharing observations about how they apply, so each one of us can become an effective, caring leader.

THE HUMAN BEING, THE HUMAN SPIRIT, AND HUMAN RELATIONSHIPS

Nursing theories unanimously describe humans as multidimensional beings and endorse complex, holistic approaches to understanding health, illness, and healing. Watson's earliest works (1979) acknowledged strongly the spiritual reality of human experience. The 10th original carative factor reminded persons using the theory to allow for existential-phenomenological-spiritual forces in their relationships with clients. In later writings, Watson (1988, 1989, 1997) continued to explicate the relationship between caring and spiritual experience:

The process of human-to-human caring illuminates the mystery of humanity and the possibility of a higher power, order, or energy in the universe that can be activated through the nurse caring process that can in turn potentiate healing and health and facilitate self-knowledge, self-reverence, self-control, self-care, and possibly even self-healing . . . Universal spirit and a central cosmic unity are identified as essential to human caring. (Watson, 1989, p. 220)

I have come to believe that the spiritual dimension of human existence provides the most useful guidance in understanding human relationships and whether they are harmonious, productive, and fulfilling. Seaward (1995) asserts that human spirituality is the very core of wellness (p. 165).

Seaward, in a later work (1997), differentiates the human spirit from the human soul as follows. He says the human spirit provides each of us with a connection to the universal. It is a universal energy that draws us toward our greater potential. Curtin (1997, p. 7) says, "[T]his universal energy is what Camus referred to when he said, 'When I choose for myself, I choose for all mankind.' It is what the Taoists mean when they say, 'If you cut a single blade of grass, the universe trembles.' And it is what Jesus Christ meant when he said, 'Whatsoever you do . . . you do unto me.'" Curtin was emphasizing that all the world's great religious traditions recognize the wholeness of the universe and the reality of a spiritual energy.

The human soul, on the other hand, is that internal energy that is unique for each individual (Seaward, 1997). The soul evolves and changes over a lifetime. Seaward states that the evolution of the human soul is the pure essence of spirituality. He goes on to say that the evolution of the soul is gauged entirely by our capacity to love. Thus, when we talk about caring for the soul in the workplace, we are concerned with creating environments where caring and love can flourish.

Watson (1997, p. 50) emphasized that humans cannot be treated as objects, cannot be separated from self, other, nature, and the larger universe. Transpersonal caring, she continues, leads participants to "an alignment of intentionality, consciousness and one's being in action, seeking an authentic presence, an integration of mindbodyspirit which is healing" (p. 51). In addition to being descriptive of conditions that support healing, these concepts apply to circumstances desirable for meaningful and fulfilling lives.

To nurture the soul(s) of those in the workplace (or any other environment), a caring leader will seek to honor the need for harmony and "alignment" in his or her own life as well as those of coworkers and others. As Watson discusses in the first part of this chapter, in her expanded perspective, the 10th carative factor becomes "opening and attending to spiritual-mysterious, and existential dimensions of one's own life-death; soul care for self and the one-being-cared-for."

> **Health implies harmony and balance among the various dimensions of human experience.**

Watson (1997, p. 51) suggests that nurses or practitioners using caring theory

> cultivate a daily practice for self. Practices such as centering, meditation, breath work, yoga, prayer, connections with nature and other forms of daily contemplation are essential to the theory's authenticity and success. In other words, if one is to work from a caring-healing paradigm, one must live it out in daily life. Thus, living authentically requires a commitment to self-care at that deep level of personal practice and discipline, which in turn is honoring one's own embodied spirit, taking time for soul care.

I believe the above words apply whether the person practicing on the basis of caring theory is an individual nurse seeking to promote caring-healing with a client or is a person seeking to provide leadership to "nurture the souls" of coworkers.

HEALTH/HEALING

In order to appreciate the relationship between using the philosophy and science of human caring as a basis for nursing and providing leadership in an organization, it is useful to consider the nature of health/healing. When the human being is considered from a holistic perspective, health implies harmony and balance among the various dimensions of human experience—physical, emotional, mental, spiritual, and so on. Because physical wholeness is not always achievable, other energies of one's existence (mental, emotional, spiritual, etc.) often grow to compensate and achieve harmony on a different level. Belanger (1996, p. 221) describes her understanding of healing based on her own experience as a cancer patient: "My healing journey has led me to see the pro-

cess as movement toward wholeness. I am convinced that the source of healing lives inside us."

THE DENVER NURSING PROJECT IN HUMAN CARING (THE CARING CENTER)

The Denver Nursing Project in Human Caring (DNPHC) provided continuous service to individuals with HIV/AIDS from 1988 to 1996 (Astorino, et al., 1994; Lennerts, Koehler, & Neil, 1996; Neil, 1994). This nurse-directed health-care facility was founded on a conscious commitment to Watson's philosophy and science of human caring. During those years, the staff developed many insights into how the theory "looks" and "works" in the practice setting.

In reflecting on the DNPHC experience, I now believe that the most essential characteristic of the center was its attention to the soul and spirit of all the people it touched, along with the ability of the participants in the center's life (including staff, clients, and volunteers) to express love. The following paragraphs describe some of the values and practices that enabled this process to flourish organizationally.

Hecomovich (see Astorino, et al., 1994, pp. 20–21) wrote: "When we first started working together at the Denver Nursing Project, we did not just sit down and decide that our ways of working together were going to be different from other settings we had known. But over time, the unique combination of our *setting* and *ourselves* has contributed to a very special and satisfying team experience. . . . We all value our spirituality, and though we may use

> **The Denver Nursing Project was much more than a workplace and a facility.**

different language to describe our belief systems, we do believe our work has a meaning beyond the concrete here and now."

The Denver Nursing Project was much more than a workplace for its staff and a facility where the clients came for a large variety of treatments, services, information, and support. It emerged, over time, to be a caring community. As expressed in an essay written by a client, "In this little red brick building, all these special people have become an extension to each other as one big family" (Neil, 1994, p. 36). Shared beliefs and values included respect for the dignity of each person, honor of the right and responsibility of each person to make informed choices concerning health, faith that individuals possess inner resources to support their own growth and healing, and belief that authentic caring relationships contribute to healing and health (Neil, 1994, p. 37). We believed that these human characteristics were common to staff, clients, and others with whom we had contact during the years of the center's life.

Kerfoot (1997) writes that the role of a leader is to create a sense of community in the workplace where people can feel a strong sense of unity and a fellowship of caring. She goes on to say that successful leaders realize that caring is the basis of any spirit of community (p. 50). At the Denver Nursing Project, leadership was definitely a shared function. As we learned to communicate honestly and openly with each other and reveal our individual values, hopes, and fears, we were able to decide together on a shared mission that took precedence over personal needs and wants. Most often, clients were partners with the staff in working toward the center's mission.

Two questions people commonly ask about the Denver Nursing Project experience are:

1. Was it easier or harder to "bring Caring Theory to life" with the HIV/AIDS population than it would have been with another population?
2. How did the nurses and other staff avoid burnout with such a high death rate among the client population?

I will respond to each of these questions by offering my observations and opinions, many of which were shaped by reflective discussion with center staff, clients, other nurses, students, and visitors.

Question 1. Caring Theory was a perfect fit to guide how we approached our work with the HIV/AIDS population. Since there wasn't, and still isn't, a cure for HIV/AIDS, Caring Theory and practices, with their emphasis on spiritual energy, connectedness, and inner healing, were the most realistic and honest approaches we could offer.

> **Leadership was definitely a shared function.**

Tronto, in writing about care with an elderly (i.e., vulnerable) population, offered these interesting suggestions about the status of caring in Western society. We are unwilling to acknowledge that we all have needs for care. She believes, "in part, the unwillingness to recognize the role of care in our lives stems from our inability to comprehend death. No matter how successfully we care for ourselves or others, human life ends in death" (Tronto, 1998, p. 19). Tronto believes that if we interpret the certitude of death as

evidence of vulnerability, we fail to embrace care as an important part of human life. She states, "[R]ecognizing its role in creating interconnections and relationships of receiving and giving over a lifetime . . . may provide us with a way to rethink some of the ways in which we now seem unable to cope with human vulnerability" (Tronto, 1998, p. 19).

Question 2. The above comments in response to the first question also provide part of the answer to the second question. In addition, I offer the following observations.

Staff at the Denver Nursing Project came to recognize and honor the profound experience of sharing the spiritual journey of clients who accepted that their diagnosis would lead to physical death, but who chose to live as fully as possible until that death occurred. Staff learned not to place distance between themselves and clients with whom they were in relationship. Staff persons and client shared their vulnerability, and thus gained from one another (each was transformed).

Even as project director, I was involved in close relationships with many clients. I want to share Jason's (not his real name) story here because it illustrates many of the ideas about spiritual growth discussed throughout this chapter. It is one example among hundreds of authentic caring relationships that were lived at the center.

Jason was a client at the Caring Center for about 3 years. When we first met him, he was a handsome, intelligent, successful, and somewhat arrogant man. His message to us then was, "I'm going to beat AIDS. It won't get me." But that wasn't to be.

Jason had unusually bad luck with adverse effects from one after another of the antiviral drugs that were introduced (necessitating numerous blood transfusions), many serious opportunistic infections, painful and debilitating peripheral neuropathy, and, finally, severe "wasting syndrome." As his health began to deteriorate noticeably, he changed his message to, "Maybe I won't beat this, but I'll never let it progress far enough to make me dependent on others for my basic life needs." We interpreted that as meaning that Jason planned to take his own life, and we expected that that would happen. It didn't. Eventually, Jason had to move into his 76-year-old mother's home, which was extremely stressful for them both. Eventually his daily needs were being attended to by his mom and by visiting nurses.

I visited him at home about a week before he died. I asked him (telling him as I asked, that if the question was too intrusive, he didn't have to answer) how it was that, after his earlier pronouncements about "staying in control" and "beating the disease,"

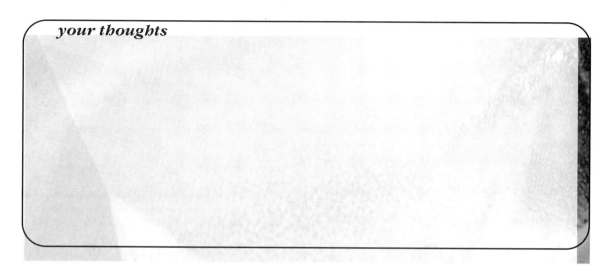

your thoughts

things had come to this. (He was, by then, bedfast and wholly dependent on others.)

He smiled; he knew the meaning of my question. He said, "First, I began to notice that as I lost one ability, I would find I had 'another,' which I'd never seen before. . . . Then, during the past few months, my mom and I have made peace, which is a good feeling . . . I decided not to commit suicide because I didn't want to leave Mark [his beloved 4-year-old nephew] with that memory. . . . And, finally, I began to feel like an observer—watching my life continue on—and it got to be interesting and I wanted to stay to see what would happen next."

Jason had spent much time during his last months at the Caring Center. His mom brought him as long as he could get out of the house. Often he spent most of his time "just dozing" on the dayroom sofa, but he was thinking and redesigning his life. He accepted his inevitable death. He came to value authentic caring. He died spiritually healthy. He "wanted to stay to see what would happen next"—not with a desire or need to control, but with a sense of acceptance and peace.

Nurses and staff at DNPHC paid attention to their own spiritual journeys and respected and supported each other's. A variety of specific strategies—including mountain retreats, creative art activities, physical exercise, journaling, body therapies, and more—were used and shared over the years to encourage open communication and mutual support.

When I left the Denver Nursing Project in Human Caring and moved into a totally different kind of role, I wondered whether and how I would be able to sustain the experience of being part of a caring community in my new position. The next section of this chapter summarizes "how it is going" and suggests new directions and uses for nursing theory in the future.

CARING THEORY IN NEW CONTEXTS

In 1996, I assumed the responsibility of being project coordinator for the National Resource Center for Health and Safety in Child Care. Our mission is to provide resource and referral information to a diverse audience, including child care administrators, regulatory agencies, consumers, media personnel, and others. We provide this service by way of our World Wide Web site, E-mails, toll-free telephone access, and participation in workshops and conferences across the country. The Resource Center is sponsored through a collaborative agreement with the Maternal and Child Health Bureau.

Besides me, our work team consists of a project director (who is involved in major policy decisions but not day-to-day operation), a resource librarian, an administrative assistant, and graduate student research assistants. As was true at the Denver Nursing Project, an important strategy in creating a fulfilling work environment is believing in our mission. The opportunity to contribute to improved practice in out-of-home child care settings is easy enough to believe in, especially as we recognize that nearly 70% of children under the age of 6 (in the United States) spend at least part of their time in child care settings.

Because none of us was experienced in child care issues prior to joining the project, we all accepted the responsibility to become as knowledgeable as possible in a short period of time. An important part of being truly caring is being competent and worthy of trust from those being cared for—the constituents we serve.

We have developed a collaborative model of decision making and value creativity in finding solutions to specific assignments that have come to us during the life of the project. (For instance, we currently are coordinating the review and update of a major publication that has more than 100 contributors from across the country. Developing systems for managing all the relevant communication and documenting decision making has provided exciting challenges for us all and given us ways to grow in respect for one another's contributions.) We have become more than coworkers; we have become people who care about one another.

Having had the opportunity to "live" Watson's theory at the Denver Nursing Project with clients facing profound life transitions, I came to know and respect its truth and value on a deep, personal level. The strength of the human spirit and evolution of the human soul during times of crisis are inspirational lessons in the common human quest for wholeness and health. Once one has experienced the beauty and growth that occur during those transpersonal caring moments, one continues to strive for reciprocity, respect, and mutuality in other human relationships.

> The opportunity we have as nurses is to share the nursing/caring model with other disciplines as well as with the public in general.

Summary

The purpose of this chapter has been to share reflections about applying Watson's Caring Theory in a unique practice setting and to suggest applications of the theory as a basis for leadership in organizations or work groups. The concept of caring community is especially relevant in both instances.

The opportunity that we have as nurses, I believe, is to share the nursing/caring model with individuals from other disciplines as well as with the public in general. Although our own application of caring knowledge is often during times of a major life transition or extreme health challenge, we recognize that the quality of human interaction in all settings is improved by caring beliefs and actions. It is encouraging to note the trends in the leadership literature that place a new focus on the need to care for the human spirit in the workplace. Let us hope that appreciation of this truth will become evident in the lives of increasing numbers of people in all settings.

References

Astorino, G., et al. (1994). The Denver nursing project in human caring. In Watson, J. (Ed.), *Applying the art and science of human caring.* (pp. 19-37). New York: National League for Nursing.

Belanger, T. W. (1996). Leadership in a healing environment. *Seminars for Nurse Managers, 4*(4), 218-223.

Curtin, L. L. (1997). [Editorial]. Whatsoever you do . . . *Nursing Management, 28*(6), 7-8.

Kerfoot, K. (1997). Leadership—The courage to care. *Nursing Economics, 15*(1), 50-51.

Lennerts, M. H., Koehler, J. A., & Neil, R. M. (1996). Nursing care models increase care quality while reducing costs. *Journal of the Association of Nursing in AIDS Care 7(4),* 37-46.

Morris, T. (1997). *If Aristotle ran General Motors: The new soul of business.* New York: Henry Holt & Co.

Neil, R. M. (1994). Authentic caring: The sensible answer for clients and staff dealing with HIV/AIDS. *Nursing Administration Quarterly,18*(2), 36-40.

Seaward, B. L. (1995). Reflections on human spirituality for the worksite. *American Journal of Health Promotion, 9*(3), 165-168.

Seaward, B. L. (1997). *Stand like a mountain, flow like water: Reflections on stress and human spirituality.* Deerfield Beach, FL: Health Communications, Inc.

Tronto, J. C. (1998). An ethic of care. *Generations, 22*(3), 15-20.

Watson, J. (1979). *Nursing: Philosophy and science of human care.* Norwalk, CT: Appleton-Century-Crofts.

Watson, J. (1988). New dimensions of human caring theory. *Nursing Science Quarterly, 1*(4), 175-181.

Watson, J. (1989). Watson's philosophy and theory of human caring in nursing. In Riehl-Sisca, J. (Ed.), *Conceptual models for nursing practice,* (3rd ed., pp. 219-236). Norwalk, CT: Appleton & Lange.

Watson, J. (1997). The theory of human caring: Retrospective and prospective. *Nursing Science Quarterly, 10*(1), 49-52.

Whyte, D. (1994). *The heart aroused: Poetry and the preservation of the soul in corporate America.* New York: Doubleday.

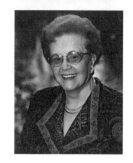

Chapter *21* Part 1

Madeleine M. Leininger
Theory of Culture Care Diversity and Universality

Madeleine M. Leininger

INTRODUCING THE THEORIST

Madeleine Leininger is the founder and leader of the field of transcultural nursing, focusing on comparative human care theory and research, and is founder of the worldwide Transcultural Nursing Society. Dr. Leininger's initial nursing education was at St. Anthony School of Nursing in Denver, Colorado. Her undergraduate degree is from Mt. St. Scholastic College in Atchison, Kansas, and her master's degree was earned at the Catholic University of America in Washington, D.C. She completed her Ph.D. in social and cultural anthropology at the University of Washington. Dr. Leininger was dean and professor of nursing at the Universities of Washington and Utah and helped initiate and direct doctoral programs in nursing at the Universities of Utah and Washington, and at Wayne State University. She facilitated the development of similar programs in other American and overseas institutions. Dr. Leininger is a fellow and distinguished living legend of the American Academy of Nursing. She is professor emeritus of the College of Nursing at Wayne State University (in Detroit, Michigan) and adjunct professor at the University of Nebraska, College of Nursing (in Omaha, Nebraska). She continues to be active as an internationally known theorist, educator, author, administrator, distinguished lecturer, researcher, and consultant in transcultural nursing from her home in Omaha, Nebraska.

> Caring for people of many different cultures seemed inevitable, and yet nurses and other health professionals were not prepared to meet this challenge.

Dr. Leininger is the author and/or editor of 27 books, has published over 200 articles, and has given more than 1100 public lectures throughout the United States and abroad. Some of her well-known books include *Basic Psychiatric Concepts in Nursing* (Leininger & Hofling, 1960), *Caring: An Essential Human Need* (1981), *Care: The Essence of Nursing and Health* (1984), *Care: Discovery and Uses in Clinical and Community Nursing* (1988), *Care: Ethical and Moral Dimensions of Care* (1990), and *Culture Care Diversity and Universality: A Theory of Nursing* (1991). Some of her books were the first in that area of nursing to be published. *Nursing and Anthropology: Two Worlds to Blend* (1970) was the first to bring together nursing and anthropology, *Transcultural Nursing: Concepts, Theories, and Practices* (1978) was the first in transcultural nursing, and *Qualitative Research Methods in Nursing*

(1985) was the first qualitative research book in nursing.

Her published works reflect four decades of cumulative transcultural work with many cultures throughout the world. In 1989, Dr. Leininger initiated the *Journal of Transcultural Nursing,* which was the first transcultural nursing journal.

Dr. Leininger conducted a pioneering field study of the Gadsup of the eastern highlands of New Guinea in the early 1960s, and has subsequently studied many other Western and non-Western cultures. During her 50 years in nursing, Dr. Leininger has been instrumental in several breakthroughs in nursing, including focusing on human care as the essence of nursing, new domains of inquiry, transcultural nursing, comparative care, and the qualitative ethnonursing research method; she also provided new ways to provide culturally competent health care. She was the first nurse and anthropologist to promote the idea of "culture-specific" and "culturally congruent care." She also initiated the concept of generic (folk, lay, or complementary) health care to be contrasted with professional health services. In 1987, she initiated the idea of worldwide certification in transcultural nursing to protect and respect the needs and lifeways of people of diverse cultures. This futuristic idea is only now being considered along with other globally sound modes of transcultural education, practice, and certification.

As a pioneering nurse educator, leader, theorist, and administrator, Dr. Leininger has been a risk taker, futurist, and innovator, never afraid to bring forth new directions in education and service. Her persistent leadership has made transcultural nursing and human care central to nursing and respected as formal areas of study and practice. She has been called the "Margaret Mead of the health field." Dr. Leininger's genuine interest and enthusiasm for whatever she pursues is contagious, inspiring, and challenging. She continues to be viewed as a transcultural leader who is "ahead of her time." Dr. Leininger encourages others to be compassionate and caring in order to help people live peaceful and healthy lives in our complex and diverse world.

CULTURE CARE DIVERSITY AND UNIVERSALITY: A WORLDWIDE NURSING THEORY
by Madeleine M. Leininger

Culturally based care can significantly contribute to human health and well-being, and transcultural nursing care can provide such meaningful and therapeutic outcomes. One of the most significant trends in the twentieth century has been the development of transcultural nursing concepts, principles, theories, and research-based knowledge to guide, challenge, and explain nursing practices. The use of transcultural nursing theories has been a critical means to open the door to advance new scientific and humanistic dimensions of caring for people of diverse and similar cultures. It has been the use of transcultural theories and research-based knowledge in teaching and clinical practices that has greatly expanded our ways of thinking and helping people in diverse cultures.

> Care is the essence and central domain of nursing; it is the unique and dominant attribute of nursing.

Transcultural nursing was first conceived of in the mid-1950s and began to be developed in the United States. The Theory of Culture Care Diversity and Universality also began to be developed in order to establish a knowledge base to guide nurses in transcultural nursing practices. It was at this time that I foresaw that nurses would need transcultural knowledge and practices to function by the year 2000 (Leininger, 1970, 1978). This was the post–World War II period, when many new immigrants and refugees—people from many places—came to America, and also migrated to other countries. Caring for people of many different cultures seemed inevitable, yet nurses and other health professionals were not prepared to meet this challenge. Instead, nursing and medicine were focused on using new technologies and on studying biomedical diseases and symptoms. Shifting to a transcultural perspective in order to understand and care for people of many different cultures was not seen as a critical need. Thus, a whole new world of knowledge discovery and practice related to transcultural nursing and health had yet to be developed, valued, and put into practice.

In this chapter, an overview of the Theory of Culture Care Diversity and Universality will be presented, along with the purpose, goal, assumptions, theoretical hunches, and related general features of the theory, as well as future uses. In addition, theory terms will be defined and the Sunrise Model will be explained. The reader is encouraged to explore other articles on the theory and to use definitive primary literature to gain accurate knowledge of the theorist's perspectives on this important subject (Leininger, 1970, 1981, 1989a, 1989b, 1990a, 1990b, 1991, 1995).

FACTORS LEADING TO THE THEORY

A frequent question often posed to me is, What led you to develop your theory? This is an important question for any theorist to answer. What inspires and motivates most theorists is generally related to the desire to discover the unknown or limitedly known. Initially, the idea for the Theory of Culture Care came to me while I was functioning as a clinical child nurse specialist in a child guidance home in a large midwestern city. From my focused observations and daily nursing experiences, I became aware that the children in the guidance home were from many different cultures. These children were different in their nursing care needs, responses, and expectations. The children were Anglo-Caucasian, African, and Jewish, representing Appalachian and many other cultures. The ways in which these children's parents responded to the children, and the parents' expectations of care and treatment modes were different. This was in the early 1950s. I had not been prepared to care for people of diverse cultures, nor were other nurses, physicians, social workers, and health professionals in the health services prepared to respond therapeutically in a knowing and competent way with clients from different cultures and cultural backgrounds (Leininger, 1970, 1978, 1991, 1995). I experienced cultural shock and felt helpless to care for both children and adults of diverse cultures. It soon became evident to me that I needed cultural knowledge with my psychiatric and general nursing care insights and experiences. To remedy this major knowledge deficit, I decided to pursue doctoral studies in anthropology. While in the anthropology program, I discovered a wealth of potentially valuable knowledge that could be most helpful if used within a nursing perspective. The challenge before me was to link or interface anthropological insights with nursing knowledge and to go beyond the physical and emotional needs of clients.

At this time, I was questioning what made nursing a distinct and legitimate profession. I also wondered about medicine and other disciplines about their unique knowledge and skill focus to help serve people. Surely not all disciplines were the same. Nurses had not addressed the cultural care focus with theory and research. I therefore declared in the mid-1950s that care is (or should be) the essence and central domain of nursing. However, most nurses resisted this idea, because they thought care was not important and was too feminine, too soft and vague and could never explain nursing (Leininger, 1970, 1977, 1981, 1984). Nonetheless, I firmly held to the claim and began to teach, study, and write about care as the essence of nursing, its unique and dominant attribute (Leininger, 1970, 1977, 1981, 1984). From an anthropological and nursing perspective I held that care and caring is a basic and essential need for human growth, development, and survival (Leininger, 1977, 1981). I argued that what humans need most to survive from birth to old age, or when ill or well, is human caring. But caring phenomena needed to be explicated, and had to fit the cultural needs of human beings in order to be scientific and useful. Clients had often said it was nursing care that helped them (the acutely or chronically ill) to recover and be healed.

My next step in the theory was to conceptualize selected cultural perspectives derived from anthropology and evolving care perspectives as nursing statements or assumptions related to culture care in order to establish a new knowledge base for transcultural nursing. Synthesizing or interfacing culture and care was the real challenge to establishing the new Theory of Culture Care Diversity and Universality (Leininger, 1976, 1978, 1990a, 1990b, 1991). Formulating such knowledge was essential to support the discipline of transcultural nursing and to use this knowledge to care for people of different cultures. Because culture care knowledge had not been explicated and linked together as an integral part of nursing education, research, and practice in the mid-1950s, much work still lay ahead. It was this new and promising paradigm to serve clients of diverse cultures. Indeed, care or caring had largely been the invisible and unknown phenomenon in nursing even though nurses frequently use words or phrases such as "I gave care to X," "My nursing care was appreciated by the family," and "I coordinated nursing care on this unit." These statements and similar linguistic uses of the word "care" were taken largely for granted or assumed to be understood by nurses, clients, and the public (Leininger, 1981, 1984). Moreover, the meaning of "care" from the perspective of different cultures was unknown.

In the 1950s there were no theories explicitly focused on care and culture in nursing environments, let alone research studies to explicate care meanings and phenomena in nursing (Leininger, 1981, 1990a, 1991, 1995). Theoretical and practice meanings of care in relation to specific cultures had not been studied, especially from a comparative cultural perspective. I became excited as I envisioned a whole new body of essential knowledge related to transcultural nursing care that was awaiting our discovery and which could be used in nursing. This was exciting to me, yet very troublesome, as nurses needed to shift their thinking and attitudes from largely medical symptoms and treatments to that of knowing and valuing culturally based care. To refocus nursing to a new theory and mode of practice would be difficult. The culture care theory, which looks for universals (or commonalties) along with differences (diversities), was viewed as "too idealistic and impossible" for many nurses. But by the mid-1980s the theoretical and clinical ideas became known, used, and valued by many nurses.

> Transcultural nursing uses research-based knowledge to provide safe, responsible, meaningful care to people of different cultures, supporting their health needs and dealing with illness, disabilities, or death.

RATIONALE FOR TRANSCULTURAL NURSING: SIGNS AND NEED

Despite the above challenges, the need for transcultural nursing with a theoretical and research knowledge base was tenaciously pursued as essential to providing quality-based care to people of diverse cultures both now and in the future (Leininger, 1978, 1989a, 1990b). Signs of critical needs became evident by the 1970s to support this position for the future survival of nursing education and practice. Several of these factors are briefly stated below (Leininger, 1970, 1978, 1984, 1989a, 1990a, 1995):

1. There were signs of increased numbers of global migrations of people from virtually every place in the world due to modern electronics, transportation, and communication.
2. There were signs of cultural stresses and cultural conflicts as nurses tried to care for strangers from many Western and non-Western cultures.
3. There were cultural indications of consumer fears and resistance to health personnel as they used new technologies and treatment modes without cultural knowledge or understanding of the people being served.
4. There were signs that clients from different cultures were angry, frustrated, and misunderstood by health personnel due to cultural ignorance of the clients' beliefs, values, and expectations along with the misdiagnosis and mistreatment of clients from unknown cultures.
5. There were signs of nurses, physicians, and other professional health personnel becoming quite frustrated and upset when clients failed to cooperate or respond quickly to them in treatment

regimes. Culture care factors were seldom recognized or understood by professional staff until nearly the late 1980s.

6. There were signs that consumers of different cultures, whether in the home, hospital, or clinic, were being treated in ways that did not satisfy them and their recovery was thwarted or unsuccessful.

7. There were many indications of intercultural conflicts and cultural pain of clients when nurses, physicians, and staff failed to respect important cultural taboos and values of clients.

8. There were evidences of culturally unrepresented (minority) cultures of clients and staff in health settings.

9. Last but not least, there were signs that nurses working in foreign countries in the military and as missionaries were having great difficulty in understanding and caring for clients of diverse cultures, due largely to a lack of knowledge about the people and their cultural beliefs and lifeways—some even encountered threats to their lives.

For these reasons and many others, it was evident in the 1960s and beyond that nurses and other health professionals urgently needed transcultural knowledge and skills to work with people of diverse cultures. Nursing and other health-care professionals were clearly not understanding and serving people of different cultures in therapeutic ways. Cultural ignorance and the unintentional mistreatment of immigrants and others had potential for major legal suits and for unfavorable client recovery processes, or even threats to the clients' lives.

It is interesting that while anthropologists are clearly experts about cultures, many were not interested in nurses' work, in nursing as a profession, or in the study of human care phenomena in the early 1950s. Most anthropologists in those early days were far more interested in medical diseases, archaeological findings, and in physical and cultural anthropology. So, as the first graduate (master's prepared) professional nurse anthropologist, I held that nurses and nursing needed to understand cultures and caring in order to provide culturally safe and congruent care practices with beneficial and therapeutic outcomes. I encouraged many nurses to take cultural and physical anthropology courses in order to obtain background supporting knowledge until transcultural nursing courses and programs were established. Unfortunately, some nurses who heeded this advice never returned to nursing and remained "wed" to anthropology, as they had no transcultural nursing framework to use the knowledge gained. Gradually transcultural nursing undergraduate and graduate courses and programs were initiated and became available to nurses by the 1970s. This was essential to prepare and help nurses remain in the transcultural nursing field (Leininger, 1970, 1978, 1989a, 1989b, 1995).

Most importantly, nurses were the largest and most direct health-care providers, so great opportunities existed for them to change health care for culturally congruent care practices—this was the ultimate goal of transcultural nursing. Nurses and those in other health-care disciplines urgently needed to become transculturally prepared to meet a growing multicultural world by the year 2000, as an essential requirement for human services worldwide to func-

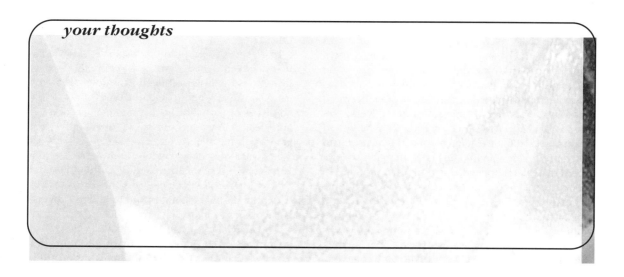

your thoughts

tion with many different people in the world. This predictive need has already occurred today as nurses try to function as practitioners, consultants, teachers, and researchers in diverse cultures, often without transcultural knowledge and skills. This has led to many problems and frustrations that often cause people to leave nursing, or cause dissatisfaction with current health-care systems.

As more courses and programs in transcultural nursing were offered to educate nurses in its basic concepts, principles, and practices, the interest of nurses grew to learn about the Theory of Culture Care Diversity and Universality. *Transcultural nursing* became meaningful, and was defined as "a formal area of study (education and research) and practice focused on the cultural care (caring) values, beliefs, and practices of individuals or groups from a particular culture in order to provide culture-specific and congruent care to people of diverse cultures" (Leininger, 1978, 1984, 1995). The central purpose of transcultural nursing is to use research-based knowledge to help nurses give safe, responsible, and meaningful care to people of different cultures to meet their care needs and to deal with illnesses, disabilities, or dying. Today the culture care theory with research-based knowledge has become recognized as essential to help guide nurses in the care of clients, families, and communities of different cultures or subcultures.

> Forms, expressions, patterns, and processes of human care vary among all cultures of the world.

MAJOR THEORETICAL TENETS

In developing the Theory of Culture Care Diversity and Universality, there were major predictive tenets or premises that were essential for nurses and others using the theory to consider. One of the principal tenets was that cultural care diversities and similarities (or commonalities) exist within and between cultures worldwide (Leininger, 1991). Nurse researchers needed to discover this knowledge to guide nurses' thinking, judgements, and decisions in order to provide therapeutic outcomes. It was predicted that such knowledge could be a gold mine to help nurses assess, plan, and provide care to people of different cultures. Providing *culture-specific care* that fit the beliefs, values, and lifeways of cultures would be a major new approach to nursing, as this was a major missing dimension of traditional nursing. Human beings are born, live, and die with their spe-

cific cultural values and beliefs, as well as with their historical and environmental context, which includes language considerations. Transcultural nursing knowledge needed to be shared with other nurses as the substantive and essential knowledge for all nursing decisions and actions. It was predicted that discovering which elements of care were culturally universal and which were different would drastically revolutionize nursing and ultimately transform the health-care systems and practices (Leininger, 1978, 1990a, 1990b, 1991).

Another predictive tenet of the theory was that the worldview and social structure factors—including religion (and spirituality), political and economic considerations, kinship (family ties), education, technology, language expressions, the environmental context, and cultural history—are essential to understand and are powerful influences on care outcomes (Leininger, 1991). This broad holistic perspective, which included specific knowledge, was imperative if one was to grasp the world of the client and family and help them. Such research-based knowledge was predicted to influence the health, well-being, sickness, and disability or dying patterns of clients from different cultures. Social structure and other influences on human care from specific cultures had not been systematically studied by nurses or used explicitly in their teaching, learning, and clinical practices. These important factors, along with ethnohistorical, language, and environmental factors, had to be discovered in order to create the theory and to bring about beneficial outcomes. Such factors would not only influence the clients' recovery and healing process, but would also disclose ways to help clients remain well. This holistic cultural knowledge needed to be documented and understood in order to guide nurses' decisions in arriving at culturally congruent care—which was the goal of the theory.

To discover such holistic yet specific knowledge, nurses needed a theory and research methods to explicate these cultural influences on the care of human beings. No longer could nurses rely only on bits and pieces of partial or fragmented medical and psychological knowledge, as these were only small glimpses of the clients' cultural world. Nurses needed to be aware of social structure knowledge, cultural history, and environmental factors in order to understand these factors when using the theory. Thus, transcultural nursing courses and programs provided instruction and mentoring experiences in these areas to appreciate and use the theory fully.

One major and predicted tenet of the theory was that there are both care differences and similarities with regard to professional and generic (traditional or indigenous folk) care knowledge and practices (Leininger, 1991). These differences were also predicted to influence the health and well-being of clients. In fact, it was predicted that there would be significant differences between generic care and that of professionally learned nursing knowledge. Again, these findings would influence the recovery (healing), health, and well-being of clients from other cultures, and had to be considered. Marked unresolved cultural conflict differences between generic and professional care providers were predicted to lead to serious client-nurse conflicts, potential illnesses, and even death (Leininger, 1978, 1991).

Finally, I theorized that if three new modalities of care were used, they would lead to culturally congruent care if based on data obtained from the culture. The three modalities postulated were (1) culture care preservation or maintenance, (2) culture care accommodation or negotiation, and (3) culture care restructuring or repatterning (Leininger, 1991, 1995). These three modes were very different from traditional nursing actions, processes, or interventions, as they were focused on ways to facilitate congruent care to fit clients' particular cultural needs. To use these modalities and arrive at culturally appropriate care, the nurse has to draw upon culture care emic knowledge discovered from the people along with the use of appropriate professional scientific and humanistic knowledge that fits with the clients' needs. Using nursing interventions would not be appropriate, as they lead to cultural imposition and cultural tensions and conflicts. These three modalities were entirely new breakthroughs in nursing, as was the idea of providing culturally congruent care. Nurses had to shift from focusing mainly on treating diseases and symptom management from their etic views to those of a holistic culture and care based on a client emic perspective. Although some learned nursing and medical knowledge might be appropriate, such knowledge was often inappropriate or did not fit the client's needs (Leininger, 1991, 1995).

With the theory, the primary focus remained on caring for people within a cultural care context or environment. Discovering environmental and cultural beliefs and values of humans was much broader, yet it was a specific approach that was unique to transcultural nursing practices. As new kinds of transcultural nursing knowledge were forthcoming, culturally based care was evident to prevent illness, maintain health, and to live in reasonably peaceful relationships with others. A life-cycle perspective and historical patterns related to care were predicted to be valuable in helping nurses to arrive at meaningful and therapeutic nursing care outcomes. This theory was the new post–Nightingale and post–World War II paradigm for new nursing practices worldwide to value and use as professional nurses.

Theoretical Assumptions: Purpose, Goal, and Definitions of the Theory

The purpose of the theory was, therefore, to discover, document, analyze, and interpret cultural and caring factors influencing human beings in health, sickness, or dying, in order to advance and improve nursing practices. The theory was developed with much thought to incorporate ideas related to the above tenets or predictive premises of the theorist. Discovery of the largely unknown, covert, and missing cultural care factors related to transcultural nursing was the primary focus and a critical need to pro-

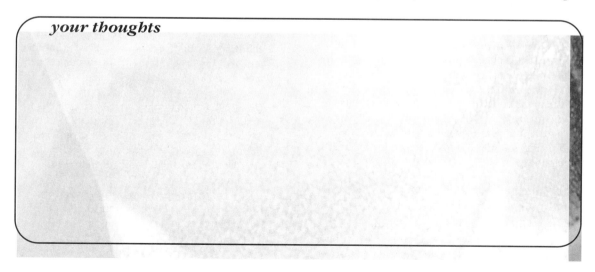

your thoughts

vide safe, meaningful, and congruent care to clients or to work effectively with families and in institutional settings.

The goal of the theory was to use research-based knowledge in order to provide culturally congruent, safe, and beneficial care to people of diverse or similar cultures for their health and well-being or for meaningful dying experiences. This goal of arriving at culturally congruent care was predicted to promote the health and well-being of clients, or to help clients face disability or death in culturally meaningful and satisfying ways. Thus, the ultimate and primary goal of the theory was to provide culturally congruent care that fit or was tailor-made for the lifeways and values of people (Leininger, 1991, 1995).

Assumptions of the Theory

Several assumptions served as the basic beliefs related to the theoretical tenets and predictive hunches of the culture care theory. They are as follows (Leininger, 1970, 1977, 1981, 1984, 1991, 1997a):

1. Care is essential for human growth, development, and survival, and when facing death.
2. Care is essential to curing and healing; there can be no curing without caring.
3. Forms, expressions, patterns, and processes of human care vary among all cultures of the world.
4. Every culture has generic (lay, folk, or naturalistic) care, and usually professional care practices.
5. Culture care values and beliefs are embedded in religious, kinship, social, political, cultural, economic, and historical dimensions of the social structure and in language and environmental contexts.
6. Therapeutic nursing care can only occur when client culture care values, expressions, and/or practices are known and used explicitly to provide human care.
7. Differences between caregiver and care receiver expectations need to be understood in order to provide beneficial, satisfying, and congruent care.
8. Culturally congruent, specific, or universal care modes are essential to the health or well-being of people whom nurses serve worldwide.
9. Nursing is a transcultural care profession and discipline.

Orientational Theory Definitions

1. *Culture Care Diversity:* Refers to variability and/or differences in meanings, patterns, values, lifeways, or symbols of care within or between collectivities that are related to assistive, supportive, or enabling human care expressions (Leininger, 1991, p. 47).
2. *Culture Care Universality:* Refers to the common, similar, or dominant uniform care meanings, patterns, values, lifeways, or symbols that are manifest among many cultures and reflect assistive, supportive, facilitative, or enabling ways to help people (Leininger, 1991, p. 47).
3. *Care:* Refers to abstract and concrete phenomena related to assisting, supporting, or enabling experiences or behaviors toward or for others with evident or anticipated needs to ameliorate or improve a human condition or lifeway. "Caring" refers to care actions and activities (Leininger, 1991, p. 46).
4. *Culture:* Refers to the learned, shared, and transmitted values, beliefs, norms, and lifeways of a particular group that guides their thinking, decisions, and actions in patterned ways (Leininger, 1991, p. 47).
5. *Culture Care:* Refers to the subjectively and objectively learned and transmitted values, beliefs, and patterned lifeways that assist, support, facilitate, or enable another individual or group to maintain their well-being and health, to improve their human condition and lifeway, or to deal with illness, handicaps, or death (Leininger, 1991, p. 47).
6. *Professional Care:* Refers to formally taught, learned, and transmitted professional care, health, illness, wellness, and related knowledge skills that prevail in professional institutions usually with multidisciplinary personnel to serve consumers (largely etic or outsiders' views) (Leininger, 1995, p. 106).
7. *Generic (Folk and Lay) Care:* Refers to culturally learned and transmitted indigenous (or traditional, folk, lay, or home-based) knowledge or skills used to provide assistive, supportive, enabling, or facilitative acts toward or for another individual or group, or in an institution (largely emic or insiders' views) (Leininger, 1995, p. 106).
8. *Health:* Refers to a state of well-being that is culturally defined, valued, and practiced, and reflects the ability of individuals (or groups) to perform their daily role activities in culturally expressed, beneficial, and patterned ways (Leininger, 1995, p. 106).
9. *Culture Care Preservation or Maintenance:* Refers to those assistive, supporting, facilitative, or enabling professional actions and decisions that help people of a particular culture to retain and/or preserve relevant care values so that they

can maintain their well-being, recover from illness, or face handicaps and/or death (Leininger, 1991, p. 48).

10. *Culture Care Accommodation or Negotiation:* Refers to those assistive, supporting, facilitative, or enabling creative professional actions and decisions that help people of a designated culture to adapt to, or to negotiate with others for, a beneficial or satisfying health outcome with professional care providers (Leininger, 1991, p. 48).

11. *Culture Care Repatterning or Restructuring:* Refers to those assistive, supporting, facilitative, or enabling professional actions and decisions that help clients reorder, change, or greatly modify their own lifeways for new, different, and beneficial health-care patterns while respecting the client(s)' cultural values and beliefs and providing more beneficial and healthy lifeways than those that existed before the changes were coestablished with the clients (Leininger, 1991, p. 49).

12. *Ethnohistory:* Refers to those past facts, events, instances, and experiences of individuals, groups, cultures, and institutions that are primarily people-(ethno)centered and describe, explain, and interpret human lifeways within particular cultural contexts and over short or long periods of time (Leininger, 1991, p. 48).

13. *Environmental Context:* Refers to the totality of an event, situation, or particular experience that gives meaning to human expressions, interpretations, and social interactions in particular physical, ecological, sociopolitical, and/or cultural settings (Leininger, 1991, p. 48).

14. *Worldview:* Refers to the way in which people tend to look out on the world or their universe to form a picture or value stance about their life or world around them (Leininger, 1991, p. 47).

15. *Kinship and Social Factors:* Refers to family intergenerational linkages and social interactions based on cultural beliefs, values, and recurrent lifeways over time.

16. *Religion and Spiritual Factors:* Refers to the supernatural and natural beliefs and practices that guide individual and group thoughts and actions toward the good or to improve one's lifeways.

17. *Political Factors:* Refers to authority and power over others that regulates or influences another's actions, decisions, or behavior.

18. *Technological Factors:* Refers to the use of electrical, mechanical, or physical (nonhuman) objects used in the service of humans.

19. *Education Factors:* Refers to formal and informal modes of learning or acquiring knowledge about specific and diverse subject matter domains.

20. *Economic Factors:* Refers to the production, distribution, and use of negotiable material or consumable productions held valuable to humans or in need by humans.

21. *Environmental Factors:* Refers to the totality of one's living context within a geographic or ecological area.

22. *Culturally Congruent Care:* Refers to the use of culturally based care knowledge and action modes with individuals or groups in beneficial and meaningful ways for the client's health and well-being, or in order to face illness, disabilities, or death.

These definitions are referred to as orientational rather than operational, as they permit the researcher to discover generally and naturally the informant's local or emic (insiders') cultural perspectives rather than focusing on the researcher's etic (outsiders') specific variables and particular views. Orientational terms are congruent with the qualitative ethnonursing discovery method, which is focused on *how people know and experience their world with their cultural knowledge and lifeways* (Leininger 1985, 1991).

SUNRISE MODEL: A CONCEPTUAL GUIDE TO KNOWLEDGE DISCOVERY

The Sunrise Model (Figure 21–1) was developed to give a holistic and comprehensive conceptual picture of the major factors held as important to the Theory of Culture Care Diversity and Universality (Leininger, 1995, 1997a). The model is a conceptual visual guide depicting multiple factors predicted to influence culturally congruent care with people of different cultures. The model essentially serves as a cognitive guide for the researcher to visualize and reflect on different factors predicted to influence culturally based care in the discovery process. The Sunrise Model has also been used as a valuable guide for doing culturalogical health-care assessment of clients' health needs. As the researcher uses the model, the different factors depicted in the model are kept in mind in relation to discovering culture care phenomena. Gender and sexual orientation, race, class factors, biomedical condition, and the extent of acculturation are all an integral part of the model and theory. The factors tend to be embedded in social structure, worldview, and other dimensions identified in the Sunrise Model and are usually not

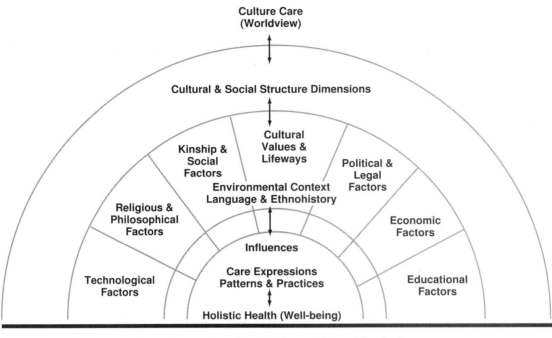

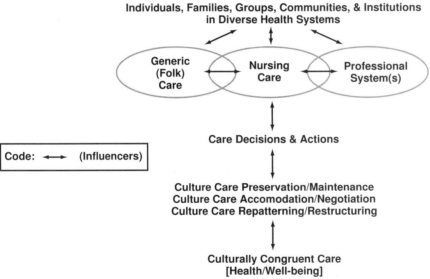

Figure 21–1 *Leininger's Sunrise Model depicts dimensions of the Theory of Culture Care Diversity and Universality. Reprinted with permission of author and National League for Nursing, New York.*

quickly identifiable. Hence, they are *not* isolated variables but are lodged in their natural and meaningful cultural context, yet are important discovery areas within the theory.

According to the researcher's interests and skills, one can begin the discovery at any place in the model except with the three modes of action and decisions, which are studied last or after drawing upon

data collected in the upper part of the model. All factors in the model need to be studied to obtain comprehensive or holistic data in order to arrive at an accurate picture of culturally based care. Some researchers may want to start with generic and professional care, whereas others may begin with the worldview and social structure dimensions. There is flexibility in the discovery process to fit the informant's interest and level of comfort as well as the researcher's goals, domains of inquiry, and research skills.

Because three modes of action and decision (in the lower part of the model) are studied and formulated with informants after the researcher has obtained data in the upper part of the model, the nursing actions or decisions become evident. The researcher involves informants in the discussion to arrive at appropriate actions, decisions, or plans. Throughout this discovery process, the researcher holds his or her own etic views, presuppositions, and biases in abeyance, so that the informants' cultural ideas will come forth, because they, rather than the researcher's views, are important and are the reason for the study. Transcultural nurses are taught, guided, and mentored in ways to withhold and deal with their biases and prejudices through formal courses and clinical experiences in transcultural nursing.

As the researcher carefully documents the different factors influencing care, he or she focuses on a specific and explicit domain of inquiry. For example, the researcher may focus on a *domain of inquiry* (DOI) such as "culture care of Mexican-American mothers caring for their children in their home." Every word in the domain statement is important to study, using the Sunrise Model and theory tenets. The researcher may have hunches about the domain, but holds them back until all data have been studied with the theory tenets. Full documentation of the informant's viewpoints, experiences, and actions is

> **The Sunrise Model is a valuable guide for culturalogical care assessment of clients' health needs.**

pursued. Generally, informants select what they first want to talk about with the researcher and then the researcher moves with informants to cover all aspects of the model and theory tenets. During the in-depth study of the domain of inquiry, all areas of the model are covered and discussed and confirmed with the informants. The informants remain active participants throughout the discovery process and in a manner that they feel is their unique and rich contribution.

The meanings, beliefs, values, and practices related to culture and care are studied in-depth and with respect to differences and similarities among key and general informants being studied. Both the differences and similarities are important to document the theory predictions. Such differences are often noted and observed with the historical, environmental, and social structure factors (i.e., religion, family, and economic, political, legal, or other factors) that influence human caring. The nurse researcher always reflects on professionally learned nursing knowledge, but always remains focused on the informants' views and their stories and experiences. Most important, the researcher is careful not to impose his or her own ideas on the informant or on the findings. Sometimes informants ask about the researcher and his or her views, which must be carefully and sparsely shared. The researcher keeps in mind the fact that some informants may want to please the researcher by talking about their professional medicines and treatments in order to get help or satisfy the researcher. Professional ideas, however, generally often cloud or mask the client's real interests and views. If this occurs, the researcher must be alert to such tendencies and keep the focus on the informants and the domain of inquiry. The informant's

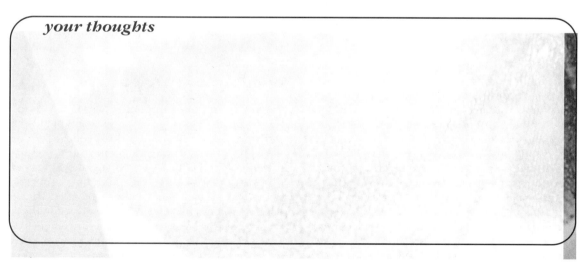

your thoughts

knowledge must always be kept central to the discovery process about culture care, health, and well-being. Factors that are unfamiliar to the researcher, such as kinship, economics, and political and other considerations depicted in the model and with the theory, may be difficult to discuss unless the nurse is prepared and understands these areas. In general, it is the informant's emic (insider's) views, beliefs, and practices that are central to studying the theory, and the researcher's views are put on a back burner in order to arrive at appropriate modes of action or decisions (Leininger, 1985, 1991, 1995, 1997a).

Throughout the study and use of the theory, the meanings, expressions, and patterns of culturally based care are important ideas to keep in mind. The researcher listens attentively to informants' accounts or stories, which include how they live, what they believe, and how they practice care or caring in their culture. Learning and documenting ideas from the informant's emic viewpoint is critical to arrive at accurate culturally based care. Unknown care meanings, such as the concepts of protection, respect, and love, and many other care constraints need to be teased out and explored in depth as informants share their ideas and experiences. These care areas of knowledge are essentially new in nursing when linked to culture. Moreover, these care meanings and expressions are often found to be lodged in religion, kinship (family), cultural values and beliefs, environment, and historical practices over time and are not always readily known. Sometimes informants are reluctant to share social structure and other ideas with nurses as they feel they are only interested in medical facts, techniques, and services and not in their religion, kinship ties, and other factors. Informants may also fear their cultural ideas will not be accepted or will be misunderstood by health personnel if they are partially known. But the cultural care ideas usually found hidden in generic (folk or indigenous) knowledge has to be teased out from the informant by showing a genuine interest in whatever they share. Such generic care must be appropriately integrated into professional knowledge and practices for quality-based health-care services (Leininger, 1981, 1984, 1990c, 1991). Generic and professional care complement each other for therapeutic nursing practices.

In identifying culturally based care knowledge with the three modalities, one will discover which of the three modes (or all) fit with the informant's care for therapeutic outcomes such as discussed in the second part of this chapter and from other transcultural nursing research reports. Informants actively participate to discover which care modes are needed to be maintained (or preserved), accommodated, structured, or repatterned to arrive at meaningful transcultural nursing care practices. Sometimes several care modes may be tailor-made to fit different cultural needs of individuals and groups. Professional knowledge may or may not be relevant or appropriate to use with some cultures.

The Sunrise Model was developed with the idea of "letting the sun enter the researcher's mind" and discovering generally unknown care factors for nurses related to the cultural values and care needs of cultures. The model depicts letting the sun "rise and shine" to get fresh and new insights. A wealth of new and unexpected nursing knowledge can be discovered with the model that has never been known and used in traditional nursing for present-day nursing and medical services.

The ethnonursing qualitative research method was specifically designed for the theory to facilitate the discovery of complex culture care phenomena. It is the only nursing research method that specifically teases out culturally based care as related to the theory (Leininger, 1985, 1990c, 1991, 1995, 1997a, 1997b). The ethnonursing method focuses primarily on discovering the people's care knowledge and lifeways rather than those of the researchers. This method will be discussed in the second part of this chapter, where Marilyn McFarland will show how the ethnonursing method is used in relation to the theory with a specific domain of inquiry, research questions, and special "enablers" to tease out the informant's data. Thus, the ethnonursing method is a method that was tailor-made to fit the theory (Leininger, 1990c, 1991, 1997a, 1997b). The reader is encouraged to read more on the theory and findings from use of the theory and ethnonursing method over the past four decades, and to discover the wealth of new transcultural care knowledge available to him or her for nursing practice (Leininger, 1991, 1995, 1997a, 1997b).

CURRENT STATUS OF THE THEORY

Currently, the Theory of Culture Care Diversity and Universality is being used in many schools of nursing and several clinical practice sites worldwide. The theory has grown in recognition and value for several reasons. First, the theory is the only nursing theory that focuses explicitly and in depth on discovering the meaning, uses, and patterns of culture care within and between specific cultures. Second, the theory looks for comparative culture care differences and similarities among and within cultures in order to expand nurses' knowledge about care in diverse cultures as essential to new nursing knowledge and practices. Third, the theory has a built-in and tailor-made ethnonursing nursing research method that was uniquely designed for the theory; it is different than ethnography and other research methods. The ethnonursing method remains unique and valuable to tease out largely covert, complex, and generally hidden care knowledge in cultures or subcultures. It was the first specific research method in nursing to fit a theory rather than the other way around; previously, nurse researchers typically used other borrowed and often inadequate research methods to study nursing phenomena.

Fourth, the theory of culture care is the only theory that searches for comprehensive and holistic social structure and worldview factors related to culture and caring to predict the health and well-being of people. The theory focuses on the totality of lifeways of individuals, families, groups, communities, and/or institutions related to culture and care phenomena to grasp a more comprehensive picture of humans in their real lifeworld. In the past, the culture of nursing has often focused on limited variables or medical symptoms and phenomena, which led to fragmented ideas about human living, beliefs, and values about maintaining wellness and preventing illnesses. Discovering the totality of living with a caring ethos in a culture has provided a wealth of new knowledge about the clients' lifeworld.

Fifth, the theory has both abstract and practical dimensions, which helps nurse researchers to discover what exists, or has the potential to be known and used for human caring and health practices. New theories are providing data of what exists and does not exist, and what has the potential for future discoveries. Moreover, some theories deal only with abstract phenomena, but this theory has both abstract and practical realities for nurses.

Sixth, the theory of culture care with the ethnonursing method and enablers has already provided a wealth of many new insights, knowledge areas, and valuable ways to work with people of diverse cultures in therapeutic or different ways than in the past. These transcultural nursing research findings are the new knowledge holdings that need to be incorporated into nursing, medicine, and other areas. They are the "gold nuggets" to change or transform in beneficial ways the current practices with clients of diverse cultures. Studies reported in the *Journal of Transcultural Nursing* and other transcultural nursing books and journals are valuable and support these claims (Leininger, 1991, 1995, 1997a, 1997b).

Seventh, the theory and its research findings have stimulated nursing faculty and clinicians to try different teaching and research approaches. Transcultural nursing findings are slowly beginning to be used in several schools of nursing to teach transcultural nursing and change outdated unicultural practices. Nursing administrators in service and academia have also been encouraged to use transcultural nursing findings and approaches with students, faculty, clients, and colleagues of different cultures and with faculty of other institutional disciplines and cultures. Nurse consultants are finding the theory is highly relevant for effective consultation services in different countries. They often use the theory for culturalogical assessments in different consultation situations to get to the problems. Transcultural nursing concepts, findings, and policies are being used with many worldwide health consultants in different disciplines. Many interdisciplinary health personnel are finding the theory and transcultural nursing research findings of great help in their work and are seeking workshops to learn more about the theory and its uses.

Eighth, and most important, informants of diverse cultures are often very pleased with the use of the theory and the ethnonursing method because it explicitly focuses on entering their world and learning from them about their culture, their health, and their care. Informants generally like having the opportunity to "tell their story" and to guide the research from what they personally believe is important for health and for their significant others. Informants speak of being more comfortable with this research and theory approach than the impersonal, nonculturally focused, and narrowly focused studies on numbers, variables, and short instant responses. Reflective thinking with the theory and multiple dimensions are valued. The theory encourages the researcher or clinician to learn from cultural informants and to let them be in control of ideas, a fact that is usually valued by informants. Many nurses who have been prepared in transcultural nursing and have used the theory and method say, "I love it and do not want to use traditional nursing research methods and theories that have failed to search for the holistic lifeways of people and their meanings."

Ninth, nurses who have used the theory and findings over time often speak of how much they have learned about cultures and caring. They realize that ethnocentric professional biases and prejudices influence quality of care to people of different cultures. Ethnocentrism and racial biases and prejudices have been reduced with transcultural nurses with the use of the theory and research method and findings. Searching for differences and similarities among cultures has expanded nurses' worldviews and deepened their appreciation of human beings and diverse cultures. The use of the theory has encouraged nursing students, staff, and faculty to become immersed in transcultural nursing, to grow intellectually, and to appreciate compassionate perspectives of past and current historical changes among cultures over time in accessing and receiving health care.

Finally, the strength of the theory is that it can be used in any culture and at any time and with most disciplines if modified slightly to fit the major and unique interest and goals of a specific discipline besides nursing. This fact makes the theory valuable and a major model and contribution from transcultural nursing and the nursing profession to other disciplines. Several disciplines, including dentistry, medicine, social work, and pharmacy, are now focusing on culturally congruent care in education and practice. Most encouraging is the fact that the concept of "culturally congruent care" (a term that I coined in the early 1960s) has become a major goal for United States government and accrediting groups in recent years. The concept is growing in use and is becoming imperative in the United States and overseas.

In general, the theory of culture care (launched in the mid-1950s) has today become well known in the past three decades and is now being used by many nurses and other health disciplines worldwide (Leininger, 1995, 1997a, 1997b). It is a theory of global interest and significance as we continue to understand cultures and their care needs and practices worldwide. As transcultural nursing concepts, principles, theory, and findings became fully incorporated into all health professional areas of teaching, practice, consultation, and research, one can anticipate many encouraging new and different health-care services from the past practices. Unquestionably, the theory will continue to grow in relevance and use as our world continues to become more intensely multicultural, especially in the twenty-first century. Indeed, nurses and other health professionals are expected in the future to function competently to meet the health-care needs of people from many diverse and similar cultures, to avoid racially destructive practices and prejudices, and to function in beneficially or therapeutic ways within and between cultures and with professional staff and students.

FUTURE OF THE CULTURE CARE THEORY

In looking to the future, one can predict that the Theory of Culture Care Diversity and Universality will be in increasing demand and highly relevant as world conflicts and tensions increase and the world becomes increasingly multicultural. Religious, business, education, and other occupations and institutions will need transcultural knowledge and practices. Already, global, transcultural, international, and culturally diverse linguistic terms and practices are common in communication and popular media. More and more, we are realizing that we are truly living in one global world with many diverse cultures and subcultures. Accordingly, worldview, social structure, and historical lifeways will be essential to assess as one works with people of different cultural lifeways in virtually every place in the world. Healthcare, business, and government entrepreneurs worldwide will increasingly promote, sell, and function with transcultural or global worldwide "products" and interests in the twenty-first century. Many transcultural research findings and the theory will be found useful in marketing and explaining outcomes.

After the launching transcultural nursing in the mid-1950s, the concept of "cultural awareness" has finally taken hold in nursing education and practice. The concept of "culturally congruent care" has gained recognition and continues to grow in use in health education and practices. It was, indeed, fortuitous and futuristic to have launched the field of transcultural nursing four decades ago and to lay the foundation for transculturalism in nursing and other fields. The full meaning and values of transcultural nursing, however, will become more evident in education, research, consultation, and practice in the third millennium, and our world will become intensely globally oriented in all spheres of birth, living, and dying.

It is reasonable to predict that the theory of culture care will become more relevant to nurses and other health-care providers as they move into working in foreign cultures and market nursing worldwide with diversities and universalities. Discovering differences and similarities worldwide in nursing is still a goal to be reached. The theory and ethnonursing method will be of great help toward attaining this goal. Indeed, the ethnonursing research method will become important so nurses can grasp how multicultural groups of immigrants and others live together, maintain health, and become ill. The theory will be important in helping to prevent community-based intercultural conflicts, violence, and crime, because the sources of these tension areas can be identified with the help of the theory. One can predict a major shift in the twenty-first century from the present dominance of the biomedical and psychology foci to culturalogical models and factors to prevent illnesses and maintain health in different environments and ecological niches. The culture care theory, along with diverse qualitative research methods, will be extremely helpful for this new future thrust in health-care, business, and educational settings. Computer models will rely on holistic data for an accurate and complete picture of culturalogical and environmental factors.

Summary

In summary, there are several major reasons why the Theory of Culture Care Diversity and Universality and research-based findings will be in demand and used worldwide. They are summarized below:

1. Global migration and movement of people worldwide will be rapidly increasing due to modern transportation, communication, and electronic media.

2. Use of electronic data and other communication modes will markedly increase, bringing more cultures closer together in Western and non-Western worlds almost instantly.

3. There will be a marked increase in demand for transcultural health-care services in education and practice by consumers worldwide.

4. Transcultural research findings in health-care services will be imperative to support, justify, and respond to meaningful health-care services.

5. There will be a marked increase in the use of human life experiences, religious ideas, spiritual beliefs, and historical data and environmental knowledge for food and well-being.

6. Transcultural ethical and moral issues will markedly increase as nurses, physicians, ethicists, and other disciplines struggle with justice, human rights, birth, death, and many genetic engineering issues.

7. Transcultural health education, consultation, and clinical practices will necessitate becoming a reality due to demands from diverse cultures.

8. Transcultural health-care and treatment policies will be essential to attract and retain consumers in using future health-care services.

9. As hospital services decrease by the year 2015 and new community services increase, transcultural control and regulation by cultural consumers will be evident.

10. Transworld corporations will become active in marketing transcultural health services and other products by the year 2010.

11. Many underrepresented (or "minority") cultures today will become majority cultures in the decades to come, which will necessitate major changes in education, research, and practice.

12. Transcultural distance in learning, consultation, and educational policies will significantly increase within countries but also across countries to remote places in the world. While electronic communication modes will be important, one will find that many cultures will want to promote peace and have fewer intercultural wars.

13. Theory development will change from a present-day reliance on a few variables to multiple holistic theories. Mini- and middle-range theories will decrease as they will be viewed as too limited to deal with complex and holistic data. Qualitative paradigmatic research will increase in value and uses with computer models to handle large amounts of rich transcultural findings.

References

Leininger, M. (1970). *Nursing and anthropology: Two worlds to blend.* New York: John Wiley and Sons.

Leininger, M. (1976). Transcultural nursing presents an exciting challenge. *The American Nurse, 5*(5), 6–9.

Leininger, M. (1977). Caring: The essence and central focus of nursing. *Nursing Research Foundation Report, 12*(1), 2–14.

Leininger, M. (1978). *Transcultural nursing: Concepts, theories, and practices.* New York: John Wiley and Sons.

Leininger, M. (1981). *Caring: An essential human need.* Thorofare, NJ: Slack.

Leininger, M. (1984). *Care: The essence of nursing and health.* Thorofare, NJ: Slack.

Leininger, M. (1985). *Qualitative research methods in nursing* (pp. 33–73). Orlando, FL: Grune & Stratton Co.

Leininger, M. (1988). *Care: Discovery and uses in clinical and community nursing.* Detroit: Wayne State University Press.

Leininger, M. (1989a). Transcultural nursing: Quo vadis (where goeth the field)? *Journal of Transcultural Nursing, 1*(1), 33–45.

Leininger, M. (1989b). Transcultural nurse specialists and generalists: New practitioners in nursing. *Journal of Transcultural Nursing, 1*(1), 4–16.

Leininger, M. (1990a). Transcultural nursing: A worldwide necessity to advance nursing knowledge and practices. In McCloskey, J. & Grace, H. (Eds.), *Current issues in nursing.* St. Louis: Mosby.

Leininger, M. (1990b). Culture: The conspicuous missing link to understand ethical and moral dimensions of human care. In Leininger, M. (Ed.), *Ethical and moral dimensions of care.* Detroit: Wayne State University Press.

Leininger, M. (1990c). Ethnomethods: The philosophic and epistemic basis to explicate transcultural nursing knowledge. *Journal of Transcultural Nursing, 1*(2), 40–51.

Leininger, M. (1990d). *Care: Ethical and moral dimensions of care.* Detroit: Wayne State University Press.

Leininger, M. (1991). *Culture care diversity and universality: A theory of nursing.* New York: National League for Nursing Press.

Leininger, M. (1995). *Transcultural nursing: Concepts, theories, research, and practice.* Columbus, OH: McGraw Hill College Custom Series.

Leininger, M. (1997a). Overview of the theory of culture care with the ethnonursing research method. *Journal of Transcultural Nursing, 8*(2), 32–53.

Leininger, M. (1997b). Transcultural nursing research to transform nursing education and practice: 40 years. *Image: Journal of Nursing Scholarship, 29*(4), 341–347.

Leininger, M., & Hofling, C. (1960). *Basic psychiatric concepts in nursing.* Philadelphia: Lippincott.

Chapter 21 Part 2

The Ethnonursing Research Method and the Culture Care Theory: Implications for Clinical Nursing Practice

Marilyn R. McFarland

The purpose of the second part of Chapter 21 is twofold. The first part will include an overview of the ethnonursing research method, which was designed to study the Theory of Culture Care Diversity and Universality. The second part will present a discussion of the implications of the culture care theory and related ethnonursing research findings for clinical nursing practice. Many nursing theories are rather abstract and do not focus on how practicing nurses might use the research findings related to a theory. However, with the culture care theory, along with the ethnonursing method, there is a purposeful built-in action means to discover and confirm data with informants in order to make nursing actions and decisions meaningful and culturally congruent (Leininger, 1991a).

THE ETHNONURSING RESEARCH METHOD

The ethnonursing research method was specifically designed by Leininger (1985, 1991b) to study the culture care theory. This was the first research method designed to study a nursing theory and related nursing phenomena. The method facilitates the discovery of people care knowledge and culturally based care related to the theory. Leininger (1991b, p. 79) has defined the *ethnonursing research method* as "a qualitative research method using naturalistic, open discovery, and largely inductively derived emic modes and processes with diverse strategies, techniques, and enabling tools to document, describe, understand, and interpret the people's meanings, experience, symbols, and other related aspects bearing on actual or potential nursing phenomena."

Qualitative Paradigm and Quantitative Paradigm

In order to grasp an understanding of the qualitative ethnonursing research method, it is important to understand the major philosophical differences between the qualitative and quantitative paradigms. Leininger has described *qualitative paradigmatic research* as "characterized by naturalistic and open inquiry methods and techniques focused on systematically documenting, analyzing, and interpreting attributes, patterns, characteristics, and meanings of specific domains and gestaltic (or holistic) features of phenomena under study within designated environmental or living contexts" (Leininger, 1997). She has described quantitative research as "characterized by a focus on an empirical and objective analysis of dis-

crete and preselected variables that have been derived *a priori* and as theoretical statements or hypotheses in order to determine causal and measurable relationships among the variables being tested" (Leininger, 1997, p. 43). In qualitative research there is no control of informant ideas or manipulation of data or variables by the researcher; only open inquiry prevails to obtain data directly and naturally from informants in their own homes, communities, or other natural environmental contexts. In contrast, in quantitative research precise measurements are obtained and specific causal relationships among variables are sought. Leininger has stated that the quantitative and qualitative paradigms should not be mixed as they violate the philosophy, purposes, and integrity of each paradigm. The ethnonursing method is a unique and essential qualitative method to study caring and healing practices, beliefs, and values in diverse cultural and environmental contexts and is a major holistic method specifically designed to fit the culture care theory.

> The ethnonursing method is a unique qualitative method to study caring and healing practices and beliefs in diverse cultural contexts. It is designed specifically for the culture care theory.

Purpose and Philosophical Features

Leininger developed the ethnonursing research method from a nursing and cultural care perspective to discover largely unknown phenomena held essential to practice nursing. She has stated that ethnonursing method is used (1985, 1991b) to "systematically document and gain greater understanding and meaning of the people's daily life experiences related to human care, health, and well-being in different or similar environmental contexts" (1991b, p. 78). The central purpose of the ethnonursing research method is "to establish a naturalistic and largely emic open inquiry method to explicate and study nursing phenomena especially related to the Theory of Cultural Care Diversity and Universality" (1991b, p. 75). The term "ethnonursing" was purposefully coined for this method. The prefix *ethno* comes from the Greek word *ethos* and refers "to the people," while the suffix *nursing* is essential to focus the research on the phenomena of nursing, particularly human care, well-being, and health in different environments and cultural contexts (Leininger, 1991b).

The ethnonursing research method has philosophical and research features that fit well with the culture care theory. Philosophically, the ethnonursing method has been grounded with the people (Leininger, 1991b) and has supported the discovery of people truths in human living contexts (Leininger, 1988). This research method was designed to tease out complex, elusive, and largely unknown nursing dimensions from the local people's viewpoints of human care, well-being and health, and environmental contexts. The terms "emic" and "etic" were important concepts chosen for foci with the ethnonursing method. Ethnonursing focuses largely on the importance of emic (insiders' or local peoples') views but does not neglect etic (the nonlocal or outsiders') views to obtain a holistic view. For instance, one ethnonursing researcher gathered emic data from elderly retirement home residents on their ideas and experiences with care but also gathered etic data focused on the professional perspectives of the nursing staff (McFarland, 1997). The culture care theory has been developed to be congruent with the ethnonursing method and requires the researcher to move into familiar and naturalistic people settings to discover human care and the related nursing phenomena of health (well-being), illness, and other phenomena within an environmental context (Leininger, 1991b, p. 85).

Domain of Inquiry

A *domain of inquiry* is the major focus of the ethnonurse researcher's interests. A domain of inquiry is broad and yet focused to obtain specific care and health outcomes of a culture with a nursing perspective. With the ethnonursing method, problem statements are not used because a researcher does not know whether there is a *people* problem or more of a researcher's problem of selected (and possibly biased) views of the people (Leininger, 1997). For example, some domains of inquiry in ethnonursing studies using the culture care theory have been: (1)

the care meanings and experiences of Lebanese Muslims living in the United States in a designated urban context (Luna, 1994), (2) the cultural care of elderly Anglo- and African-American residents within the environmental context of a long-term care institution (McFarland, 1997), and (3) the care of Mexican-American women during pregnancy (Berry, 1999).

Key and General Informants

Key and general informants are important in the ethnonursing research method. The research using this method does not have subjects, but works with informants. In an ethnonursing study of the culture care of Anglo- and African-American elderly residents of a retirement home (McFarland, 1997), the researcher worked with the elders and nursing staff members as key and general informants. They told the researcher about themselves and the cultural care within the environmental context of a retirement home. Key informants were carefully and purposefully selected (often by the people themselves, e.g., elderly residents suggested other residents for the researcher to observe, interview, and study about care, health, and well-being). These informants were most knowledgeable about the domain of inquiry and could give details to the nurse researcher. General informants usually are not as fully knowledgeable about the domain of inquiry as the key informants. They have general ideas about the domain, however, and can offer data from their emic and etic views. For instance, general informants can reflect on how similar and/or different their ideas are from those of the key informants when asked by the researcher.

Enablers

In order to discover the people's (or informant's) innermost world of knowing, Leininger developed sev-

TABLE 21-1	*Leininger's Ethnonursing Observation-Participation-Reflection Phases*			
Phases	1	2	3	4
Description	Primary observation and active listening (no active participation)	Primary observation with limited participation	Primary participation with continued observations	Primary reflection and reconfirmation of findings with informants

Source: Leininger, M. (1997). Overview and reflection of the Theory of Culture Care and the Ethnonursing Research Method. *Journal of Transcultural Nursing, 8*(2), 32–51.

TABLE 21-2	*Leininger's Stranger to Trusted Friend Enabler Guide*		

The purpose of this enabler is to facilitate the researcher (or clinician, who can also use it) to move from a mainly distrusted stranger to a trusted friend in order to obtain authentic, credible, and dependable data or establish favorable relationships as a clinician. The user assesses himself or herself by reflecting on the indicators as he or she moves from stranger to friend.

Indicators of Stranger (Largely etic or outsider's views)	Date Noted	Indicators of a Trusted Friend (Largely emic or insider's views)	Date Noted
Active to protect self and others. They *are gatekeepers* and guard against outside intrusions. Suspicious and questioning.		Less active to protect self. More trusting of researchers (their *gatekeeping is down or less*). Less suspicious and less questioning of researcher.	
Actively watch and are attentive to what researcher does and says. Limited signs of trusting the researcher or stranger.		Less watching of the researcher's words and actions. More signs of trusting and accepting a new friend.	
Skeptical about the researcher's motives and work. May question how findings will be used by the researcher or stranger.		Less questioning of the researcher's motives, work, and behavior. Signs of working with and helping the researcher as a friend.	
Reluctant to share cultural secrets and views as private knowledge. Protective of local lifeways, values, and beliefs. Dislikes probing by the researcher or stranger.		Willing to share cultural secrets and private world information and experiences. Offers most local views, values, and interpretations spontaneously or without probes.	
Uncomfortable to become a friend or to confide in stranger. May come late, be absent, and withdraw from researcher at times.		Signs of being comfortable and enjoying friends and a sharing relationship. Gives presence, is on time, and gives evidence of being a *genuine friend*.	
Tends to offer inaccurate data. Modifies *truths* to protect self, family, community, and cultural lifeways. Emic values, beliefs, and practices are not shared spontaneously.		Wants research *truths* to be accurate regarding beliefs, people, values, and lifeways. Explains and interprets emic ideas so researcher has accurate data.	

Source: Leininger, M. (1991). *Culture care diversity and universality: A theory of nursing.* New York: National League for Nursing, p. 82.

eral enablers to tease out data bearing on cultural care related to specific domains of study. As the word denotes, enablers help ease out ideas from informants in meaningful and natural ways. Leininger (1997) specifically makes the point that enablers are different than tools, scales, or measurement instruments used in quantitative studies, which tend to cut off natural flow of informant ideas. Some of the enablers that serve as important guides to obtain data naturalistically and holistically are: (1) Leininger's observation participation reflection enabler (Table 21-1); (2) the stranger to trusted friend enabler (Table 21-2); (3) Leininger's acculturation enabler (Leininger, 1991b); and (4) specific enablers developed by the researcher to tap ideas of informants related to the specific domain of inquiry (Figure 21-2).

The Sunrise Model (see Part 1 of this chapter by Dr. Leininger and the discussion under the Three Care Modes later in this chapter) can also be viewed as an enabler since it assists and guides the researcher to tease out culture care and health data within each dimension of the Sunrise Model to provide holistic and yet specific cultural findings (Leininger, 1997).

The observation participation reflection enabler (Table 21-1) guides the nurse researcher to be an active observer and listener before being a participant in any research context. Researchers have found it most helpful to observe informants and their environmental contexts before and after the researcher becomes an active participant. This is quite different from the traditional participant observation method

<table>
<tr><td colspan="2" align="center">**ETHNODEMOGRAPHICS**</td></tr>
<tr><td>Name:</td><td>Religious affiliation:</td></tr>
<tr><td>Informant #:</td><td>Years of formal education:</td></tr>
<tr><td>Sex:</td><td>Cultural background:</td></tr>
<tr><td>Age:</td><td>Previous occupation:</td></tr>
<tr><td>Place of Residence or Institution:</td><td>Dates of contact:</td></tr>
<tr><td>Years in home:</td><td>Languages spoken:</td></tr>
</table>

I. CARE

1. I am interested in learning from you about the care here from your own experiences at this place. What does care mean to you from your own experiences here?

2. Did you come to this place because you needed care? If so, tell me about the care that you needed as you entered and while you have been here over time. How does your care meet your expectations?

3. Tell me about the care you receive here during a typical day and night.

4. What statement, words, or ideas describe care in this home?

5. For you, then, care means _____?

Figure 21–2 *Cultural care of Anglo-American and African-American elders: Resident Open Inquiry Guide. Reprinted with permission of McFarland, M. (1995).* Cultural care of Anglo- and African-American elderly residents within the environmental context of a long-term care institution. (*UMI No. 9530568*). Ann Arbor, MI: UMI Microfilm.

used in anthropology, because the process is reversed (Leininger, 1997). Nurses who are used to doing something actively for or with clients must stop and observe before actively participating with informants with this method.

The stranger to trusted friend enabler (Table 21-2) has been extremely helpful as a researcher enters and remains in a strange and unfamiliar environment. The researcher moves from being a stranger to a trusted friend and can eventually obtain accurate, honest, credible, and in-depth data from informants. Several ethnonurse researchers have found that when informants considered the researcher a trusted friend, the findings were very different from those found by a stranger (Berry, 1999; Luna, 1994; McFarland, 1997). Being a trusted friend leads to informants sharing their cultural secrets and their insights and experiences. For instance, the author used the stranger friend enabler to assess her relationship with elderly residents and the staff in a study of cul-

ture care in a retirement home. She used this enabler to enter the informant's world and get close to the people who were being studied (McFarland, 1997). Initially the researcher worked with a staff nurse while observing and interviewing the informants for the first few weeks she was in the institution. The staff nurse was friendly and acted as a guide but also watched the researcher and planned her day in a general way. The researcher knew she had moved from being a stranger to a trusted friend when the director of nursing said, "You are on your own today; you know several residents really look forward to your visits." After the researcher had been at the research site for several months, an elderly Anglo-American resident informant said to her, "I'm really revealing myself to you today," and then went on to describe her negative feelings about the increasing numbers of African-Americans coming to live at the retirement home. The researcher had moved from a stranger to a trusted friend; the informant revealed meaningful

Chapter 21 *Marilyn R. McFarland Implications of Ethnonursing Research Method* **381**

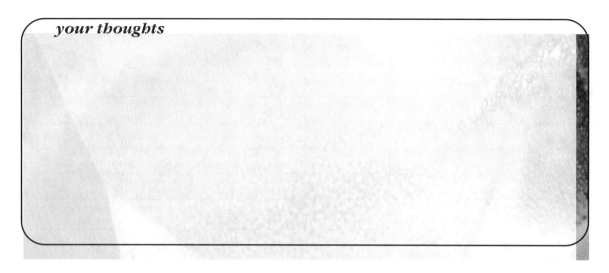

and sensitive information to her, and the informant felt safe and trusted the researcher. This enabler is invaluable to gauge one's relationship with informants as the study progresses.

Leininger's acculturation enabler (Leininger, 1991b) has been used in many ethnonursing studies to identify traditional and nontraditional beliefs, values, and general lifeways of informants. This enabler is useful with all informants, but especially with immigrant groups undergoing rapid cultural changes. The Sunrise Model was also developed as an enabler to help researchers discover multiple and diverse holistic lifeways related to culture care experiences and practices. It is unique as a guide for holistic yet specific factors influencing care in cultures under study within an ethnohistory, language, social structure, and environmental context (Leininger, 1991b, 1995, 1997).

In addition to the four enablers just discussed, the ethnonurse researcher develops a *special enabler* that fits with the specific domain of inquiry under study, such as the care meanings and experiences of Lebanese Muslims (Luna, 1989), the culture care of Anglo- and African-American elders (McFarland, 1997), and the culture care of pregnant Mexican-American women (Berry, 1996). These enablers were specifically designed by the researchers to help tease out in-depth specific details of culture care phenomena related to the theoretical assumptions and the domain of inquiry of the study. Examples of special enablers can be found in the studies mentioned above and in other ethnonursing research studies listed in the references at the end of this chapter and in the *Journal of Transcultural Nursing* (1989 to 1999). The complete text of an enabler, *The Experience of Mexican Americans Receiving Profes-*

sional Care: An Open Inquiry Guide, has been published in the *Journal of Transcultural Nursing* (Zoucha, 1998, pp. 42–44).

Qualitative Criteria to Evaluate Ethnonursing Studies

Leininger has developed specific criteria to evaluate qualitative research, including ethnonursing studies. Because qualitative studies have very different meanings and purposes, goals, and outcomes from quantitative studies, the nurse researcher is required to use qualitative criteria to evaluate ethnonursing research studies (Leininger, 1991b, 1995). Leininger's (1997) succinct definitions of qualitative criteria are as follows:

1. *Credibility:* Refers to direct evidence from the people and the environmental context as *truths* to the people.
2. *Confirmability:* Refers to documented verbatim evidence from the people who can firmly and knowingly confirm the data or findings.
3. *Meaning-in-Context:* Refers to meaningful or understandable findings that are known and relevant to the people within their familiar and natural living environmental contexts.
4. *Recurrent Patterning:* Refers to documented evidence of repeated patterns, themes, and acts over time reflecting consistency in lifeways or patterned behaviors.
5. *Saturation:* Refers to in-depth evidence of taking in all that can be known or understood about phenomena or a domain of inquiry under study by the informants.
6. *Transferability:* Refers to whether the findings from the study will have similar (not identical)

TABLE 21-3

TABLE 21-3 *Leininger's Phases of Ethnonursing Analysis for Qualitative Data*

Fourth Phase
Major Themes, Research Findings, Theoretical Formulations, and Recommendations

This is the highest phase of data analysis, synthesis, and interpretation. It requires synthesis of thinking, configurations, analysis, interpreting findings, and creative formulations from data of the previous phases. The researcher's task is to abstract and present major theses, research findings, recommendations, and sometimes theoretical formulations.

Third Phase
Pattern and Contextual Analysis

Data are scrutinized to discover saturation ideas and recurrent patterns of similar or different meanings, expressions, structural forms, interpretations, or explanations of data related to the domain of inquiry. Data are examined to show patterning with respect to meanings-in-context and along with further credibility and confirmation of findings.

Second Phase
Identification and Categorization of Descriptors and Components

Data are coded and classified as related to the domain of inquiry and sometimes the questions under study. Emic or etic descriptors are studied within context and for similarities and differences. Recurrent components are studied for their meanings.

First Phase
Collecting, Describing, and Documenting Raw Data (Use of Field Journal and Computer)

The researcher collects, describes, records, and begins to analyze data related to the purpose, domain of inquiry, or questions under study. This phase includes recording interview data from key and general informants; making observations and having participatory experiences; identifying contextual meanings; making preliminary interpretations; identifying symbols; and recording data related to the phenomena under study, mainly from an emic focus, but attentive to etic ideas. Field data from the condensed and full field journal are processed directly into the computer and coded.

Source: Leininger, M. (1991). *Culture care diversity and universality: A theory of nursing* New York: National League for Nursing (p. 95).

meanings and relevance in a similar situation or context (pp. 44–45).

Each of these criteria needs to be used thoughtfully and explicitly in a systematic and continuous process while obtaining data or observing informants over periods of time.

Four Phases of Ethnonursing Analysis for Qualitative Data

Leininger (1997) has developed the phases of ethnonursing qualitative data analysis (Table 21–3). The four phases provide for systematic ongoing data analysis, which is from the beginning of data collection until the final analysis and completion of the written report of the research findings. The Leininger Templin Thompson (LTT) Qualitative Software Data Program (or a similar one) can be used to process the qualitative data. The first two phases of data analysis are focused on obtaining raw data and beginning indicators of the phenomena under study. The third phase of data analysis requires that the researcher identify recurrent patterns, and in the fourth phase the focus is on developing and synthesizing major themes derived from the previous sequential three phases. A research mentor skilled in the ethnonursing method can help the researcher to reflect on the major phases and to meet the qualitative evaluation criteria. Themes must be clearly stated to provide guidance to assist nurses in providing culturally congruent and relevant care for people from diverse cultures or subcultures. Themes are the dominant finding from the analysis, and thematic statements require much critical and analytic thinking to accurately reflect the emic and etic raw data and holistic findings.

The Steps in the Ethnonursing Research Process

The general research process of conducting an ethnonursing study is presented as a guide. The process may be modified to fit with the research setting or

your thoughts

context. The research process needs to be flexible so the researcher can move with the people and be open to make allowances or change plans in accord with naturalistic developments. As the researcher moves from stranger to friend to collect and process research data, modifications in the research plan often become necessary. The phases of the ethnonursing research method developed by Leininger (1991b, p. 105) are as follows:

1. Identify the general intent or purpose(s) of your study with a focus on the domain(s) of inquiry phenomenon under study, area of inquiry, or research questions being addressed.
2. Identify the potential significance of the study to advance nursing knowledge and practice.
3. Review available literature on the domain or phenomena being studied.
4. Conceptualize a research plan from the beginning to the end with the following general phases or sequence of factors in mind:
   a. Consider the research site, community, and people to study the phenomena.
   b. Deal with the informed consent expectations.
   c. Explore and gradually gain entry (with essential permissions/informed consent) to the community, hospital, or country where the study is being done.
   d. Anticipate potential barriers and facilitators related to getekeepers' expectations, language, political leaders, location, and other factors.
   e. Select and appropriately use the ethnonursing enablers with the research process; for example, Leininger's Stranger-Friend Guide, Observation-Participation-Reflection Guide, and others. The researcher may also develop enablers as guides for their study.

f. Chose key and general informants.
g. Maintain trusting and favorable relationships with the people conferring with ethnonurse research experts to prevent unfavorable developments.
h. Collect and confirm data with observations, interview, participant experiences, and other data. (This is a continuous process from the beginning to the end and requires the use of qualitative research criteria to confirm findings and credibility factors.)
i. Maintain continuous data processing on computer and with field journals, depicting active analysis and reflections and discussions with research mentor(s). Computer processing with Leininger Templin Thompson's software is a helpful means of handling large amounts of qualitative data.
j. Frequently present and reconfirm findings with the people studied to check credibility and confirmability of findings.
k. Make plans to leave the field site, community, and informants in advance.
5. Do final analysis and writing of research findings soon after completing the study.
6. Prepare published findings in appropriate journals.
7. Help implement the findings with nurses interested in findings.
8. Plan future studies related to this domain or other new ones.

Again, there is flexibility with the ethnonursing data processing, but the above steps help to conceptualize the process to do a systematic investigation that has credibility and meets other qualitative evaluation criteria.

CULTURE CARE THEORY AND NURSING PRACTICE

Over the past four decades, the culture care theory, along with the ethnonursing method, have been used by nurse researchers to discover knowledge that can and has been used in nursing practice. Nurses can use such knowledge not only to care for individual clients, but also to focus on care practices for families, groups, communities, cultures, and institutions that are beneficial. Our multicultural world has made it imperative that nurses understand different cultures to work and care for people who have diverse and similar values, beliefs, and ideas about nursing, health, caring, wellness, illness, death, and disabilities (Leininger, 1991a, 1995). As stated in the first part of this chapter by Dr. Leininger, the goal of the Theory of Culture Care Diversity and University is to improve or maintain health and well-being by providing culturally congruent care to people that is beneficial and fits with the lifeways of the client, family, or cultural group. The Sunrise Model serves as a cognitive map depicting the seven culture and social structure dimensions that influence care, which in turn influences the health and/or illness of clients.

The culture care theory and the Sunrise Model include what is similar (universal) and different (diverse) between generic (or folk) care and professional care and provides a focus on both types of care for the provision of culturally congruent care for clients in diverse nursing practice settings. Leininger predicted that if culturally congruent care was evident, this would prevent cultural clashes, cultural illnesses, and other unfavorable human conditions under human control (Leininger, 1991a). These general ideas are kept in mind as one uses findings related to the theory in clinical practice.

> The term "nursing intervention" often implies to clients from different cultures that the nurse is imposing his or her views, which may not be helpful.

The Three Care Modes and the Sunrise Model

To provide a different focus from traditional nursing, Leininger developed the unique three modes of care to incorporate theory findings (Sunrise Model, Figure 21–1). To review, the three modes are: (1) culture care preservation or maintenance, (2) culture care accommodation or negotiation, and (3) culture care repatterning or restructuring. The theorist predicts that the researcher can use ethnoresearch findings to guide nursing judgements, decisions, and actions related to providing culturally congruent care (Leininger, 1991a). Leininger prefers not to use the phrase "nursing intervention" because this term often implies to clients from different cultures that the nurse is imposing his or her (etic) views, which may not be helpful. Instead, the term "nursing actions and decisions" is used, but always with the clients helping to arrive at whatever actions or decisions are implemented. The modes fit with the clients' or peoples' lifeways and yet are therapeutic and satisfying for them. The nurse can draw upon scientific nursing, medical, and other knowledge with each mode.

Data collected from the upper and lower parts of the Sunrise Model provide culture care knowledge for nurse researchers to discover and establish useful ways to provide quality care practices. Active participatory involvement with clients is essential to arrive at culturally congruent care with one or all of the three action modes in order to meet clients' care needs in their particular environmental contexts. The use of these modes in nursing care is one of the most creative and rewarding features of transcultural and general nursing practice with clients of diverse cultures.

It is most important (and a shift in nursing) to carefully focus on the holistic dimensions as depicted in the Sunrise Model to arrive at therapeutic culture care practices. All the factors in the Sunrise Model (which include worldview, and technological, religious, kinship, political/legal, economic, and educational factors, as well as cultural values and lifeways, environmental context, language, ethnohistory, and generic [folk] and professional care practices) (Leininger, 1991a) must be considered to arrive at culturally congruent care. Only when the nurse in clinical practice (in a community, home, or institutional context) becomes fully aware of and explicitly uses knowledge generated from the theory and ethnonursing method will care become safe, congruent, meaningful, and beneficial to clients. The culture care theory, along with the ethnonursing method, are a powerful means for new directions and practices in nursing. Incorporating culture-specific care into clients' care is essential today and in the future to practice professional care and to be licensed as registered nurses. Culture-specific care is the safe means to ensure culturally based holistic care to fit the client's culture—a major new challenge for nurses who practice and provide services in all health-care settings.

The Use of Culture Care Research Findings

Over the past four decades, Dr. Leininger and other research colleagues have used the culture care theory and the ethnonursing method to focus on the meanings and lived experiences of 87 cultures, and discovered 187 care constructs in Western and non-Western cultures (Leininger, 1998), as reported in the *Journal of Transcultural Nursing* (1989 to 1999). Leininger listed the 11 most dominant constructs of care in priority ranking, with the most universal or frequently discovered first: (1) respect for/about (most universal care construct); (2) concern for/about; (3) attention to/with anticipation of; (4) helping, assisting, and facilitative acts; (5) active listening; (6) giving presence (being there physically); (7) understanding the cultural beliefs, values, and lifeways of clients; (8) being connected to/relatedness; (9) protection of/for some gender and kin differences; (10) touching (how, where, and when varied); and (11) providing comfort measures. These care constructs are the most critical and important universal or common findings to consider in nursing practice, but care diversities must also be considered. Although many of these dominant care constructs may be found in certain cultures, diversities will also be found. The ways in which culture care is applied and used in specific cultures will reflect both similarities and differences among (and sometimes within) different cultures. Next, three ethnonursing studies will be reviewed with a focus on the findings, which have implications for nursing practice.

Culture Care of Lebanese Muslims in the United States

In the late 1980s, Luna conducted an ethnonursing study of the culture care of Arab Muslim cultural groups in a large urban community in the midwestern United States. In 1989, she published the findings relevant to the culture care of Lebanese Muslim Americans using Leininger's three modes of nursing decisions and actions to provide culturally congruent and responsible care. The study focused on the care for Lebanese Muslims in the hospital, clinic, and home-community contexts. She stated: "[An] understanding [of] the cultural context in which Lebanese Muslims attempt to adapt, survive, and practice their faith in America necessitates a look into the community into which they migrate" (Luna, 1994, p. 15). Luna's research findings and the nursing practice implications related to the home and community context in the late 1980s remain important today as health care shifts from hospital care services to home or community settings. Luna discovered that attending a clinic in an urban context (in the midwestern United States) was often a new and different approach to health care for Lebanese Muslim women, especially during pregnancy and childbirth. Luna's study revealed that many women relied on the traditional midwife in Lebanon for home deliveries. The routine of monthly and weekly visits to the prenatal clinic was incongruent with what the client had experienced in her home country. In the United States, prenatal care in the clinic context involved long waiting periods with the husband missing work to take his wife to the clinic. Examination by a male physi-

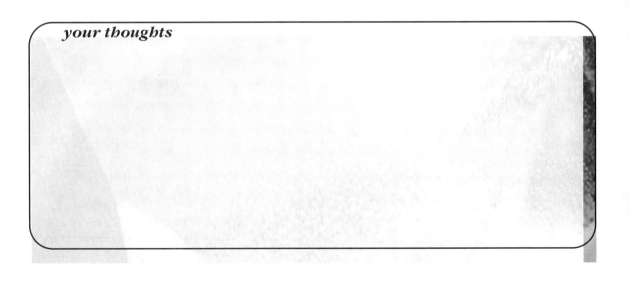

your thoughts

cian was culturally incongruent for the women, so *culture care negotiation and repatterning* was essential for culturally congruent care. Luna described the clinic as *culturally decontextualized* for clients and their families because the prenatal care and the environmental clinic context in which the care was provided were not congruent with the clients' cultural values, beliefs, and practices (Luna, 1989).

Luna discovered the dominant and universal care constructs for Lebanese Muslim men, which included surveillance, protection, and maintenance of the family. For Lebanese women, the dominant and universal care constructs included emphasizing the positive attributes of educating the children and maintaining a family caring environment according to the precepts of Islam. A number of generic or folk care practices were discovered related to these care constructs that should be recognized, preserved, and maintained by nurses to enhance the health and well-being of clients. For instance, the female network in the Lebanese Muslim culture is very important at the time of birth; Lebanese women come together to care for each other and offer practical and emotional assistance for new immigrants who are struggling to survive in a new cultural context such as the United States. Hence, by recognizing the benefits of this network and by allowing women flexibility in their visiting and presence in the hospital and clinic contexts, the nurse would use culture care preservation to maintain these generic care practices for the health and well-being of clients.

Luna found that female modesty was an important cultural care value for Lebanese women; this was reflected in requests by female clients to have only female nurses, physicians, and other caregivers. Culture care accommodation of this generic care practice was accomplished by nurses negotiating for these women to have female caregivers whenever possible, which would promote health, well-being, and client satisfaction with care. Including Lebanese Muslim men in health teaching and discharge planning was a way Luna discovered to use culture care preservation that recognized the family as a unit, rather than focusing on the individual. Luna recognized that the patriarchal organization of the family should be preserved as a social structure feature, which acknowledges males for their roles in family care continuity rather than being narrowly interpreted as males always being in control. Negative stereotypes about the Arab male's reluctance to participate in the birth process were discovered often to be a barrier in giving nursing care. To counter this, Luna suggested the nurse could use culture care preservation to maintain and support the generic culture care practices of men, which included surveillance, protection, and maintenance of the family.

Still another finding from Luna's study was the discovery of the importance of religious rituals to many Muslim clients as an essential component of providing care within their cultural context (Luna, 1989, 1994). Luna found that some Muslims pray three to five times a day, and others do not pray at all. During the culturalogical assessment (in the hospital context), Luna suggested the nurse should ask about the client's wishes regarding prayer, and could practice cultural care accommodation by negotiating for time and a private place for prayer which for many Muslims is an important cultural expression for their health and well-being. She also suggested that nurses should practice cultural care accommodation for clients by negotiating with a social service organization which served Arab clients in order to gather written and video materials in the Arabic language related to health to be used in the hospital and clinic settings. Luna (1989) identified culture care repatterning to improve attendance at the prenatal clinic for Lebanese Muslim women. Nurses should avoid direct confrontation and spend considerable time during the first clinic visit to educate women regarding the benefits of regular prenatal care, including emphasizing the health and well-being of both the mother and the baby.

Culture Care of Elderly Anglo- and African Americans

In the mid-1990s the theory of culture care was used to guide a study of the culture care of Anglo- and African-American elders in a long-term care institution (McFarland, 1997). This study revealed care implications for nurses who practice in retirement homes, nursing homes, apartments for the aged, and other long-term care settings. Many residents from both cultural groups participated in the care of their fellow residents. Residents assisted other residents to the dining room, checked on others who did not appear for meals in the dining room (care as surveillance of others), and assisted in ambulation of those who were not able to walk independently. This focus on other care versus only self-care was a form of cultural congruent care that residents desired in order to maintain healthy and beneficial lifeways in an institutional setting. Culture care preservation was practiced by nursing staff as these generic care practices were integrated into professional nursing care.

Within the retirement home, both Anglo- and African-American residents desired spiritual or religious care and had some diverse aspects of such care rooted in their respective cultures. The findings of both universality and diversity within the pattern of religious or spiritual care supported Leininger's theory, which states that "culture care concepts, meanings, expressions, patterns, processes, and structural forms of care are different (diversity) and similar (toward universality) among all cultures of the world" (Leininger, 1991a, p. 45). African-American residents received care from church friends who ran errands, did banking, paid bills, did laundry, visited, and brought communion to them. Anglo-American residents received a more formal type of care from their churches, such as a minister coming to the retirement home to do a worship service or a church choir traveling to the retirement home to entertain the residents. The nurses at the retirement home practiced culture care preservation by maintaining the involvement of churches in the daily lives of both cultural groups to help residents face living in a retirement home with increasing disabilities related to aging and handicaps, and even with the prospect of death. With an increase in the numbers of elderly from both the Anglo- and African-American cultural groups being admitted to long-term care institutions, the knowledge of culture-specific care for both Anglo- and African-American elders is important to nurses who practice in these settings.

The generic care pattern of families helping their elderly relatives enhanced the health and lifeways of both Anglo- and African-American elders in the retirement home setting. Anglo-American residents received help from their spouses and/or adult children. In contrast with the Anglo-American findings, African-American spouses and children, extended family members, and nonkin who were considered family reflected the care pattern of families helping elderly residents. Grandchildren, great-grandchildren, nieces, nephews, grandnieces, and grandnephews, as well as church members or friends who were considered family and referred to as brothers, sisters, or daughters, were involved in caring for African-American elders. The nursing staff recognized the importance of family involvement in the care of residents and practiced culture care preservation to maintain culture-specific family care practices for residents from each cultural group.

The care pattern of protection was important to African-American residents but not to Anglo-American residents. Most African-American residents had left homes that were in unsafe neighborhoods and had moved in part for that reason. African-American

nursing staff recognized the importance of protective care and often accompanied African-American residents when they wanted to go outside. The nursing staff made efforts to practice culture care accommodation by negotiating to take the residents outside to sit on the small grass strip around the perimeter of the parking lot of the home. McFarland (1997) also discovered that the nursing care and the lifeways of elderly residents in the nursing home setting were less satisfying than in the apartment setting within the retirement home context. Professional nurses need to be involved in culture care repatterning as coparticipants with elders to restructure lifeway practices, care routines, and the environmental context of nursing homes (including room designs and privacy considerations). Culture care restructuring of these care-related concerns can only be accomplished by nurses assuming an advocacy role for the elderly residents and working with governmental and private agencies that provide the funding and make the rules and regulations that affect long-term care. The culture care theory, along with the ethnonursing method, assisted the researcher in this study to discover action and decision modes that were culturally specific for Anglo- and African-American elders residing in a long-term care institution.

Culture Care of Mexican-American Pregnant Women

In the late 1990s, Berry studied the generic and professional nursing care of pregnant Mexican-American women in an urban area of southern California. Cultural care values and practices related to religion, family, respect, and generic care were found to be of particular importance to the informants (Berry, 1999). Spiritual beliefs and the extended family network were major sources of strength and provided support for Mexican-American women throughout pregnancy. There was a universal pattern among both key and general Mexican-American informants that revealed a fatalistic worldview in which individuals did not have control over their lives but had faith that God would protect them. Berry discovered that assisting in the provision of religious advisors and providing time for prayer when desired in the hospital context would demonstrate culture care maintenance by preserving the cultural values and practices related to religion for this cultural group.

Involvement of the Mexican-American family in care during pregnancy was a universal cultural care value and practice, which demonstrated the care pattern of concern for pregnant women. Berry discovered that it was important that nurses practice culture care accommodation by negotiating for family participation in the care of pregnant women in both clinic and hospital contexts. Berry found that some male partners in the Mexican-American culture may want to be present during the birth process to provide care as protection and support, but may not want to be actively involved in direct care practices. Mexican-American women often also desired female family members such as mothers and sisters to be present (care as presence), which may be counter to the usual hospital labor room practice of limiting participants in the United States. Berry suggested that nurses could provide culturally congruent care through the practice of culture care accommodation by negotiating with family and staff to arrange for multiple family members to be present in the delivery area as well as on the postpartum units.

Berry discovered that the Spanish language was an important part of cultural care for Mexican-American women. As a sign of respect, bilingual nurses could practice culture care accommodation by offering a choice of languages when speaking with clients, and developing enablers with common phrases in Spanish and English with pictures could greatly facilitate communication. Health-care institutions with large Latino populations might consider culture care accommodation by offering a course on the Spanish language for the nurses.

There was little need for professional nurses to use the mode of culture care repatterning or restructuring for childbearing Mexican-American women, because the majority of generic care practices for pregnancy in this culture, such as herbal remedies, activity levels, or the wearing of metal during an eclipse, were either discovered to be health promoting or not harmful. However, Berry discovered that, although many Mexican-American foods and eating patterns are healthy, some, such as the belief that large food consumption during pregnancy is necessary, could contribute to obesity and medical or obstetrical complications. Nurses could practice culture care restructuring by helping Mexican-American women to repattern their dietary consumption by considering culturally congruent alternatives. For example, educational emphasis could be placed on the Mexican-American cultural belief that one should eat well for the health of the baby when discussing an appropriate diet for pregnancy.

Summary

The purpose of the culture care theory has been to discover culture care (along with the ethnonursing method) with the goal of using the knowledge to combine generic and professional care to provide culturally congruent nursing care (using the three modes of nursing actions and decisions) that is meaningful, safe, and beneficial to people of similar and diverse cultures worldwide (Leininger, 1991a, 1995). The clinical use of the three major care modes (culture care preservation or maintenance, culture care accommodation or negotiation, and culture care repatterning or restructuring) by nurses to guide nursing judgements, decisions, and actions is essential in order to provide culturally congruent care that is beneficial, satisfying, and meaningful to the people nurses serve. The studies of the four cultures just reviewed (Lebanese Muslim, Anglo-American, African-American, and Mexican-American) substantiate that the three modes are care-centered and based on the use of generic care (emic) knowledge along with professional care (etic) knowledge obtained from research using the culture care theory along with the ethnonursing method. This chapter has reviewed only a small selection of the culture care findings from ethnonursing research studies conducted over the past four decades. There is a wealth of additional findings of interest to practicing nurses who care for clients of all ages from diverse and similar cultural groups in many different institutional and community contexts around the world. More in-depth culture care findings along with the use of the three modes can be found in the *Journal of Transcultural Nursing* (1989 to 1998) and in the numerous books and articles by Dr. Madeleine Leininger. Nurses in clinical practice are advised to consult a list of research studies and doctoral dissertations conceptualized within the culture care theory for additional detailed nursing implications for clients from diverse cultures (Leininger, 1998, p. 24).

The Theory of Culture Care Diversity and Universality is one of the most comprehensive yet practical theories to advance transcultural and general nursing knowledge with concomitant ways for practicing nurses to establish or improve care to people. Nursing students and practicing nurses have remained the strongest advocates of the culture care theory (Leininger, 1997). The theory focuses on a long-neglected area in nursing practice—that of culture care—which is most relevant to our multicultural world now and in the new millennium.

For practicing nurses, the depiction of the Theory of Culture Care Diversity and Universality, the Sunrise Model, is a rising sun. This metaphor is particularly apt as the future of the culture care theory shines brightly indeed because it is holistic, comprehensive, and fits discovering care related to different cultures, contexts, and ages of people in familiar and naturalistic ways. Not only is the theory useful to nurses and nursing, but also to professionals in other disciplines, such as medicine and pharmacy. Healthcare practitioners in other disciplines are beginning to use this theory because they also need to become knowledgeable about and sensitive and responsible to people of diverse cultures who need care (Leininger, 1997).

References

Berry, A. (1996). *Culture care expression, meanings, and experiences of pregnant Mexican American women within Leininger's culture care theory.* (UMI No. 9628875). Ann Arbor, MI: UMI Microfilm.

Berry, A. (1999). Mexican American women's expressions of the meaning of culturally congruent prenatal care. *Journal of Transcultural Nursing 103,* 203–212.

Leininger, M. (1985). *Qualitative research methods in nursing.* Orlando, FL: Grune & Stratton, Inc.

Leininger, M. (1988). *Care: Discovery and uses in clinical and community nursing.* Detroit: Wayne State University Press.

Leininger, M. (1991a). The Theory of Culture Care Diversity and Universality. In Leininger, M. (Ed.), *Culture care diversity and universality: A theory of nursing* (pp. 5–68). New York: National League for Nursing Press.

Leininger, M. (1991b). Ethnonursing: A research method with enablers to study the theory of culture care. In Leininger, M. (Ed.), *Culture care diversity and universality: A theory of nursing* (pp. 73–118). New York: National League for Nursing Press.

Leininger, M. (1995). *Transcultural nursing: Concepts theories, research, and practice.* Blacklick, OH: McGraw-Hill College Custom Series.

Leininger, M. (1997). Overview and reflection of the theory of culture care and the Ethnonursing Research Method. *Journal of Transcultural Nursing, 8*(2), 32–51.

Leininger, M. (1998). Special research report: Dominant culture care (emic) meanings and practice findings from Leininger's theory. *Journal of Transcultural Nursing, 9*(2), 44–47.

Luna, L. (1989). *Care and cultural context of Lebanese Muslims in an urban U.S. community: An ethnographic and ethnonursing study conceptualized within Leininger's theory.* (UMI No. 9022423). Ann Arbor, MI: UMI Microfilm.

Luna, L. (1994). Care and cultural context of Lebanese Muslim immigrants with Leininger's theory. *Journal of Transcultural Nursing, 5*(2), 12–20.

McFarland, M. (1995). *Cultural care of Anglo- and African American elderly residents within the environmental context of a long-term care institution.* (UMI No. 9530568). Ann Arbor, MI: UMI Microfilm.

McFarland, M. (1997). Use of culture care theory with Anglo- and African American elders in a long-term care setting. *Nursing Science Quarterly, 10*(4), 186–192.

Zoucha, R. (1998). The experiences of Mexican-Americans receiving professional nursing care: An ethnonursing study. *Journal of Transcultural Nursing, 9*(2), 33–43.

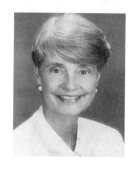
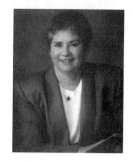

Chapter 22 Part 1

Anne Boykin and
Savina O. Schoenhofer
Nursing as Caring

❖ Introducing the Theorists

❖ Nursing as Caring: An Overview of
a General Theory of Nursing

❖ Relevance of Nursing as Caring in Various Nursing Roles

❖ Questions Nurses Ask about the Theory of Nursing as Caring

❖ Nursing as Caring: Historical Perspective and Current
Development

❖ References

**Anne Boykin and
Savina O. Schoenhofer**

INTRODUCING THE THEORISTS

Anne Boykin

Anne Boykin is dean and professor of the College of Nursing at Florida Atlantic University. She is director of the Christine E. Lynne Center for Caring, which is housed in the College of Nursing. This center was created for the purpose of humanizing care through the integration of teaching, research, and service. She has demonstrated a long-standing commitment to the advancement of knowledge in the discipline, especially regarding the phenomenon of caring.

Positions she has held within the International Association for Human Caring include: president-elect (1990 to 1993), president (1993 to 1996), and member of the nominating committee (1997 to 1999). As immediate past president, she served as co-editor of the journal *International Association for Human Caring,* from 1996 to 1999.

Her scholarly work is centered in caring as the grounding for nursing. This is evidenced in her co-authored book, *Nursing as Caring: A Model for Transforming Practice* (1993), and the book *Living a Caring-based Program.* The latter book illustrates how caring grounds the development of a nursing program from creating the environment for study through evaluation. In addition to these books, Dr. Boykin is co-editor of *Power, Politics and Public Policy: A Matter of Caring* (1994), and *Caring as Healing: Renewal through Hope.* She has also authored numerous book chapters and articles. She serves as a consultant locally, regionally, nationally, and internationally on the topic of caring.

Dr. Boykin is a graduate of Alverno College in Milwaukee, Wisconsin; she received her master's degree from Emory University in Atlanta, Georgia and her doctorate from Vanderbilt University in Nashville, Tennessee.

Savina O. Schoenhofer

Savina Schoenhofer was born the second child and eldest daughter in a family of nine children, and spent her formative years on the family cattle ranch in Kansas. She is named for her maternal grandfather, who was a classical musician in Kansas City, Missouri. She has a daughter, Carrie, and granddaughter, Emma. Schoenhofer spent 3 years in the Amazon region of Brazil in the 1960s, working as a volunteer in community development. Her initial nursing study was at Wichita State University, where she earned undergraduate and graduate degrees in nursing, psychology, and counseling. She completed a Ph.D. in educational foundations and administration at Kansas

State University in 1983. In 1990, Schoenhofer co-founded *Nightingale Songs,* an early venue for communicating the beauty of nursing in poetry and prose. In addition to her work on caring, she has written on nursing values, primary care, nursing education, support, touch, personnel management in nursing homes, and mentoring. Her career in nursing has been significantly influenced by three colleagues: Lt. Col. Ann Ashjian (Ret.), whose community nursing practice in Brazil presented an inspiring model of nursing; Marilyn E. Parker, Ph.D., a faculty colleague who mentored her in the idea of nursing as a discipline, the academic role in higher education, and the world of nursing theories and theorists; and Anne Boykin, Ph.D., who introduced her to caring as a substantive field of nursing study.

NURSING AS CARING: AN OVERVIEW OF THE GENERAL NURSING THEORY

by Anne Boykin and Savina O. Schoenhofer

This chapter is intended as an overview of the Theory of Nursing as Caring, a general theory, framework, or disciplinary view of nursing. A general theory or framework of nursing presents an abstract, integrated, comprehensive picture of nursing as a practiced discipline. The Theory of Nursing as Caring offers a view that permits a broad, encompassing understanding of any and all situations of nursing practice (Boykin & Schoenhofer, 1993). This theory serves as an organizing framework for nursing scholars in the various roles of practitioner, researcher, administrator, teacher, and developer.

Initially, we will present the theory in its most abstract form, addressing assumptions and key themes. We will then discuss the meaning of the theory in relation to practice and other nursing roles. In the second part of this chapter, Danielle Linden further describes the theory by illustrating its use as a guide to practice.

Assumptions

Certain fundamental beliefs about what it means to be human underlie the Theory of Nursing as Caring. These assumptions, which will be illustrated later, reflect a particular set of values that provide a basis for understanding and explicating the meaning of nursing, listed as follows:

1. Persons are caring by virtue of their humanness.
2. Persons are whole and complete in the moment.

3. Persons live caring from moment to moment.
4. Personhood is a way of living grounded in caring.
5. Personhood is enhanced through participation in nurturing relationships with caring others.
6. Nursing is both a discipline and a profession.

Caring

Caring is an altruistic, active expression of love, and is the intentional and embodied recognition of value and connectedness. Caring is not the unique province of nursing. However, as a discipline and a profession, nursing uniquely focuses on caring as its central value, its primary interest, and the direct intention of its practice. The full meaning of caring cannot be restricted to a definition, but is illuminated in the experience of caring and in reflection on that experience.

> The focus of nursing . . . is person as living in caring and growing in caring.

Key Themes

Focus and Intention of Nursing

Disciplines as identifiable entities or "branches of knowledge" grow from the holistic "tree of knowledge" as need and purpose develop. A discipline is a community of scholars with a particular perspective on the world and what it means to be in the world. The disciplinary community represents a value system that is expressed in its unique focus on knowledge and practice. The *focus of nursing,* from the perspective of the Theory of Nursing as Caring, is person as living in caring and growing in caring. The general *intention of nursing* as a practiced discipline is nurturing persons living caring and growing in caring.

Nursing Situation

The practice of nursing, and thus the practical knowledge of nursing, lives in the context of person-with-person caring. The *nursing situation* involves particular values, intentions, and actions of two or more persons choosing to live a nursing relationship. Nursing situation is understood to mean the shared lived experience in which caring between nurse and nursed enhances personhood. Nursing is created in the "caring between." All knowledge of nursing is created and understood within the nursing situation. Any single nursing situation has the potential to illuminate the depth and complexity of nursing knowledge. Nursing situations are best communicated through aesthetic media to preserve the lived meaning of the situation and the openness of the situation as text. Storytelling, poetry, graphic arts, and dance are effective modes of representing the lived experience and allowing for reflection and creativity in advancing understanding.

Personhood

Personhood is understood to mean living grounded in caring. From the perspective of the Theory of Nursing as Caring, personhood is the universal human call. A profound understanding of personhood communicates the paradox of person-as-person and person-in-communion all at once.

Call for Nursing

"A call for nursing is a call for acknowledgment and affirmation of the person living caring in specific ways in the immediate situation" (Boykin & Schoenhofer, 1993, p. 24). *Calls for nursing* are calls for nurturance through personal expressions of caring. Calls for nursing originate within persons as they live out caring uniquely, expressing personally meaningful dreams and aspirations for growing in caring. Calls for nursing are individually relevant ways of saying "Know me as caring person in the moment and be with me as I try to live fully who I truly am." Intentionality and authentic presence open the nurse to hearing calls for nursing. Because calls for nursing are unique situated personal expressions, they cannot be predicted, as in a "diagnosis." Nurses develop sensitivity and expertise in hearing calls through intention, experience, study, and reflection in a broad range of human situations.

Nursing Response

As an expression of nursing, "caring is the intentional and authentic presence of the nurse with another who is recognized as living [in] caring and growing in caring" (Boykin & Schoenhofer, 1993, p. 25). The nurse enters the nursing situation with the intentional commitment of knowing the other as a caring person, and in that knowing, acknowledging, affirming, and celebrating the person as caring. The nursing response is a specific expression of caring nurturance to sustain and enhance the "other" as he or she lives caring and grows in caring in the situation of concern. Nursing responses to calls for caring evolve as nurses clarify their understandings of calls

> The "caring between" is the source and ground of nursing.

through presence and dialogue. Nursing responses are uniquely created for the moment, and cannot be predicted or applied as preplanned protocols. Sensitivity and skill in creating unique and effective ways of communicating caring are developed through intention, experience, study, and reflection in a broad range of human situations.

The "Caring Between"

The "caring between" is the source and ground of nursing. It is the loving relation into which nurse and nursed enter and cocreate by living the intention to care. Without the loving relation of the caring between, unidirectional activity or reciprocal exchange can occur, but nursing in its fullest sense does not occur. It is in the context of the *caring between* that personhood is enhanced, each expressing self and recognizing the other as caring person.

Lived Meaning of Nursing as Caring

Abstract presentations of assumptions and themes lay the groundwork and provide an orienting point. However, the lived meaning of nursing as caring can best be understood by the study of a nursing situation. The following poem is one nurse's expression of the meaning of nursing, situated in one particular experience of nursing and linked to a general conception of nursing.

I CARE FOR HIM

My hands are moist,
My heart is quick,
My nerves are taut,
He's in the next room,
I care for him.

The room is tense,
It's anger-filled,
The air seems thick,

I'm with him now,
I care for him.

Time goes slowly by,
As our fears subside,
I can sense his calm,
He softens now,
I care for him.

His eyes meet mine,
Unable to speak,
I feel his trust,
I open my heart,
I care for him.

It's time to leave.
Our bond is made,
Unspoken thoughts,
But understood,
I care for him!

—J. M. Collins (1993)

Each encounter—each nursing experience—brings with it the unknown. In Collins's reflections, he shares a story of practice that illuminates the opportunity to live and grow in caring.

In the nursing situation that inspired this poem, the nurse and nursed live caring uniquely. Initially, the nurse experiences the familiar human dilemma, aware of separateness while choosing connectedness as he responds to a yet unknown call for nursing: ["My] hands are moist,/my heart is quick/my nerves are taut . . . I care for him." As he enters the situation and encounters the patient as person, he is able to "let go" of his presumptive knowing of the patient as "angry." The nurse enters with the guiding perspective that all persons are caring. This allows him to see past the "anger-filled" room and to be "with him"

your thoughts

(Stanza 2). As they connect through their humanness, the beauty and wholeness of other is uncovered and nurtured. By living caring moment to moment, hope emerges and fear subsides. Through this experience, both nurse and nursed live and grow in their understanding and expressions of caring.

In the first stanza, the nurse prepares to enter the nursing relationship with the formed intention of offering caring in authentic presence. Perhaps he has heard a report that the person he is about to encounter is a "difficult patient" and this is a part of his awareness; however, his nursing intention to care reminds him that he and his patient are, above all, caring persons. In the second stanza, the nurse enters the room, experiences the challenge that his intention to nurse has presented, and responds to the call for authentic presence and caring: "I'm with him now,/I care for him." Patterns of knowing are called into play as the nurse brings together intuitive, personal knowing, empirical knowing, and the ethical knowing that it is right to offer care, creating the integrated understanding of aesthetic knowing that enables him to act on his nursing intention (Boykin, Parker, & Schoenhofer, 1994; Carper, 1978). Mayeroff's (1971) caring ingredients of courage, trust, and alternating rhythm are clearly evident.

Clarity of the call for nursing emerges as the nurse begins to understand that this particular man in this particular moment is calling to be known as a uniquely caring person, a person of value, worthy of respect and regard. The nurse listens intently and recognizes the unadorned honesty that sounds angry and demanding and is a personal expression of a heartfelt desire to be truly known and worthy of care. The nurse responds with steadfast presence and caring, communicated in his way of being and of doing. The caring ingredient of hope is drawn forth as the man softens and the nurse takes notice.

In the fourth stanza, the "caring between" develops and personhood is enhanced as dreams and aspirations for growing in caring are realized: "His eyes meet mine . . . I open my heart." In the last stanza, the nursing situation is completed in linear time. But each one, nurse and nursed, goes forward newly affirmed and celebrated as caring person, and the nursing situation continues to be a source of living caring and growing in caring.

Assumptions in the Context of the Nursing Situation

In this poem, the power of the basic assumption that all persons are caring by virtue of their humanness enabled the nurse to find the courage to live his intentions. The idea that persons are whole and complete in the moment permits the nurse to accept conflicting feelings and to be open to the nursed as a person, not merely as an entity with a diagnosis and superficially understood behavior. The nurse demonstrated an understanding of the assumption that persons live caring from moment to moment, striving to know self and other as caring in the moment with a growing repertoire of ways of expressing caring. Personhood, a way of living grounded in caring that can be enhanced in relationship with caring other, comes through in that the nurse is successfully living his commitment to caring in the face of difficulty and in the mutuality and connectedness that emerged in the situation. The assumption that nursing is both a discipline and a profession is affirmed as the nurse draws on a set of values and a developed knowledge of nursing as caring to actively offer his presence in service to the nursed.

> Nursing is . . . always unfolding and guided by intention.

RELEVANCE OF NURSING AS CARING IN VARIOUS NURSING ROLES

Nursing Practice

The commitment of the nurse practicing nursing as caring is to nurture persons living caring and growing in caring. This implies that the nurse comes to know the other as caring person in the moment. "Difficult to care" situations are those that demonstrate the extent of knowledge and commitment needed to nurse effectively. An everyday understanding of the meaning of caring is obviously challenged when the nurse is presented with someone for whom it is difficult to care. In these extreme (though not unusual) situations, a task-oriented, non–discipline-based concept of nursing may be adequate to assure the completion of certain treatment and surveillance techniques. Still, in our eyes that is an insufficient response—it certainly is not the nursing we advocate. The Theory of Nursing as Caring calls upon the nurse to reach deep within a well-developed knowledge base that has been structured using all available patterns of knowing, grounded in the obligations inherent in the commitment to know persons as caring. These patterns of knowing may develop knowledge as intuition; scientifically quantifiable data emerging from research; and related knowledge from a variety of disciplines, ethical beliefs, and many other types of knowing. All knowledge held by the nurse that may be relevant to understanding the situation at hand is drawn forward and integrated into practice in particular nursing situations (aesthetic knowing). Although the degree of challenge presented from situation to situation varies, the commitment to know self and other as caring persons is steadfast.

The Nursing as Caring theory, grounded in the assumption that all persons are caring, has as its focus a general call to nurture persons as they live caring uniquely and grow as caring persons. The challenge for nursing, then, is not to discover what is missing, weakened, or needed in another, but to come to know the other as caring person and to nurture that person in situation-specific, creative ways. We no longer understand nursing as a "process" in the sense of a complex sequence of predictable acts resulting in some predetermined desirable end product. Nursing, we believe, is inherently a process, in the sense that it is always unfolding and guided by intention.

The nurse practicing within the caring context described here will most often be interfacing with the health-care system in two ways: first, communicating nursing so that it can be understood; and second, articulating nursing service as a unique contribution within the system in such a way that the system itself grows to support nursing.

Nursing Administration

From the viewpoint of Nursing as Caring, the nurse administrator makes decisions through a lens in which the focus of nursing is on nurturing persons as they live caring and grow in caring. All activities in the practice of nursing administration are grounded in a concern for creating, maintaining, and supporting an environment in which calls for nursing are heard and nurturing responses are given. From this point of view, the expectation arises that nursing administrators participate in shaping a culture that evolves from the values articulated within Nursing as Caring.

Although often perceived to be "removed" from the direct care of the nursed, the nursing administrator is intimately involved in multiple nursing situations simultaneously, hearing calls for nursing and participating in responses to these calls. As calls for nursing are known, one of the unique responses of the nursing administrator is to enter the world of the nursed either directly or indirectly, to understand special calls when they occur, and to assist in securing the resources needed by each nurse to nurture persons as they live and grow in caring (Boykin & Schoenhofer, 1993). All administrative activities

should be approached with this goal in mind. Here, the nurse administrator reflects on the obligations inherent in the role in relation to the nursed. The presiding moral basis for determining right action is the belief that all persons are caring. Frequently, the nurse administrator may enter the world of the nursed through the stories of colleagues who are assuming another role, such as that of nurse manager. Policy formulation and implementation allow for the consideration of unique situations. The nursing administrator assists others within the organization to understand the focus of nursing and to secure the resources necessary to achieve the goals of nursing.

Nursing Education

From the perspective of Nursing as Caring, all structures and activities should reflect the fundamental assumption that persons are caring by virtue of their humanness. Other assumptions and values reflected in the education program include knowing the person as whole and complete in the moment and living caring uniquely; understanding that personhood is a way of living grounded in caring and is enhanced through participation in nurturing relationships with caring others; and, finally, affirming nursing as a discipline and profession.

The curriculum, the foundation of the education program, asserts the focus and domain of nursing as nurturing persons living caring and growing in caring:

> All activities of the program of study are directed toward developing, organizing, and communicating nursing knowledge, that is, knowledge of nurturing persons living caring and growing in caring.
>
> The model for organizational design of nursing education is analogous to the dancing circle. . . . Members of the circle include administrators, faculty, colleagues, students, staff, community, and the nursed. What this circle represents is the commitment of each dancer to understand and support the study of the discipline of nursing. The role of administrator in the circle is more clearly understood when the origin of the word is reflected upon. The term "administrator" derives from the Latin *ad ministrare,* to serve (according to Webster's, cited in Guralnik, 1976). This definition connotes the idea of rendering service. Administrators within the circle are by nature of [their] role obligated to ministering, to securing, and to providing resources needed by faculty, students, and staff to meet program objectives. Faculty, students, and administrators

dance together in the study of nursing. Faculty support an environment that values the uniqueness of each person and sustains each person's unique way of living and growing in caring. This process requires trust, hope, courage, and patience. Because the purpose of nursing education is to study the discipline and practice of nursing, the nursed must be in the circle. The community created is that of persons living caring in the moment and growing in personhood, each person valued as special and unique. (Boykin & Schoenhofer, 1993, pp. 73–74)

In teaching Nursing as Caring, faculty assist students to come to know, appreciate, and celebrate both self and "other" as caring persons. Students, as well as faculty, are in a continual search to discover greater meaning of caring as uniquely expressed in nursing. Examples of a nursing education program based on values similar to those of Nursing as Caring are illustrated in the book *Living a Caring-based Program* (Boykin, 1994).

Nursing Research and Development

The roles of researcher and developer in nursing take on a particular focus when guided by the Theory of Nursing as Caring. The assumptions and focus of nursing explicated in the theory provide an organizing value system that suggests certain key questions and methods. Research questions lead to exploration and illumination of patterns of living caring personally (Schoenhofer, Bingham, & Hutchins, 1998) and in nursing practice (Schoenhofer & Boykin, 1998b). Dialogue, description, and innovations in interpretative approaches characterize research methods. De-velopment of systems and structures (e.g., policy formulation, information management, nursing delivery, and reimbursement) to support nursing necessitates sustained efforts in reframing and refocusing familiar systems as well as creating novel configurations (Schoenhofer, 1995; Schoenhofer & Boykin, 1998a).

QUESTIONS NURSES ASK ABOUT THE THEORY OF NURSING AS CARING

How Does the Nurse Come to Know Self and Other as Caring Persons?

Nursing practice guided by the Theory of Nursing as Caring entails living the commitment to know self and other as living caring in the moment and growing in caring. Living this commitment requires intention, formal study, and reflection on experience. Mayeroff's (1971) caring ingredients offer a useful starting point for the nurse committed to knowing self and other as caring persons. These ingredients include knowing, alternating rhythm, honesty, courage, trust, patience, humility, and hope. Roach's (1992) five C's—commitment, confidence, conscience, competence, and compassion—provide another conceptual framework that is helpful in providing a language of caring. Coming to know self as caring is facilitated by:

- Trusting in self; freeing self up to become what one can truly become, and valuing self.
- Learning to let go, to transcend—to let go of problems, difficulties, in order to remember the interconnectedness that enables us to know self

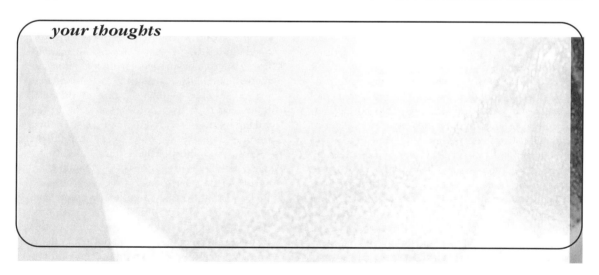

your thoughts

and other as living caring, even in suffering and in seeking relief from suffering.

- Being open and humble enough to experience and know self to be at home with one's feelings.
- Continuously calling to consciousness that each person is living caring in the moment and we are each developing uniquely in our becoming.
- Taking time to fully experience our humanness, for one can only truly understand in another what one can understand in self.
- Finding hope in the moment.

(Schoenhofer & Boykin, 1993, pp. 85–86)

Must I Like My Patients to Nurse Them?

The simple answer to this question is "yes." In order to know the other as caring, the nurse must find some basis for respectful human connection with the person. Does this mean that the nurse must like everything about the person, including personal life choices? Perhaps not; however, the nurse as nurse is not called upon to judge the "other," only to care for the other. A concern with judging or censuring another's actions is a distraction from the real purpose for nursing—that is, coming to know the other as caring person, as one with dreams and aspirations of growing in caring, and responding to calls for caring in ways that nurture personhood.

What about Nursing a Person for Whom It Is Difficult to Care?

Related to the previous dilemma, this question presents the crucible within which one's commitment to the assumptions and themes of Nursing as Caring is tested to the limit. The underlying question is, "Does the person to be nursed deserve or merit my care?" Again, as before, the simple answer is "yes." All persons are caring, even when not all chosen actions of the person live up to the ideal to which we are all called by virtue of our humanness. In discussions of hypothetical situations involving child molesters, serial killers, and even political figures who have attempted mass destruction and racial annihilation, certain ethical systems permit and even call for making judgements. However, when such a person as described above presents to the nurse for care, the nursing ethic of caring supersedes all other values. The Theory of Nursing as Caring asserts that it is *only* through recognizing and responding to the other as a caring person that nursing is created and personhood enhanced in that nursing situation. This question and the previous one make it clear that caring is

much more than "sweetness and light"; caring effectively in "difficult to care" situations is the most challenging prospect a nurse can face. It is only with sustained intention, commitment, study, and reflection that the nurse is able to offer nursing in these situations. Falling short in one's commitment does not necessitate self-deprecation nor warrant condemnation by others; rather, it presents an opportunity to care for self and other and to grow in personhood. Making real the potential of such an opportunity calls for seeing with clarity, reaffirming commitment, and engaging in study and reflection, individually and in concert with caring others.

Is it Impossible to Nurse Someone Who Is in an Unconscious or Altered State of Awareness?

The key point here is the "caring between" that *is* the nursing creation:

> When nursing a person who is unconscious, the nurse lives the commitment to know the other as caring person. How is that commitment lived? It requires that all ways of knowing be brought into action. The nurse must make self as caring person available to the one nursed. The fullness of the nurse as caring person is called forth. This requires use of Mayeroff's caring ingredients: the alternating rhythm of knowing about the other and knowing the other directly through authentic presence and attunement; the hope and courage to risk opening self to one who cannot communicate verbally, patiently trusting in self to understand the other's mode of living caring in the moment; honest humility as one brings all that one knows and remains open to learning from the other. The nurse attuned to the other as person might for example experience the vulnerability of the person who lies unconscious from surgical anesthetic or traumatic injury. In that vulnerability, the nurse recognizes that the one nursed is living caring in humility, hope, and trust. Instead of responding to the vulnerability, merely "taking care of" the other, the nurse practicing Nursing as Caring might respond by honoring the other's humility, by participating in the other's hopefulness, by steadfast trustworthiness. Creating caring in the moment in this situation might come from the nurse resonating with past and present experiences of vulnerability. Connected to this form of personal knowing might be an ethical knowing that power as a reciprocal of vulnera-

bility can develop undesirable status differential in the nurse-patient role relationship. As the nurse sifts through a myriad of empirical data, the most significant information emerges—this is a *person* with whom I am called to care. Ethical knowing again merges with other pathways as the nurse forms the decision to go beyond vulnerability and engage the other as caring person, rather than as helpless object of another's concern. Aesthetic knowing comes in the praxis of caring, in living chosen ways of honoring humility, joining in hope, and demonstrating trustworthiness in the moment (Schoenhofer & Boykin, 1993, pp. 86–87).

How Does Nursing Process Fit with This Theory?

Process, as it is understood in the term "nursing process," connotes a systematic and sequential series of steps resulting in a predetermined, specifiable product. Nursing process, as introduced into nursing by Orlando (1961), is a linear stepwise decision-making tool based on rational analysis of empirical data, known in other disciplines as the problem-solving process, and is a key structural theme of many nursing theories developed in past decades. Proponents of the Theory of Nursing as Caring view nursing not as a process with an endpoint, but as an ongoing process; that is, as dynamic and unfolding, guided by intention although not directed by a preenvisioned outcome or product. Nursing responses of care arise in aesthetic knowing, the creative and evolving patterns of appreciation and understanding, in the context of a shared lived experience of caring. Instead of preselected and quantifiable outcomes, the value of nursing to the nursed and to others is that which is experienced as valuable arising in and evolving through the "caring between" of the nursing situation. Much of that value is

neither measurable nor empirically verifiable. That which is measurable and empirically verifiable is relevant in the situation, however, and may be called upon at any time to contribute to and through the nurse's empirical knowing. Information which the nurse has available becomes knowledge within the nursing situation. Knowing the person directly is what guides the selection and patterning of relevant points of factual information in a nursing situation. That is, any fact or set of facts from nursing research or related bodies of information can be considered for relevance and drawn into the supporting knowledge base. This

knowledge base remains open and evolving as the nurse employs an alternating rhythm of scanning and considering facts for relevance while remaining grounded in the nursing situation. (Schoenhofer & Boykin, 1993, pp. 89–90)

In addition to empirical knowing, knowing for nursing purposes also requires personal knowing, including intuition and ethical knowing, all converging in aesthetic knowing within each unique nursing situation.

How Practical Is This Theory in the Real World of Nursing?

Nurses are frequently heard to say they have no time for caring, given the demands of the role. All nursing roles are lived out in the context of a contemporary environment. At the beginning of the twenty-first century the environment for practice, administration, education, and research is fraught with many challenges. Some of these challenges are:

- technological advancement and proliferation that can promote routinization and depersonalization on the part of the caregiver as well as the one seeking care;
- demands for immediate and measurable outcomes that favor a focus on the simplistic and the superficial;
- organizational and occupational configurations that tend to promote fragmentation and alienation; and
- economic focus and profit motive ("time is money") as the apparent prime institutional value.

Nurses express frustration when evaluating their own caring efforts against an idealized, rule-driven conception of caring. Practice guided by the Theory of Nursing as Caring reflects the assumption that caring is created from moment to moment and does not demand idealized patterns of caring. Caring in the moment (and moment to moment) occurs when the nurse is living a committed intention to know and nurture the other as caring person. No predetermined ideal amount of time or form of dialogue is prescribed. A simple example of living this intention to care is the nurse who goes to the IV or the monitor *through* the person, rather than going directly to the technology, and failing to acknowledge the person. When the nurse goes *to* the person, it becomes clear that the use of technology is one way the nurse expresses caring *for the person*. In proposing his model of machine technologies and caring in nursing, Locsin (1995) distinguishes between mere technological competence and technological competence as an intentional expression of caring in nursing. Simply avowing an intention to care is not sufficient; the committed intention to care is supported by serious study of caring and ongoing reflection if nurses are to communicate caring effectively from moment to moment. As Locsin (1995, p. 203) so aptly states:

[A]s people seriously involved in giving care know, there are various ways of expressing caring. Professional nurses will continue to find meaning in their technological caring competencies, expressed intentionally and authentically, to know another as a whole person. Through the harmonious coexistence of machine technology and caring technology the practice of nursing is transformed into an experience of caring.

The nurse administrator is subject to challenges similar to those of the practitioner and often walks a very precarious tightrope between direct caregivers and corporate executives. The nurse administrator, whether at the executive or managerial level of the organization chart, is held accountable for "customer satisfaction" as well as for "the bottom line." Nurses who "move up the executive ladder" may be suspected of disassociating from their nursing colleagues, on one hand, and of not being sufficiently cognizant of the harsh realities of fiscal constraint, on the other hand. Administrative practice guided by the assumptions and themes of Nursing as Caring can enhance eloquence in articulating the connection between caregiver and institutional mission: the person seeking care. Nursing practice leaders who recognize their care role, indirect as it may be, are in an excellent position to act on their committed intention to promote caring environments. Participating in rigorous negotiations for fiscal, material, and human resources and for improvements in nursing practice calls for special skill on the part of the nurse administrator, skill in recognizing, acknowledging, and celebrating the other (e.g., CEO, CFO, nurse manager, or staff nurse) as a caring person. The nurse administrator who understands the caring ingredients (Mayeroff, 1971) recognizes that caring is neither soft nor fixed in its expression. A developed understanding of the caring ingredients helps the nurse administrator mobilize the courage to be honest with self and "other," to trust patience, and to value alternating rhythm with true humility while living a hope-filled commitment to knowing self and "other" as caring persons.

Nurse educators guided by Nursing as Caring struggle with similar challenges. Mentoring students as colearners and creating caring learning environments while concomitantly accepting responsibility for summative evaluation calls for the integrated foundation provided by the guiding intention to know and nurture persons as caring. This intention helps the nurse to transcend limiting historical practices while creatively inventing ways to inspire. The humility of unknowing, joined with courage and hope, helps the nurse educator to guide the study of nursing as a commitment to knowing and nurturing persons as caring. Many nurse educators are struck with the incongruity of instilling a commitment to nursing as an opportunity to care through means that seem to view the student as an object and the discipline as a preexisting set of operating rules. Nursing education practiced from the perspective of Nursing as Caring opens the way for faculty to truly value the discipline and the student.

Nurses in research and development roles carry out their work facing environmental pressures similar to those experienced by the practitioner, the administrator, and the educator. Research and development in nursing require disciplinary-congruent values and perspective, freely ranging thought, openness, and creativity. Institutional systems and structures often seem to favor values and practices that are incongruent with the values of the discipline of nursing, patterned thought, rigidity, and conformity. Researchers and developers guided by the assumptions and themes of Nursing as Caring are empowered to create novel methods in the search for understanding and meaning and to articulate effectively the value, purpose, and relevance of their work.

NURSING AS CARING: HISTORICAL PERSPECTIVE AND CURRENT DEVELOPMENT

The Theory of Nursing as Caring developed as an outgrowth of the curriculum development work in the College of Nursing at Florida Atlantic University, where both authors were among the faculty group revising the caring-based curriculum. When the revised curriculum was in place, each of us recognized the potential and even the necessity of continuing to develop and structure ideas and themes toward a comprehensive expression of the meaning and purpose of nursing as a discipline and a profession. The point of departure was the acceptance that caring is the end, rather than the means, of nursing, and the intention of nursing rather than merely its instrument. This work led to the statement of focus of nursing as "nurturing persons living caring and growing in caring." Further work to identify foundational assumptions about nursing clarified the idea of the nursing situation, a shared lived experience in which the caring between enhances personhood, with personhood understood as living grounded in caring. The clarified focus and the idea of the nursing situation are the key themes that draw forth the meaning of the assumptions underlying the theory and permit the practical understanding of nursing as both a discipline and a profession. As critique of the theory and study of nursing situations progressed, the notion of nursing being primarily concerned with health was seen as limiting, and we now understand nursing to be concerned with human living.

Three bodies of work significantly influenced the initial development of Nursing as Caring. Roach's (1987/1992) basic thesis that caring is the human mode of being was incorporated into the most basic assumption of the theory. We view Paterson and Zderad's (1988) existential phenomenological Theory of Humanistic Nursing as the historical antecedent of Nursing as Caring. Seminal ideas such as "the between," "call for nursing," "nursing response," and "personhood" served as substantive and structural bases for our conceptualization of Nursing as Caring. Mayeroff's (1971) work, *On Caring,* provided a language that facilitated the recognition and description of the practical meaning of caring in nursing situations. In addition to the work of these thinkers, both authors are long-standing members of the community of nursing scholars whose study focuses on caring, and who are supported and undoubtedly influenced in many subtle ways by the members of this community and their work.

Fledgling forms of the Theory of Nursing as Caring were first published in 1990 and 1991, with the first complete exposition of the theory presented at a theory conference in 1992 (Boykin & Schoenhofer, 1990, 1991; Schoenhofer & Boykin, 1993), followed by the work, *Nursing as Caring: A Model for Transforming Practice,* published in 1993 (Boykin & Schoenhofer, 1993).

Research and development efforts at this writing are concentrated on expanding the language of caring by uncovering personal ways of living caring in everyday life (Schoenhofer, Bingham, & Hutchins, 1998), reconceptualization of nursing outcomes as "value experienced in nursing situations" (Boykin & Schoenhofer, 1997; Schoenhofer & Boykin, 1998a, 1998b), and in consultation with graduate students, nursing faculties, and health-care agencies who are using aspects of the theory to ground research, teaching, and practice.

References

Boykin, A. (Ed.). (1994). *Living a caring-based program.* New York: National League for Nursing Press.

Boykin, A., Parker, M. E., & Schoenhofer, S. O. (1994). Aesthetic knowing grounded in an explicit conception of nursing. *Nursing Science Quarterly, 7,* 158-161.

Boykin, A., & Schoenhofer, S. O. (1990). Caring in nursing: Analysis of extant theory. *Nursing Science Quarterly, 3*(4), 149-155.

Boykin, A., & Schoenhofer, S. O. (1991). Story as link between nursing practice, ontology, epistemology. *Image, 23,* 245-248.

Boykin, A., & Schoenhofer, S. O. (1993). *Nursing as caring: A model for transforming practice.* New York: National League for Nursing Press.

Boykin, A., & Schoenhofer, S. O. (1997). Reframing outcomes: Enhancing personhood. *Advanced Practice Nursing Quarterly, 3*(1), 60-65.

Carper, B. A. (1978). Fundamental patterns of knowing in nursing. *Advances in Nursing Science, 1*(1), 13-24.

Collins, J. M. (1993). I care for him. *Nightingale Songs, 2*(4), 3.

Gaut, D., & Boykin, A. (Eds.). 1994. Caring as healing: Renewal through hope. New York: National League for Nursing Press.

Guralnik, D. (1976). Webser's new world dictionary of the American language. Cleveland: William Collings & World Publishing Co.

Locsin, R. C. (1995). Machine technologies and caring in nursing. *Image, 27,* 201-203.

Mayeroff, M. (1971). *On caring.* New York: Harper & Row.

Orlando, I. (1961). *The dynamic nurse-patient-relationship: Function, process and principles.* New York: G. P. Putnam's Sons.

Paterson, J. G., & Zderad, L. T. (1988). *Humanistic nursing.* New York: National League for Nursing Press.

Roach, S. (1987/1992). *The human act of caring.* Ottawa, Canada: Canadian Hospital Association.

Roach, M. S. (1992). *The human act of caring: A blueprint for the health professions* (rev. ed.). Ottawa, Canada: Canadian Hospital Association Press.

Schoenhofer, S. O. (1995). Rethinking primary care: Connections to nursing. *Advances in Nursing Science, 17*(4), 12-21.

Schoenhofer, S. O., Bingham, V., & Hutchins, G. C. (1998). Giving of oneself on another's behalf: The phenomenology of everyday caring. *International Journal for Human Caring, 2*(1), 23-29.

Schoenhofer, S. O., & Boykin, A. (1993). Nursing as caring: An emerging general theory of nursing. In Parker, M. E. (Ed.), *Patterns of nursing theories in practice* (pp. 83-92). New York: National League for Nursing Press.

Schoenhofer, S. O., & Boykin, A. (1998a). The value of caring experienced in nursing. *International Journal for Human Caring, 2*(3), 9-15.

Schoenhofer, S. O., & Boykin, A. (1998b). Discovering the value of nursing in high-technology environments: Outcomes revisited. *Holistic Nursing Practice, 12*(4), 31-39.

Chapter 22 Part 2

The Lived Experience of Nursing as Caring

Danielle Linden

Anne Boykin and Savina Schoenhofer have developed a theory of nursing that "suspends the traditional past" and offers nursing a new lens with which to view "other"—the one nursed. This nontraditional perspective transforms the way one comes to know "other" and creates an endless array of new possibilities for nursing.

I have been invited to share the experience of nursing from the theoretical perspective of the book *Nursing as Caring: A Model for Transforming Practice*. The application of Nursing as Caring in my practice has been fulfilling both professionally and personally. Professionally, every day poses a new challenge. Nursing as Caring requires the nurse to use many different ways of knowing to come to know "other" in the fullness of one's existence. Each domain contains a vast amount of knowledge. The nurse must be knowledgeable of each and artfully apply this knowledge in an effort to transcend the physical boundaries of the human body to come to know "other's" complex existence. Personally, this effort is rewarded by enhancing who I am as a person. I grow with each encounter.

> Nursing as Caring guides the nursing situation, serving as a framework in my patient encounters.

CURRENT PRACTICE AS AN ADVANCED PRACTICE NURSE

The application of the theory of Nursing as Caring is a unique practice perspective. Nursing as Caring guides the use of knowledge generated from within and borrowed from other disciplines. The theory embodies all of the knowledge that is brought into the nursing situation and all that is generated therein. It is through this theory that I have come to know new possibilities for nursing practice.

As an Advanced Registered Nurse Practitioner (ARNP) in family practice, I see patients in a primary care setting. Grounded in Nursing as Caring, I borrow knowledge from other disciplines, such as pathophysiology, microbiology, pharmacology, and philosophy, and use this knowledge to come to know "other" in each moment of our visit. Some patients have acute needs that need to be addressed immediately. Some of them have chronic problems that require maintenance therapy. All of them need to be recognized as holistic and complex human beings with a unique existence in this world, living in car-

ing and growing in caring. I am a facilitator of this process and risk entering into another's world with the intent of living caring in that nursing situation.

I enjoy my role as a primary care provider. In practice, I emphasize wellness and prevention. Nursing as Caring guides the nursing situation, serving as a framework in my patient encounters. I walk in the room with the intent of coming to know "other" as a holistic being with a body, mind, and spirit. The call for nursing then begins to unfold and reveals itself to me. My presence with "other" is authentic and there exists a genuine responsiveness to come to know "other." Authentic presence allows one to know that which is not spoken. A person can speak one's mind. A physical assessment can reveal an ailment. The spirit, however, must be attended to as well. Everything is revealed in one's spirit. When you are in authentic presence with "other," the call for nursing unfolds before you. These are the profound encounters that never leave you.

> Authentic presence allows one to know that which is not spoken.

Then there are the more frequent encounters where reflection becomes a useful tool to uncover the deeper meaning behind these chance nursing situations. Sometimes the patients' call for nursing is physical. I recognize it and treat accordingly. Reflection allows me to answer these questions: Was I nursing? What did I do differently from another healthcare provider? My answer is the perspective from which I practice. I walked into the room with the willingness to come to know "other," whatever may have been revealed in that moment. It was the way I touched the patient, my tone of voice, my unhurried pace, and my smile—all the tools I use to convey to "other" that I am here for you and I care about you. The goal is to enhance "other" as he or she live and grow in caring. Boykin and Schoenhofer's theory puts forth a framework for reflection: Reflection, in their view, serves as a form of "personal theorizing about caring experiences, trusting that each person will examine the content of those experiences as a sequence of more or less meaningful events—meaningful both in themselves and in the patterns of their occurrence" (Boykin & Schoenhofer, 1993, p. xxiii).

I take time regularly to reflect upon the profound and not so profound nursing situations in my life. Reflection uncovers those hidden meanings that are not readily apparent in the moment. It is also a time for self-growth and validation—a process of coming to know self and others as caring persons.

APPLICATION OF THE THEORY

Another form of reflection is the sharing of nursing situations with others. There are many different ways one can present a nursing situation, such as case presentations, poems, projects, and various other art forms. When one shares a nursing situation with others, new possibilities for knowing "other" unfold exponentially. Each practitioner brings the wealth of his or her education and experiences. New revelations come to life.

I would like to share with you a nursing situation presented in the traditional medical model of case presentation and then in the form of a story from a nursing perspective grounded in the Nursing as Caring theory. It is my intent that through comparison, the lived experience of both of these models will make clearer the difference between practice perspectives.

Nursing Situation: As a Case Presentation

The following is a case presentation of a person I had the privilege of caring for.

E. S. was a 76-year-old white female patient who came to the office with the complaint of a lump in her abdomen. By her own admission, she remarked that she did not like going to the doctor and had neglected to have any checkups in quite a few years. A comprehensive history and physical exam was unremarkable with the exception of her abdomen, which revealed a small, palpable, nontender mass in the right lower quadrant.

I ordered blood tests, all of which were unremarkable with the exception of the Ca125, which was

625, well above normal parameters. My suspicion for ovarian cancer was confirmed.

Three days after our initial visit, I asked her to return to the office so we could discuss the results. She did so, and with her, she brought a gift. She said I had done so much for her in our visit, she wanted to share with me a precious gift the Lord had given her—her voice. There, in the office, I sat with her labs in my lap as she serenaded me with a song. I don't remember the name of the song, but the verse told me Jesus was calling her home and she was not afraid.

When she was done, we discussed the findings. I advised her that although the blood test was not diagnostic, the possibility of cancer did exist and she needed to see an oncological gynecologist. Tears were shed and hugs exchanged.

After a month of invasive testing at the family's prompting, exploratory surgery and biopsies confirmed the diagnosis of ovarian cancer with extensive metastasis. The patient underwent a total abdominal hysterectomy and bilateral salapingo-oophorectomy with debulking, and died shortly thereafter.

There is a lot one can learn from a case presentation such as this one, but it does not reflect the essence of what occurred between the nurse and the one nursed. The reader is left wondering what the nurse did that prompted such a special present in return.

Nursing Situation: As a Story

I invite you now to relive this nursing situation as I have chosen the form of a story to illustrate the application of Nursing as Caring to help others understand what it is to nurse from this perspective.

As the morning rolled along I began to dream. I dreamed I was a tree. My roots entwined deep within the foundation upon which I stood. I took from the Earth what I needed to nourish and strengthen me. My roots drank from the spring of knowledge beneath me. I felt strong. I grew tall. My arms outstretched, reached for the sun, found the sky, and in it, a gentle breeze that surrounded and calmed me. I stood in awe of the sun's beauty as its rays poured over me and warmed my spirit. I felt connected. I felt whole.

I saw a glow on the horizon, unlike the sun and different from the moon and stars. An ember, the residual of a fire that has burned through the night, tirelessly, to provide warmth. I was drawn to it. Unafraid that my branches might catch fire and burn, I reached for her abdomen. I searched. As my hands pressed on, I began to feel the Earth slipping from the sky. I reached upward, grasping for the restoration of harmonious interconnectedness, but in the sky, there is nothing to grab onto. You may grow into it, enjoy its beauty, bask in its breezes, and breathe in its life-giving oxygen, but you cannot hold onto it or possess it.

My arms grew weary, my leaves were wilted, so I drank from the spring beneath my foundation. My roots nourished me with courage, patience, trust, and humility. She reached for my hand. Her spirit filled me and strengthened me as she ascended toward the sky. I began to feel stronger and reached toward the sky, hoping to catch one last glimpse of her ember and saw her reflection in the sun. Her rays poured over me and warmed my spirit. I felt whole once again.

This nursing story is a reflection of a nursing situation grounded in caring. It demonstrates the perspective of enhancing "other" as one lives and grows in caring, which subsequently results in the enhancement of self as the nurse lives and grows in caring.

I chose this story as the medium with which to share. Boykin and Schoenhofer encourage nurses to choose various art forms as media for sharing and reflection. This is aesthetic knowing. It is the artful integration of all the ways of knowing to create a meaningful, caring moment that is born in a nursing situation.

> **Nursing theory sets apart what nurse practitioners do from any other profession.**

Personal knowing is that which is known intuitively by encountering self and "other." Authentic presence is a key component for my intuitive experiences when I just know. The patient trusted me and humbled herself to ask me to validate her concern that the mass in her belly was of grave concern. The patient knew, intuitively, before I laid my hands on her. There is a lot to be gained by learning to trust our intuition, and we can "know" more by engaging in authentic presence. Authentic presence, for me, removes all physical boundaries to my coming to know "other." It is a spiritual connectedness that has no time limits or physical boundaries. It is a feeling of interconnectedness with the patient that reverberates beyond the room, city, state, country, world, and galaxy. It brings with it the wisdom of the universe.

The first three basic assumptions inherent in Nursing as Caring facilitate the lived experience of authentic presence in this moment. The assumption that this person is a caring person by virtue of her humanness, complete in that moment, gave me the courage to enter into authentic presence to come to know her as a complete, caring person in that moment. As the moment unfolded, our mutual trust enhanced and supported who we were as we lived and grew in that caring encounter.

The patient's need to share with me a special gift was validation that she felt it, too. The fifth basic assumption of the theory of Nursing as Caring is personhood, which is enhanced through participation in nurturing relationships. As the patient demonstrated in the words of her song, she knew that the end of her physical existence was coming to an end and she was not afraid. There was a mutual knowingness that was unspoken, even without the lab work or biopsies. Her lack of fear and her courage allowed her spirit to soar free in the open sky, giving me a glimpse of the spiritual existence.

This is not to devalue the importance of empirical knowledge. It, too, is an important part of coming to know "other." Empirical knowledge is the information that is organized into laws and theories to describe, explain, or predict phenomena. This knowledge is acquired through the senses. Based in the sciences, it is our understanding of anatomy and physiology, diagnostic processes, and treatment regimens. For me, it is the concrete form of the foundation upon which my practice is built.

Empirical knowledge is essential to be recognized as a profession. The sixth assumption of Nursing as Caring is that nursing is both a discipline and a profession. The scientific evidence that lends theory-based knowledge to our profession gives us the diagnostic reasoning we need to address the physical needs that people have. In this particular situation, the laboratory findings confirmed that which we knew personally. Oftentimes the bereaved loved ones need a diagnosis to help cope with the grief of losing a family member.

This brings us to ethical knowing—the patience and compassion to be with grieving family members when they are not ready to let go of a loved one who is ready to die. Ethical knowing is also the recognition that these family members are caring persons as well, coping in the only way they know how, through their experiences. Humility has allowed me to come to know and respect the family's perspective. Patience is needed to allow "other" to come to know hope in the moment a loved one is diagnosed with a terminal illness. Hope for a spiritual existence beyond this world was revealed to me in this nursing situation.

Each of these patterns of knowing—aesthetic, personal, empirical, and ethical—is borrowed from Carper (1978). They serve as conceptual tools to help us understand and implement the theory of Nursing as Caring. These tools lend organization to the theory, helping us to examine ways of knowing the whole of a nursing situation, with caring as the central focus.

BROAD APPLICATION FOR ADVANCED PRACTICE NURSING

Nursing as Caring provides a theoretical perspective with an organizing framework that guides practice and allows for the generation of new knowledge. In addition, it lends a methodologic process to define, explain, and verify this knowledge. This theory reaches beyond the received view of traditional science. Nursing as Caring guides the use of nursing knowledge and information from other disciplines in ways appropriate to nursing. Through the application of this theory, I have come to know new possibilities for nursing practice.

I believe now, more than ever, that, with the advancing roles of nurses, we need to be clear on what it is that we do that is different from other practitioners. As Advanced Practice Nurses (APNs) and ARNPs, assume more responsibilities and perform tasks that were traditionally reserved for those of the medical profession, the overlapping further blurs the boundaries of our professions. We need to maintain our nursing perspective. As nurse practitioners continue to be lumped into categories with other midlevel practitioners, we need to demonstrate to our patients that our profession was born of a need from society, a need that only nurses can fill. If there is no call to nursing, our profession will dissolve into the sea of midlevel practitioners.

Nursing theory sets apart what nurse practitioners do from any other profession. To ensure that our practice maintains its identity, the practice must be built upon research-based nursing theory. The Theory of Nursing as Caring is one such theory. I hope that by sharing how I live and practice Nursing as Caring, I will lend understanding to applying something that can seem abstract.

The call for nursing can be spoken in many different languages. If you use only your ears, you may not hear it.

References

Boykin, A., & Schoenhofer, S. O. (1993). *Nursing as caring: A model for transforming practice.* New York: National League for Nursing Press.

Carper, B. A. (1978). Fundamental patterns of knowing in nursing. *Advances in Nursing Science, 1*(1), 13–24.

Section IV

Nursing Theory: Illustrating
Processes of Development

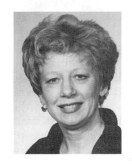

Chapter 23

Kristen M. Swanson
A Program of Research
on Caring

Kristen M. Swanson

This chapter has turned out to be somewhat autobiographical. In writing it, I have tried to answer the questions of graduate students who were interested in learning more about how my research on caring came to be. I have attempted to situate myself as a nurse and woman so that the history of my scholarship, particularly as it pertains to caring, may be chronicled. I consider myself to be a "second-generation" nursing scholar. I was taught by first-generation nursing scientists (that is, nurses who received their doctoral education in fields other than nursing). My struggle for identity as a woman and as an academician was, like that of other women of my era (the baby boomers), and continues to be, a reflective process of self-discovery. Third-generation nursing scholars (those taught by nurses whose doctoral preparation is in nursing) may find my "yearning" somewhat naive and adolescent given their struggle for identity. To those who are wont to offer critique about the egocentricity of my pondering, I offer the defense of having been brought up during an era in which nurses dealt with such struggles as, "Are we a profession? Have we a unique body of knowledge? Are we entitled to a space in the full (i.e., Ph.D.-granting) academy?" As we enter a new century, I fully appreciate that questions of uniqueness and entitlement have not completely disappeared. Rather, they have faded as a backdrop to the weightier concerns of making a significant contribution to the health of all, working collaboratively with consumers and other scientists and practitioners, embracing pluralism, and acknowledging the socially constructed power differentials associated with gender, race, and class.

> I believe that the key to my research is that I have studied human responses to a specific health problem in a framework that assumed from the start that a clinical therapeutic had to be defined.

TURNING POINT

In September 1982 I had no intention of studying caring; my goal was to study what it was like for women to miscarry. However, my dissertation chairperson, Dr. Jean Watson, had quite a different idea. Given her devotion to studying caring, I suppose I should not have been very surprised that when I approached her to chair my committee, she immediately struck a deal that included the need for me to examine the meaning of caring in the context of miscarriage. In truth, I said "yes" because, having been a student at that point for 20 of my 29 years, I readily recognized the difference between a negotiable and a nonnegotiable request. As it turned out, Dr. Watson's advice proved sage, and to this day I am grateful for her firmness and wisdom. I believe that the key to my research is that I have studied human responses to a specific health problem (miscarriage) in a framework (caring) that assumed from the start that a clinical therapeutic had to be defined. So, hand in glove, the research has constantly gone back and forth between "what's wrong and what can be done about it," "what's right and how can it be strengthened," and "what's real to women who miscarry and how might care be customized to that reality." The back-and-forth nature of this line of inquiry has resulted in insights about the nature of miscarrying and caring that might otherwise have remained elusive. Because the caring theory was developed empirically and from a clinical perspective, it is my hope that the theory has merit for guiding practice, education, and research even beyond the perinatal contexts from which it was originally derived.

PREDOCTORAL EXPERIENCES

My preparation for studying caring-based therapeutics from a psychosocial perspective began, ironically, in a cardiac critical care unit. After receiving my BSN at the University of Rhode Island, I was wisely coached by Dean Barbara Tate to pursue a job at the brand-new University of Massachusetts Medical Center (U. Mass.) in Worcester, Massachusetts. I was drawn to that institution because of the nursing administration's clear articulation of how nursing could and should be. It was so exciting to be there from day one. We were all essential players in shaping the institutional vision for practice. Within 6 months of opening, the hospital was ready to launch a cardiac surgery program, and with that I shifted from the floor to the unit (and I do mean "the" in both cases, because we literally had one of each). It was a phenomenal experience to witness myself and my friends (nurses, physicians, respiratory therapists, and housekeepers) make a profound difference in the lives of those people we served. However, what I learned most from that experience came from the patients and their families. I realized that there was a powerful force that people could call upon to get themselves through incredibly difficult times. Watching patients move into a space of total dependency and come out the other side restored was like witnessing a miracle unfold. Sitting with spouses in the waiting room while they entrusted the heart (and lives) of their partner to the surgical team was awe-inspiring. It was encouraging to observe the inner reserves family members could call upon in order to hand over that which they could not control. It warmed my heart to be so privileged as to be invited into the spaces that patients and families created in order to endure their transitions through illness, recovery, and, in some instances, death. It also both humbled and filled me with gratitude for all that I was learning.

After a year and a half at U. Mass., I was still a fairly new nurse and very unclear about what all of these emotional insights had to do with nursing. I really saw all of it as more of something about my spiritual beliefs and me than about my profession. At that point, what mattered most to me as a nurse was my emerging technological savvy, understanding of complex pathophysiological processes, and desire to convey that same information to other nurses. Hence, I applied to graduate schools with the intention of focusing on teaching and care of the acutely ill adult. Approximately 2 years after completing my baccalaureate degree, I enrolled in the Adult Health and Illness Nursing program at the University of Pennsylvania.

> Caring consisted of five basic processes: knowing, being with, doing for, enabling, and maintaining belief.

While I was at Penn, I served as the student representative to the graduate curriculum committee and, as such, was invited to attend a 2-day retreat to revise the master's program. I distinctly remember when, having just caught myself daydreaming, I made myself focus on the speaker, Dr. Jacqueline Fawcett. As I tuned in, I could not believe what I was hearing. She was talking about such concepts as health, environments, persons, and nursing and claiming that these four concepts were the stuff that really comprises nursing. It was like hearing someone give voice to the inner stirrings I had kept to myself back in Massachusetts. It really impressed me that there were actually nurses who studied in such arenas. Shortly after the retreat, I received my MSN and was hired at Penn on a temporary basis to teach undergraduate medical-surgical nursing. I immediately enrolled as a post-master's student in Dr. Fawcett's new course on the conceptual basis of nursing. It proved to be one of the best decisions I had ever made, primarily because it helped me to figure out an answer to that constant question, "Why doesn't a smart girl like you enter medicine?" I finally knew that it was because nursing, a discipline that I was now starting to understand from an experiential and personal as well as an academic point of view, was more suited to my beliefs about serving people who were moving through the transitions of illness and wellness. I suppose it is safe to say that I was beginning to understand that my "gifts" lie not in the diagnosis and treatment of illness but in the ability to understand and work with people going through transitions of health, illness, and healing.

DOCTORAL STUDIES

Such insights made me want more; hence, I applied for doctoral studies and was accepted into the graduate program at the University of Colorado. My area of study, psychosocial nursing, emphasized such concepts as loss, stress, coping, caring, transactions, and person-environment fit. Having been supported by a National Institute of Mental Health (NIMH) traineeship, one requirement of our doctoral program was a hands-on experience with the process of undergoing a health promotion activity. Our faculty offered us the opportunity to carry out the requirement by enrolling ourselves in some type of support or behavior change program of our own choosing. Four weeks into the same semester in which I was required to complete that exercise, my first son was born. I decided to enroll in a cesarean birth support group as a way to deal with the class assignment and the unexpected circumstances surrounding his birth. It so happened that an obstetrician had been invited to speak to the group about miscarriage at the first meeting I ever attended. I found his lecture informative with regard to the incidence, diagnosis, prognosis, and medical management of spontaneous abortion. However, when the physician sat down and the women began to talk about their personal experiences with miscarriage and other forms of pregnancy loss, I was suddenly overwhelmed with the realization that there had been a one-in-five chance that I could have miscarried my son. Up until that point, it had never occurred to me that anything could have gone wrong with something so central to my life. I was 29 years old and believed, quite naively, that anything was possible if you were only willing to work hard at it.

Two profound insights came to me from that meeting. First, I was acutely aware of the American Nurses' Association social policy statement, namely, "Nursing is the diagnosis and treatment of human responses to actual and potential health problems" (1980, p. 9). It was so clear to me that whereas the physician had talked about the health problem of spontaneously aborting, the women were living the human response to miscarrying. Second, being in my last semester of course work, I was desperately in need of a dissertation topic. From that point on it became clear to me that I wanted to understand what it was like to miscarry. The problem, of course, was that I was a critical care nurse and knew very little about anything having to do with childbearing. An additional concern was that during the early 1980s although there was a very strong emphasis on epistemology, ontology, and the methodologies to support multiple ways of understanding nursing as a human science, our methods courses were very traditionally quantitative. Luckily, two mentors came my way. Dr. Jody Glittenberg, a nurse anthropologist, agreed to guide me through a predissertation pilot study of five women's experiences with miscarriage in order that I might learn about interpretive methods. Dr. Colleen Conway-Welch, a midwife, agreed to supervise my trek up the psychology of pregnancy learning curve.

Dissertation: Caring and Miscarriage

Twenty women who had miscarried within 16 weeks of being interviewed agreed to participate in my phenomenological study of miscarriage and caring. The results of this inquiry have been published in greater depth elsewhere (Swanson-Kauffman, 1985, 1986, 1991). Through that investigation, I proposed that caring consisted of five basic processes: knowing, being with, doing for, enabling, and maintaining belief. At that time, the definitions were fairly awkward and definitely tied to the context of miscarriage. In addition to naming those five categories, I also learned some important things about studying caring: (1) if you directly ask people to describe what caring means to them, you force them to speak so abstractly that it is hard to find any substance; (2) if you ask people to list behaviors or words that indicate that others care, you end up with a laundry list of "niceties"; (3) if you ask people for detailed descriptions of what it was like for them to go through an event (i.e., miscarrying) and probe for their feelings and what the responses of others meant to them, it is much easier to unearth instances of people's caring and noncaring responses; and finally, (4) I learned that although my intentions were to gather data, many of my informants thanked me for what I did for them. As it turned out, a side effect of accomplishing my agenda to gather detailed accounts of the informants' experiences was that women felt, heard, understood, and attended to in a nonjudgmental fashion. In later years, this insight would actually become the grist for a caring-based intervention study.

At the completion of the dissertation, and in the years following, I have often been asked if my re-

search was an application of Jean Watson's Theory of Human Caring (Watson, 1979/1985, 1985/1988). Neither Dr. Watson nor I have ever seen my research program as an application of her work per se, but we do agree that the compatibility of our scholarship lends credence to both of our claims about the nature of caring. I have come to view her work as having provided a research tradition that other scientists and I have followed. Watson's research tradition asserts that caring is (1) a central concept in nursing, (2) values multiple methodologies for inquiry, and (3) honors the importance of nurses (and others) studying caring so that it may be better understood, consciously claimed, and intentionally acted upon to promote, maintain, and restore health and healing.

POSTDOCTORAL STUDY

Postdoctoral Study #1: Providing Care in the NICU

Approximately 9 months after I completed the dissertation, my second son was born. This child had a difficult start on life and spent a few days in the newborn intensive care unit (NICU). Through this event, I became aware that in my later childbearing loss (having a not-well child at birth), I, too, wished to receive the kinds of caring responses that my miscarriage informants had described. Hence, my next study, an individually awarded National Research Service Award postdoctoral fellowship (1989–1990), was inspired. Dr. Kathryn Barnard, at the University of Washington, agreed to sponsor this investigation and ended up opening doors for me that still continue to open. With her guidance, I spent over a year "hanging out" in the NICU at the University of Washington Medical Center (the staff gave me permission to acknowledge them and their practice site when discussing these findings).

The question I answered through the NICU phenomenological investigation was, "What is it like to be a provider of care to vulnerable infants?" In addition to my observational data, I did in-depth interviews with some of the mothers, fathers, physicians, nurses, and other health-care professionals who were responsible for the care of five infants. The results of this investigation are published elsewhere (Swanson, 1990). With respect to understanding caring, there were three main findings:

1. Although the names of the caring categories were retained, they were grammatically edited and somewhat refined so as to be more generic (specific words having to do with miscarrying were replaced with more general language).

2. It was evident that care in a complex context called upon providers to simultaneously balance *caring* (for self and "other"), *attaching* (to people and roles), *managing responsibilities* (self-, other-, and society-assigned), and *avoiding bad outcomes* (for self, "other," and society).

3. What complicated everything was that each NICU provider (parent or professional) knew only a portion of the whole story surrounding the care of any one infant. Hence, there existed a strong potential for conflict stemming from misunderstanding the behaviors of others and second-guessing each other's motives.

While I was presenting the findings of the NICU study to a group of neonatologists, I received a very interesting comment. One young physician told me that it was the caring and attaching parts of his vocation that brought him into medicine, yet he was primarily evaluated on and made accountable for the aspects of his job that dealt with managing responsibilities and avoiding bad outcomes. Such a schism in his role performance expectations and evaluations had forced him to hold the caring and attaching parts of doing his job inside. Unfortunately, it was his experience that those more person-centered aspects of his role could not be "stuffed" for too long and that they oftentimes came hauntingly into his consciousness at about 3 A.M. His remarks left me to wonder if the true origin of burnout is the failure of professions and care delivery systems to adequately value, monitor, and reward practitioners whose comprehensive care embraces *caring, attaching, managing responsibilities,* and *avoiding bad outcomes*.

Postdoctoral Study #2: Caring for Socially At-Risk Mothers

While I was still a postdoctoral scholar, Dr. Barnard invited me to present my research on caring to a group of five master's-prepared public health nurses. As I did the presentation, I noticed that there was a lot of head nodding going on. When I finished, the five of them became quite excited and claimed that the model I had just described was a good description of what it had been like for them to care for a group of socially at-risk new mothers. As it turned out, about 4 years prior to my meeting them, these five advanced practice nurses had participated in Dr. Barnard's Clinical Nursing Models Project (Barnard et al., 1988). They had provided care to 68 socially at-risk expectant mothers for approximately 18 months (from shortly after conception until their babies were 12 months old). The purpose of the intervention had been to help the mothers take control of

themselves and their lives so that they could ultimately take care of their babies. As I listened to these nurses endorsing the relevance of the caring model to their practice, I began to wonder what the mothers would have to say about the nurses. Would the mothers (1) remember the nurses, and (2) describe the nurses as caring?

I was able to locate 8 of the original 68 mothers (a group of women with highly transient lifestyles). They agreed to participate in a study of what it had been like to receive an intensive long-term advanced practice nursing intervention. The result of this phenomenological inquiry was that the caring categories were further refined and a definition of caring was finally derived.

Hence, as a result of the miscarriage, NICU, and high-risk mothers studies, I began to call the caring model a middle-range theory of caring. I define *caring* as a "nurturing way of relating to a valued "other," toward whom one feels a personal sense of commitment and responsibility" (Swanson, 1991, p. 162). "Knowing," striving to understand an event as it has meaning in the life of the other, involves avoiding assumptions, focusing on the one cared for, seeking cues, assessing thoroughly, and engaging the self of both the one caring and the one cared for. "Being with" means being emotionally present to the "other." It includes being there, conveying availability, and sharing feelings while not burdening the one cared for. "Doing for" means doing for the "other" what he or she would do for himself or herself if it were at all possible. The therapeutic acts of doing for include anticipating needs, comforting, performing competently and skillfully, and protecting the "other" while preserving their dignity. "Enabling" means facilitating the "other's" passage through life transitions and unfamiliar events. It involves focusing on the event, informing, explaining, supporting, allowing and validating feelings, generating alternatives, thinking things through, and giving feedback. The last caring category is "maintaining belief," which means sustaining faith in the other's capacity to get through an event or transition and face a future with meaning. This means believing in the "other" and holding him or her in esteem, maintaining a hope-filled attitude, offering realistic optimism, helping find meaning, and going the distance or standing by the one cared for, no matter how his or

> I define caring as a nurturing way of relating to a valued "other," toward whom one feels a personal sense of commitment and responsibility.

her situation may unfold (Swanson, 1991, 1993, 1999a, 1999b).

THE MISCARRIAGE CARING PROJECT

As my postdoctoral studies were coming to an end, Dr. Barnard suggested that I should apply for a new investigator award from the National Institutes of Health. I told her I had been thinking about another phenomenological study on loss and caring. In her straightforward fashion, she looked at me and said, "I think you've described caring long enough. It's time you did something with it!" We then proceeded to talk about the fact that data-gathering interviews were so often perceived by study participants as caring. Together we realized that, at the very least, open-ended interviews involved aspects of knowing, being with, and maintaining belief. We suspected that if doing-for and enabling interventions specifically focused on common human responses to health conditions were added, it would be possible to transform the techniques of phenomenological data gathering into a caring intervention. That conversation ultimately led to my design of a caring-based counseling intervention for women who miscarried.

The next thing I knew, I was writing a proposal for a Solomon four-group randomized experimental design (Swanson, 1999a,b). It was funded by the National Institute of Nursing Research and the University of Washington Center for Women's Health Research. The primary purpose of the study was to examine the effects of three 1-hour-long, caring-based counseling sessions on the integration of loss (miscarriage impact) and women's emotional well-being (moods and self-esteem) in the first year subsequent to miscarrying. Additional aims of the study were to (1) examine the effects of early versus delayed measurement and the passage of time on women's healing in the first year after loss, and (2) develop strategies to monitor caring as the intervention/process variable.

An assumption of the caring theory was that the recipient's well-being should be enhanced by receipt of caring from a provider who is informed about common human responses to a designated health problem (Swanson, 1993). Specifically, it was proposed that if women were guided through in-depth discussion of their experience and felt understood, informed, provided for, validated, and believed in, they would be better prepared to integrate miscarrying into their lives. Content for the three counseling sessions was derived from the miscarriage model, a phenomenologically derived model that summarized the common human responses to miscarriage (Swanson, 1999b; Swanson-Kauffman, 1983, 1985, 1986a, 1986b, 1988).

Women were randomly assigned to two levels of treatment (caring-based counseling and controls) and two levels of measurement ("early"—completion of outcome measures immediately, 6 weeks, 4 months, and 1 year post loss; or "delayed"—completion of outcome measures at 4 months and 1 year only). Counseling took place at 1, 5, and 11 weeks postloss. ANOVA was used to analyze treatment effects. Outcome measures included self-esteem (Rosenberg, 1965); overall emotional disturbance, anger, depression, anxiety, and confusion (McNair, Lorr, & Droppleman, 1981); and overall miscarriage

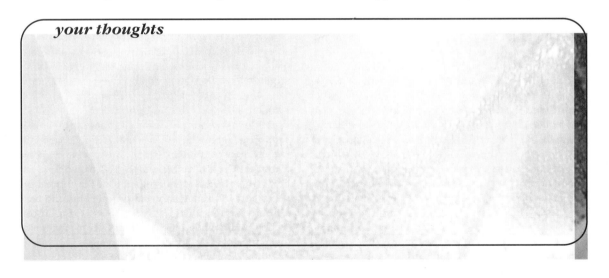

your thoughts

impact, personal significance, devastating event, lost baby, and feeling of isolation (investigator-developed Impact of Miscarriage Scale).

A more detailed report of these findings is published elsewhere (Swanson, 1999a). There were 242 women enrolled, of which 185 completed. Participants were within 5 weeks of loss at enrollment; 89% were partnered, 77% were employed, 94% Caucasian. Over 1 year, main effects included the following: (1) caring was effective in reducing overall emotional disturbance, anger, and depression; and (2) with the passage of time, women attributed less personal significance to miscarrying, and realized increased self-esteem and decreased anxiety, depression, anger, and confusion. There were no interactive effects of treatment and time over that first year. Between 4 months and 1 year, the following main effects were determined: (1) treated women had less anger; (2) delayed-measured women (those who completed no outcome measures until 4 months after loss) had higher anger and were less likely to identify their loss as a baby; and (3) time passing led to diminished impact of miscarriage and personal significance of loss, increased self-esteem, and decreased overall emotional disturbance, anxiety, depression, anger, and confusion. Between 4 months and 1 year there were also the following interactive effects: (1) the healing effect of time on the personal significance attributed to miscarrying was greater for treated women; (2) the healing effects of treatment on the assessment of miscarriage as personally significant and as a devastating event were greater for delayed-measured women; and (3) the healing effects of time on overall miscarriage impact and assessment of miscarriage as a devastating event were greater for women in the delayed-measured groups.

In summary, the Miscarriage Caring Project provided evidence that, although time had a healing effect on women after miscarrying, caring did make a difference in the amount of anger, depression, and overall disturbed moods that women experienced after miscarriage. This study was unique in that it employed a clinical research model to determine whether or not caring made a difference. I believe that its greatest strength lies in the fact that the intervention was based both on an empirically derived understanding of what it is like to miscarry and on a conscientious attempt to enact caring in counseling women through their loss. Of course, the greatest limitation of that study is that I derived the caring theory, developed from the intervention, and conducted most of the counseling sessions. Hence, it is unknown whether similar results would be derived

under different circumstances. My work is further limited by the lack of diversity in my research participants. Over the years, I have predominantly worked with middle-class, married, educated Caucasian women. I am currently making a concerted effort to try to rectify this situation and to examine what it is like for diverse groups of women to experience both miscarriage and caring.

Monitoring Caring as an Intervention Variable

Monitoring caring as an intervention variable was the second specific aim of the Miscarriage Caring Project. The project was an attempt to monitor the intervention variable and document that caring had indeed occurred, as claimed. Three strategies were employed. First, approximately 10% of the total intervention sessions were transcribed. Analysis was done by Research Associate Katherine Klaich, RN, Ph.D. Dr. Klaich, having also been one of the counselors in the study, found she could not approach analysis of the transcripts naively—that is, with no preconceived notions, as would be expected in the conduct of phenomenologic analysis. Hence, she employed both deductive and inductive content analytic techniques to render the transcribed counseling sessions meaningful. She began with the broad question, "Is there evidence of caring as defined by Swanson [1991] on the part of the nurse counselors?" The unit of analysis was each emic phrase that was used by the nurse counselor. Phrases were coded, for which (if any) of the five caring processes were represented by the emic utterances. Each counselor statement was then further coded, for which subcategory of the five processes was represented by the phrase. Twenty-nine subcategories of the five major processes were defined. With few exceptions (social chitchat) every therapeutic utterance of the nurse counselor could be accounted for by one of the subcategories.

The second way in which caring was monitored was through the completion of paper-and-pencil measures. Before each session, the counselor completed a Profile of Mood States (McNair, Lorr, & Droppleman, 1981) in order to document her presession moods (thus enabling examination of the association between counselor presession mood and self or client postsession ratings of caring). After each session, women were asked to complete the Caring Professional Scale (investigator-developed). Women, having been left alone to complete the measure, were asked to place the evaluations in a sealed envelope. In the meantime, in another room, the counselor wrote out her counseling notes and completed the Counselor Rating Scale, a brief five-item rating of how well the session went.

The Caring Professional Scale originally consisted of 18 items on a five-point Likert-type scale. It was developed through the Miscarriage Caring Project and was completed by participants in order to rate the nurse counselors who conducted the intervention and to evaluate the nurses, physicians, or midwives who took care of the women at the time of their miscarriage. The items included: "Was the health-care provider that just took care of you understanding, informative, aware of your feelings, centered on you, etc.?" The response set ranged from 1— "yes, definitely" to 5—"not at all." The items were derived from the caring theory. Three negatively worded items (abrupt, emotionally distant, and insulting) were dropped due to minimal variability across all of the data sets. For the counselors at 1, 5, and 11 weeks postloss, Chronbach alphas were .80, .95, and .90 (sample sizes for the counselor reliability estimates were 80, 87, and 76). The lower reliability estimates were because the counselors' caring professional scores were consistently high and lacked variability (mean item scores ranged from 4.52 to 5.0).

Noteworthy findings include the following:

1. Each counselor had a full range of presession feelings, and those feelings/moods were, as might be expected, highly intercorrelated.
2. For the most part, counselor presession mood was not associated with postsession evaluations.
3. The caring professional scores were extremely high for both counselors indicating that, overall, the clients were pleased with what they got and, as claimed, caring was "delivered" and "received."

4. One of the counselors was a psychiatric nurse by background. She knew very little about miscarriage prior to participating in this study and had recently experienced a death in her family. The only time her presession moods (in this case, depression and confusion) were significantly associated ($p \leq .05$) with any of the postsession ratings (both client caring professional score and counselor self-rating) was in Session I. During Session I, women discussed in depth what the actual events of miscarrying felt like. It is possible that the counselor was so touched by and caught up in the sadness of the stories that her own vulnerabilities were a bit less veiled.

5. Session II, in which the two topics addressed were relationship-oriented (who the woman could share her loss with and what it felt like to go out in public as a woman who had miscarried), was the only session in which the other counselor's vulnerabilities came through. This counselor, having just gone through a divorce, was probably least able to hide her presession moods (depression ($p \leq .05$) and low vigor, confusion, fatigue, and tension (all at $p \leq .01$), as was evident in the significant associations with her own postsession self-rating. Also, most notably, there was an association between this counselor's presession tension and the client's caring professional rating ($p \leq .05$).

A LITERARY META-ANALYSIS OF CARING

My most recent study about caring was an in-depth review of the literature. This literary meta-analysis is published elsewhere (Swanson, 1999). Approximately

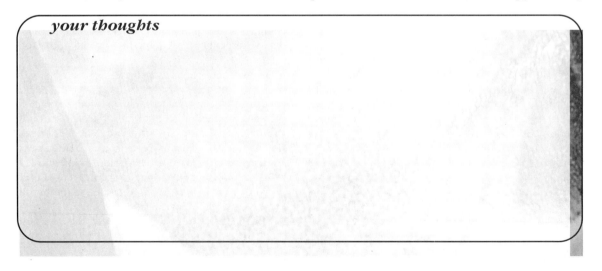

your thoughts

130 data-based publications on caring were reviewed for this state of the science paper. Developed was a framework for discourse about caring knowledge in nursing. Proposed were five domains (or levels) of knowledge about caring in nursing. I believe that these domains are hierarchical and that studies conducted at any one domain (e.g., Level III) assumes the presence of all previous domains (e.g., Levels I and II). The first domain includes descriptions of the capacities or characteristics of caring persons. Level II deals with the concerns and/or commitments that lead to caring actions. These are the values nurses hold that lead them to practice in a caring manner. Level III describes the conditions (nurse, patient, and organizational factors) that enhance or diminish the likelihood of caring occurring. Level IV summarizes caring actions. This summary consisted of two parts. In the first part, a meta-analysis of 18 quantitative studies of caring actions was performed. It was demonstrated that the top five caring behaviors valued by patients were that the nurse helps the patient to feel confident that adequate care was provided; knows how to give shots and manage equipment; gets to know the patient as a person; treats the patient with respect; and puts the patient first, no matter what. By contrast, the top five caring behaviors valued by nurses were: listens to the patient, allows expression of feelings, touches when comforting is needed, is perceptive of the patient's needs, and realizes the patient knows himself/herself best. The second part of the caring actions summary was a review of 67 interpretive studies of how caring is expressed (the total number of participants was 2314). These qualitative studies were classified under Swanson's caring processes, thus lending credibility to caring theory. The last domain was labeled "consequences." These are the intentional and unintentional outcomes of caring and noncaring for patient and provider. In summary, this literary meta-analysis clarified what "caring" means, as the term is used in nursing, and validated the generalizability or transferability of Swanson's Caring Theory beyond the perinatal contexts from which it was originally derived.

Summary

Much work lies ahead. The profession has a long way to go to make a case for the education needed to support caring practices; the importance of nurses practicing in a caring manner; the essential contributions of caring to the well-being of all; and the costs of caring in terms of time, money, and personal energy expended. The discipline also has much work left to do. It is essential that nurse investigators frame nursing interventions under the framework of caring in order to tie together the essential contributions of the profession to the health of society. Finally, caring, in order to be effective, must be sensitive to those involved in caring transactions (nurses and clients), the cultural contexts in which it is performed, and the common responses that individuals, families, groups, and communities experience when living with conditions of wellness and illness.

References

American Nurses' Association. (1980). *Nursing: A social policy statement*. Kansas City, MO: American Nurses' Association.

Barnard, K. E., Magyary, D., Sumner, G., Booth, C. L., Mitchell, S. K., & Spieker, S. (1988). Prevention of parenting alterations for women with low social support. *Psychiatry, 51*, 248–253.

McNair, D. M., Lorr, M., & Droppleman, L. F. (1981). *Profile of mood states: Manual*. San Diego: Educational and Industrial Testing Service.

Rosenberg, M. (1965). *Society and the adolescent self-image*. Princeton: Princeton University Press.

Swanson, K. M. (1990). Providing care in the NICU: Sometimes an act of love. *Advances in Nursing Science, 13*(1), 60–73.

Swanson, K. M. (1991). Empirical development of a middle-range theory of caring. *Nursing Research, 40*, 161–166.

Swanson, K. M. (1993). Nursing as informed caring for the well-being of others. *Image, 25*, 352–357.

Swanson, K. M. (1999). What's known about caring in nursing science: A literary meta-analysis. In Hinshaw, A. S., Feetham, S., & Shaver, J. (Eds.), *Handbook of clinical nursing research*. Thousand Oaks, CA: Sage.

Swanson, K. M. (1999a). The effects of caring, measurement, and time on miscarriage impact and women's well-being in the first year subsequent to loss, *Nursing Research, 48*, 6, 288–298.

Swanson, K. M. (1999b). Research-based practice with women who miscarry. *Image: Journal of Nursing Scholarship, 31*, 4, 339–345.

Swanson-Kauffman, K. M. (1983). The unborn one: The human experience of miscarriage (Doctoral dissertation, University of Colorado Health Sciences Center, 1983). *Dissertation Abstracts International, 43*, AAT8404456.

Swanson-Kauffman, K. M. (1985). Miscarriage: A new understanding of the mother's experience. *Proceedings of the 50th anniversary celebration of the University of Pennsylvania School of Nursing*, 63–78.

Swanson-Kauffman, K. M. (1986a). A combined qualitative methodology for nursing research. *Advances in Nursing Science, 8*(3), 58–69.

Swanson-Kauffman, K. M. (1986b). Caring in the instance of unexpected early pregnancy loss. *Topics in Clinical Nursing, 8*(2), 37–46.

Swanson-Kauffman, K. M. (1988). The caring needs of women who miscarry. In Leininger, M. M. (Ed.), *Care: Discovery and uses in clinical and community nursing*. Detroit: Wayne State University Press.

Watson, M. J. (1979/1985). *Nursing: The philosophy and science of caring*. Boulder, CO: Colorado Associated Press.

Watson, M. J. (1985/1988). *Nursing: Human science and human care*. New York: National League for Nursing.

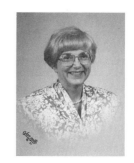

Chapter 24 Part 1

Marilyn Anne Ray
The Theory of
Bureaucratic Caring

Marilyn Anne Ray

INTRODUCING THE THEORIST

Marilyn A. Ray, RN, PhD, CTN, CNAA, is a professor at Florida Atlantic University, College of Nursing, in Boca Raton, Florida. She holds a bachelor's of science in nursing and a master's of science from the University of Colorado in Denver, Colorado, a master's of arts in cultural anthropology from McMaster University in Hamilton, Canada, and a doctorate from the University of Utah. She recently retired as a colonel after 30 years of service with the U.S. Air Force Reserve Nurse Corps. As a certified transcultural nurse, she has published widely on the subjects of caring in organizational cultures, caring theory and inquiry development, transcultural caring, and transcultural ethics. She is associate editor of the *Journal of Transcultural Nursing.* Dr. Ray's research has revolved around technological and economic issues related to caring in complex organizations. Her current research, which uses both qualitative and quantitative research methods, relates to the study of the nurse-patient relationship as an economic resource and how the economics of health and managed care are affecting the practice and administration of nursing. She is active in local and national political and educational activities. She was recently elected vice president of Floridians for Health Care, Inc., and is a charter member of the Nurses' Network for a National Health Care Program.

THE THEORY OF BUREAUCRATIC CARING REVISITED: FROM GROUNDED THEORY TO HOLOGRAPHIC THEORY

by Marilyn Anne Ray

Theory is the intellectual life of nursing (Levine, 1995): "Scientific theories in the discipline of nursing have developed out of the choices and assumptions a particular theorist believes about nursing, what the basis of nursing's knowledge is, and what nurses do or how they practice in the real world" (Ray, 1998, p. 91). Van Manen (1982) refers to theory as "wakefulness of mind" or the pure viewing of truth. *Truth* in the Greek sense is not the property of consensus among theorists but the disclosure of the essential nature or the good of things. In essence, truth refers to contemplating the good (van Manen, 1982). Collectively, theories in nursing have focused on the good of nursing—what nursing is and what it does or should do. Based on the assumptions of nursing as serving the good, the locus of the discipline centers

on caring for others, caring in the human health experience (Newman, 1992; Newman, Sime, & Corcoran-Perry, 1991). A theory of nursing actually must edify—direct or enlighten the good. Theories such as the classical grand theories in nursing demonstrate a variety of integrated approaches to nursing based on the worldview of an individual theorist. Ongoing research through testing and evaluation has supported the validity and reliability of the theories. Grounded or middle-range theories, however, focus on particular aspects of nursing practice and are commonly generated from nursing practice. As such, some intellectuals view middle-range theories as more relevant and useful to nursing than the application of grand theories (Cody, 1996). Newer approaches to theory, such as holographic theory/complexity theory (Battista, 1982; Davidson & Ray, 1991; Harmon, 1998; Wheatley, 1994; Wilbur, 1982), center on the multiple interconnectedness and relational reality of all things, the interdependence of all human communities, and the concept of choice.

Levine (1995) pointed out that one of nursing's most recent innovations, nursing theory, has already received its share of criticism and skepticism from educators and practitioners. Many schools of nursing pride themselves on taking a theoretical approach and believe that nursing theory is not a part of nursing's consciousness and professional life. This thinking often results from the way in which some nurses view theory—as abstract, esoteric, or distant from everyday life. Frequently critics say that after all the research, theory has contributed little to guide nursing's practical tasks and responsibilities. The criticism persists, especially because of the strength of the varying worldviews or paradigms of organizational social systems, such as the power of the current economic system, which impact nursing's professional practice. Given the interpretive nature of consciousness or wakefulness, this author holds the position that nurses do operate within a theory or theories by integrating their knowledge and experience. These theories, whether positive or negative, are established by the way in which nurses interpret their world and in the context where nursing is played out. Theories in this sense are philosophies or ideologies that serve a practical purpose. The Theory of Bureaucratic Caring illuminated in this chapter is a theory with a practical purpose that emerged from the worldviews of health professionals and clients in practice (Ray, 1989). This chapter will present a discussion of contemporary nursing culture, share theoretical views related to the author's developmental theoretical vision of nursing, and discuss the Theory of Bureaucratic Caring as grounded theory.

> Newer approaches to theory, such as holographic theory, center on multiple interconnectedness and relational reality of all things.

After revisiting the theory in the contemporary age, the author will elucidate bureaucratic caring theory as a holographic theory to further the good of nursing by illustrating the significance of spiritual and ethical caring in relation to the structural dimensions of complex organizations and societal cultures.

CONTEMPORARY NURSING PRACTICE

The Current Context: Organizational Cultures as Bureaucracies

The practice of nursing occurs in organizations that are generally bureaucratic or systematic in nature. Organizational culture has a rich heritage and has been studied both formally and informally since the 1930s in the United States (Smircich, 1985). Informal organization or the integration of codes of conduct encompassing commitment, identity, character, coherence, and a sense of community was considered essential to the successful functioning or the administering of power and authority in the formal organization. Political, economic, legal, and technical systems comprise the formal organization. What distinguishes organizations as culture from other paradigms, such as organizations as machines, brains, or other images (Morgan, 1997) is its foundation in anthropology or the study how people act in communities or formalized structures, and the significance or meaning of work life (Louis, 1985). Organizational cultures, therefore, are viewed as social constructions, symbolically formed and reproduced through interaction (Smircich, 1985). The beliefs about work show up in organizational policy statements. A nation's prevailing tenets and expectations about the nature of work, leisure, and employment are pivotal to the work life of people; hence, there is an interplay between the macrocosm of a national/global culture and the microcosm of specific organizations (Eisenberg & Goodall, 1993). In recent years, economics has been a potent contestant in macro- and microcultures. Now there is an ever greater concentration of economic and political power in a handful of corporations, which separate their interests—which are usually profit-driven—from the interests of human beings, which are life-centered (Korten, 1995). Health care and its activities are tightly inter-woven into the social and economic fabric of nations. In the past decade, impacted by issues of cost and profit, health-care systems have undergone immense change, particularly in the United States. Confidence in major health-care institutions and their leaders has fallen so low as to put their legitimacy at risk. Rather than working for the good of everyone, these institutions are working for only a relative few, such as chief executive officers and other financially oriented administrators. Work life in all sectors has been redefined by economic, business, technological, and political issues. Little account is taken by formal organizations of the spiritual and ethical dimensions of human beings. The actual work of health care professionals, especially that of registered nurses—such as caring for the needy or sick—is undervalued in terms of both cost and worth. Human caring work is viewed as unimportant and generally neglected. The conflict between health care as a business and health care as a human need has resulted in a crisis for health-care organizations. Rather than professional nurse caring work valued as an expression of one's soul or an expression of one's creative self, work in health-care organizations is increasingly business and machinelike.

Bureaucracy, considered by some as a machine-like metaphor, plays a significant role in the meanings and symbols of organizations (Ray, 1989). Weber, (1999) actually predicted that the future belonged to the bureaucracy and not to the working class. Weber, who saw bureaucracy as an efficient and superior form of organizational arrangement, predicted that bureaucratization of enterprise would dominate the world (Bell, 1974; Weber, 1999). This, of course, can be witnessed by the current globalization of commerce. Recent acquisitions and mergers of industrial firms and even health-care systems, especially in the United States, are larger and hold more power than some world governments. The concept of bureaucratization is thus a worldwide phenomenon (Ray, 1989). Britain and Cohen (1980) stated that, "Like it or not, humankind is being driven to a bureaucratized world whose forms and functions, whose authority and power must be understood if they are ever to be even partially controlled" (p. 27).

The characteristics of bureaucracies are as follows: a fixed division of labor, a hierarchy of offices, a set of general rules that govern performances, a separation of the personal from the official, a selection of personnel on the basis of technical qualifications, equal treatment of all employees or standards of fairness, employment viewed as a career by participants, and protection of dismissal by tenure (Eisenberg & Goodall, 1993). Bureaucracy, while condemned by some as associated with red tape and inflexibility, continues to provide the most reasonable way in which to view systems and facilitate the preservation of organizations, particularly under the current mergers and acquisitions mentality. In the past two decades there has been a call for decentralization and the "flattening" of organizational structures—to become less bureaucratic and more participative. Many firms have begun to hold to new principles that honor creativity and imagination (Morgan, 1997). Even nursing has advanced in a more collaborative or decentralized manner by its focus on primary nursing in hospitals and more decentralized control from administration (Nyberg, 1998). But reengineering and restructuring views have taken hold as economics has swept the globe. Authoritarian models have replaced the short-lived participative movement toward decentralization and the building of workplace communities. Power has been put back into the hands of a few, and authoritarianism governs by global economics and the market rules (Korten, 1995). As a result, the concept of bureaucracy does not seem as bad as was once thought. It can be considered as much less radical than the new business paradigm, which focuses on response to market forces, subsequently eradicating standards of fairness for human beings in the workplace. This can be witnessed by the actions taken to ignore the public interests for equity in employment, health security, sufficient environmental protection, and so forth. Defending and institutionalizing the rights of the economically powerful to do whatever best serves their immediate interests without public accountability for consequences seems to be the order of the day (Korten, 1995). As such, the author joins with Perrow (1986), who defended bureaucracy as a superior

social tool because of its focus on rationality over other forms of organization in the contemporary workplace. Rationality from the author's interpretation relates to the "Greek sense of 'logos' or rationality as genesis: as that which brings things into being" (van Manen, 1982, p. 45)—what makes human community possible and what is edifying to our spiritual and intellectual lives.

Caring as the Unifying Focus of Nursing

Caring in nursing brings things into being. It is humane and rational. As such, caring is considered by many nurse scholars to be the essence of nursing (Boykin & Schoenhofer, 1993; Leininger, 1981, 1991, 1997; Morse, Solberg, Neander, Bottorff, & Johnson, 1990; Ray, 1989, 1994a, 1994b; Swanson, 1991; Watson, 1985, 1988, 1997). Although not uniformly accepted, Newman, Sime, and Corcoran-Perry (1991; Newman, 1992) characterized the social mandate of the discipline of nursing as caring in the human health experience. Caring thus is an influential concept, and the expression "caring" in the human health experience emphasizes the social mandate to which nursing has responded throughout its history and encompasses the extent of the discipline. Caring, however, is manifested in different and complex ways in the nursing discipline and profession (Morse et al., 1990; Newman, 1992). Various paradigms that enfold the care and caring ideal exist in nursing. A *paradigm* signifies a cluster of basic assumptions that form a worldview, a way of screening knowledge and experience to bring forth a new way of understanding the life world (Smircich, 1985). The totality (Fawcett, 1993), the simultaneity (Parse, 1987) and the unitary-transformative (Newman, 1992) paradigms have been the prevailing worldviews in nursing and

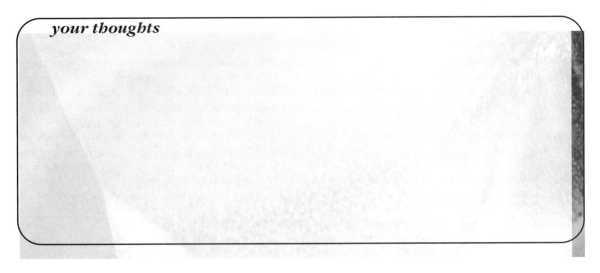

your thoughts

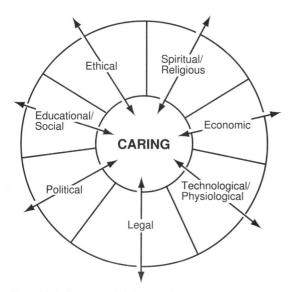

Figure 24–1. *The grounded theory of bureaucratic caring.*

have directed nursing theories. The totality paradigm demonstrates that nursing, person, society, environment, and health characterize the nature of nursing. The simultaneity paradigm illuminates the human-environment integral nature of nursing. The unitary-transformative paradigm states that what constitutes nursing's reality is the view that the human being is unitary and evolving as a self-organizing field embedded in a larger self-organizing field identified by pattern and interaction with the larger whole. Health is considered expanded consciousness, and caring in the human health experience is the focus of the discipline (Newman, 1986, 1992; Newman, Sime, & Corcoran-Perry, 1991). Many caring theories correspond to one or all of these paradigms (Morse, Solberg, Neander, Bottorff, & Johnson, 1990). The Theory of Bureaucratic Caring has its roots in all these paradigms by its synthesis of caring and the organizational context (see Figure 24-1).

Bureaucratic Caring Theory: Emergent Grounded Theory

The Theory of Bureaucratic Caring originated as a grounded theory from a study of caring in the organizational culture and appeared in the literature in 1989. In the qualitative study of caring in the institutional context, the research revealed that nurses and other professionals struggled with the paradox of serving the bureaucracy and serving human beings, especially clients, through caring. The discovery of bureaucratic caring resulted in both substantive and formal theories (Ray, 1984, 1989). The substantive

theory emerged as differential caring and showed that caring in the complex organization of the hospital was complex and differentiated itself in terms of meaning by its context—dominant caring dimensions related to areas of practice or units wherein professionals worked and clients resided. Differential Caring Theory showed that different units espoused different caring models based on their organizational goals and values. The formal Theory of Bureaucratic Caring symbolized a dynamic structure of caring which was synthesized from a dialectic between the thesis of caring as humanistic, social, educational, ethical, and religious/spiritual (elements of humanism), and the antithesis of caring as economic, political, legal, and technological (elements of bureaucracy) (Ray, 1989).

Although the model demonstrates that the dimension are equal, the research revealed that the economic, political, technical, and legal dimensions were dominant in relation to the social and ethical/spiritual dimensions. The theory reveals that nursing and caring are contextual and are influenced by the social structure or the culture (normative system) that is given in the organization. Interactions and symbolic systems of meaning are formed and reproduced from the constructions or dominant values held within the organization. In some respect, "we are the organization," which is analogous to Wittgenstein's (1969) adage, "we are our language."

The theory has been embraced by researchers, nursing administrators, and clinicians, who, after witnessing changes in health-care policy in the past decade, have begun to appreciate how the context—micro- and macrocultures—influence's nursing. Moving away from centering on patient care to the economic justification of nursing and health-care systems has prompted professionals to desire a fuller understanding of how to preserve humanistic caring within the business or corporate culture (Miller, 1989; Nyberg, 1989, 1991, 1998). The theory also has been used in part as a foundation for additional research studies of the nurse-patient relationship as an economic resource and its importance as financially dominated integrated health-care systems have grown (Ray & Turkel, 1998; Turkel, 1997).

PRACTICE THEORY REVIEWED: EVOLUTION OF THEORY DEVELOPMENT

Organizations are not working well today. In health care, registered nurses are disillusioned with the total disregard for their honorable services and for the profession dedicated to the well-being of others. Everything is increasingly complex. Expectations for success are diminished to such a point that nurses are escaping hospitals, yet not fully realizing that wherever they go they will be haunted by bureaucracies, some functional, most problematic. What, then, is the deeper reality of nursing practice? The following is a presentation of theoretical views that relate to bureaucratic caring theory, culminating in a vision for understanding the deeper reality of nursing life.

Substantive and Formal Theory

Glaser and Strauss (1967; Glaser, 1978; Strauss & Corbin, 1998) were the first social scientists to present the perspective of social theory, both substantive and formal, discovered from inductive research processes. Substantive and formal theories emerge from in-depth qualitative studies of social processes—action and interaction associated with the social world. Social categories and their properties are generated from simultaneous processing of collecting, coding, and categorizing empiric data from interviews and observations. The researcher considers evidence about how one event affects another and explains the things observed and recorded by developing theoretical relationships about the data. Theoretical sampling (Glaser, 1978) refines, elaborates, and exhausts conceptual categories so that an actual integration of descriptors and categories can facilitate the discovery of substantive theory. The discovery of a basic social process is the foundation for substantive theory. The formal theory is generated from both the inductive process, based on substantive knowledge/theory, and deductive approaches, which draw upon cumulative knowledge from the social world to examine the initial propositions advanced. A formal theory reflects the structure of both processes.

In nursing, grounded theory has been used to generate theories from and in practice. Qualitative nurse researchers seek to identify and reveal the social (nursing) processes related to participation and interaction with caregivers and clients, and depth of living in the world of health care. On occasion, methods are mixed to give more richness to the research. For example, ethnography, which is informed by the knowledge of culture, or phenomenology, which is informed by the philosophical knowledge related to the study of the meaning of experience, can be used to advance theory (Ray, 1989). Substantive and formal theories generated from practice convey the essential characteristics of nursing to form a social process related to nursing practice. A structure is arranged related to the specific concepts of the theory or theories (Chinn & Kramer, 1995).

The Theory of Bureaucratic Caring integrated knowledge from data that is associated with researching the meaning and action of caring in the institutional culture of a hospital, which resulted in a substantive theory of differential caring. Narrative responses to the meaning of caring reported by different health-care professionals and patients produced varied beliefs and values, ranging from humanistic definitions such as empathy, love, and ethical-religious delineations to legal, political-economic descriptions. The formal theory evolved as a result of using the Hegelian dialectical process of examining and connecting codetermining polar opposites of the humanistic dimensions as the thesis of caring in relation to the dimensions of economics, politics, law, and technology of the bureaucracy as the antithesis of caring. The process was synthesized into a dialectical, formal Theory of Bureaucratic Caring. The laws of the dialectic—codetermination of polar opposites, negation of each of the separate codetermining opposites, and synthesis of conceptualizations toward transformation and change—demonstrated that the understanding of institutional caring as a whole, or the Theory of Bureaucratic Caring, is simply a representation of its integral nature in contemporary organizational culture. The theory shows that caring reached its completeness through the process of its own relevance (Ray, 1989).

> The Theory of Bureaucratic Caring originated from a study of caring in the organizational culture of a hospital and led to a substantive theory of differential caring.

Middle-Range Theory

Middle-range theory deals with a relatively broad scope of phenomena but does not cover the full range of phenomena of a discipline, as do grand theories that encompass the fullest range or the most global phenomena in the discipline (Chinn & Kramer, 1995). As such, middle-range theories are generally considered narrower in scope than grand theories, and to some extent narrower than formal theory from the grounded theory tradition. There is a paradox in caring as middle-range theory. Caring in nursing, for example, may be considered by some intellectuals in the discipline as having a narrow scope or a foundation for a middle-range theory. However, others who have adopted Newman's (1992) paradigmatic view regarding the focus of the discipline of nursing as caring in the human health experience, or who have seriously studied caring, may see it as a broad enough concept to capture the nature of nursing.

Is the Theory of Bureaucratic Caring a middle-range theory as well as a grounded theory? Middle-range theories are abstract enough to extend beyond data generated in a specific space, place, and time, but specific enough to allow for testing the theory in different arenas or permitting interventions for practice to transform nursing practice (Moody, 1990). The initial dialectical theory showed that "living caring in organizational life" with the meaning and symbols in an institutional culture reflects the culture of the macro or dominant culture. The meaning of "caring" in the organization showed that that meaning was constituted within a larger pattern of significance. Organizations are representations of our humanity (Smircich, 1985). Social forms and social arrangements reflect the interplay between cultural systems of thought and organization. The system reflected the symbols of political and economic power and authority and psychodynamics of caring in human experience. Middle-range theory embodies the perspective that these theories fall between the concrete world of practice and the grand theories that guide nursing research and practice (Moody, 1990). Bureaucratic caring reflects the concrete world of practice and responds to the caring ideal that is unique to nursing. Therefore, the Theory of Bureaucratic Caring is not only a grounded theory but also a middle-range theory; it could also be considered a grand theory because of the ubiquitousness of the constructs of caring and culture.

Holographic Theory

The holographic paradigm in science recognizes that the ontology or "what is" of the universe or creation is the interconnectedness of all things, that the epistemology or knowledge that exists is in the relationship rather than in the objective world or subjective experience, that uncertainty is inherent in the relationship because everything is in process, and that information holds the key to grasping the holistic and complex nature of the meaning of holography or the whole (Battista, 1982; Harmon, 1998). *Holography* means that the implicit order (the whole) and explicit order (the part) are interconnected, that everything is a holon in the sense that everything is a whole in one context and a part in another—each part being in the whole and the whole being in the part (Harmon, 1998; Wilbur, 1982). It is the relational aspect of information that makes it a holistic rather than a mechanistic construct.

Ray (1998) states: "Complexity theory is a scientific theory of dynamical systems collectively referred to as the sciences of complexity" (p. 91). Complexity theory has replaced other theories, such as Newtonian physics and even Einstein's beliefs that the physical world is governed by law and order. New scientific views state that phenomena that are antithetical actually coexist—determinism with uncertainty, and reversibility with irreversibility (Nicolis & Prigogine, 1989). Thus, both linear and nonlinear and simple (e.g., gravity) and complex (economic and cultural) systems exist together. One of the tools in the studies of complexity is chaos theory. Chaos deals with life at the edge, or the notion that the concept of order exists within disorder at the system communication or choice point phases or where old patterns disintegrate or new patterns evolve (Ray, 1994a, 1998). This new science, which signifies interrelationship of mind and matter, interconnectedness and choice, carries with it moral re-

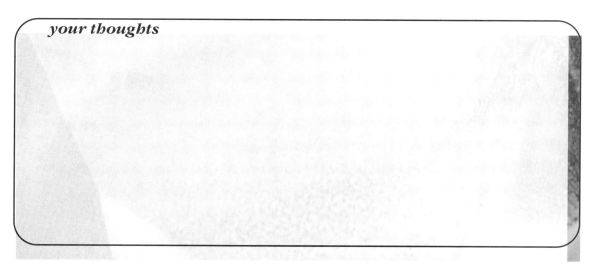

your thoughts

sponsibility and the quest toward wisdom which includes awareness and creativity (Fox, 1994). Certain nursing theorists have embraced the notion of nursing as complexity in which consciousness, caring, and choice making are central to nursing (Davidson & Ray, 1991; Newman, 1986, 1992; Ray, 1994, 1998).

REVISIONING THE THEORY OF BUREAUCRATIC CARING AS HOLOGRAPHIC THEORY

Can the Theory of Bureaucratic Caring be viewed as a holographic theory? The theory arose initially from the decisions that were made about the structure of organization (consciousness), the caring transactions that were engaged in (caring), and the effective negotiations or ability to make choices and reconcile the system demands with the humanistic client care needs (choice making). The theoretical processes of awareness of viewing truth or seeing the good of things (caring), and communication, are central to the theory. The dialectic of caring (the implicit order) in relation to the various structures (the explicit order) illustrates that there is room to consider the theory as holographic. The synthesis of Bureaucratic Caring Theory shows that everything is interconnected with caring and the system in a microcosm of the whole of culture.

How can knowledge of caring interconnectedness motivate nursing to continue to embrace the human dimension within the current economic and technologic environment of health care? Can higher ground be reclaimed for the twenty-first century? Higher ground requires that we make excellent choices. It is therefore imperative that spiritual and ethical caring thrive in complex systems. Figure 24–2, the Holographic Theory of Bureaucratic Caring, illustrates that through spiritual/ethical caring as the choice point for communication in relation to the complexity of the sociocultural system, nursing can reclaim higher ground.

Reflections on the Theory as Holographic

Freeman (in Appell & Triloki, 1988) pointed out that human values are a function of the capacity to make choices, and called for a paradigm giving recognition to awareness and choice. As noted, a revision toward this end is taking place in science based on the new holographic scientific worldview. Nursing has the capacity to make creative and moral choices for a preferred future. Nursing theory can focus on the capacity to continue to direct the good. Nursing is being

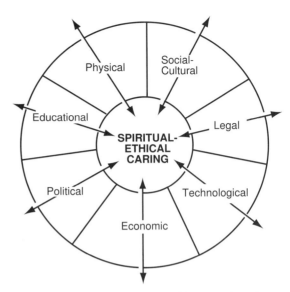

Figure 24–2. *The holographic theory of bureaucratic caring.*

shaped by the historical revolution going on in science, social sciences, and theology (Harmon, 1998; Newman, 1992; Ray, 1998; Reed, 1997; Watson, 1997; Wheatley, 1994). In these new approaches, constructs of consciousness and choice are central and demonstrate that phenomena of the universe, including society, arise from the choices that are or are not made (Freeman cited in Appell & Triloki, 1988; Harmon, 1998). In the social sciences, the critical task is to comprehend the relationship between what is given in culture (the jural order) and what is chosen (the moral and spiritual), between destiny and decision. In nursing, the unitary-transformative paradigm and the various theories of Newman, Leininger, Parse, Rogers, and the Holographic Theory of Bureaucratic Caring are challenging nursing to comprehend a similar relationship. The unitary-transformative paradigm of nursing and their holographic tenets are consistent with the changing images of the new science despite the reality that nursing continues to be threatened by the business model over its long-term human interests for facilitating health and well-being (Davidson & Ray, 1991; Ray, 1994a, 1998; Reed, 1997; Vicenzi, White, & Begun, 1997). The creative, intuitive, ethical, and spiritual mind is unlimited, however. Through "authentic conscience" (Harmon, 1998), we must find hope in our creative powers.

In the revised theoretical model, everything is infused with spiritual/ethical caring (the center of the model) by its integrative and relational connection to the structures of organizational life. Spiritual/ethical caring is both a part and a whole, and every part secures its purpose and meaning from each of the parts that can also be considered wholes. In other words, the model shows how spiritual/ethical caring is involved with qualitatively different processes or systems; for example, political, economic, technological, and legal. The systems, when integrated and presented as open and interactive, are a whole and must operate as such by conscious choice, especially by the choice making of nursing, which always has, or should have, the interest of humanity at heart.

The model presents a vision, but it is based on the reality of practice. The model emphasizes a direction toward the unity of experience. Spirituality involves creativity and choice and refers to genuineness, vitality, and depth. It is revealed in attachment, love, and community and comprehended within as intimacy and spirit (Harmon, 1998; Secretan, 1997). Secretan (p. 27) states: "Most of us have an innate understanding of soul, even though each of us might define it in a very different and personal way."

Fox (1994) calls for the theology of work—a redefinition of work. Because of the crisis of our relationship to work, we are challenged to reinvent it. For nursing, this is important because work puts us in touch with others, not only in terms of personal gain, but also at the level of service to humanity or the community of clients and other professionals. Work must be spiritual, with recognition of the creative spirit at work in us.

> The synthesis of the Theory of Bureaucratic Caring shows that everything is interconnected with caring and that the system is a microcosm of the whole culture. The model presents a vision based on the reality of practice.

Thus, nurses must be the "custodians of the human spirit" (Secretan, 1997, p. 27).

The ethical imperatives of caring that join with the spiritual relate to questions or issues about our moral obligations to others. The ethics of caring as edifying the good through communication involve never treating people simply as a means to an end or as an end itself, but rather as beings who have the capacity to make choices. Ethical content—as principles of doing good, doing no harm, allowing choice, being fair, and promise-keeping—functions as the compass in our decisions to sustain humanity in the context of political, economic, and technological situations within organizations. Roach (1992) pointed out that ethical caring is operative at the level of discernment of principles, in the commitment needed to carry them out, and in the decisions or choices to uphold human dignity through love and compassion. Furthermore, Roach (1987) remarked that health is a community responsibility, an idea that is rooted in ancient Hebrew ethics. The expression of human caring as an ethical act is inspired by spiritual traditions that emphasize charity. Spiritual/ethical caring for nursing does not question whether or not to care in complex systems, but intimates how sincere deliberations and ultimately the facilitation of choices for the good of others can or should be accomplished. The scientist Sheldrake (1991, p. 207) remarks:

> Transformation can occur even in the businesslike atmosphere of today if nurses reintroduce the spiritual and ethical dimensions of caring.

> The recognition that we need to change the way we live [work] is now very common. It is like waking up from a dream. It brings with it a spirit of repentance, seeing in a new way, a change of heart. This conversion is intensified by the sense that the end of an age is at hand.

Summary

As the millennium has arrived, nursing in organizations have to arrive as well. There must be an end to the age of bureaucratic control where powerlessness and helplessness have reigned. As the Theory of Bureaucratic Caring has demonstrated, caring is the primordial construct and consciousness of nursing. Revisioning the theory as holographic shows that through creativity and imagination, nursing can build the profession it wants. Nurses are calling for expression of their own spiritual and ethical existence. The new scientific and spiritual approach to nursing theory as holographic will have positive effects. The union of science, ethics, and spirit will engender a new sense of hope for transformation in the work world. This transformation can occur even in the businesslike atmosphere of today if nurses reintroduce the spiritual and ethical dimensions of caring. The deep values that underlie choice to do good for the many will be felt both inside and outside organizations. We must awaken our consciences and act on this awareness to no longer surrender to injustices and oppressiveness of systems that focus primarily on the good of a few. "Healing a sick society [work world] is a part of the ministry of making whole" (Fox, 1994, p. 305). The Holographic Theory of Bureaucratic Caring—idealistic, yet practical; visionary, yet real—can give direction and impetus to lead the way.

References

Appell, G., & Triloki, N. (Ed.). 1988. *Choice and morality in anthropological perspective*. Albany: State University of New York Press.

Battista, J. (1982). The holographic model, holistic paradigm, information theory, and consciousness. In Wilber, K. (Ed.), *The holographic paradigm and other paradoxes* (pp. 143-150). Boulder, CO: Shambhala.

Bell, D. (1974). *The coming of post-industrial society*. New York: Basic Books.

Boykin, A., & Schoenhofer, S. (1993). *Nursing as caring: A model for transforming practice*. New York: National League for Nursing Press.

Britain, G., & Cohen, R. (1980). *Hierarchy and society: Anthropological perspectives on bureaucracy*. Philadelphia: ISHI.

Chinn, P., & Kramer, M. (1995). *Theory and nursing: A systematic approach* (4th ed.). St. Louis: Mosby.

Cody, W. (1996). Drowning in eclecticism. *Nursing Science Quarterly, 9*, 96-88.

Davidson, A., & Ray, M. (1991). Studying the human-environment phenomenon using the science of complexity. *Advances in Nursing Science, 14*(2), 73-87.

Eisenberg, E., & Goodall, H. (1993). *Organizational communication*. New York: St. Martin's Press.

Fawcett, J. (1993). From a plethora of paradigms to parsimony in worldviews. *Nursing Science Quarterly, 6*, 56-58.

Fox, M. (1994). *The reinvention of work*. San Francisco: Harper.

Glaser, B. (1978). *Theoretical sensitivity*. Mill Valley, CA: The Sociology Press.

Glaser, B., & Strauss, A. (1967). *The discovery of grounded theory: Strategies for qualitative research*. Hawthorne, NY: Aldine de Gruyter.

Harmon, W. (1998). *Global mind change* (2nd ed.). San Francisco: Berrett-Koehler Publishers, Inc.

Korten, D. (1995). *When corporations rule the world*. San Francisco: Berrett-Koehler Publishers, Inc.

Leininger, M. (Ed.). (1981). *Caring: An essential human need*. Thorofare, NJ: Slack.

Leininger, M. (1991). *Culture care diversity and universality: A theory of nursing*. New York: National League for Nursing Press.

Leininger, M. (1997). Transcultural nursing research to transform nursing education and practice: 40 years. *Image: Journal of Nursing Scholarship, 29*, 341-354.

Levine, M. (1995). The rhetoric of nursing theory. *Image: Journal of Nursing Scholarship, 27*, 11-14.

Louis, M. (1985). An investigator's guide to workplace culture. In Frost, P., Moore, L., Louis, M., Lundberg, C., & Martin, J. (Eds.), *Organizational culture* (pp. 73-93). Beverly Hills: Sage.

Matteson, M., & Ivancevich, J. (Eds.). *Management and organizational behavior classics* (7th ed.). Chicago: Irwin McGraw-Hill.

Miller, K. (1989). The human care perspective on nursing administration. *Journal of Nursing Administration, 25*(11), 29-32.

Moody, L. (1990). *Advancing nursing science through research*. Newbury Park, CA: Sage.

Morgan, G. (1997). *Images of organization* (2nd ed.). Thousand Oaks: Sage.

Morse, J., Solberg, S., Neander, W., Bottorff, J., & Johnson, J. (1990). Concepts of caring and caring as a concept. *Advances in Nursing Science, 13*, 1-14.

Newman, M. (1986). *Health as expanding consciousness*. St. Louis: Mosby.

Newman, M. (1992). Prevailing paradigms in nursing. *Nursing Outlook, 40*, 10-14.

Newman, M., Sime, A., & Corcoran-Perry, S. (1991). The focus of the discipline of nursing. *Advances in Nursing Science, 14*(1), 1-6.

Nicolis, G., & Prigogine, I. (1989). *Explaining complexity*. New York: W. H. Freeman.

Nyberg, J. (1989). The element of caring in nursing administration. *Nursing Administration Quarterly, 13*, 9-16.

Nyberg, J. (1991). Theoretical explanations of human care and economics: Foundations of nursing administration practice. *Advances in Nursing Science, 13*(1), 74-84.

Nyberg, J. (1998). A caring approach in nursing administration. Niwot, CO: University Press of Colorado.

Parse, R. (1987). *Nursing science: Maps, paradigms, theories, and critiques*. Philadelphia: Saunders.

Perrow, C. (1986). *Complex organizations: A critical essay* (2nd ed.). Glenview, IL: Scott, Foresman.

Ray, M. (1984). The development of a nursing classification system of caring. In Leininger, M. (Ed.), *Care the essence of nursing and health* (pp. 95-112). Thorofare, NJ: Slack.

Ray, M. (1989). The Theory of Bureaucratic Caring for nursing practice in the organizational culture. *Nursing Administration Quarterly, 13*(2), 31-42.

Ray, M. (1994a). Complex caring dynamics: A unifying model of nursing inquiry. *Theoretic and applied chaos in nursing, 1*(1), 23-32.

Ray, M. (1994b). Communal moral experience as the starting point for research in health care ethics. *Nursing Outlook, 41*, 104-109.

Ray, M. (1998). Complexity and nursing science. *Nursing Science Quarterly, 11*, 91-93.

Ray, M., & Turkel, M. (1998). Economic analysis of the nurse-patient relationship. Unpublished raw data.

Reed, P. (1997). Nursing: The ontology of the discipline. *Nursing Science Quarterly, 10*, 76-79.

Roach, M. S. (1992). The human act of caring: A blueprint for the health professions (rev. ed.). Ottawa, Canada: Canadian Hospital Association Press.

Secretan, L. (1997). *Reclaiming higher ground*. New York: McGraw-Hill.

Sheldrake, R. (1991). *The rebirth of nature*. New York: Bantam.

Smircich, L. (1985). Is the concept of culture a paradigm for understanding organizations and ourselves? In Frost, P., Moore, L., Louis, M., Lundberg, C., & Martin, J. (Eds.), *Organizational culture*. Beverly Hills: Sage.

Strauss, A., & Corbin, J. (1998). *Basics of qualitative research* (2nd ed.). Newbury Park, CA: Sage.

Swanson, K. (1991). Empirical development of a middle-range theory of caring. *Nursing Research, 40,* 161–166.

Turkel, M. (1997). *Struggling to find a balance:A grounded theory study of the nurse-patient relationship in the changing health care environment.* Unpublished doctoral dissertation, University of Miami, Florida. Microfilm # 9805958.

van Manen, M. (1982). Edifying theory: Serving the good. *Theory Into Practice, 31,* 45–49.

Vicenzi, A., White, K., & Begun, J. (1997). Chaos in nursing: Make it work for you. *American Journal of Nursing, 97,* 26–32.

Watson, J. (1985). *Human science, human care:A theory of nursing.* Norwalk, CT: Appleton & Lange.

Watson, J. (1988). New dimensions of human caring theory. *Nursing Science Quarterly, 1,* 175–181.

Watson, J. (1997). The theory of human caring: Retrospective and prospective. *Nursing Science Quarterly,* 175–181.

Weber, M. (1999). The ideal bureaucracy. In Matteson, M., & Ivancevich, J. (Eds.), *Management and organizational behavior classics* (7th ed.). Chicago: Irwin McGraw-Hill.

Wheatley, M. (1994). *Leadership and the new science.* San Francisco: Berrett-Koehler Publishers, Inc.

Wilbur, K. (Ed.). (1982). *The holographic paradigm and other paradoxes.* Boulder, CO: Shambhala.

Wittgenstein, L. (1969). *On certainty.* New York: Harper & Row.

Chapter 24 Part 2

Applicability of Bureaucratic Caring Theory to Contemporary Nursing Practice: The Political and Economic Dimensions

❖ Current Context of Health-Care Organizations

❖ Review of the Literature: Political and Economic Constraints of Nursing Practice

❖ Economic Implications of Theory of Bureaucratic Caring: Research in Current Atmosphere of Health-Care Reform

❖ Political/Economic Implications of Bureaucratic Caring

❖ Summary

❖ References

Marian C. Turkel

Ray (1989, p. 31) warned that the "transformation of America and other health care systems to corporate enterprises emphasizing competitive management and economic gain seriously challenges nursing's humanistic philosophies and theories, and nursing's administrative and clinical policies." Approximately 10 years later, in the current managed care environment, there is an intense focus on operating costs and the bottom line, and caring is often not valued within the corporate culture. However, nurse researchers, nurse administrators, and nurses in practice can use the political and/or economic dimensions of the Theory of Bureaucratic Caring as a framework to guide practice and decision making. Use of these dimensions of the theory integrates the constructs of politics, economics, and caring within the health-care organization.

The purpose of this chapter is to illuminate the notion of political/economic caring in the current health-care environment. Ray's (1989) original Theory of Bureaucratic Caring included political and economic entities as separate and distinct structural caring categories. However, the revised Theory of Bureaucratic Caring is represented as a complex holographic theory. Given this philosophical framework, the political and economic dimensions of bureaucratic caring as portrayed in this chapter are illuminated as interrelated constructs.

The political dimension of bureaucratic caring encompasses health-care reform at the national level, and the economic dimension refers to the economic impact of these changes at the institutional level. The chapter includes sections on the current context of health-care organizations, review of the literature related to the political and economic constraints of nursing practice, economic caring research, political and economic implications of bureaucratic caring, and visions for the future.

CURRENT CONTEXT OF HEALTH-CARE ORGANIZATIONS

In the wake of the controversial health-care reform process that is currently being debated in the United States, the central thesis in today's economic health-care milieu in both the for-profit and not-for-profit sectors is managed care (Kongstvedt, 1997). Managed care is an economic concept based on the premise that purchasers of care, both public and private, are unwilling to tolerate the substantial growth of the last several years in health-care costs. Managed care involves managed competition, an economic concept that is based on the premise that health-care

prices will fall if hospitals and providers are forced to compete on the basis of cost and quality, like other industries (Kenkel, 1992). Within traditional complex health-care organizations, community or public health agencies, or alternative health systems such as health maintenance organizations, financing in relation to managed care and managed competition is becoming a topic of heated discussion in the development of operational goals. This new form of health-care financing, based on the ratio of benefits over costs or the "highest quality services at the lowest available cost" (Prescott, 1993a, p. 192), challenges the old ways of competing for and paying for health-care services. Cost-saving measures integrating patient outcomes are paramount to health-care organizational survival and the economic viability of professional nursing practice.

> The human dimension of health care is missing from the economic discussion.

As the United States is in the midst of radical health-care changes, the entire debate focuses on the concept of economics. From an economic perspective, health-care organizations are a business. The competition for survival among organizations is becoming stronger and cost controls are becoming tighter. However, the human dimension of health care is missing from the economic discussion.

In the economic debate, the belief in caring for the patients as the goal of health-care organizations has been lost. Ray (1989) questioned how economic caring decisions are made related to patient care in order to enhance the human perspective with a corporate culture. When patients are hospitalized, it is the caring and compassion of the registered nurse that the patients perceive as quality care and making a difference in their recovery (Turkel, 1997). The concerns of patients are not about costs or health-care finance.

However, in a climate increasingly focused on economics, it has become difficult to quantify the economic value of caring. Consequently, newer cost systems, such as managed care, do not look at human caring or the nurse-patient relationship when allocating resource dollars for reimbursement.

Historically, nursing care delivery has not been financed or costed out in terms of reimbursement as a single entity. The prospective payment system of diagnostic related groups (DRGs) connected nursing services to the bed rate for patients (Shaffer, 1985). The current reimbursement systems, including health maintenance organizations (HMOs), managed care, Medicare, Medicaid, and private insurers, are reimbursing hospitals at a flat capitated rate. Subsequently, it is hospital administrators who must determine how these resource dollars will be allocated within their respective institutions.

Thus, it is necessary for caring nursing interactions to be viewed as having value as an economic resource. When professional nursing salary dollars are viewed as an economic liability that limits the potential profit margins of organizations, they are examined closely, and in many instances the number of registered nurses has been significantly reduced (Ketter, 1995). Hospital executives attribute these workforce reductions to the declining reimbursements of a managed care environment. It is imperative to the future of professional nursing practice that the economic value of caring be studied and documented, so human caring is not subsumed by the economics of health care.

REVIEW OF THE LITERATURE: POLITICAL AND ECONOMIC CONSTRAINTS OF NURSING PRACTICE

In order to use the economic dimension of the Theory of Bureaucratic Caring to guide research, nursing administration, and clinical practice, it is necessary to understand both the way in which health care has been financed and the current reimbursement system. Nurses, who understand the economics of health-care organizations, will be able to synthesize this knowledge into a framework for practice that integrates the dimensions of economics and human caring.

Nursing had its origins in poorly paid domestic work and charitable religious organizations (Dolan, 1985). Prior to the establishment of Medicare and Medicaid in 1965, the health-care system was not profitable for hospitals. Nursing students subsidized hospitals, and hospital-based nursing care was not considered an expense or source of revenue (Lynaugh & Fagin, 1988).

Nursing students provided the labor, and hospital administrators made no attempt to identify the real cost of nursing care. As nursing education moved away from the hospital setting to universities in the late 1950s and the role of the student nurse was reformed, hospital administrators began to account for the actual cost and revenue of hospital nursing care (Lynaugh & Fagin, 1988). However, the retrospective reimbursement of Medicare and Medicaid in 1965 allowed for hospital profitability and the issue of nursing care costs was not confronted.

During this era of retrospective reimbursement (1965 to 1983), the actual cost of nursing care was unknown because it was embedded in the daily hospital room charge. However, acute care hospitals had been under scrutiny because of the rapidly escalating costs of health care. A 1976 report from the National Council on Wage and Price Stability reported that during the period of 1965 to 1976, hospital costs and physicians' fees rose more than 50% faster than the overall cost of living (Walker, 1983). Hospital administrators were under considerable pressure to control costs.

Nursing service represented the largest hospital department and was singled out as a major cost in operating expenditures (Porter-O'Grady, 1979). It was assumed that the rising costs of health care were due to nurses' salaries and the number of registered nurses (Walker, 1983). Yet nursing costs as a percent of hospital charges could not be identified, because historically they had been tied to the room rate.

During the late 1970s and early 1980s, health-care costs continued to rise. Health-care costs did not follow traditional economic patterns. Cost-based reimbursement altered the forces of supply and demand. In the traditional economic marketplace, when the price of a product or service goes up, the demand decreases and consumers seek alternatives at lower prices (Mansfield, 1991). However, in the health-care marketplace, consumers did not seek an alternative as the price of hospital-based care continued to rise (DiVestea, 1985). This imbalance of the supply and demand curve occurred because consumers paid little out-of-pocket expense for health care. Government expenditure for the cost-based reimbursement system was predicted to bankrupt Social Security by 1985 unless changes were made (Gapenski, 1993). In an attempt to control hospital costs, the prospective payment system based on DRGs was instituted.

As a result of the change to the prospective payment system, hospital administrators were pressured to increase efficiency, reduce costs, and maintain quality. Consequently, nursing administrators needed to develop systems to gather information relative to nursing costs and productivity. Research was conducted in order to examine the costs associated with nursing (Bargagliotti & Smith, 1985; Curtin, 1983; McCormick, 1986; Walker, 1983). Common to all these studies was the use of a patient classification system that was time-based, and a predictor of the level of care needed for each class of patient. Data derived from these studies were used to calculate nursing costs per DRG, to predict expenditures, and to determine nursing productivity.

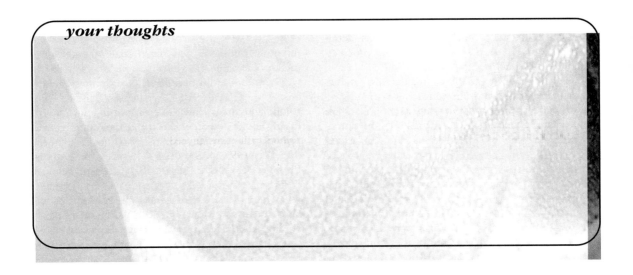

These studies identified the amount of times nurses spent doing specific interventions, but underrepresented the wide variations and clinical complexity of nursing care. Nor did this cost-accounting process include the humanistic, caring behaviors of nurses; consequently, the costs associated with the humanistic caring behaviors were not determined.

Foshay (1988) investigated 20 registered nurses' perceptions of caring activities, and the ability of patient classification systems to measure these caring activities. Findings from this study revealed that patient classification systems could not address the emotional needs of patients, the needs of the elderly, or unpredictable events that required intensive nursing interventions (Foshay, 1988). Specific caring behaviors that could not be measured included giving a reassuring presence, attentive listening, and providing information.

Other research of this time period focused on the cost and outcomes of all registered nurse staffing patterns (Dahlen & Gregor, 1985; Glandon, Colbert, & Thomasma 1989; Halloran, 1983; Minyard, Wall, & Turner, 1986). These studies showed that nursing units staffed with more registered nurses had decreased costs per nursing diagnosis, increased patient satisfaction, and decreased length of stay.

Helt and Jelinek (1988) examined registered nurse staffing in five different hospitals over 2 years. During this time period, the hospitals had increased their nursing skill mix from 60% to 70% registered nurses. It was shown that, although the acuity of hospitalized patients increased, the average length of stay dropped from 9.2 to 7.3 days (Helt & Jelinek, 1988). Nursing productivity improved and quality of care scores increased with the increased registered nurse staffing. The higher costs of employing registered nurses was offset by the productivity gains, and the hospitals netted an average of 55% productivity savings (Helt & Jelinek, 1988).

Hospital administrators had made budgeting and operating decisions based on the undocumented belief that nursing care accounted for 30 to 60% of patient charges. Thus, as stated earlier, nursing services were considered to be a major cost for hospitals. However, documented nursing research showed this assumption to be in error. A study conducted at Stanford University Hospital found that actual nursing costs constituted only 14 to 21% of total hospital charges (Walker, 1983). Similarly, the Medicus Corporation funded a study in which data were collected from 22 hospitals and 80,000 patient records. Direct nursing care costs represented on average only 17.8% of the Medicare reimbursement for each of the top 40 DRGs (McCormick, 1986). In a study of Medicare reimbursement and operating room nursing costs, nursing represented only 11% of the total operating costs (Jennings, 1991).

By the time nursing researchers had demonstrated the difficulty of costing out caring activities with patient classification systems, and the effectiveness of registered nurse staffing on patient outcomes, patient satisfaction, and mortality, the move toward managed care had already started. With the introduction of managed care and increased corporatization of health care, the economic environment was changing faster than nurse researchers could document the impact of these changes on clinical practice. In a managed care environment, reimbursement to hospitals had been further constrained. As a response to shrinking operating budgets, many hospital administrators have instituted registered nurse staff reductions or used unlicensed nursing assistants to replace registered nurses.

ECONOMIC IMPLICATIONS OF BUREAUCRATIC CARING THEORY: RESEARCH IN CURRENT ATMOSPHERE OF HEALTH-CARE REFORM

Investigation of the economic dimension of bureaucratic caring is being explicated in part in nursing research studies. Findings from these research studies have been valuable when linking the concepts of politics, economics, caring, cost, and quality in the new paradigm of health-care delivery. Although caring and economics may seem paradoxical, contemporary health-care concerns emphasize the importance of understanding the cost of caring in relation to quality.

Miller (1987, 1995), Nyberg (1990, 1991), Ray (1987, 1989, 1997), Ray and Turkel (1997, 1998), and Valentine (1989, 1991) have examined the paradox between the concepts of human caring and economics. It was a challenge for nurses to combine the science and art of caring within the economic context of the health-care environment. However, according to Nyberg (1990), human care is what patients want from the nursing profession.

Nyberg (1990) examined human care and economics in the hospital nursing environment. The Nyberg Caring Assessment Scale was used to determine which caring attributes were important to nurses and how often they used these caring attributes in practice. At the end of the questionnaire, four open-ended questions were asked: Two concerned economics and two concerned caring. One hundred and thirty-five nurses from seven hospitals participated in the study. Interviews were conducted with the nurse executives of each hospital. The executives were asked to define "human care" and "economics."

There was little significant difference in which caring attributes were important to nurses among the seven hospitals. However, correlation studies indicated that the ability to use these caring attributes in practice was positively correlated to the number of nursing hours per patient day used at the various hospitals.

Open-ended questions suggested that nurses were extremely frustrated over the economic pressures of the past 5 years, but that human care was present in nurses' day-to-day practice. According to Nyberg (1989, p. 17), "[T]oday's economic environment constrains human care, but nurses see human care as their responsibility and goal." Nurse executives agreed that care and economics must be viewed as interdependent. One nurse administrator proposed "caring as the mission of the hospital with economic and management as supporting facets" (p. 14). Although human care is the goal of nursing, economics cannot be ignored.

Miller (1995, p. 30) used Nyberg's Caring Assessment Tool to evaluate nurses' ability to care on eight different pediatric nursing units in seven Colorado hospitals. Although there were organizational differences, results showed a high correlation of caring attributes among the various settings. Interviews conducted with nurses indicated a concern that their "ability to be caring was in jeopardy." Some of the responses they gave included "financial pressure on the hospital distracts us from our mission of caring" and "managed care emphasizes the efficiency of nursing tasks over caring" (p. 30). These nurses felt that the practice of caring was being seriously threatened by the economic pressure associated with health-care changes.

Ray (1997) interviewed six nurse administrators to study the art of caring in nursing administration. The theme, economic-political-ethical valuing and its three attributes of exchanging commodity values, negotiating the politics, and valuing the ethic of caring, showed that the caring expressions of nurse administrators are bound to the economics and politics of the organization (Ray, 1997). Narrative examples of the attribute, exchanging commodity values, were "making caring tangible" and "patient care is a commodity (economic good or value)." Narrative examples of the attribute negotiating the politics were "the nurse administrator is a system coordinator, nurses are the system and know what impinges on them," and "nurses are political beings (powerful in the organization)." Narrative examples of the attribute, valuing the ethics of caring, were "the nurse administrator needs to be caring and shouldn't be like other administrators," and "value of nursing is to care holistically." Findings from this research study validate the interwoven relationship among caring, economics, and politics within organizational culture.

What is the role of professional nursing in the current atmosphere of health care economic reform? How are nurses preparing for changes, especially external control over the discipline and practice of nursing? Concern by nurses for humanistic caring and the preservation of the nurse-patient relationship in all aspects of clinical practice is growing.

In an attempt to answer these questions, nursing inquiry over the last 2 decades has firmly established that the focus of nursing is caring in the human health experience (Boykin & Schoenhofer, 1993; Leininger, 1981; Newman, Sime, & Corcoran-Perry, 1991; Ray, 1994; Watson, 1985). Caring between nurse and patient occurs within the realm of the nurse-patient relationship.

A recent nursing study demonstrated that high-quality care is located in the reciprocal actions of the interpersonal nurse-patient relationship (Hoggard-Green, 1995). Turkel (1993) used an ethnographic approach to study nurse-patient interactions in the critical care environment. The subsequent theme generated among all categories of interaction was the nurse-patient relationship. In a qualitative study, Price (1993) examined the meaning of quality nursing care from the perspective of parents of hospitalized children. A key category that emerged from the data was a positive relationship between quality of care and parents' perspectives. In the wake of workplace restructuring as a result of health-care reform and managed care, nurses are finding themselves in a period of transition, moving from traditional inpatient hospital practice to community-based practice. In a research study conducted by Turkel, Tappen, and Hall (1999), the development of a positive nurse-patient relationship was shown to be seen as a reward for nurses undergoing change in practice roles.

The foregoing studies identified the critical nature of the nurse-patient relationship. However, these studies did not merge economic concepts into nursing research or theory. As the nursing practice environment has continued to change, new research is needed to explore how nurses can continue to provide humanistic care with limited economic resources.

Challenge to Researchers

The challenge to articulate the economic value of the nurse-patient relationship as a commodity, just as goods, money, and services are viewed in traditional economics, is imperative. Foa (1971), an exchange theorist, designed an economic theory that could bridge the gap between economic and noneconomic resources. In this model, noneconomic resources (love, status, and information) were correlated with economic resources (money, goods, and services). According to Ray (1987, p. 40), "[T]he inclusion of these resources is necessary and will require a major effort on the part of nurses and patients to see that they become an integral part of the health care economic analysis."

In order to appraise the nurse-patient relationship as an economic interpersonal resource, it is neces-sary to conduct qualitative and quantitative research studies to describe this unique relationship as an economic exchange process and economic resource. The philosophical framework of the economic dimension of bureaucratic caring has served in part as the basis for this type of needed nursing research. Turkel (1997) interviewed nurses, patients, and administrators from the for-profit sector to examine the process involved in the development of the nurse-patient relationship as an economic resource. No other published research has included the perspective of nonnursing hospital administrators when studying the nurse-patient relationship. In addition, this research was conducted as managed care penetration was having an enormous impact on the current health-care delivery system.

Interviewing participants was the primary source of data collection for Turkel's (1997) grounded theory study. Participants' descriptions of their experiences provided the researcher with rich data for simultaneous data analysis. The initial interviews began with a general open-ended question. Nurses, for example, were asked, "Tell me about a typical day on your unit. Start with "I come to work. . . ." Patients were asked, "Tell me about a day in the hospital." Administrators were asked, "How would you describe a typical day for a nurse from your understanding of the experience?"

As the interview process proceeded, more specific questions were asked, including inquiries about specific nurse-patient interactions and the costs and benefits associated with these interactions. Use of the word "costs" was consistent with the challenge to nurse researchers by Buerhaus (1986) to conduct interviews that provide economic or dollar value data in relation to caring nursing interactions.

The researcher examined the data for relationships among categories for each group of participants: nurses, patients, and administrators. Subsequent relationships were also discovered by looking at similarities and differences among these three groups. The combined analysis of the responses of nurses, patients, and administrators described the process of establishing the nurse-patient relationship within the ever-changing health-care environment. Results from this research study were characterized by the categories of sustaining the caring ideal while simultaneously facing a new reality controlled by costs.

Despite the economic changes of the current health-care environment, all three groups of participants talked about the importance of a positive nurse-patient relationship. The concept of caring between the nurse and the patient was recognized and valued by the nurses, patients, and administrators. *Sustaining the caring ideal* was operationally defined as "acknowledging the relationship and differentiating caring."

The economic changes in health care brought about a new reality for practice controlled by costs. Nurses, patients, and administrators were affected by these changes and the subsequent impact on nursing care delivery within the hospital. *Facing a new reality* was defined as "enduring chaos, calculating the costs, and anticipating future concerns."

> The economic changes in health care brought about a new reality for practice controlled by costs.

Diminishing health-care resources was the basic social problem encountered by nurses, patients, and administrators. The basic social process of the nurse-patient relationship as an economic resource was struggling to find a balance, which referred to sustaining the caring ideal in a new reality controlled by costs.

In a study conducted by Ray and Turkel (1997), qualitative interviews were accomplished in not-for-profit and military sectors of the health-care delivery system. The purpose of this research was to continue the study of the nurse-patient relationship as an economic interpersonal resource. Findings from this study identified that the nurse-patient relationship was both outcome and process. Categories, which emerged during data analysis, included relationships, caring, and costs.

In the study, a formal theory of the nurse-patient relationship as an economic resource was generated from the qualitative research. The formal theory emerged as relationship (set of variables). The formal theory consisted of two parts: (1) relationship as a function of interactions or the intentionality and actions of nurses and patients; and (2) the value of the interactions, or what are the important interactions. Although this theory is described as a linear process, the process is dynamic and holistic, and is considered both outcome and process. Relationship is intentional, action-oriented, and characterized by both economic and caring dimensions. As testing of this theory continues via quantitative research, it is highly probable that this new theory will fall in the category of nonlinear dynamic theory development.

Continued Research on Economics and Caring

In order to measure the nurse-patient relationship as an economic resource and to refine and test the theory, Ray and Turkel (1998) developed the Nurse-Patient Relationship Resource Analysis (NPRRA) Questionnaires (patient and professional). It is anticipated that this research will facilitate understanding of the value of nursing in the health-care system. Research conducted in practice settings provides an integrated link for theory, research, and practice.

Tool Development

The NPRRA Questionnaires are a 45-item instrument for patients and professionals designed from qualitative research (Ray & Turkel, 1997) and validated and established as reliable through quantitative research (Ray & Turkel, 1998). Research questions were asked of participants by means of interviews to elicit information describing benefits of the nurse-patient relationship and perceived costs related to this interaction. Patterns of interaction and knowledge of cost parameters of the nurse-patient relationship were the foundation for the construction of the questionnaire. Three central categories of relationships, caring, and costs, with related subscales and properties, served as the basis for the items of the questionnaire. Initially, the instrument response set was a Likert-type scale with six response choices; now there are five response choices. Initial instrument testing included assessment of the level of readability and review by a panel of experts. At the outset, the initial questionnaire consisted of 89 items; however, after a prepilot cluster analysis was conducted, the questionnaire was made into two and the number of items was reduced to 60, which was further reduced to 45 items after a pilot study. The questionnaire was then redistributed to a sample of over 300 nurses, patients, and administrators from the for-profit, not-for-profit, and military settings. Reliability of .81 was established using Cronbach's alpha and test/retest. Validity was determined by the Index of Context Validity and factor analysis.

At this time, Ray and Turkel are in the process of administering the questionnaires to over 600 respondents on a national level. Findings from this research in process will use regression analysis to determine whether or not there is a correlation between the nurse-patient relationship and patient outcomes such as health, well-being, satisfaction, and cost. The long-term goal of this research is to establish the nurse-patient relationship as an economic interpersonal resource. In order to successfully merge economics and caring, it is necessary for researchers to examine the dynamic patterns of interpersonal relationships as economic resources and their subsequent effect on health, healing, nurse-patient satisfaction, and costs.

POLITICAL/ECONOMIC IMPLICATIONS OF BUREAUCRATIC CARING

Findings from current nursing research on the economic dimension of bureaucratic caring can be used to guide administrative practice within health care organizations. As a dimension of her 1997 research, Turkel (1997) interviewed eight top-level hospital and corporate-level administrators to gain an understanding of how they viewed the experiences of nurses and patients in the hospital setting. Administrators were chosen to be interviewed because they make the ultimate decision on how to allocate scarce human and economic resources within the organizational setting.

Administrator participants explained the value and importance of the nurse-patient relationship. They discussed receiving letters from patients, scoring high on surveys, and getting positive verbal feedback from patients as indicators of caring nurse-patient interactions. One administrator shared the following with the researcher (Turkel, 1997, p. 148):

> Lying in a bed like that, people feel vulnerable and are vulnerable, and they want to know that someone is there for them and will share with them what's going on. And it has to do with the caring. I hear [patients say] that my nurse cared, she listened, and she kept me informed. I would say that more than half of the positive comments I receive from patients have to do with the nurses being caring. What comes back to me is they cared about me, they took time to talk to me, they were kind to me.

Health Care and Nursing Administration

The results of Turkel's (1997) study showed that administrators value caring and high-quality care. However, their actions and the action of other administrators must then reflect these values to ensure that the caring philosophy of the hospital remains in the forefront of organizational profit-making or economics. The issue of time constraints and inadequate staffing has been identified as problematic. Nurses and patients view lack of time as a hindrance to forming a caring nurse-patient relationship. This points out the need for administrators to restructure the organization so that the maximum of nursing time is focused on direct nurse-patient interactions. Hospital administrators desire high levels of quality care and see financial benefits from return business when patients are satisfied with nursing care. To maintain this standard, administrators must maintain adequate staffing

ratios in order to allow time for nurses to be with their patients.

There has been limited published literature studying the nurse-patient relationship from a nonnursing administrator perspective (Ray & Turkel, 1997; Turkel, 1997). However, the changing health-care environment has been addressed from an organizational perspective (Hammer & Champy, 1993; Iglehart, 1993; Korten, 1995; O'Donnell & Sampson, 1994). The organizational focus was on maximizing efficiency, making a profit, and economic survival.

In the research conducted by Ray and Turkel (1997), administrator participants confirmed the above, but also discussed the concomitant need for maintaining care and quality. The challenge facing administrators in a managed care environment is the simultaneous management of costs, care, and quality. Ray (1989) asserted that this can be accomplished if administrators consider both the tangible and intangible benefits of services provided within the organization.

Administrators need to recognize caring as a value-added interaction. From this point of view, the benefits of the interaction outweigh the expense of the registered nurse. Caring can be viewed as an "opportunity cost" or the cost of doing it right. This concept is applicable to contemporary health-care organizations. If people don't come back to a hospital (because of poor care), "you've lost an opportunity."

Administrative/Nursing Education

The Theory of Bureaucratic Caring is being used to guide curriculum development in the master of science in nursing administration program at Florida Atlantic University in Boca Raton, Florida. The revised nursing administration track is entitled "Administrative and Financial Leadership in Nursing and Health Care." Caring and humanizing of the health-care delivery system are key concepts in the cognate and concentration courses. Issues impacting caring, administrative roles, leadership, organizational culture, health-care delivery systems, health-care policy, and health-care finance are explored from ethical, spiritual, economic, technological, legal, political, and social perspectives.

The economic dimension of bureaucratic caring is a central component of the courses entitled "Health Care Delivery Systems," "Health Care Policy," and "Health Care Finance." In "Health Care Delivery Systems," students are challenged to analyze the current economic and reimbursement structure of health care from the perspective of a caring lens. Throughout the course, students develop strategies to challenge the present economic structure and shape the future by advancing caring as a central component of health-care delivery systems. The course culminates in the creation of a futuristic model for humanizing the health-care delivery system through the convergence of caring and economics.

In the course entitled "Health Care Policy," the economic and political dimensions of bureaucratic caring are explored. Emphasis is placed on the role of the professional nurse on influencing the policy-making process in terms of policy redesign. Students are encouraged to dialogue with members of the legislature and discuss both the economic and political impact of humanizing the health-care delivery system.

The "Health Care Finance" course is integral to the students' understanding of the synergy between nursing and finance within organizational cultures. As students prepare budgets and review financial statements, they validate how health-care organizations respond to "being known for caring" and still remain financially viable. Given today's environment, it is important for students to understand the fiscal and resource constraints imposed by managed care. Students synthesize acquired knowledge grounded in the perspective of caring to create a balance between caring and finance within organizations.

Nursing Practice

The economic dimension of bureaucratic caring can be used to guide practice. A common yet challenging goal of health-care organizations is to reduce cost while simultaneously improving quality patient care. Now is the time for professional nurses to become proactive and use theory-based practice to shape their future instead of having the future dictated by others outside the discipline. Staff nurses can hold

close their core value that caring is the essence of nursing, and still retain a focus on meeting the bottom line.

Recent quantitative studies have demonstrated that higher registered nurse staffing ratios are linked to better patient outcomes and decreased lengths of stay (Blegen & Vaughn, 1998; Blegen, Goode, & Reed, 1998; Brooten & Naylor, 1995; Duffy, 1990). Other studies have linked nurse caring to increased patient satisfaction and improved patient outcomes (Duffy, 1992; Larson & Ferketich, 1993; Valentine, 1989, 1991, 1993).

Numerous qualitative studies have documented the relationship between caring and positive patient outcomes (Duffy, 1992; Eriksson, 1997; Ray & Turkel, 1997; Valentine, 1998; Zerwekh, 1997). In these studies, the definition of "outcomes" was expanded from the traditional measures of process and product of care, mortality, morbidity, and adverse effects. Examining outcomes from the perspective of caring involved vivid descriptions and stories of how nurses transformed their patients' lives.

In a slight departure from other qualitative studies, Boykin and Schoenhofer (1997) explored outcomes within the theoretical context of enhancing personhood. The value and richness of nursing as caring was explicated via a nursing situation. Outcomes drawn from this nursing situation included one each for the nursed (patient), one for the nurse, and one for the health-care agency. The following is an example of outcome statements derived from the nursing situations: "[a]ffirmation of self as loving father, sense of personal connectedness, and demonstration of agency services as valuable and culturally competent" (Boykin & Schoenhofer, 1997, pp. 63–64).

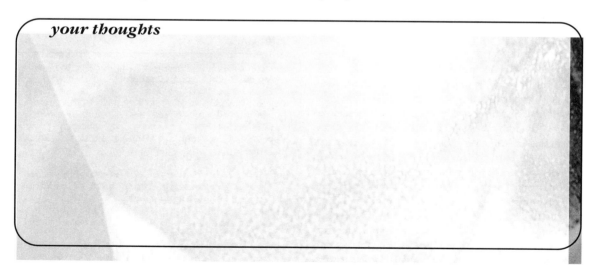

your thoughts

Nyberg's recent (1998) research has focused on the issue of equating patient outcomes with caring. This demonstration project is designed to measure caring outcomes after nurses receive education about caring and caring/healing treatments. The purpose of the research is "to obtain the objective measures of caring as required by today's health care evaluation systems (p. 97)."

These empirical studies have firmly established a link between caring and positive patient outcomes. Positive patient outcomes are needed for organizational survival in this competitive era of health care. Given this, professional nursing practice must embrace and illuminate the caring philosophy.

Staff nurses describe the essence of nursing as the caring relationship between nurse and patient (Trossman, 1998). However, nurses are practicing in an environment where the economics and costs of health care permeate discussions and clinical decisions. The focus on costs is not a transient response to shrinking reimbursement; instead, it has become the catalyst for change within corporate health-care organizations.

Nurses are continuing to struggle with economic changes. With a system goal of decreasing length of stay and increasing staffing ratios, nurses need to establish trust and initiate a relationship during their first encounter with a patient. As this relationship is being established, nurses need to focus on being, knowing, and doing all at once, (Turkel, 1997) and being there from a patient perspective. For the nurses, this means completing a task while simultaneously engaging with a patient. This holistic approach to practice means viewing the patient as a person in all his or her complexity and then identifying the needs for professional nursing as they arise.

must be integrated into staff development curricula. Nurses need to search continually for different approaches to professional practice that will incorporate caring in an increasingly technical and cost-driven environment. Doing more with less no longer works; nurses must move outside of the box to create innovative practice models based on nursing theory.

Administrative nursing research needs to continue to study the relationship among staff nursing caring, patient outcomes, and organizational economic outcomes. Further research is required to firmly establish the nurse-patient relationship as an economic resource in the new paradigm of health-care delivery. Findings from these research studies will continue to validate the Theory of Bureaucratic Caring as a middle-range holographic practice theory.

Nurses need repeated exposure to the economics and costs associated with health care. Lack of knowledge in this area means others outside of nursing will continue to make the political and economic decisions concerning the practice of nursing. Having an in-depth knowledge of the economics of health care will allow nurses to challenge and change the system. A new theory-based model can be created for nursing practice that supports human caring in relation to the organization's economic and political values. The political and economic dimensions of bureaucratic caring serve as a philosophical/theoretical framework to guide both contemporary and futuristic theory-based nursing practice.

> Knowledge of the economics of health care will allow nurses to challenge and change the system.

Summary

The foundation for professional caring is the blending of the humanistic and empirical aspects of care. In today's environment, the nurse needs to integrate caring, knowledge, and skills all at once. Given political and economic constraints, the art of caring cannot occur in isolation from meeting the physical needs of patients. When caring is defined solely as science or as art, it is not adequate to reflect the reality of current practice.

Nurses need to be able to understand and articulate the politics and the economics of nursing practice and health care. Classes that examine the environment of practice generally, and the politics and the economics of health care in relation to caring,

References

Bargagliotti, L. A., & Smith, M. (1985). Patterns of nursing costs with capitated reimbursement. *Nursing Economics, 3*(5), 270–275.

Blegen, M. A., Goode, C. J., & Reed, L. (1998). Nurse staffing and patient outcomes. *Nursing Research, 47*(1), 43–50.

Blegen, M. A., & Vaughn, T. (1998). A multisite study of nurse staffing and patient outcomes. *Nursing Economics, 16*(4), 196–203.

Boykin, A., & Schoenhofer, S. (1993). *Nursing as caring: A model for transforming practice.* New York: National League for Nursing.

Boykin, A., & Schoenhofer, S. (1997). Reframing outcomes: Enhancing personhood. *Advanced Practice Nursing Quarterly, 3*(1), 60–65.

Brooten, D., & Naylor, M. D. (1995). Nurses' effect in changing patient outcomes. *Image, 27*(2), 95–99.

Buerhaus, P. (1986). The economics of caring: Challenges, and new opportunities for nursing. *Topics in Clinical Nursing, 8*(2), 13-21.

Curtin, L. (1983). Determining costs of nursing service per DRG. *Nursing Management, 14*(4), 16-20.

Dahlen, A. L., & Gregor, J. R. (1985). Nursing costs by DRG with an all RN staff. In Shaffer, F. A. (Ed.), *Costing out nursing: Pricing our product* (pp. 113-122). New York: National League for Nursing.

DiVestea, N. (1985). The changing health care system: An overview. In Shaffer, F. A. (Ed.), *Costing out nursing: Pricing our product* (pp. 29-36). New York: National League for Nursing.

Dolan, J. (1985). *Nursing in society: A historical perspective*. Philadelphia: W. B. Saunders.

Duffy, J. (1990). *The relationship between nurse caring behaviors and selected outcomes of care in hospitalized medical and/or surgical patients*. Unpublished doctoral dissertation, Catholic University of America, Washington, DC.

Duffy, J. (1992). The impact of nurse caring on patient outcomes. In D. A. Gaut (Ed.), *The presence of caring in nursing* (pp. 113-136). New York: National League for Nursing.

Eriksson, K. (1997). Understanding the world of the patient, the suffering human being: The new clinical paradigm from nursing to caring. *Advanced Practice Nursing Quarterly, 3*(1), 8-13.

Foa, U. (1971). Interpersonal and economic resources. *Science, 171*(29), 345-351.

Foshay, M. C. (1988). *Professional nurses' perceptions of their caring activities and their perceptions of the ability of patient classification systems to measure their caring activities*. Unpublished master's thesis, University of Southern Maine, Portland.

Gapenski, L (1993). *Understanding health care financial management: Text, cases, and models*. Ann Arbor, MI: Health Administration Press.

Glandon, G., Colbert, K., & Thomasma, M. (1989). Nursing delivery models and RN mix: Cost implications. *Nursing Management, 20* (5), 30-33.

Halloran, E. J. (1983). Nursing workload, medical diagnosis related groups, and nursing diagnosis. *Research in Nursing and Health, 8*(4), 421-433.

Hammer, M., & Champy, J. (1993). *Reengineering the corporation*. New York: HarperCollins.

Helt, E., & Jelinek, R. (1988). In the wake of cost cutting, nursing productivity, and quality improvement. *Nursing Management, 19*(6), 36-38, 42, 46-48.

Hoggard-Green, J. (1995). *A phenomenological study of a consumer's definition of quality health care*. Unpublished doctoral dissertation, University of Utah, Salt Lake City.

Iglehart, J. (1993). *Debating health care reform*. Bethesda, MD: Health Affairs, Project Hope.

Jennings, T. (1991). Medicare reimbursement deficits: Are nursing care costs to blame? *Today's OR Nurse, 13*(9), 13-17.

Kenkel, P. (1992). Latest study a boost for managed competition. *Modern Health Care, 22*(15), 76-78.

Ketter, J. (1995, May). Re-engineering the workforce. *The American Nurse, 27*(3), 1, 14.

Kongstvedt, P. (1997). *Essentials of managed health care* (2nd ed.). Gaithersburg, MD: Aspen.

Korten, D. (1995). *When corporations rule the world*. San Francisco: Berrett-Koehler Publishers.

Larson, P., & Ferketich, S. (1993). Patients' satisfaction with nurses' caring during hospitalization. *Western Journal of Nursing Research, 15*(6), 690-707.

Leininger, M. (1981). The phenomenon of caring: Importance, research questions and theoretical considerations. In Leininger, M. (Ed.), *Caring: An essential human need* (pp. 3-15). Thorofare, NJ: Slack.

Lynaugh, J., & Fagin, C. (1988). Nursing comes of age. *Image, 20*(4), 184-190.

Mansfield, E. (1991). *Microeconomics* (7th ed.). New York: Norton.

McCormick, B. (1986). What's the cost of nursing care? *Hospitals, 60,* 48-52.

Miller, K. (1987). The human care perspective in nursing administration. *Journal of Nursing Administration, 17*(2), 10-12.

Miller, K. (1995). Keeping the care in nursing care. *Journal of Nursing Administration, 25*(11), 29-32.

Minyard, K., Wall, J., & Turner, R. (1986). RNs may cost less than you think. *Journal of Nursing Administration, 16*(5), 29-34.

Newman, M., Sime, M., & Corcoran-Perry, S. (1991). The focus of the discipline of nursing. *Advances in Nursing Science, 14*(1), 1-6.

Nyberg, J. (1989). The element of caring in nursing administration. *Nursing Administration Quarterly, 13,* 9-16.

Nyberg, J. (1990). The effects of care and economics on nursing practice. *Journal of Nursing Administration, 20*(5), 13-18.

Nyberg, J. (1991). Theoretical explorations of human care and economics: Foundations of nursing administration practice. *Advances in Nursing Science, 13*(1), 74-84.

Nyberg, J. (1998). *A caring approach in nursing administration*. Niwot, CO: University Press of Colorado.

O'Donnell, K., & Sampson, E. (1994). The pivotal link in the creation of a new health care delivery system. *Journal of Health Care Finance, 21*(2), 74-86.

Porter-O'Grady, T. (1979). Financial planning: Budgeting for nurses, part I. *Supervisor Nurse, 10,* 35-38.

Prescott, P. (1993). Nursing: An important component of hospital survival under a reformed health care system. *Nursing Economics, 11*(4), 192-199.

Price, P. (1993). Parents' perceptions of the meaning of quality nursing care. *Advances in Nursing Science, 16*(1), 33-41.

Ray, M. (1987). Health care economics and human caring in nursing: Why the moral conflict must be resolved. *Family Community Health, 10*(1), 35-43.

Ray, M. (1989). The Theory of Bureaucratic Caring for nursing practice in the organizational culture. *Nursing Administration Quarterly, 13*(2), 31-42.

Ray, M. (1994). Complex caring dynamics: A unifying model of nursing inquiry. *Theoretic and Applied Chaos in Nursing, 1*(1), 23-32.

Ray, M. (1997). The ethical theory of existential authenticity: The lived experience of the art of caring in nursing administration. *Canadian Journal of Nursing Research, 29*(1), 111-126.

Ray, M., & Turkel, M. (1997). [Nurse-patient relationship patterns: An economic resource]. Unpublished raw data.

Ray, M., & Turkel, M. (1998). [Econometric analysis of the nurse-patient relationship]. Unpublished raw data.

Shaffer, F. (1985). *Costing out nursing: Pricing our product.* New York: National League for Nursing.

Trossman, S. (1998, September/October). The human connection: Nurses and their patients. *The American Nurse, 30*(5), 1, 8.

Turkel, M. (1993). *Nurse-patient interactions in the critical-care setting.* Manuscript submitted for publication.

Turkel, M. (1997). Struggling to find a balance: A grounded theory study of the nurse-patient relationship within an economic context (Doctoral dissertation, University of Miami, 1997). *Dissertation Abstracts International.*

Turkel, M., Tappen, R., & Hall, R. (1999). Moments of excellence. *Journal of Gerontological Nursing, 25*(1), 7–12.

Valentine, K. (1989). Caring is more than kindness: Modeling its complexities. *Journal of Nursing Administration, 19*(11), 28–34.

Valentine, K. (1991). Comprehensive assessment of caring and its relationship to outcome measures. *Journal of Nursing Quality Assurance, 5*(2), 59–68.

Valentine, K. (1993). Development of a nurse compensation system. In Gaut, D. A. (Ed.), *A global agenda for caring* (pp. 329–345). New York: National League for Nursing.

Valentine, K. (1998). *A convincing argument for effectiveness: Is caring more than nice people doing nice things?* Paper presented at Communicating Caring, the Essence of Nursing, International Association for Human Caring, Philadelphia, PA.

Walker, D. (1983). The cost of nursing care in hospitals. *Journal of Nursing Administration, 13*(3), 13–18.

Watson, J. (1985). *Nursing: Human science and human care.* East Norwalk, CT: Appleton-Century-Croft.

Zerwekh, J. (1997). Making the connection during home visits: Narratives of expert nurses. *International Journal for Human Caring, 1*(1), 25–29.

Appendix

Evaluating Nursing Theory Resources

❖ Why Evaluate Resources for Nursing Inquiry Research?

❖ Evaluation of Resources for Nursing Inquiry and Research

❖ Preparing to Initiate a Search

❖ A Search Example with Strategies

❖ Summary

❖ References

Marguerite J. Purnell

The study of nursing theory is a rich and exciting journey into the heart and intention of nursing. Reflective appreciation of theory offers a fascinating living connection both to the history of nursing and to its future. Through the development and use of theory, nursing is able to reflect upon itself and respond purposefully to human need. The distilled nursing knowledge that is captured as essence in theory plainly speaks of nursing that is lived.

WHY EVALUATE RESOURCES FOR NURSING INQUIRY AND RESEARCH?

Previous chapters have addressed evaluation of nursing theory. This appendix offers guidelines to help establish credibility of nursing resources used in inquiry and research. Resources that support development and dissemination of knowledge must themselves be consistent with the intent of nursing theory and congruent with values expressed in reflective inquiry and research. Resources in nursing should be authoritative, accurate, and current, and characterized by rich content. The guiding framework for evaluation of resources presented in these pages moves toward a realistic understanding of the applicability and utility of the resource. Practical pointers for application of these guidelines, a search example with strategies, and a way to synthesize evaluation findings should help inquiring individuals maintain a confident relationship with the resources that undergird inquiry and research in nursing.

Theory as Guiding Framework for Evaluation

Theory-based practice provides nurses with a perspective (Raudonis & Acton, 1997), and expresses the essential activity of nursing caring in the enacting, adapting, and adding to the nursing human knowledge base. The framework for practice also becomes a framework for education, research, and administration (Boykin & Schoenhofer, 1993). Nursing theory is integrated and lived out in the personhood of the nurse, continuing to shape, guide, and focus the nurse in all activities.

Ways of studying nursing are also becoming more creative and reflect rapid changes in nursing practice and in embedded and expressed societal values. The thoughtful study of nursing theory includes not only consideration of works contributed by the theorist, but also those works contributed by practitioners and critics of the theory present in multiple, complex forms of media.

The Confluence of Computer Technology and Nursing

The rapid advance and integration of technology has not only affected practice, but has also affected ways in which nurses investigate, evaluate, and think about practice (Turley, 1996). Computers increasingly dominate familiar environments (Brennan, 1996) and create their own electronic substitutes, such as websites on the Internet. Ways of inquiry and research have seemingly become more simple and less laborious, yet are paradoxically more complex, with linked and interlinking infrastructures of communication webs and bibliographic databases.

Major emphasis has been placed on evaluating electronic media for the simple reason that electronic media and the Internet dominate communications, data processing, and storage, and the dissemination of knowledge. Riddlesperger et al. (1996, p. 599) observe that the last 20 years have witnessed the electronic domain becoming the "primary method for academic and professional communication of research and information." A new science called "nursing information science" has evolved (Graves & Corcoran-Perry, 1996). Hard copy from libraries is routinely being uploaded onto the Internet for online dissemination. Books and journals themselves are less attractive to many who now prefer the accessibility and convenience of electronic media and the redefined or reinvented electronic book or journal.

Other forms of media, such as magnetic tape, audiotape, and microfiche, are falling into disuse at varying speeds. Just like outmoded theories, they too are being replaced by new types of media that can accommodate greater and more complex information. Databases—vast electronic repositories of information—have allowed the capture and expression of the lives of millions of humans on a microchip, and provided the storage, sifting, and retrieval of generations of knowledge and living encapsulated in the convenience of a small desktop or laptop computer.

In nursing, also, new ways of searching the literature have transferred the library of the building to the convenience of a computer hard drive. Time invested in library research has been dramatically reduced through the use of electronic tools. Multiple databases of nursing literature, once confined to hand-typed reference cards, can be accessed, sorted, and published simultaneously and immediately through electronic computer interfaces. In most libraries, a thorough literature search can now no longer be accomplished without a computer. As the indispensable technology of a pioneer electronic generation in nursing, computers provide portals to nursing science and to the artifacts of the world. It is through these same portals we venture in our examination of flow to evaluate resources for inquiry and research.

EVALUATION OF RESOURCES FOR NURSING INQUIRY AND RESEARCH

Theory—Conceptual Transformation

Conceptual frameworks in the mind of the nurse provide the means of interfacing and transforming values of the contrived artifice of the electronic data bit (Carlton, Ryan, & Siktberg, 1998). Located in the intransigence of the electronic nanosecond, virtual data are fleeting, and only as permanent as the source of power. Explicit and implicit claims to truth and reality in electronic media, storage or otherwise, cannot be easily disputed. To whom or to what does one respond or carry concerns? A framework of virtual values is thus engineered and deeply embedded in electronic information technologies. The challenge for the nurse is to analyze, evaluate, and transform electronic frameworks of values into a conceptual framework of human values that are realized in theory and actualized in practice. The ubiquitous website—the most numerous, frequent, and transient of electronic data or resource locators to which information seekers turn—is, for the most part, unregulated. It exists at the will of the website "owner." Claims of "authority" and ownership of those claims often cannot be traced or are unprovable. Hebda, Czar, and Mascara (1998) refer to the necessity for authority of websites to be validated, and feel it is a problem unless the source can be traced to a reputable institution, such as in education or government. Table Appendix-1, detailing Internet sites where website addresses of educational institutions all over the world may be located, begins to address that particular challenge.

In order to evaluate and substantiate resources for nursing inquiry such as theorist home pages and nursing information websites, layers of electronic in-

---

TABLE APPENDIX-1 *General Resources*

College and University Home Pages

http://www.mit.edu:8001/people/cdemello/univ.html

This is a website that will enable you to search efficiently for college and university home pages by geographical region, alphabetically, nationally, and internationally. One home page per college or university is available. Several thousand entries are listed.

American Universities Home Pages

http://www.clas.ufl.edu/CLAS/american-universities.html

This is a linked site to College and University Home Pages. One home page per college or university is available.

In searching for information on theory or theorists, the web address of the "home" university or academic institution is frequently elusive. The above websites should facilitate the beginning of the search process for nursing theory information.

The Nursing Theory Page

http://www.ualberta.ca/~jrnorris/nt/theory/html

This is a site at the University of Alberta that serves as a general "clearinghouse," where theorists listed are linked back to their home pages. Some newer, lesser known models and theories are listed. The Nursing Theory Page is created by the Nursing Theory Page Development Group, whose members are listed with E-mail addresses on this site.

Searching Bibliographic Databases for Nursing Theory

http://www.ualberta.ca/~irnorris/nt/CINAHL/allen.html

Also at the University of Alberta, this page, which is authored by Margaret (Peg) Allen, MLS, AHIP, provides useful, detailed information for searching CINAHL. Several links are provided to other useful search resource sites on the Internet.

---

formation must be peeled back to reveal those authoritative nurse scholars, scientists, and practitioners who are the source of disseminated nursing knowledge. Since no two nursing information resources are exactly alike, guidelines for evaluation should remain flexible and adaptable. Conceptual frameworks for nursing practice become meaningful when lived out in the reflective, intentional application of theory in the exchange and transfer of knowledge. The nursing research tool of electronic information must affirm the values both of the nurse offering and the nurse receiving the transfer of knowledge. In nursing, a call for nursing is a call for transforming information; the response from nursing should be a response with clarity and humility, regardless of the medium used. The consistent evaluation of resources is therefore an affirmation of the values grounding the practice of nursing.

A Guiding Framework for Evaluation of Resources

The questions following provide for flexible assessment and insightful evaluation of nursing theory resources. Although these questions emphasize electronic media, they are also applicable in the evaluation of books, journals, physical archives, and other resources.

Reflective Preparations:

- What do you want to know?
- What are your expectations of the resource? How complex do you expect the information to be?
- How comprehensive do you intend your analysis and evaluation to be?
- Will you share the results of your evaluation with colleagues?

Focus on Authority:

- Who are authoritative sources for information about development, evaluation, and use of the theory you are inquiring about? Are they contributors to the website or media you are evaluating? For example, who speaks authoritatively for continuing development for theorists such as Martha Rogers, Hildegard Peplau, or Dorothy Johnson?
- Who are nursing authorities who speak, write about, and use the theory? Who are the practitioners? Are they contributors to this website or media?
  - What are the professional attributes of these persons?

- What are the attributes of authorities, and how does one become one?
- Which other nurses should be considered authorities? Why?
- What are major resources, other than the one you are now evaluating, that are authoritative sources on the theory?
  - Books? Articles? Audiovisual media? Electronic media?
  - What nursing societies share and support work of the theory? Do they also have a website?
- What service and academic programs are authoritative sources?

Focus on Content:

- What is the purpose of the resource?
- Is the resource dedicated to the work of one theorist, or is it a general resource for the work of many theorists?
- Do sources for authoritative information show their credentials on the webpage or provide links to pages that do?
- Does the website or media provide accurate information in a logical and easily accessible manner?
  - Is there clear reference to source data?
  - Where possible, are there specific HTML links to that data?
- Does the website or media provide comprehensive information?
  - How detailed is the information presented? Does it cover nursing research, administration, and education?
  - Do related resources present the information in greater depth?
- Is the information presented even in quality and quantity?
- Is the information current? What evidence is presented to verify currency?

Focus on the website:

- Is the website or media well maintained? Are you able to contact the Webmaster from an onsite address?
- Are there links to other, similar, websites? Are these links active addresses? Are you informed when you are seamlessly transferred to another website?
- Are there fees to access information?

- Is the website or media aesthetically pleasing? What unique characteristics enhance your understanding and appreciation of the theorist's work?

Listed in Table Appendix-2 are authoritative resources with which to begin a study of nursing theorists and their theories, and include home pages for theorists such as Martha Rogers, Dorothea Orem, and Rosemarie Parse. Home pages and websites are listed where they are available. Use the guidelines offered to evaluate these websites. It will be helpful to search out and evaluate other sites dedicated to nursing theory and compare your findings.

Table Appendix-1 lists some useful general information on websites which can give you access to a vast repertoire of nursing information resources through educational institutions. These sites can also be evaluated using the above guidelines. The information noted in this chapter is not intended to provide a compendium of websites, facilities, or venues of information, but rather to facilitate and guide reflective evaluation of nursing theory and other nursing knowledge information resources.

PREPARING TO INITIATE A SEARCH
Begin at the Beginning with Yourself

Organizing and purposefully attending to self before undertaking research will affirm the intention and focus of your philosophical perspective. Theoretical frameworks become blueprints for action. Frustrations inherent in new methodologies, new technologies, and virtual information will be less able to deflect your nursing intention to uncover and integrate nursing knowledge if you are prepared. Attending to self in ways that are meaningful to you will quiet, focus, and center reflective inquiry.

Connecting with a Computer

If you are new to a computer search of nursing literature, be prepared to spend many, many hours searching for information. When first becoming acquainted with the electronic world, be prepared to accept that you will forget where you are on this electronic highway: It takes practice and intense focus to remain on the elusive information trail. Forgive yourself if you accomplish little, and forgive the computer if you are "dropped" from a key theorist website and don't remember where it was or who the theorist was. Practice self-care by becoming organized and remaining within the parameters of your inquiry.

Lingering in the Library

In order to conserve time and effort, it is beneficial to know how to access the library computers to search for locations of nursing journals, books, videos, microfiches, and databases *before* commencing your search. Seek the help of experts *before* you attempt the impossible and end up frustrated. Time spent browsing books and journals because they are interesting (yet irrelevant to your investigation) also means time spent returning to the library on another day to return all the books you don't have time to read.

Aging in the Archives

Unless you have already used a computer to identify a specific holding or collection in the archives that you wish to investigate, engage the help of the archivist to clarify and expedite your search. A "hands-on" search of archived records involves painstaking handling, lengthy and careful perusing, and hours of time. Search nursing archives only if you are unable to access the information elsewhere: The pleasure of the spirit and feel of nursing history in its tangible artifacts is enhanced without the constraints of time. Resolve to spend unpressured leisure time in the nursing archives. In your goal-directed endeavors to balance time, effort, and outcome, however, it is preferable to reserve time-restricted activities for electronic inquiries.

How to Become Organized

- **Define the reason for your search:**
  - Is your search preparation for creation of a manuscript? What is the scope of the manuscript topic?
  - Is your search the beginning of formal research? What is the scope of the formal research?
  - Is your search simply because you would like to know more about a theorist or theory to apply to your practice?
- **How much time will you be prepared to invest?**
- **Construct a preliminary time line and begin a countdown:**
  - When is the absolute deadline for producing the end product—for example, manuscript or formal research dissemination?
  - When is the absolute deadline for completion of research activities?

Theorists:	**Anne Boykin**
	Savina Schoenhofer

Theory:	Theory of Nursing as Caring
Website	The Caring Archives of the Christine E. Lynn Center for Caring
	http://www.fau.edu/

This is the home page of Florida Atlantic University. Choose "Colleges" and then "Nursing." A link is provided from the College of Nursing Home Page to the home page of The Caring Archives of the Christine E. Lynn Center for Caring at FAU College of Nursing.

These archives were recently instituted for the purpose of humanizing health care through the global dissemination of caring nursing knowledge. The Caring Archives is beginning to accumulate a database of full text documents of caring literature as well as a Signature Collection of multimedia information on the nursing theorists and their theories. Special collections, such as the Nursing Poetry Collection, will house significant contributions to caring in nursing. Access to this database is free. Watch this growing site for updates and special announcements.

A further link is provided from this website to the International Association for Human Caring (I. A. H. C.)

Theorist:	**Virginia Avenel Henderson**

Theory:	Basic Care Components
Videotape:	Celebrating Virginia Henderson
	Available from: Center for Nursing Press,
	550 West North Street, Indianapolis, IN 46202
Website:	Virgina Henderson International Nursing Library
	http://www_son.hs.washington.edu/vhl.html

The Virginia Henderson International Nursing Library provides innovative data, information, and knowledge about nursing research. These resources are provided through two electronic research subscription services: the Registry of Nursing Research, and the Online Journal of Knowledge Synthesis for Nursing. Both services are maintained by Sigma Theta Tau. The Online Journal of Knowledge Synthesis for Nursing is free to Sigma Theta Tau members. For more information about the online services, contact Sigma Theta Tau International at (317) 634-8171 (Library Department), or E-mail: library@ stti-sun.iupui.edu

Theorist:	**Imogene King**

Theory:	Theory of Goal Attainment
Archive:	Being developed by the Oakland University School of Nursing
Organization:	King International Nursing Group

Theorist:	**Myra Levine**

Theory:	Levine's Conservation Model
Website:	Allentown College
	http://www.allencol.edu

Select: Karen Schaefer's home page, and you can choose the link to Levine's Conservation Model. Currently, there exists an up-to-date journal and book reference list. Future changes will include model updates, suggestions, and summaries of the model.

Select: Shelly Yeager's home page, and a summary of key theorists, including Myra Levine, can be found.

Theorist:	**Betty Neuman**
Theory:	The Neuman Systems Model
Website:	http://www3.bc.sympatico.ca/neuman99/
Organization:	The Neuman Systems Model Trustees Group, Inc. Neuman College, c/o Director of Library Media and Archives Neuman College One Neuman Drive Aston, Pennsylvania 19014

Individuals interested in using the Neuman Systems Model may be interested in associate membership in order to communicate and collaborate with trustees. Each member receives the *Neuman News* newsletter, and is included in the mailing list for Call for Abstracts and Symposia brochure. Each member has access to the Neuman data base, and also receives discounted fees for the Neuman Biennial Symposia.

The Biennial International Neuman Systems Model Symposia provide accumulated information about the model and ample opportunities to work with people worldwide who are using the model.

Archives:	**Neuman Archival Collection** Neuman College

Theorist:	**Margaret Neuman**
Theory:	Health as Expanding Consciousness
Website:	http://www.tc.umnj.edu/~hoyin003/

This site at University of Minnesota details current works emanating from the Theory of Health as Expanding Consciousness.

Theorist:	**Florence Nightingale**
Website:	Clendening History of Medicine Library Kansas University Medical Center
	http://kumc.edu/service/clendening/florence/florence.html

This is a fascinating collection of Miss Nightingale's letters, published online in the original text.

Website:	American Association for the History of Nursing (AAHN)
	http://www.aahn.org/ P.O. Box 175 Lanoka Harbor, NJ 08734

This interesting website offers "Gravesites of Prominent Nurses," in which Florence Nightingale and other historically significant nurses' gravesites are featured. Links connect with other sites of interest, including the Florence Nightingale Museum Trust.

E-mail:	AAHN@AAHN.org
Organization:	Florence Nightingale International Nurses' Association

Theorist:	**Dorothea Orem**

Theory:	Self-Care Deficit Nursing Theory
Website:	http://www.hsc.missouri.edu/~son/scdnt/scdnt.html

This site advises of the Dorothea Orem International Self-Care Deficit Conferences, in addition to publishing the Orem Society Newsletters. A case study of advanced practice using the Self-Care Deficit Nursing Theory (SCDNT) is available online. A linked site at Georgetown University School of Nursing provides information on a conceptual framework developed using Dorothea Orem's Self-Care Theory.

Discussion List:	Subscribe through the home website.
Organization:	The International Orem Society for Nursing Science and Scholarship S428 School of Nursing University of Missouri Columbia, MO 65211 Fax: (573) 884-4544 E-mail: K. Renpenning, <104072@compuserve.com>

Theorist:	**Rosemarie R. Parse**

Theory:	The Human Becoming School of Thought
Website:	The Parse Page http://www.utoronto.ca/icps
List server:	Parse-L is an online discussion group. To subscribe, send an E-mail to the server at: listserv@listserv.utoronto.ca

In the body of the note, say ONLY "sub parse-L Yourfirstname Yourlastname." For further information, E-mail Pat Lyon at plyon@gpu.utcc.utoronto.ca

Videotapes:	The Human Becoming Theory: Living True Presence in Nursing Practice (½" VHS and PAL formats). Parse's Theory of Human Becoming: A Learning Guide. Videos are available from: Pat Lyon, Rehabilitation Institute of Toronto 550 University Avenue, Toronto, Ontario, Canada M5G 2A2. E-mail: plyon@gpu.utcc.utoronto.ca
CD-ROM:	Nurse Theorists: Portraits of Excellence: Rosemarie Rizzo Parse Available from FITNE, Inc. Telephone: 1–800–691–8480 Website: www.ev.net/fitne E-mail: fitne@fitne.ev.net

- When would you prefer to complete your research activities?
- How much time do you realistically have for inquiry or research? Count the hours you have available and list days on which they are available, then reassess.
- Produce a detailed, realistic schedule of time available.

- **Define the focus of your search:**
  - Will your inquiry center on one theory only?
  - Will your inquiry also concern the nursing theorist and be an additional focus?
  - Will your inquiry center only on the life of the theorist?

Theorist:	**Hildegard E. Peplau**
Theory:	Interpersonal Theory of Nursing
Website:	http://www.uwo.ca/nursing/homepg/peplau.html

This is the Hildegard Peplau Home Page at the University of Western Ontario School of Nursing.

Videotape:	The Nurse Theorists: Portraits of Excellence: Hildegard Peplau (1988)
	The video is available from: Fuld Video Project, Studio III, 370 Hawthorne Avenue, Oakland, CA 94609
Audiotape:	Life of an Angel: Interview with Hildegard Peplau (1998). Hatherleigh Co.
	The audiotape is available from the American Psychiatric Nurses Association, http://www.apna.org/items/htm

Theorist:	**Martha Rogers**
Theory:	Rogers' Science of Unitary Human Beings
Website:	Martha Rogers Home Page
	http://www.uwcm.ac.uk/uwcm/ns/martha/homepage.html
Organizations:	The Martha E. Rogers Center for the Study of Nursing Science Division of Nursing, New York University 429 Shimkin Hall, 50 West 4th Street, New York, NY 10012–1165

New York University also cosponsors the Rogerian Conferences, held every 2 to 3 years.

	The Society of Rogerian Scholars, Inc. Canal Street Station, P.O. Box 1195, New York, 10013–0867

The Society of Rogerian Scholars, Inc. publishes the referred journal *Visions: The Journal of Rogerian Nursing Science* and the newsletter *Rogerian Nursing Science News.*

List server:	NYU Division of Nursing, Martha E. Rogers Listserv:
	To subscribe, send an E-mail to: listproc@lists.nyu.edu
List server:	Nurse-Rogers Listerv:
	http://www.mailbase.ac.uk/lists/nurse-rogers/join.html
	To subscribe, send an E-mail to: mailbase@mailbase.ac.uk
	For further information contact: Francis C. Biley E-mail: BILEY@cardiff.ac.uk University of Wales College of Medicine Cardiff, Wales, UK

- Will your inquiry center only on practice implications?
- **Define the scope of your search— acknowledge limits:**
  - Will your search include critiques by other nurses and articles from other disciplines?
- Will your search be limited by time, lack of computer, location of computer, or location of library?
- What topics or focus will you *not* include?

Based on the answers to these questions, decide the most convenient physical location where you will base your search, and turn to consider the informa-

Theorist:	**Sr. Callista Roy**
Theory:	The Roy Adaptation Model
Website:	http://www2.bc.edu/~royca/
	http://www.bc.edu/bc_org/avp/son/theorist/nurse-theorist.html
Organization:	Boston Based Adaptation Research in Nursing Society (BBARNS)

The purpose of this society is to advance nursing practice by developing basic and clinical knowledge based on the model. It also provides scholarly colleagueship for knowledge development and research, and the dissemination of research.

Theorist:	**Jean Watson**
Theory:	The Theory of Human Caring
Website:	University of Colorado
	http://www.uchsc.edu
	Go to centers/institutes, then to Center for Human Caring/International Center for Integrative Caring Practices.
Listserv:	Carenet—an international discussion group.
	To subscribe, send an E-mail message to: <listerv@sco.georcoll.on.ca>
	In the body of the message, place the line SUBSCRIBE CARENET Your full_name.
Video:	Applying the Art and Science of Human Caring (1988)

A video and monograph. New York: National League for Nursing Press.

Theorist:	**Ernestine Wiedenbach**
Theory:	Wiedenbach's Prescriptive Theory
Archived videotapes:	Historical Perspective of Nursing Midwifery

Videotaped interview, Ernestine Wiedenbach and Therese Gesse.

> Audiotaped Interviews with Ernestine Wiedenbach (3).
> Susan Nickel and Ernestine Wiedenbach.
> Tape 1: October 20, 1980; Tape 2: February 2, 1981; Tape 3: May 22, 1981.
> Copies in University of Miami School of Nursing Archives,
> 5801 Red Road, Miami, Florida 33124
> Telephone: (305) 284–1624.

tion media you will use. Expect your search to yield surprising results, and accept that only experience will assist you to sift through this process smoothly. Expect also that during this journey you will transform expectations of yourself and of your inquiry. The search example below will serve to outline a typical initial inquiry beginning from home or office, which are both locations where computers have become commonplace. Basic strategies and alternative approaches are designed to be helpful by acknowledging the absence of linearity in this process of experience and growth.

A SEARCH EXAMPLE WITH STRATEGIES

Beginning from Home or Office— a Basic Literature Search

You decide to begin your preliminary search with *a survey of the nursing literature* from your home or office via the Internet. You access your library, and then through your library you access CINAHL, the nursing literature data base. From the abstracts you find in CINAHL, you decide that you would like to *review the literature more closely* with specific search words highlighted.

Relocating the Physical Search from Your Home to the Library

Because the CINAHL database that is accessed from the library computers has search words (finding aids) highlighted, you choose to *physically relocate your search to the library* itself, where you have access to microfiches as well as the full text of nursing journals and books. You are reminded that there are other sources of information available in the library, such as newspapers, conference proceedings, government studies, microfiches, and so on.

Continuing the Literature Search from Your Home or Office

However, you realize that part of the preliminary search conducted from your home could have included a time-saving strategy—a visit to the nurse theorist's home page on the Internet. You did not realize that nurse theorist home pages are most often located at the university of their academic "home."

It is a tacit assumption that the theorist's home page is kept current, with the latest publications and updated biographical information, including practice and research, available. This, however, is frequently not the case: The date on the home page noted by the Webmaster as the last date of modification simply records a visit to the home page data file, with or without an update.

Continuing and Extending the Literature Search from Your Home or Office

You decide that you would like access to different perspectives concerning the nursing theorist as well as information concerning other nurses who practice using this theory. You discover by "browsing" with search engines such as Infoseek and Lycos that you can retrieve many "hits" (Sparks & Rizzolo, 1998)

in your search for schools and colleges of nursing with websites dedicated to nursing theorists. You also discover that all websites are not created equal: Although some sites are exciting to visit, the information is less dense or less specific on some nursing theorist websites than on others. Given the multitude of websites, you wonder how you can evaluate which sites are the most accurate sources of information in the electronic domain. You also wonder about the credibility of website information used as a scholarly, authoritative reference.

Results of the Beginning Search

After considerable investment of time and energy in your search, you have rapidly acquired growing familiarity with computers and databases. The results of your initial efforts, however, can be seen in the abstracts of nursing journals extracted from your search of CINAHL, and in the multitudes of website addresses for nursing theory home pages and other sites captured along the information trail. Unsubstantiated information worries you. There is little to show for your efforts except experience. It occurs to you that the information authority on some nursing theory webpages may be tenuous and may constitute a weak link in your research methodology. You conclude that evaluation of nursing theory resources, electronic or otherwise, is of major importance in laying the groundwork for consistent, credible, and authoritative research findings.

This is a good time to reflect and

- clarify and adjust your expectations
- clarify and adjust your needs
- clarify and adjust your methods

Now turn to the Guiding Framework for Evaluating Resources (p. 448) and choose, as an exemplar for evaluation, a website from a theorist such as Rosemarie Parse, Martha Rogers, or Dorothea Orem, detailed in Table Appendix-2. Begin evaluating this theorist website, and as you thoughtfully consider each question, assess whether or not the information you gather from the resource meets the criteria. Remember that not all questions will apply to all websites, and may be modified by the purpose of the website. When you have answered as many questions as you are able to, use the following evaluation summary to synthesize your findings (Table Appendix-3). Compare your findings with other websites you have located. Which websites hold up under critical evaluation? Which website can you use as a model?

TABLE APPENDIX–3	*Nursing Resource—Evaluation Summary*

Resource:

Date Evaluated:

❏	Authoritative sources are known.	Yes/No/Some
❏	Nursing authorities contribute to the website.	Yes/No
❏	Practitioners of nursing contribute to the website.	Yes/No

Comments:

❏	Information presented is accurate.	Yes/No
❏	Information is comprehensive.	Yes/No
❏	Information is clear.	Yes/No

Comments:

❏	The website is easy to use and well organized.	Yes/No
❏	The website has unique characteristics.	Yes/No
❏	The website is satisfying to visit and use.	Yes/No
❏	I will recommend this website to colleagues.	Yes/No

Comments:

❏	This nursing theory resource will ground my inquiry as a credible, authoritative, and accurate source of information.	Yes/No

Nursing information resources, such as theorist home pages and databases, are continually being developed and evolving. You are ultimately the one deciding the outcome of your evaluation. Regular evaluation of the resource each time you wish to use it will assure accuracy, credibility, currency, and stability of the information that contributes to your learning and scholarly practice. See Table Appendix–2 for general resources.

Summary

The ability to access information freely and to contribute freely to knowledge in nursing is not only a gift, but a responsibility without dimensions. Our endeavors as nurses always come with the reminder that change is a constant, and that sometimes adapting to change takes superhuman effort. The twentieth century has seen unparalleled change, especially in nursing. The compassionate endeavors of nursing have meshed with commercial endeavors of business megaliths. There is no return to "old ways" anymore. The twenty-first century greets us with a challenge: Nursing must expertly know, use, and control all contemporary knowledge and technology that affects its domain, yet remain true to the values that define it and give it reason for being. This appendix on the evaluation of nursing resources holds the answer to this challenge.

References

Boykin, A., & Schoenhofer, S. (1993). *Nursing as caring: A model for transforming practice.* New York: National League for Nursing Press.

Brennan, P. F. (1996). The future of clinical communication in an electronic environment. *Holistic Nursing Practice, 11*(1), 97–104.

Carlton, K. H., Ryan, M. E., & Siktberg, L. L. (1998). Designing courses for the Internet. *Nurse Educator, 23*(3), 45–50.

Graves, J. R., & Corcoran-Perry, S. (1996). The study of nursing informatics. *Holistic Nursing Practice, 11*(1), 15–24.

Hebda, T., Czar, P., & Mascara, C. (1998). *Handbook of informatics for nurses and health care professionals.* Menlo Park, CA: Addison-Wesley.

Raudonis, B. M., & Acton, G. J. (1997). Theory-based nursing practice. *Journal of Advanced Nursing, 26,* 138–145.

Riddlesperger, K. L., Beard, M., Flowers, D. L., Hisley, S., Pfeifer, K. A., & Stiller, J. J. (1996). CINAHL: An exploratory analysis of the current status of nursing theory construction as reflected by the electronic domain. *Journal of Advanced Nursing, 24,* 599–606.

Sparks, S., & Rizzolo, M. A. (1998). World Wide Web search tools. *Image: Journal of Nursing Scholarship, 30*(2), 161–171.

Turley, J. (1996). Nursing decision making and the science of the concrete. *Holistic Nursing Practice, 11*(1), 6–14.

Index

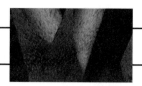